全国高等中医药院校中药学类专业双语规划教材
Bilingual Planned Textbooks for Chinese Materia Medica Majors in TCM Colleges and Universities

中药药剂学

Pharmaceutics of Traditional Chinese Medicine

（供中药学、药学、药物制剂、制药工程及相关专业使用）
(For Chinese Materia Medica, Pharmacy, Pharmaceutics Technology, Pharmaceutical Engineering and other related majors)

主　审　谢秀琼　黄庆娴

主　编　傅超美　刘中秋

副主编　贾永艳　桂双英　廖　婉　刘文龙　严国俊

编　者（以姓氏笔画为序）

王　芳（江西中医药大学）　王　芳（广东药科大学）
王　莹（新疆医科大学）　王艳宏（黑龙江中医药大学）
付　强（成都大学）　兰　卫（新疆医科大学）
庄　婕（上海健康医学院）　刘中秋（广州中医药大学）
刘文龙（湖南中医药大学）　孙　琴（西南医科大学）
孙　黎（安徽中医药大学）　严国俊（南京中医药大学）
杨军宣（重庆医科大学）　李　文（成都中医药大学）
李　玲（西华大学）　张　臻（成都中医药大学）
张纯刚（辽宁中医药大学）　周　宁（河南中医药大学）
郑勇凤（成都中医药大学）　柯　瑾（云南中医药大学）
桂双英（安徽中医药大学）　贾永艳（河南中医药大学）
章津铭（成都中医药大学）　傅超美（成都中医药大学）
曾　锐（西南民族大学）　廖　婉（成都中医药大学）
颜　红（湖南中医药大学）

编写秘书　郑勇凤

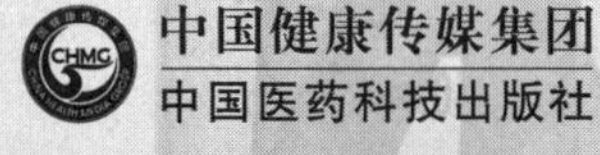

中国健康传媒集团
中国医药科技出版社

内容提要

本教材是“全国高等中医药院校中药学类专业双语规划教材”之一，以中医药理论为指导，将中药药剂学的配制理论、生产技术、质量控制和合理应用等基本理论知识作为核心主线，以案例导入为创新特色，从“理论”到“实践”呈现中药药剂学学科体系。全书分二十二章论述，主要概述了中药药剂学的性质、中药药剂工作的依据、中药制剂共性技术，论述了中药各类常用剂型及新剂型、中药制剂的稳定性、生物药剂学与药物动力学在中药制剂中的应用等内容。本教材在体现科学性、系统性、先进性、准确性、实用性及“全、新、准、精、特”基础上，强调中药制剂特色，系统介绍传统剂型“膏丹丸散”的经典制剂理论及特有制备技术，重点介绍中医临床主要的给药形式“汤剂”的制备关键环节，内容更加丰富，形式更加多样，并采用书网结合模式，使教学资源更加立体化。

本教材主要适用于全国高等院校中药学、药学、药物制剂、制药工程及相关专业教学使用，也可作为国家执业中药师资格考试的重要参考用书。

图书在版编目（CIP）数据

中药药剂学：汉英对照 / 傅超美，刘中秋主编 .—北京：中国医药科技出版社，2020. 10

全国高等中医药院校中药学类专业双语规划教材

ISBN 978-7-5214-1891-0

Ⅰ. ①中… Ⅱ. ①傅… ②刘… Ⅲ. ①中药制剂学 – 双语教学 – 中医学院 – 教材 – 汉、英 Ⅳ. ① R283

中国版本图书馆 CIP 数据核字（2020）第 100513 号

美术编辑 陈君杞

版式设计 辰轩文化

出版 **中国健康传媒集团** | 中国医药科技出版社

地址 北京市海淀区文慧园北路甲 22 号

邮编 100082

电话 发行：010-62227427 邮购：010-62236938

网址 www.cmstp.com

规格 889 × 1194 mm $^{1}/_{16}$

印张 33$^{3}/_{4}$

字数 929 千字

版次 2020 年 10 月第 1 版

印次 2020 年 10 月第 1 次印刷

印刷 三河市万龙印装有限公司

经销 全国各地新华书店

书号 ISBN 978-7-5214-1891-0

定价 99.00 元

获取新书信息、投稿、为图书纠错，请扫码联系我们。

出版说明

近些年随着世界范围的中医药热潮的涌动，来中国学习中医药学的留学生逐年增多，走出国门的中医药学人才也在增加。为了适应中医药国际交流与合作的需要，加快中医药国际化进程，提高来中国留学生和国际班学生的教学质量，满足双语教学的需要和中医药对外交流需求，培养优秀的国际化中医药人才，进一步推动中医药国际化进程，根据教育部、国家中医药管理局、国家药品监督管理局等部门的有关精神，在本套教材建设指导委员会主任委员成都中医药大学彭成教授等专家的指导和顶层设计下，中国医药科技出版社组织全国50余所高等中医药院校及附属医疗机构约420名专家、教师精心编撰了全国高等中医药院校中药学类专业双语规划教材，该套教材即将付梓出版。

本套教材共计23门，主要供全国高等中医药院校中药学类专业教学使用。本套教材定位清晰、特色鲜明，主要体现在以下方面。

一、立足双语教学实际，培养复合应用型人才

本套教材以高校双语教学课程建设要求为依据，以满足国内医药院校开展留学生教学和双语教学的需求为目标，突出中医药文化特色鲜明、中医药专业术语规范的特点，注重培养中医药技能、反映中医药传承和现代研究成果，旨在优化教育质量，培养优秀的国际化中医药人才，推进中医药对外交流。

本套教材建设围绕目前中医药院校本科教育教学改革方向对教材体系进行科学规划、合理设计，坚持以培养创新型和复合型人才为宗旨，以社会需求为导向，以培养适应中药开发、利用、管理、服务等各个领域需求的高素质应用型人才为目标的教材建设思路与原则。

二、遵循教材编写规律，整体优化，紧跟学科发展步伐

本套教材的编写遵循“三基、五性、三特定”的教材编写规律；以“必需、够用”为度；坚持与时俱进，注意吸收新技术和新方法，适当拓展知识面，为学生后续发展奠定必要的基础。实验教材密切结合主干教材内容，体现理实一体，注重培养学生实践技能训练的同时，按照教育部相关精神，增加设计性实验部分，以现实问题作为驱动力来培养学生自主获取和应用新知识的能力，从而培养学生独立思考能力、实验设计能力、实践操作能力和可持续发展能力，满足培养应用型和复合型人才的要求。强调全套教材内容的整体优化，并注重不同教材内容的联系与衔接，避免遗漏和不必要的交叉重复。

三、对接职业资格考试，“教考”“理实”密切融合

本套教材的内容和结构设计紧密对接国家执业中药师职业资格考试大纲要求，实现教学与考试、理论与实践的密切融合，并且在教材编写过程中，吸收具有丰富实践经验的企业人员参与教材的编写，确保教材的内容密切结合应用，更加体现高等教育的实践性和开放性，为学生参加考试和实践工作打下坚实基础。

四、创新教材呈现形式，书网融合，使教与学更便捷更轻松

全套教材为书网融合教材，即纸质教材与数字教材、配套教学资源、题库系统、数字化教学服务有机融合。通过“一书一码”的强关联，为读者提供全免费增值服务。按教材封底的提示激活教材后，读者可通过PC、手机阅读电子教材和配套课程资源（PPT、微课、视频等），并可在线进行同步练习，实时收到答案反馈和解析。同时，读者也可以直接扫描书中二维码，阅读与教材内容关联的课程资源，从而丰富学习体验，使学习更便捷。教师可通过PC在线创建课程，与学生互动，开展在线课程内容定制、布置和批改作业、在线组织考试、讨论与答疑等教学活动，学生通过PC、手机均可实现在线作业、在线考试，提升学习效率，使教与学更轻松。此外，平台尚有数据分析、教学诊断等功能，可为教学研究与管理提供技术和数据支撑。需要特殊说明的是，有些专业基础课程，例如《药理学》等9种教材，起源于西方医学，因篇幅所限，在本次双语教材建设中纸质教材以英语为主，仅将专业词汇对照了中文翻译，同时在中国医药科技出版社数字平台“医药大学堂”上配套了中文电子教材供学生学习参考。

编写出版本套高质量教材，得到了全国知名专家的精心指导和各有关院校领导与编者的大力支持，在此一并表示衷心感谢。希望广大师生在教学中积极使用本套教材和提出宝贵意见，以便修订完善，共同打造精品教材，为促进我国高等中医药院校中药学类专业教育教学改革和人才培养做出积极贡献。

全国高等中医药院校中药学类专业双语规划教材
建设指导委员会

数字化教材编委会

主　　审　谢秀琼　黄庆娴

主　　编　傅超美　刘中秋

副 主 编　贾永艳　桂双英　廖　婉　刘文龙　严国俊

编　　者（以姓氏笔画为序）

王　芳（江西中医药大学）　王　芳（广东药科大学）

王　莹（新疆医科大学）　王艳宏（黑龙江中医药大学）

付　强（成都大学）　兰　卫（新疆医科大学）

庄　婕（上海健康医学院）　刘中秋（广州中医药大学）

刘文龙（湖南中医药大学）　孙　琴（西南医科大学）

孙　黎（安徽中医药大学）　严国俊（南京中医药大学）

杨军宣（重庆医科大学）　李　文（成都中医药大学）

李　玲（西华大学）　张　臻（成都中医药大学）

张纯刚（辽宁中医药大学）　周　宁（河南中医药大学）

郑勇凤（成都中医药大学）　柯　瑾（云南中医药大学）

桂双英（安徽中医药大学）　贾永艳（河南中医药大学）

章津铭（成都中医药大学）　傅超美（成都中医药大学）

曾　锐（西南民族大学）　廖　婉（成都中医药大学）

颜　红（湖南中医药大学）

编写秘书　郑勇凤

前 言

中药药剂学是中药学及相关专业的主干课程，是一门综合性应用技术学科。本教材为“全国高等中医药院校中药学类专业双语规划教材”之一，以中英双语编写为优势特色，为规范和提高我国高等中医药院校中药学类专业双语教学和来华中医药专业留学生的教育质量，培养高素质、国际化视野的中药学专业优秀人才，促进中医药文化的国际化传播、交流与学习，推动中医药国际化进程奠定基础。

本教材将中药药剂的配制理论、生产技术、质量控制和合理应用等基本理论知识作为核心主线，以案例导入为特色创新，从“理论”到“实践”呈现中药药剂学学科体系，着重强调中药制剂特色，同时结合中药药剂学自身规律及教学特点，将内容共分二十二章论述。第一章为“绪论”，主要概述中药药剂学的性质、任务及其发展，药物剂型的分类，中药剂型选择的基本原则以及中药药剂工作的依据等内容，第二、三章介绍“中药调剂及制药卫生”，主要介绍中药处方调配、配伍变化及制药环境卫生、灭菌方法与无菌操作等内容，第四到六章介绍“中药制剂共性技术”，包括中药粉碎、筛析、混合、制粒，中药浸提、分离与纯化、浓缩与干燥等技术，第七到十八章介绍“中药常用剂型”，各剂型下以“含义－特点－分类－制法－质量检查”为主线，按浸出药剂、液体、半固体、固体、气体和其他剂型顺序编写，第十九到二十二章介绍“药物制剂新技术与新剂型及其他”，分为药物制剂新技术与新剂型、中药制剂的稳定性、中药制剂的配伍变化、生物药剂学与药物动力学在中药制剂中的应用。本教材系统介绍了传统剂型“膏丹丸散”的经典制剂理论及特有制备技术，重点介绍了中医临床主要的给药形式“汤剂”的制备关键环节。主要适用于全国高等院校中药学、药学、药物制剂、制药工程及相关专业教学使用，也可作为国家执业中药师资格考试的重要参考用书。

为充分体现行业特色，体现药学与临床的结合、基础理论与中药产业的结合、中医药与现代药学的结合，全面反映中药药剂学的发展水平，本教材在体现科学性、系统性、先进性、准确性、实用性及“全、新、准、精、特”基础上，还具备以下特色。

1. 严格按照中药药剂学教学大纲和教材编写的基本原则，充分吸收各版《中药药剂学》教材成功的编写经验和内容精华，同时紧密结合现行版《中国药典》《药品生产质量管理规范》等国家有关最新法规以及中医药本科教学的最新要求，体现了继承传统药剂与发展现代剂型相结合的编写特点。

2. 特设“案例导入”模块，选取经典实用的案例，将理论与实践相融合，帮助学生系统理解中药药剂的关键知识与技能，提高学生的分析能力，启发学生的综合创新能力。设立“学习目标”模块，一般分为掌握、熟悉、了解3个层次，帮助读者厘清学习重点。

3. 根据学科特点，对中药药剂的工艺、技术等内容大部分以图表形式表达，使抽象的概念形象化、复杂的流程条理化，便于学生更好地理解、掌握和应用，体现内容的科学性、时代性和适用性。

4. 创新教材呈现形式，书网融合，将纸质版教材与数字化教材资源（PPT、题库）有机融合。通过“一书一码”的强关联，为读者提供增值服务。限于篇幅，“岗位对接”“重点小结”“案例导入”，以及有些章节对应的英文内容均以“二维码”的形式呈现，通过扫描“二维码”可阅览学习。

本教材的编者均在中药药剂学领域中具有丰富的科研教学经验，多数具有双语教学经验及海外学习经历。在编写本教材过程中得到各编者所在院校领导和兄弟院校同行的大力支持，在此一并感谢。

由于编者水平所限，书中难免有不妥之处，殷切地希望读者在使用过程中提出宝贵意见，以便修订完善。

编　者

2020 年 4 月

Preface

Pharmaceutics of TCM is the main course of Chinese medicine and related majors, and a comprehensive discipline with applied technology. As one of the bilingual teaching materials for students majoring in Chinese materia medica in TCM universities and colleges, the advantage of this book is the Chinese/English bilingual writing features, whose purpose are standardizing and improving our bilingual teaching quality of Chinese medicine in TCM universities and colleges, and the educational quality of international students majoring in Chinese medicine in China. In addition, it's aimed to cultivate professional talents majoring in Chinese medicine with high quality and international foresight, to promote the international dissemination, exchange and learning of Chinese pharmacy culture, to lay a good foundation to promote the internationalization of TCM.

The core line of this textbook contains the basic theoretical knowledge of the preparation theory, production technology, quality control and rational application in *Pharmaceutics of TCM*, the introduction of cases belongs to its characteristic innovation, aiming to present the discipline system of it from "theory" to "practice" and emphasize the characteristics of TCM preparation. This book is divided into 22 chapters according to the regularity and teaching characteristics of *Pharmaceutics of TCM*. The chapter 1 is the "Introduction", which mainly summarizes the properties, tasks and development of *Pharmaceutics of TCM*, the classification of dosage forms, the basic principles for selecting dosage forms of TCM and the basis for the work of *Pharmaceutics of TCM*. The chapter 2 and 3 introduces "prescription filling of TCM and Pharmaceutical hygiene", Main content includes compatibility change of prescription preparation of TCM, hygiene of pharmaceutical environment, method of sterilization and aseptic operation, etc. Chapter 4-6 introduces "common technology of traditional Chinese medicine preparation", including traditional Chinese medicine comminution, screening, mixing, granulation, extraction, separation and purification, concentration and drying. Chapter 7-18 introduces the "commonly used dosage forms of TCM". The main line of each dosage form is "Meaning – Characteristics – Classification – Preparation - Quality inspection", which is compiled in the order of leaching agents, liquid, semi-solid, solid, gas and other dosage forms. Chapter 19-22 introduces " New technologies and new dosage forms of pharmaceutical preparations and others", including new technologies and new dosage forms of pharmaceutical preparations and others, the stability of TCM preparation, the Compatibility Changes in The TCM preparations, and application of biopharmaceutics and pharmacokinetics in the TCM preparations. This textbook systematically introduces the classical preparation theory and the special preparation technology of the traditional dosage form Gao, Dan, Wan and San, and emphatically introduces the key links in the preparation of "decoction", the main clinical drug delivery form of TCM. The book is mainly used in the undergraduate teaching of Chinese pharmacy, pharmacy, pharmaceutical engineering, pharmaceutical preparation and related majors, and it can also be used as an important reference book for the national licensed Chinese pharmacist qualification examination.

In order to fully embody the industry characteristic, manifest the combination of medicine and clinic, the combination of basic theory and industry of TCM, and the combination of TCM and modern medicine, and fully reflect the development level of *Pharmaceutics of TCM*, this textbook has the following characteristics, except for reflecting scientific, systemic, advanced, accurate, practicable and being based "overall, new, exact, accurate, special" basis.

1. Strictly according to the teaching syllabus of *Pharmaceutics of TCM* and the basic principles of planning textbooks, richly absorbing successful writing experience and essential contents of each editions of " *Pharmaceutics of TCM* " teaching materials. At the same time, it closely follows the current edition of "*Chinese Pharmacopoeia*" "*Drug Production Quality Management Standard*" and other national relevant new laws and regulations, as well as the updated and higher requirements for TCM undergraduate teaching, which reflects the writing characteristics of combination with inheriting traditional Chinese dosage forms and developing modern dosage forms.

2. Specially sitting "case introduction" column, selecting classic and practical cases, and integrating theory with practice to help students understand the key knowledge and skills of *Pharmaceutics of TCM*, improve students' analytical ability, and inspire students' comprehensive innovation ability. Setting up the "Learning goals" column, which is generally divided into three levels: mastery, familiarity and understanding. to help readers to clarify the key points of learning.

3. According to the characteristics of this subject, most contents of craft and technology of *Pharmaceutics of TCM* are expressed in the form of charts, so as to visualize the abstract concept and organize the complex process, the ultimate aim is to help students better understand, master and apply them. In addition, some new drawings of pharmaceutical machinery are added and replaced. The pictures are bilingual in Chinese and English, which reflects the scientificity, timeliness and applicability of contents.

4. Innovating the presentation form of teaching materials, integrating books with websites, and organically combining paper teaching materials with digital teaching materials (PPT, test bank, micro-course). Using the strong relevance "book code" to provide readers with value-added services. Due to the limited space, " Jobs Matched", "Key Points" and some corresponding English contents of chapters are presented in the form of " two-dimensional barcodes", which can be read and learned by scanning " two-dimensional barcodes".

The editors of this textbook have rich experience in the field of *Pharmaceutics of TCM*, most of them have bilingual teaching experience and overseas study experience. In the process of writing, we also got strong support from the leaders of colleges and universities and peers, we owe many thanks.

Due to short time and limited writing ability of editors, it's hard to avoid all inappropriate places or mistakes, we're eager our readers to give valuable advice for revision.

Editors

In April, 2020

目录 | Contents

第一章　绪论 …… 1

Chapter 1　An Introduction …… 1

第一节　概述 …… 1

1.1　Overview …… 1

一、中药药剂学的性质 …… 1

1.1.1　The Characteristics of Pharmaceutics of Traditional Chinese Medicine …… 1

二、中药药剂学的任务 …… 4

1.1.2　The Tasks of TCM Pharmaceutics …… 4

三、中药药剂学在中医药事业中的地位与作用 …… 5

1.1.3　Position and Role of TCM Pharmaceutics in Chinese Medicine …… 5

四、中药药剂学常用术语 …… 6

1.1.4　Commonly-Used Terms of TCM Pharmaceutics …… 6

第二节　中药药剂学的发展简况 …… 10

1.2　The Advancing of TCM Pharmaceutics …… 10

一、中药药剂学发展的历史回顾 …… 10

1.2.1　A Historical Review of the Development of TCM Pharmaceutics …… 10

二、新中国成立后中药药剂学的主要成就 …… 15

1.2.2　The Major Achievements after the Founding of New China …… 15

第三节　药物剂型的分类 …… 19

1.3　Classification of Drug Dosage Forms …… 19

一、按物态分类 …… 19

1.3.1　Classification by Physical States …… 19

二、按制备方法分类 …… 20

1.3.2　Classification by Processing Methods …… 20

三、按分散系统分类 …… 20

1.3.3　Classification by Dispersing System …… 20

四、按给药途径与方法分类 …… 21

1.3.4　Classification by Medication Route and Administration …… 21

第四节　中药剂型选择的基本原则 …… 22

1.4　The Essential Principles for the TCM Dosage Form Selection …… 22

一、根据防治疾病的需要选择剂型 …… 23

1.4.1　To Select the Dosage Forms in Line with the Disease Prevention and Treatment …… 23

二、根据药物性质选择剂型 …… 25

1.4.2　To Choose Dosage Form According to Drugs' Properties …… 25

三、根据原方不同剂型的生物药剂学和药代动力学特性选择剂型……26
1.4.3 Dosage Forms Selection Based on the Specialities of Biopharmaceutics and Pharmacokinetic in Different Dosage Forms of the Original Prescriptions ……26
四、根据生产条件和“五方便”的要求选择剂型……27
1.4.4 Selecting Dosage Forms in Accordance with Production Conditions and “Five Conveniences” ……27
第五节 中药药剂工作的依据 ……28
1.5 Basis of TCM Pharmaceutics Work ……28
一、药典……28
1.5.1 Pharmacopoeia ……28
二、局颁、部颁药品标准……31
1.5.2 Drug Standards Issued by Either the Administration or the Ministry ……31
三、药品管理法规……32
1.5.3 Drug Administration Rules and Regulations ……32

第二章 中药调剂 ……35
Chapter 2 Traditional Chinese Medicine Prescription Filling ……35
第一节 概述 ……35
2.1 Overview ……35
第二节 处方 ……36
2.2 Prescription ……36
一、处方的概念与种类……36
2.2.1 The Concept and Type of Prescription ……36
二、医师处方的内容……37
2.2.2 Contents of A Doctor's Prescription ……37
三、处方药与非处方药……37
2.2.3 Prescription Drugs and Over-The-Counter Drugs ……37
第三节 中药处方的调配 ……38
2.3 Allocation of Traditional Chinese Medicine Prescriptions ……38
一、处方的调配程序……38
2.3.1 Formulation Procedures ……38
二、中药“斗谱”的排列原则……40
2.3.2 The Principle of Traditional Chinese Medicine Ranking……40
第四节 中药饮片形式的沿革 ……41
2.4 History of The Forms for Pieces of Traditional Chinese Medicine ……41
一、传统中药饮片……41
2.4.1 Traditional Pieces of TCM ……41
二、新型中药饮片……41
2.4.2 New Pieces of TCM ……41

第三章 制药卫生 ……43
Chapter 3 Pharmaceutical Hygiene ……43
第一节 概述 ……43

3.1 Overview ······ 43
一、制药卫生的含义 ······ 43
3.1.1 Definition of Pharmaceutical Hygiene ······ 43
二、中药的微生物限度标准 ······ 44
3.1.2 Microbial Limit Standards of TCM ······ 44
三、预防中药制剂污染的措施 ······ 47
3.1.3 The Methods of Preventing Herbal Preparation Contamination ······ 47
第二节 制药环境的卫生管理 ······ 48
3.2 Management of the Pharmaceutical Environment ······ 48
一、中药制药环境的基本要求 ······ 48
3.2.1 The Basic Requirements of the Pharmaceutical Environment ······ 48
二、洁净室的净化标准 ······ 49
3.2.2 Purification Standards of Lean Room ······ 49
三、空气洁净技术与应用 ······ 50
3.2.3 Air Clean Technology and Application ······ 50
第三节 灭菌方法与无菌操作 ······ 51
一、灭菌方法 ······ 51
二、无菌操作法 ······ 53
三、F 与 F_0 值在灭菌中的意义与应用 ······ 53
第四节 防腐与防虫 ······ 54
3.4 Anti-Corrosion and Pest Control ······ 54
一、防腐与防虫措施 ······ 55
3.4.1 Anti-Corrosion and Pest Control Measures ······ 55
二、防腐剂 ······ 55
3.4.2 Preservatives ······ 55

第四章 粉碎、筛析、混合与制粒 ······ 57
Chapter 4 Pulverization, Sieving, Mixing and Granulation ······ 57
第一节 粉碎 ······ 58
4.1 Pulverization ······ 58
一、粉碎的含义与目的 ······ 58
4.1.1 Definition and Purpose of Pulverization ······ 58
二、常用的粉碎方法 ······ 58
4.1.2 Methods of Pulverization ······ 58
三、粉碎原则 ······ 61
4.1.3 Principle of Pulverization ······ 61
四、粉碎设备 ······ 62
4.1.4 Equipment of Pulverization ······ 62
第二节 筛析 ······ 65
一、筛析的目的 ······ 66
二、药筛和粉末的分等 ······ 66
三、影响过筛的因素 ······ 67

四、过筛和离析的设备 …… 67
第三节 混合 …… 69
4.3 Mixing …… 69
一、混合的含义与目的 …… 69
4.3.1 Definition and Purpose of Mixing …… 69
二、混合方法 …… 70
4.3.2 Mixing Method …… 70
三、混合机械 …… 70
4.3.3 Mixer …… 70
四、影响混合的因素 …… 72
4.3.4 Factors Affecting Mixing …… 72
第四节 制粒 …… 73
4.4 Granulation …… 73
一、制粒的含义与目的 …… 73
4.4.1 The Meaning and Purpose of Granulation …… 73
二、制粒的方法与设备 …… 74
4.4.2 Methods and Equipment of Granulation …… 74

第五章 散剂 …… 78

Chapter 5 Powders …… 78

第一节 概述 …… 78
5.1 Overview …… 78
一、散剂的含义 …… 78
5.1.1 The Definition of Powders …… 78
二、散剂的特点 …… 79
5.1.2 The Characteristics of Powders …… 79
三、散剂的分类 …… 79
5.1.3 The Classification of Powders …… 79
第二节 散剂的制备 …… 80
5.2 Preparation of Powders …… 80
一、一般散剂的制备 …… 80
5.2.1 Preparation of General Powders …… 80
二、特殊散剂的制备 …… 82
5.2.2 Preparation of Special Powders …… 82
第三节 散剂的质量要求与检查 …… 85
5.3 Quality Requirements and Inspections of Powders …… 85
一、散剂的质量要求 …… 85
5.3.1 Quality Requirements of Powders …… 85
二、散剂的质量检查项目 …… 86
5.3.2 Inspection Items of Powder Quality …… 86

第六章　浸提、分离与纯化、浓缩与干燥 …… 87

Chapter 6　Extraction, Separation and Purification, Concentration and Drying …… 87

第一节　概述 …… 88

6.1　Overview …… 88

一、浸提、分离与纯化的目的 …… 88

6.1.1　Purposes of Extraction, Separation and Purification …… 88

二、浓缩与干燥的目的 …… 88

6.1.2　Purposes of Concentration and Drying …… 88

三、中药成分与疗效 …… 89

6.1.3　Composition and Efficacy of TCM …… 89

第二节　浸提 …… 90

6.2　Extraction …… 90

一、浸提过程 …… 90

6.2.1　Extraction Process …… 90

二、影响浸提的因素 …… 91

6.2.2　Factors Affecting Extraction …… 91

三、常用浸提溶剂 …… 92

6.2.3　Commonly Used Extraction Solvent …… 92

四、浸提辅助剂 …… 93

6.2.4　Extraction Auxiliary …… 93

五、常用浸提方法与设备 …… 93

6.2.5　Commonly Used Extraction Method and Equipment …… 93

第三节　分离与纯化 …… 98

6.3　Separation and Purification …… 98

一、分离 …… 98

6.3.1　Separation …… 98

二、纯化 …… 100

6.3.2　Purification …… 100

第四节　浓缩 …… 103

6.4　Concentration …… 103

一、影响浓缩效率的因素 …… 104

6.4.1　Factors Affecting the Efficiency of Concentration …… 104

二、浓缩方法与设备 …… 104

6.4.2　Concentration Method and Equipment …… 104

第五节　干燥 …… 106

6.5　Drying …… 106

一、干燥的基本原理 …… 106

6.5.1　The Principle of Drying …… 106

二、影响干燥的因素 …… 107

6.5.2　Factors Affecting Drying …… 107

三、干燥方法与设备 …… 109

6.5.3 Drying Methods and Equipments ······ 109

第七章 浸出药剂 ······ 112

Chapter 7 Extractions ······ 112

第一节 概述 ······ 113

7.1 Overview ······ 113

一、浸出药剂的含义 ······ 113

7.1.1 The Definition of Extractions ······ 113

二、浸出药剂的特点 ······ 113

7.1.2 The Characteristics of Extractions ······ 113

三、浸出药剂的分类 ······ 114

7.1.3 The Classification of Extractions ······ 114

第二节 汤剂 ······ 115

7.2 Decoctions ······ 115

一、汤剂的含义 ······ 115

7.2.1 The Definition of Decoctions ······ 115

二、汤剂的特点 ······ 115

7.2.2 The Characteristics of Decoctions ······ 115

三、汤剂的制备与影响质量的因素 ······ 116

7.2.3 Preparation of Decoctions and Factors That Influence the Quality of Decoctions ······ 116

四、煎煮过程对药效的影响 ······ 119

7.2.4 Effects on the Efficacy of the Decoction Process ······ 119

第三节 中药合剂（含口服液） ······ 121

7.3 Chinese Medicinal Mixture (Oral Liquid Included) ······ 121

一、中药合剂的含义 ······ 121

7.3.1 The Definition of Chinese Medicinal Mixture ······ 121

二、中药合剂的特点 ······ 122

7.3.2 The Characteristics of Chinese Medicinal Mixture ······ 122

三、中药合剂的制法 ······ 122

7.3.3 Preparation of Chinese Medicinal Mixture ······ 122

四、中药合剂的质量要求与检查 ······ 124

7.3.4 Quality Requirements and Inspections of Chinese Medicinal Mixture ······ 124

第四节 糖浆剂 ······ 126

7.4 Syrups ······ 126

一、糖浆剂的含义 ······ 126

7.4.1 The Definition of Syrups ······ 126

二、糖浆剂的特点 ······ 126

7.4.2 The Characteristics of Syrups ······ 126

三、糖浆剂的分类 ······ 127

7.4.3 The Classification of Syrups ······ 127

四、糖浆剂的制法 ······ 127

7.4.4 Preparation of Syrups …… 127
五、糖浆剂的质量要求与检查及质量问题讨论…… 129
7.4.5 Discussion on Quality Control of Syrups …… 129
第五节 煎膏剂（膏滋）…… 132
7.5 Concentrated Decoctions …… 132
一、煎膏剂的含义…… 132
7.5.1 The Definition of Concentrated Decoctions …… 132
二、煎膏剂的特点…… 132
7.5.2 The Characteristics of Concentrated Decoctions …… 132
三、煎膏剂的制法…… 133
7.5.3 Preparation of Concentrated Decoctions …… 133
四、煎膏剂的质量要求与检查…… 135
7.5.4 Quality Requirements and Inspections of Concentrated Decoction …… 135
第六节 酒剂与酊剂 …… 137
7.6 Medicinal Wines and Tinctures …… 137
一、酒剂与酊剂的含义…… 137
7.6.1 The Definitions of Medicinal Wines and Tinctures…… 137
二、酒剂和酊剂的特点…… 138
7.6.2 The Characteristics of Medicinal Wines and Tinctures …… 138
三、酒剂与酊剂的制法…… 138
7.6.3 Preparation of Medicinal Wines and Tinctures …… 138
四、酒剂与酊剂的质量要求与检查…… 141
7.6.4 Quality Requirements and Inspections of Medicinal Wines and Tinctures …… 141
第七节 流浸膏剂与浸膏剂 …… 142
7.7 Liquid Extracts and Extracts …… 142
一、流浸膏剂及浸膏剂的含义和特点…… 142
7.7.1 The Definitions and Characteristics of Fluid Extracts and Extracts …… 142
二、流浸膏剂及浸膏剂的制法…… 142
7.7.2 Preparation of Fluid Extracts and Extracts …… 142
三、流浸膏剂与浸膏剂的质量要求与检查…… 144
7.7.3 Quality Requirements and Inspections of Fluid Extracts and Extracts …… 144
第八节 茶剂 …… 145
7.8 Medicinal Tea …… 145
一、茶剂的含义…… 145
7.8.1 The Definition of Medicinal Teas …… 145
二、茶剂的特点…… 145
7.8.2 The Characteristics of Medicinal Teas …… 145
三、茶剂的制法…… 145
7.8.3 Preparation of Medicinal Teas …… 145
四、茶剂的质量要求与检查…… 146
7.8.4 Quality Requirements and Inspections of Medicinal Teas …… 146

第九节 浸出药剂容易出现的质量问题 …… 147
7.9 Quality Problems of Extractions …… 147
一、长霉发酵 …… 147
7.9.1 Mildew and Fermentation …… 147
二、浑浊沉淀 …… 148
7.9.2 Turbidity and Precipitation …… 148
三、成分水解 …… 148
7.9.3 Hydrolysis …… 148

第八章 液体药剂 …… 150
Chapter 8 Liquid Preparations …… 150
第一节 概述 …… 151
8.1 Overview …… 151
一、液体药剂的含义与特点 …… 151
8.1.1 The Definition and Characteristics of Liquid Preparations …… 151
二、液体药剂的分类 …… 151
8.1.2 The Classifications of Liquid Preparations …… 151
三、液体药剂常用的溶剂 …… 152
8.1.3 Common Solvents for Liquid Preparations …… 152
第二节 表面活性剂 …… 153
一、表面活性剂的含义、组成与特点 …… 153
二、常用的表面活性剂 …… 154
三、表面活性剂的基本性质 …… 155
四、表面活性剂在药剂中的应用 …… 157
第三节 溶解度与增加药物溶解度的方法 …… 157
一、溶解度及其影响因素 …… 157
二、增加药物溶解度的方法 …… 158
第四节 真溶液型液体药剂 …… 158
8.4 True Solution Liquid Preparations …… 158
一、概述 …… 158
8.4.1 Overview …… 158
二、溶液剂 …… 159
8.4.2 Solution …… 159
三、芳香水剂与露剂 …… 160
8.4.3 Aromatic Water and Distillate …… 160
四、甘油剂 …… 160
8.4.4 Glycerins …… 160
五、醑剂 …… 160
8.4.5 Spirits …… 160
第五节 胶体溶液型液体药剂 …… 161
一、概述 …… 161
二、胶体溶液的性质 …… 161

三、胶体溶液的稳定性 …… 161
四、胶体溶液的制法 …… 162
第六节 乳状液型液体药剂 …… 162
8.6 Emulsion Liquid Preparations …… 162
一、概述 …… 162
8.6.1 Overview …… 162
二、常用的乳化剂种类与选用 …… 163
8.6.2 Commonly Used Emulsifiers and the Selection of Emulsifiers …… 163
三、乳剂的稳定性 …… 165
8.6.3 Stability of Emulsions …… 165
四、乳剂的制备 …… 167
8.6.4 Preparation of Emulsions …… 167
第七节 混悬液型液体药剂 …… 170
8.7 Suspension Liquid Preparations …… 170
一、概述 …… 170
8.7.1 Overview …… 170
二、影响混悬剂稳定性的因素 …… 170
8.7.2 Factors Affecting the Stability of Suspension …… 170
三、混悬剂的稳定剂 …… 172
8.7.3 Stabilizer of Suspensions …… 172
四、混悬剂的制法 …… 173
8.7.4 Preparation of Suspensions …… 173
第八节 其他液体药剂 …… 175
8.8 Other Liquid Medicinal Preparations …… 175
一、灌肠剂 …… 175
8.8.1 Enemas …… 175
二、洗剂 …… 175
8.8.2 Lotions …… 175
三、搽剂 …… 175
8.8.3 Liniments …… 175
四、滴耳剂 …… 176
8.8.4 Ear Drops …… 176
五、滴鼻剂 …… 176
8.8.5 Nasal Drops …… 176
六、含漱剂 …… 176
8.8.6 Gargarismas …… 176
第九节 液体药剂的质量要求与检查 …… 176
8.9 Quality Requirements and Inspection of Liquid Medicinal Preparations …… 176
一、口服溶液剂、口服乳剂、口服混悬剂的质量要求 …… 176
8.9.1 Quality Requirements of Oral Solutions, Emulsions and Oral Suspensions …… 176
二、口服溶液剂、口服乳剂、口服混悬剂的质量检查 …… 177
8.9.2 Quality Inspections of Oral Solutions, Emulsions and Suspensions …… 177

第十节　液体药剂的矫味、矫臭与着色 177
8.10　Taste Modifying, Odor Modifying and Coloration of Liquid Medicinal Preparations 177
一、矫味剂 178
8.10.1　Flavoring Agents 178
二、着色剂 178
8.10.2　Coloring Agents 178
第十一节　液体药剂的包装与贮藏 179
8.11　Packing and Storage of Liquid Preparations 179
一、液体药剂的包装 179
8.11.1　Packing of Liquid Preparations 179
二、液体药剂的贮藏 179
8.11.2　Storage of Liquid Preparations 179

第九章　注射剂 180

Chapter 9　Injections 180

第一节　概述 181
9.1　Overview 181
一、注射剂的含义 181
9.1.1　The Definition of the Injections 181
二、注射剂的特点 181
9.1.2　The Characteristic of the Injections 181
三、注射剂的分类 181
9.1.3　The Classification of the Injections 181
四、注射剂的给药途径 182
9.1.4　Administration Routes of Injections 182
第二节　热原 182
一、热原的含义与组成 182
二、热原的基本性质 183
三、注射剂热原的污染途径 183
四、除去注射剂中热原的方法 183
五、热原与细菌内毒素的检查方法 184
第三节　注射剂的溶剂 184
9.3　The Solvent of the Injection 184
第四节　注射剂的附加剂 189
9.4　The Additives of Injections 189
一、增加主药溶解度的附加剂 189
9.4.1　Enhancing the Solubility of the Drug Substance 189
二、帮助主药混悬或乳化的附加剂 190
9.4.2　Emulsifying Agents and Suspending Agents 190
三、防止主药氧化的附加剂 191
9.4.3　The Additives for Avoiding the Main Drug Oxidation 191

四、调整渗透压的附加剂 …… 192
9.4.4 Additives Regulating the Osmotic Pressure …… 192
五、抑制微生物增殖的附加剂 …… 195
9.4.5 An Additive that Inhibits Microbial Proliferation …… 195
六、调整 pH 的附加剂 …… 196
9.4.6 The Additives Which are Used for Adjusting the pH …… 196
七、减轻疼痛的附加剂 …… 197
9.4.7 The Additives to Alleviate Pain …… 197
第五节 注射剂的制备 …… 197
9.5 Preparation of the Injections …… 197
一、注射剂制备的工艺流程 …… 197
9.5.1 Technological Process Flow of the Preparation of Injections …… 197
二、中药注射用半成品 …… 198
9.5.2 Semi-Finished Product for TCM Injections …… 198
三、注射剂的容器与处理 …… 200
9.5.3 The Containers and Handling of Injections …… 200
四、注射剂的配液与滤过 …… 201
9.5.4 Compounding and Filtration of Injections …… 201
五、注射剂的灌封 …… 203
9.5.5 Filling/Sealing of Injections …… 203
六、注射剂的灭菌与检漏 …… 204
9.5.6 Sterilization and Leak Detection of Injections …… 204
七、注射剂的印字与包装 …… 204
9.5.7 Injections Printing and Packaging …… 204
第六节 中药注射剂的质量控制 …… 206
9.6 Quality Control of Chinese Medicine Injections …… 206
一、中药注射剂的质量控制项目与方法 …… 206
9.6.1 Quality Control Items and Methods of Chinese Medicine Injections …… 206
二、中药注射剂存在的质量问题 …… 209
9.6.2 Quality Problems of Chinese Medicine Injections …… 209
第七节 输液剂与血浆代用液 …… 211
一、输液剂的含义 …… 211
二、输液剂的特点与分类 …… 211
三、输液剂的制法 …… 212
四、输液剂质量问题讨论 …… 212
五、血浆代用液 …… 213
第八节 粉针剂与其他注射剂 …… 214
一、粉针剂 …… 214
二、混悬液型注射剂 …… 214
三、乳状液型注射剂 …… 215
第九节 眼用液体制剂 …… 216
一、概述 …… 216

二、眼用液体制剂的附加剂…… 216
三、眼用液体制剂的制法…… 217
四、眼用液体制剂的质量要求与检查…… 217

第十章 外用膏剂 …… 218
Chapter 10 External Ointments …… 218
第一节 概述 …… 218
10.1 Overview …… 218
一、外用膏剂的含义…… 218
10.1.1 The Definition of External Ointments …… 218
二、外用膏剂的特点…… 219
10.1.2 The Characteristics of External Ointments …… 219
三、外用膏剂的分类…… 219
10.1.3 The Classification of External Ointments …… 219
四、药物经皮吸收机制与影响因素…… 220
10.1.4 Drug Transdermal Absorption Mechanism and Influencing Factors …… 220
第二节 软膏剂 …… 225
10.2 Ointments …… 225
一、概述…… 225
10.2.1 Overview …… 225
二、基质…… 225
10.2.2 Bases …… 225
三、软膏剂的制法…… 231
10.2.3 Preparation Method of Ointments …… 231
四、软膏剂的质量检查…… 234
10.2.4 Ointment Quality Inspection…… 234
五、眼膏剂…… 235
10.2.5 Eye Ointments …… 235
第三节 膏药 …… 236
10.3 Plasters …… 236
一、概述…… 236
10.3.1 Overview …… 236
二、黑膏药…… 237
10.3.2 Black Plasters…… 237
三、白膏药…… 240
10.3.3 White Plasters …… 240
四、膏药的质量检查…… 240
10.3.4 Quality Inspection of Plasters …… 240
第四节 贴膏剂 …… 241
10.4 Cataplasms…… 241
一、橡胶膏剂…… 241

10.4.1 Adhesive Plasters …… 241
二、凝胶膏剂…… 244
10.4.2 Hydrogel Plasters …… 244
三、贴剂…… 246
10.4.3 Patches …… 246
四、贴膏剂的质量检查…… 248
10.4.4 Quality Inspection of Cataplasms …… 248
第五节 凝胶剂、糊剂和涂膜剂 …… 250
一、凝胶剂…… 250
二、糊剂…… 251
三、涂膜剂…… 251

第十一章 栓剂 …… 252

Chapter 11 Suppository …… 252

第一节 概述 …… 253
11.1 Overview …… 253
一、栓剂的含义…… 253
11.1.1 The Definition of Suppositories …… 253
二、栓剂的特点 …… 253
11.1.2 The Characteristics of Suppositories …… 253
三、栓剂的分类…… 254
11.1.3 The Classification of Suppositories …… 254
四、栓剂中药物的吸收途径及其影响因素…… 257
11.1.4 Drug Absorption Pathways of Suppositories and Relevant Factors Affecting Absorption …… 257
第二节 栓剂的基质与附加剂 …… 259
11.2 Bases and Additives in Suppositories …… 259
一、基质的要求…… 260
11.2.1 Requirements of Bases …… 260
二、基质的种类…… 260
11.2.2 The Classification of Bases …… 260
三、栓剂的附加剂…… 263
11.2.3 Additives in Suppositories …… 263
四、栓剂基质与附加剂的选用…… 265
11.2.4 Selection of Bases and Additives in Suppositories …… 265
第三节 栓剂的制法 …… 267
11.3 Preparation of Suppositories …… 267
一、一般栓剂的制法…… 267
11.3.1 Preparation of General Suppositories …… 267
二、特殊栓剂的制法…… 271
11.3.2 Preparation of Special Suppositories …… 271
第四节 栓剂的质量检查、包装与贮藏 …… 273

11.4 The Quality Inspection, Packaging and Storage of Suppositories ······ 273
一、栓剂的质量检查······ 273
11.4.1 Quality Inspection of Suppositories ······ 273
二、栓剂的包装与贮藏······ 274
11.4.2 The Packaging and Storage of Suppositories ······ 274

第十二章 胶剂······ 275

Chapter 12 Glues ······ 275

第一节 概述 ······ 275
12.1 Overview ······ 275
一、胶剂的含义······ 275
12.1.1 The Definition of Glues ······ 275
二、胶剂的分类······ 276
12.1.2 The Classification of Glues······ 276
第二节 胶剂的原辅料选择 ······ 277
12.2 Raw Materials Selection of Glues······ 277
一、原料的选择······ 277
12.2.1 Selection of Raw Material ······ 277
二、辅料的选择······ 278
12.2.2 Selection of Excipients ······ 278
第三节 胶剂的制法 ······ 279
12.3 Preparation of Glues ······ 279
第四节 胶剂的质量要求与检查 ······ 284
12.4 Quality Requirements and Inspections of Glues ······ 284
一、胶剂的质量要求······ 284
12.4.1 Quality Requirements of Glues ······ 284
二、胶剂的质量检查······ 284
12.4.2 Quality Inspection of Glues ······ 284

第十三章 胶囊剂 ······ 285

Chapter 13 Capsules ······ 285

第一节 概述 ······ 285
13.1 Overview ······ 285
一、胶囊剂的含义······ 285
13.1.1 The Definition of Capsules ······ 285
二、胶囊剂的特点······ 286
13.1.2 The Characteristics of Capsules······ 286
三、胶囊剂的分类······ 287
13.1.3 The Classifications of Capsules ······ 287
第二节 胶囊剂的制法 ······ 288
13.2 Preparation of Capsules ······ 288

一、硬胶囊的制法…… 288
13.2.1 Preparation of Hard Capsule …… 288
二、软胶囊的制法…… 293
13.2.2 Preparation of Soft Capsule …… 293
三、肠溶胶囊的制法…… 299
13.2.3 Preparation of Enteric Capsule …… 299
第三节 胶囊剂的质量检查、包装与贮藏 …… 300
13.3 Quality Inspection, Packaging and Storage of Capsules …… 300
一、胶囊剂的质量检查…… 300
13.3.1 Quality Inspection of Capsules …… 300
二、胶囊剂常见质量问题…… 302
13.3.2 Common Quality Problems of Capsules …… 302
三、胶囊剂的包装、贮藏…… 302
13.3.3 Packaging and Storage of Capsules …… 302

第十四章 丸剂 …… 304

Chapter 14 Pills …… 304

第一节 概述 …… 305
14.1 Overview …… 305
一、丸剂的含义…… 305
14.1.1 The Definition of Pills …… 305
二、丸剂的特点…… 305
14.1.2 The Characteristics of Pills …… 305
三、丸剂的分类及制法…… 306
14.1.3 The Classification and Preparation of Pills …… 306
第二节 水丸 …… 307
14.2 Water-bindered Pills …… 307
一、水丸的含义与特点…… 307
14.2.1 Definition and Characteristics …… 307
二、水丸的赋形剂…… 307
14.2.2 Excipients …… 307
三、水丸的制法…… 308
14.2.3 Preparation of Water-bindered Pills …… 308
第三节 蜜丸 …… 311
14.3 Honeyed Pills …… 311
一、蜜丸的含义与特点…… 311
14.3.1 Definition and Characteristics …… 311
二、蜂蜜的炼制…… 311
14.3.2 Refining of Honey …… 311
三、蜜丸的制法…… 312
14.3.3 Preparation of Honeyed Pills …… 312

四、蜜丸常见质量问题与解决措施…… 314
14.3.4 Common Quality Problems and Solutions …… 314
五、水蜜丸…… 315
14.3.5 Water-Honeyed Pills …… 315
第四节 浓缩丸 …… 316
14.4 Condensed Pills …… 316
一、概述 …… 316
14.4.1 Overview …… 316
二、浓缩丸的制法…… 317
14.4.2 Preparation of Condensed Pills …… 317
第五节 糊丸与蜡丸 …… 319
14.5 Pasted Pills and Waxed Pills …… 319
一、糊丸…… 319
14.5.1 Pasted Pills …… 319
二、蜡丸…… 320
14.5.2 Waxed Pills …… 320
第六节 滴丸 …… 320
14.6 Dripping Pills …… 320
一、滴丸的含义与特点…… 320
14.6.1 Definition and Characteristics …… 320
二、滴丸的制法…… 321
14.6.2 Preparation of Dripping Pills …… 321
三、滴丸的质量评价与影响滴丸质量的因素…… 323
14.6.3 Quality Evaluation of Dripping Pills and Its Quality Influence Factors …… 323
第七节 丸剂的包衣 …… 325
14.7 Pill Coating …… 325
一、包衣目的…… 325
14.7.1 Purpose of Pill Coating …… 325
二、包衣种类 …… 325
14.7.2 Types of Pill Coating …… 325
三、丸剂包衣的方法…… 326
14.7.3 Method of Pill Coating …… 326
第八节 丸剂的质量检查、包装与贮藏 …… 326
14.8 Quality Inspection, Packaging and Storage of Pills …… 326
一、质量检查…… 326
14.8.1 Quality Inspection …… 326
二、丸剂的包装与贮藏…… 328
14.8.2 Package and Storage of Pills …… 328

第十五章　颗粒剂 …… 329
Chapter 15　Granules …… 329
第一节　概述 …… 329
15.1　Overview …… 329
一、颗粒剂的含义与特点 …… 329
15.1.1　The Definition and Characteristics of Granules …… 329
二、颗粒剂的分类 …… 330
15.1.2　The Classification of Granules …… 330
第二节　颗粒剂的制法 …… 331
15.2　Preparation of Granules …… 331
一、颗粒剂的制备工艺流程 …… 331
15.2.1　The Preparation Process of the Granules …… 331
二、水溶性颗粒的制法 …… 331
15.2.2　Preparation of Water-Soluble Granules …… 331
三、酒溶性颗粒的制法 …… 335
15.2.3　Preparation of Alcohol-Soluble Granules …… 335
四、混悬颗粒的制法 …… 336
15.2.4　Preparation of Suspended Granules …… 336
五、泡腾颗粒的制法 …… 336
15.2.5　Preparation of Effervescent Granules …… 336
第三节　颗粒剂的质量检查 …… 337
15.3　Quality Inspection of Granules …… 337
一、外观性状 …… 337
15.3.1　Appearance …… 337
二、粒度 …… 337
15.3.2　Particle Size …… 337
三、水分 …… 337
15.3.3　Determination of Water …… 337
四、溶化性 …… 337
15.3.4　Dispersion …… 337
五、装量差异 …… 338
15.3.5　Weight Variation …… 338
六、装量 …… 338
15.3.6　Filling …… 338
七、微生物限度 …… 338
15.3.7　Microbial Limit …… 338

第十六章　片剂 …… 339
Chapter 16　Tablets …… 339
第一节　概述 …… 340
16.1　Overview …… 340

一、中药片剂的含义与特点 …… 340
16.1.1 The Definition and Characteristics of Traditional Chinese Medicinal Tablets …… 340
二、片剂的分类 …… 341
16.1.2 The Classification of Tablets …… 341
三、中药片剂的类型 …… 343
16.1.3 The Classification of Traditional Chinese Medicinal Tablets …… 343
第二节 片剂的辅料 …… 344
一、稀释剂与吸收剂 …… 344
二、润湿剂与黏合剂 …… 345
三、崩解剂 …… 346
四、润滑剂 …… 347
第三节 中药片剂的制法 …… 348
16.3 Manufacturing Operations of Traditional Chinese Medicinal Tablets …… 348
一、湿法制粒压片法 …… 348
16.3.1 Wet Granulation …… 348
二、干法制粒压片法 …… 359
16.3.2 Dry Granulation …… 359
三、粉末直接压片法 …… 359
16.3.3 Direct Compression …… 359
四、压片时可能发生的问题与解决办法 …… 360
16.3.4 Compression Issues: Causes and Remedies …… 360
第四节 片剂的包衣 …… 364
16.4 Tablets Coating …… 364
一、片剂包衣的目的、种类与要求 …… 365
16.4.1 Purpose, Types and Requirements of Tablet Coating …… 365
二、片剂包衣的方法与设备 …… 366
16.4.2 Methods and Equipments for Tablet Coating …… 366
三、片剂包衣物料与工序 …… 367
16.4.3 Tablet Coating Materials and Coating Operations …… 367
第五节 片剂的质量要求与检查 …… 376
16.5 Quality Requirements and Inspection of Tablets …… 376
一、片剂的质量要求 …… 376
16.5.1 Quality Requirements of Tablets …… 376
二、片剂的质量检查 …… 378
16.5.2 Quality Inspection of Tablets …… 378
第六节 片剂的包装与贮存 …… 380
16.6 Packaging and Storage of Tablets …… 380
一、片剂的包装 …… 380
16.6.1 Packaging of Tablets …… 380
二、片剂的贮存 …… 381
16.6.2 Storage of Tablets …… 381

第十七章　气体药剂 …… 382

Chapter 17　Gas Potion …… 382

第一节　气雾剂 …… 382

17.1　Aerosols …… 382

一、概述 …… 382

17.1.1　Overview …… 382

二、气雾剂的组成 …… 384

17.1.2　The Composition of Aerosols …… 384

三、气雾剂的制法 …… 386

17.1.3　The Preparation of Aerosols …… 386

四、气雾剂的质量要求与检查 …… 388

17.1.4　The Quality Requirements and Inspections of the Aerosols …… 388

五、气雾剂的贮存 …… 388

17.1.5　Aerosol Storage …… 388

第二节　喷雾剂与粉雾剂 …… 388

17.2　Sprays and Powder Aerosols …… 388

一、喷雾剂 …… 388

17.2.1　Sprays …… 388

二、粉雾剂 …… 390

17.2.2　Powder Aerosols …… 390

三、喷雾剂与粉雾剂的质量要求与检查 …… 391

17.2.3　Quality Requirements and Inspections of Sprays and Powder Aerosols …… 391

第十八章　其他剂型 …… 393

Chapter 18　Some Other Dosage Forms …… 393

第一节　膜剂 …… 394

18.1　Pellicles …… 394

一、概述 …… 394

18.1.1　Overview …… 394

二、膜剂常用的成膜材料与辅料 …… 395

18.1.2　The Commonly Film-Forming and Auxiliary Materials of Pellicles …… 395

三、膜剂的制备 …… 396

18.1.3　Preparation of Pellicles …… 396

四、膜剂的质量检查 …… 399

18.1.4　Quality Inspection of Pellicles …… 399

第二节　海绵剂 …… 400

18.2　Spongia Agent …… 400

一、海绵剂的含义 …… 400

18.2.1　The Definition of Spongia Agent …… 400

二、海绵剂的分类 …… 400

18.2.2　The Classifications of Spongia Agent …… 400

三、海绵剂的制法…… 400
18.2.3 The Preparation of Spongia Agent …… 400
第三节 丹药 …… 401
18.3 Dan Yao …… 401
一、丹药的含义…… 401
18.3.1 The Definition of Dan Yao …… 401
二、丹药的特点…… 401
18.3.2 The Characteristics of Dan Yao …… 401
三、丹药的分类…… 402
18.3.3 The Classification of Dan Yao …… 402
四、丹药的制法…… 402
18.3.4 The Preparation of Dan Yao …… 402
五、丹药生产过程中的防护…… 402
18.3.5 The Protective Measures During Preparation of Dan Yao …… 402
第四节 烟剂、烟熏剂、香囊（袋）剂 …… 403
18.4 Fumicants, Fumigants and Sachets …… 403
一、烟剂…… 403
18.4.1 Fumicants …… 403
二、烟熏剂…… 404
18.4.2 Fumigants …… 404
三、香囊（袋）剂…… 404
18.4.3 Sachets …… 404
第五节 离子导入剂与沐浴剂 …… 405
18.5 Ionphoretic Agent and Bath Agent …… 405
一、离子导入剂…… 405
18.5.1 Ionphoretic Agent …… 405
二、沐浴剂…… 406
18.5.2 Bath Agent …… 406
第六节 锭剂、糕剂、钉剂、线剂、条剂、灸剂、熨剂与棒剂 …… 407
18.6 Pastille, Cake Agent, Nail Agent, Thread Agent, Strip Agent, Moxibustion Agent, Compression Agent and Club Agent …… 407
一、锭剂…… 407
18.6.1 Pastille …… 407
二、糕剂…… 407
18.6.2 Cake Agent …… 407
三、钉剂…… 408
18.6.3 Nail Agent …… 408
四、线剂…… 408
18.6.4 Thread Agent …… 408
五、条剂…… 408
18.6.5 Strip Agent …… 408
六、灸剂…… 408

18.6.6 Moxibustion Agent …… 408
七、熨剂…… 409
18.6.7 Compression Agent …… 409
八、棒剂…… 409
18.6.8 Club Agent…… 409

第十九章 药物制剂新技术与新剂型 …… 410

Chapter 19 New Technologies and New Dosage Forms of Pharmaceutical Preparations …… 410

第一节 药物制剂新技术 …… 411
19.1 New Pharmaceutical Technique …… 411
一、包合技术…… 411
19.1.1 Inclusion Compounds Technology …… 411
二、固体分散技术…… 414
19.1.2 Solid Dispersion Technology…… 414
三、微囊与微球的制备技术…… 418
19.1.3 Microencapsulation Technology and Microspheres Technology …… 418
四、纳米乳与亚微乳的制备技术…… 426
19.1.4 Nano-Emulsion and Sub-Microemulsion Preparation Technology …… 426
五、纳米粒的制备技术…… 428
19.1.5 Nanoparticle Preparation Technology …… 428
六、脂质体的制备技术…… 430
19.1.6 Liposomes Preparation Technology …… 430
第二节 药物制剂新剂型 …… 433
一、缓控释制剂…… 433
二、迟释制剂…… 438
三、前体药物…… 439
四、靶向制剂…… 439

第二十章 中药制剂的稳定性…… 442

Chapter 20 The Stability of TCM Preparations …… 442

第一节 概述 …… 442
20.1 Overview …… 442
一、中药制剂稳定性的研究意义…… 442
20.1.1 Significance of Research on the Stability of TCM Preparations…… 442
二、中药制剂稳定性的研究内容…… 443
20.1.2 Research Contents on the Stability of TCM Preparations …… 443
第二节 影响中药制剂稳定性的因素及提高稳定性的方法 …… 444
20.2 Factors Affecting the Stability of TCM Preparations and Methods for Improving the Stability…… 444
一、影响中药制剂稳定性的因素…… 444

20.2.1 Factors Affecting the Stability of TCM Preparations ········ 444
二、提高中药制剂稳定性的方法 ········ 448
20.2.2 Methods for Improving the Stability of TCM Preparations ········ 448
第三节 中药制剂的稳定性考察方法 ········ 451
20.3 Methods to Test the Stability of TCM Preparation ········ 451
一、中药制剂稳定性考察要求 ········ 451
20.3.1 Requirements for the Stability of TCM Preparation ········ 451
二、中药制剂稳定性考察项目 ········ 452
20.3.2 Testing Items of the Stability of TCM Preparation ········ 452
三、中药制剂稳定性考察方法 ········ 454
20.3.3 Methods for Testing the Stability of TCM Preparation ········ 454
四、中药制剂稳定性试验应注意的问题 ········ 463
20.3.4 Problems Requiring Attention Regarding the Stability of TCM Preparations ········ 463
第四节 包装材料对制剂稳定性的影响 ········ 465
20.4 The Effect of Packaging Materials on the Stability of Preparation ········ 465
一、玻璃 ········ 466
20.4.1 Glass ········ 466
二、塑料 ········ 467
20.4.2 Plastic ········ 467
三、橡胶 ········ 467
20.4.3 Rubber ········ 467
四、金属 ········ 468
20.4.4 Metal ········ 468

第二十一章 中药制剂的配伍变化 ········ 470
Chapter 21 The Compatibility Changes in Traditional Chinese Medicine Preparations ········ 470
第一节 概述 ········ 470
21.1 Overview ········ 470
一、药物配伍的概念 ········ 470
21.1.1 The Concept of the Medical Compatibility ········ 470
二、药物配伍应用的目的 ········ 471
21.1.2 The Purposes of the Medical Compatibility Application ········ 471
三、药物配伍变化的类型 ········ 471
21.1.3 The Types of Medical Compatibility Changes ········ 471
第二节 药剂学的配伍变化 ········ 473
21.2 The Compatibility Changes in Pharmaceutics ········ 473
一、物理的配伍变化 ········ 473
21.2.1 The Physical Compatibility Changes ········ 473
二、化学的配伍变化 ········ 474
21.2.2 The Chemical Compatibility Changes ········ 474
三、注射剂的配伍变化 ········ 477
21.2.3 The Compatibility Changes of Injections ········ 477

第三节　药理学的配伍变化 479
21.3 The Pharmacological Compatibility Changes 479
一、协同作用 480
21.3.1 The Synergistic Effects 480
二、拮抗作用 480
21.3.2 The Antagonistic Effects 480
三、产生不良反应 480
21.3.3 The Adverse Reactions 480
四、制剂在体内发生的相互作用 480
21.3.4 The *in vivo* Interactions of the Preparations 480
第四节　预测配伍变化的实验方法 482
21.4 Experimental Methods for Predicting Compatibility Changes 482
第五节　配伍变化的处理原则与方法 484
21.5 The Handling Principles and Methods of the Compatibility Changes 484
一、处理原则 484
21.5.1 The Handling Principles 484
二、药剂学配伍变化的处理方法 484
21.5.2 The Handling Method of the Pharmaceutical Compatibility Changes 484

第二十二章　生物药剂学与药物动力学在中药制剂中的应用 487
Chapter 22 Application of Biopharmaceutics and Pharmacokinetics in the Preparations of Chinese Medicine 487
第一节　生物药剂学概论 488
22.1 Introduction to Biopharmaceutics 488
一、生物药剂学的含义与研究内容 488
22.1.1 Concept and Contents of Biopharmaceutics 488
二、药物的体内过程 489
22.1.2 The in *vivo* Behavior of Drugs 489
第二节　药物动力学概论 492
22.2 Introduction to Pharmacokinetics 492
一、药物动力学的含义与研究内容 492
22.2.1 Concept and Contents of Pharmacokinetics 492
二、药物动力学常用术语 493
22.2.2 Commonly used Terms in Pharmacokinetics 493
三、生物利用度与生物等效性 496
22.2.3 Bioavailability and Bioequivalence 496
第三节　中药制剂的生物药剂学与药物动力学研究 498
22.3 Biopharmaceutics and Pharmacokinetics in Chinese Medical Preparations 498
一、中药制剂的生物药剂学与药物动力学研究意义 498
22.3.1 Significance of Research on Biopharmaceutics and Pharmacokinetics of Chinese Medical Preparations 498
二、中药制剂的生物药剂学与药物动力学发展概况 499

22.3.2 Overview of the Development of Biopharmaceutics and Pharmacokinetics in Chinese Medical Preparations ········ 499
三、影响药物（中药）制剂疗效的因素 ········ 500
22.3.3 Factors Affecting the Efficacy of Pharmaceutical Preparations ········ 500

参考文献 ········ 503

第一章 绪论
Chapter 1 An Introduction

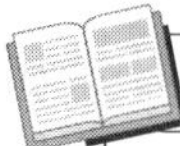

学习目标 | Learning Goals

1. **掌握** 中药药剂学的含义、性质、任务；中药剂型选择的基本原则；中药药剂工作的法定依据。

2. **熟悉** 中药药剂学常用术语的概念；中药药剂学在中医药事业中的地位与作用；药品标准。

3. **了解** 中药药剂学的发展简况、研究进展；药品管理法规；中药剂型的分类方法。

Knowledge Requirements:

1. **To master** the definition, characteristics, and tasks of Pharmaceutics of Traditional Chinese Medicine; the basic selection principles of dosage forms; the legal basis for Pharmaceutics of Chinese medicine.

2. **To be familiar with** the concepts of commonly-used terms in Pharmaceutics of Traditional Chinese Medicine; its position and role in TCM cause; and drug standards.

3.**To know** the brief history of R&D of TCM Pharmaceutics; drug management regulations; and the classification of dosage forms of TCM.

第一节 概述
1.1 Overview

一、中药药剂学的性质
1.1.1 The Characteristics of Pharmaceutics of Traditional Chinese Medicine

中药药剂学是以中医药理论为指导，运用现代科学技术，研究中药药剂的配制理论、生产技术、质量控制与合理应用等内容的综合性应用技术学科。该学科是连接中医与中药的纽带，其内容涉及中药类专业的诸多课程以及现代制药理论和技术，既具有运用多学科知识与技能的综合性，又具有紧密联系生产和临床的实用性，还具有保持传统制剂理论和现代制剂理论的统一性。该课程是高等中医药教育中药类各专业的主干课程之一。

Pharmaceutics of Traditional Chinese Medicine, with the guidance of TCM theroies, is a comprehensive application and technics discipline which studies the theories in herbal dosage preparation, productive technics, quality control and correct usage by modern scientific technology. This discipline is the tie linking Chinese medicine and Chinese pharmacy, which involves many courses in Chinese pharmacy, and modern pharmaceutical theories and technics. It covers the application of multidisciplinary knowledge and skills, utility in practical production and clinics, and reserving unity of the traditional and modern theories in dosage preparation. This course is one of the stem programs in higher education of Traditional Chinese Medicine.

中药药剂学包括中药调剂学和中药制剂学。中药调剂学是研究方剂调配技术、理论和应用的科学，除应掌握中药调配应用及毒剧药管理等技能外，还应熟悉常用药物的性能特点、用法用量、功能主治、组方配伍等相关知识，以便配合临床，指导和监督合理用药，并能开展中药临床药学的相关研究。中药制剂学主要阐述中药剂型的基本理论、特点与应用，剂型和药物传递系统设计，以及中药制剂的工艺方法、操作技术与辅料选用等。中药制剂学的内容随着中药制剂产业化、现代化的发展得以不断丰富和完善。

TCM Pharmaceutics includes Dispensing Pharmaceutics and Technological Pharmaceutics. TCM Dispensing pharmaceutics is a science of studying the technology, theories and application of formulations. The formulation and highly toxic drugs arrangement should be handled and also the commonly-used drugs' properties, application and doses, functions and indications, prescriptions prescribed should be learnt by heart so as to have them coodinated with clinics for guiding supervising rational medication and studying on clinical pharmacy. TCM Pharmaceutics focuses basic theories of dosages, characteristics and applications, design of dosage forms and drug transmitting systems and technical methods and auxiliary material selection, etc.. Along with its development of industrialization and modernization, TCM Pharmaceutics will be continuely enriched and improved.

中药药剂学是中医药学的重要组成部分，其理论和技术随中医药学的发展进程而得以产生、发展并逐步形成体系。中药药剂学应坚持以中医药理论为指导，体现制剂功能主治的特点。中药药剂学的研究发展，特别应注意以下几个方面。

TCM Pharmaceutics is an important component part of TCM, the theories and techniques of which are gradually produced, developed and then a system is gradually formed. with the advancing of TCM. TCM Pharmaceutics should adhere to the guidance of TCM theories and embody its functions and indications.

The following aspects should be take into consideration in R&D of TCM Pharmaceutics:

（1）中药制剂的处方组成必须符合中医药理论。在理、法、方、药的基础上，遵循君、臣、佐、使的制方规律，选择合适的药物组合成方，通过合理的配伍，增强或改变其原有的功用。调其偏性，制其毒性，消除或减缓其对人体的不利因素，使各具特性的药物发挥综合作用，达到增效减毒的目的。所谓“药有个性之专长，方有合群之妙用”，即是此意。

(1) The drug composition must conform to TCM theories. Based on the principles of "theories, methods, prescriptions, drugs", in accordance with the formula rules of "monarch, minister, assistant and guide(or jun chen zuo shi)", proper drugs are selected for a good prescription by thoughtful compatibility so that the original functioning is to be intensified or changed. In addition, the drug's specific property is modified, its toxicity controlled, and the poor factors to human body, eliminated or alleviated. Thus, drugs with various natures play a united role to get better effect and lesser toxicity. So, there is an interesting saying: "Each drug has its own speciality, while each formula creates its wonder".

（2）中药制剂提取与纯化的工艺研究，首先必须考虑君臣药的提取效率，以维持原方特有疗效。不仅要考虑有效成分和（或）指标性成分，而且要考虑“活性混合物”。即采用现代科学技术与评价指标深入研究能保持中医方剂特色的中药提取、纯化工艺条件与参数，达到“去粗取精”的目的，以获得体现原方剂功能主治的中药有效物质（半成品）。

(2) In technical researches on extraction and purification of TCM Pharmaceutics. It must be dwelt on first that the extraction efficiency of monarchal and ministerial drugs should keep the original curative effect. Considering not only the active ingredients and/or targeted ingredients, but the “active mixture”. That is, using modern sci-tech techniques and evaluating indicators to further study the conditions and the parameters of extraction and purification which will help the TCM formulae features maintained, so as to achieve “discarding the dross and selecting the essential”, and obtain the effective substances (semi-finished products) which embody the functions of original formulations.

（3）中药制剂成型工艺的研究，是中药制剂制备工艺研究中十分重要的环节。该工艺研究强调“方-证-剂”的理念，坚持根据疾病治疗需求与方药性质选择相应剂型的指导原则，以满足中药制剂的“三效”（速效、高效、长效）、“三小”（剂量小、副作用小、毒性小）、“五方便”（服用、携带、生产、运输、贮藏方便）要求。

(3) The molding of TCM Pharmaceutics is a very important link in the drug preparation process. This technology values the idea of “formula-certificate-agent” and sticks to the guiding principle of selecting the proper dosage form matching with the need for the treatment of diseases, and the characters of drugs in the prescription, so that to lead to the “three effects” (quick effect, high efficiency, and long-term effect), “three smalls” (small dose, a little side effects, and low toxicity)”, five conveniences (convenient to taking, carrying, producing, transporting, and storing).

（4）中药制剂是直接应用于临床的药品，衡量其质量优劣的最终指标是药品是否安全、有效、稳定、可控。中药制剂质量标准的制定，要显示中药制剂质量控制与评价标准的特点。除符合现行版《中国药典》制剂通则要求外，应首选君、臣药中的有效或活性成分作为定性鉴别和含量控制指标，同时尽量考虑以多成分作为指标，从而保证制剂处方的功能主治可控。此外，还可以探索制定中药制剂的指纹图谱。

(4) TCM preparations are directly applied in clinics, whose ultimate indicator for measuring their quality is whether they are safe, effective, stable and controllable. Making the quality standards of TCM preparations should highlight the quality control and evaluation standards. In addition to complying with the general requirements of the current *Chinese Pharmacopoeia*, the active ingredients in monarch and minister drugs are reguarded as indexes of qualitative identification and content control. Meanwhile, it is better to involve multi-components in indicators to ensure their aimed functions and indications available and controllable. In addition, the fingerprints of TCM preparations may be explored.

（5）中药制剂的药效学研究，在运用现代药理学方法及模型的同时，注重中药对机体的整体协调作用，应尽可能建立符合中医学辨证要求的动物模型，特别注意自然环境、精神状态等对疾病的发生与发展的作用。因此中医证候动物模型需要在中医理论体系指导下，体现中药的功能主治。中药制剂的药物动力学研究不仅要借鉴现代药剂学中药物动力学的研究方法，而且还应发展符合中医药传统理论和中药复方配伍特点的新的研究方法，如药理效应法、毒理效应法等。

(5) In the researching on pharmacodynamics of TCM preparations, the modern pharmacological methods and models are employed, the holistic coordination of the preperation on the organic body, is stressed, and animal models are built with TCM dialectical requirements as far as possible, attention is paid to the effect on the occurrence and development of diseases by natural environment and mindset.

Therefore, the animal models with TCM syndromes should be instructed by TCM systematic theories which will embody the functions and indications of preparations. The study of pharmacokinetics of TCM preparations should not only learn from the methods of pharmacokinetics in modern pharmacy, but also expand new methods which should conform to TCM theories and the compound compatibility features, such as pharmacological effect method, toxicological effect method and so on.

（6）中药制剂的临床应用，必须在中医药理论指导下辨证用药，方可发挥其应有的疗效。成药组方时应注重所防治病证的病因、病机、治疗法则，以病证为主体，辩证立法，以法统方，以方遣药。虽然方中药物有君、臣、佐、使之分，但药味及用量的多少，取决于病情、治法的需要。

(6) TCM preparations usage must be carried out under the guidance of TCM syndrome differentiation for its due effect. Formulating drugs should focus on the etiology, pathogenesis, and therapeutic rules of diseases, taking syndrome as the main body, to determine the treating method, choosing formula, thinking over and deciding drugs. Although there are monarch, minister, admirer and envoy, in the formation, yet the variety and quantity of drugs entirely depend on the disease and treatment of it.

任何一个药品在从原料药转化为制剂产品的过程中，即从组方与剂型选择、制剂研究以及质量标准的制定等方面，都必然涉及很多基础研究。中药药剂固然具有原料药物加工科学的属性，同时为保证加工后的药物制剂具有良好的理化性质和生理药理活性，在运用该学科本身的知识外，还需涉及中医学、中药学、方剂学、中药炮制学、有机化学、中药化学、生理学、生物化学、病理学、中药药理学、物理化学、化工原理、计算机数学、统计学等相关知识。因此学习者应该具备比较全面的中医药专业知识和现代科学知识。

To transform drug substances from active pharmaceutical ingredients(APIs) into a preparation, that is, the prescription, made, dosage form, selected, preparation studied, and quality standards formulated, necessarily all cover many basic researches. TCM preparations have the properties of raw material processing, meanwhile, to ensure that they have good properties in physics/chemistry and physiology/pharmacology after having been processed. This discipline’s knowhow is quite important besides the knowledge of Chinese medicine, Chinese Pharmacy TCM Formulae, TCM Drug Processing, Organic Chemistry, TCM Chemistry, Physiology, Biochemistry, Pathology, TCM Pharmacology, Physical Chemistry, Chemical Engineering Principles, Computer Mathematics, Statistics and other related knowledge. Therefore, learners should have a relatively comprehensive knowledge of traditional Chinese medicine and modern scientific knowledge.

二、中药药剂学的任务
1.1.2 The Tasks of TCM Pharmaceutics

中药药剂学的基本任务是研究如何根据临床用药和处方中药材的性质以及生产、贮藏、运输、携带、服用等方面的要求，将中药制成适宜的剂型，以质优价廉的制剂满足医疗卫生保健的需要。具体任务概述如下。

The main task of TCM Pharmaceutics is to study how to make drugs into proper dosages in accordance with clinical needs and drug properties in the prescription. When meeting the requirements in production, storage, transportation, carrying, taking, they will satisfy the need of health care.

The specific tasks are outlined below.

（1）继承和整理中医药学中有关药剂学的理论、技术与经验，为发展中药药剂奠定基础。中医药宝库中有关药剂的内容极其丰富，但大多散见于历代医书、方书、本草、医案等医药典籍

中。在“系统学习，全面掌握，整理提高”理念的指引下，虽已进行了部分继承和整理工作，但尚需进一步深入，以使其系统化、科学化。很多著名的传统制剂目前还缺少客观的质量控制方法与标准，以至于难以达到中药现代化的要求。

(1) Inheriting and summarizing the theories, techniques and experience of drug preparation in TCM is to lay the foundation for the development of TCM Pharmaceutics. TCM treasure house has plenty of descriptions and sayings on pharmacy, but most of them are seen in various dynasties' medical books, formulae books, herb books, case records. Under the guidance of the idea of "systematic learning, overall grasping, collating and hoisting", the work of inheritance and organization has to be carried out, further in-depth work is necessary to help it systematicized and with scientificity. Many well-known traditional preparations still lack objective quality control methods and standards, which cause difficulties to meet the requirements for TCM modernization.

（2）充分吸收和应用现代药剂学的理论知识和研究成果，实现中药剂型现代化。在中医药理论指导下，应用和推广制药新技术、新工艺、新设备和新辅料，以提高中药药剂的研究水平，改进某些传统的中药剂型，逐步创制出既具有中国传统医药特色，又与现代科学发展相适应的中药新剂型。

(2) The theoretical knowledge and research outcomes of modern pharmacy should be fully absorbed and applied to realize the modernization of TCM Pharmaceutics. With the guidance of TCM theories, drug preparation new skills, new technology, new equipments and new auxiliary materials are to be applied and spread to scale up the research level, better traditional dosage forms, and gradually to built new formulation development with both Chinese tradition and modern scientific scenario.

（3）积极寻找与开发新的药用辅料，以适应新制剂、新剂型、大品种二次开发的需要。药用辅料是指生产药品和调配处方时所用的赋形剂和附加剂。辅料不仅是原料药物制剂成型的物质基础，而且与制剂工艺过程的难易，药品的质量、稳定性与安全性，给药途径，作用方式与释药速度，临床疗效，以及新剂型、新药品的开发密切相关。故需积极寻找与开发符合中药制剂特色的新辅料，体现“药辅合一”“与药效相结合”的特色，以适应中药制剂学现代化发展的迫切需求。

(3) By actively seeking and trying new medicinal auxiliary material, the needs of new preparations, new dosage forms and secondary development of large varieties are met. Medicinal auxiliary materials refer to the excipients and additives used in the manufacturing pharmaceuticals and the formulation of prescriptions. Auxiliary materials are the material base for the formation of raw material pharmaceutical preparations.They also closely related to the preparation process, quality, stability and safety, the route of administration, the mode of action, the release rate of drugs, clinical efficacy and development of new dosage forms and new medications. Therefore, it's necessary to actively seek and develop new auxiliary materials that conform to the characteristics of TCM preparations, embody the features of "drugs and auxiliary materials in one" and "bond of effect and drugs", so as to adapt the urgent situation in modern advancing of TCM preparations.

三、中药药剂学在中医药事业中的地位与作用

1.1.3 Position and Role of TCM Pharmaceutics in Chinese Medicine

中药药剂学是专门研究中药剂型和制剂的学科，作为联系中医与中药的纽带和桥梁，在中医临床和医药工业中占有极其重要的地位。中药药剂学的发展水平在一定程度上集中体现了整个中医药行业和现代科学技术的技术水平和发展情况。

Pharmaceutics of Traditional Chinese Medicine is a discipline specializing in drug dosage forms and preparations. As a link and bridge between traditional Chinese medicine and medication, it plays an extremely important role in the clinics and medical industry. To a certain extent, the development level of TCM Pharmaceutics reflects the technical level and progress of the entire TCM industry and modern science and technology.

中药药剂学将中药基础研究与产业化发展紧密结合，是“中药研究—产业化生产—医疗实践”的关键环节。中药制剂的安全、有效、稳定和可控的程度，决定了用药效果及药品的成本和经济效益。通过合理的剂型设计、给药途径，及制备工艺等方面的研究，可实现中药制剂研究成果从实验室向产业化的转变。研究成果的转化需要不断依据生产实际情况解决工艺、技术和质量中存在的问题，并密切联系临床医疗实践，根据临床需要，改进和提高中药制剂的质量。此外，通过开展中药制剂现代化关键技术、核心问题的攻关研究，逐步解决影响中药制剂现代化发展的一系列瓶颈问题，如制剂物质基础不明确、制备工艺不合理、质量评价不完善等，才能逐渐实现中药药剂的剂型现代化、质量控制标准化和生产技术产业化，逐步提升我国制药工业的整体技术水平，发挥中药全产业链的优势与作用，增强中药在国际经济环境中的核心竞争力。

TCM Pharmaceutics is the key link of “Chinese drug researches-industrialized production-medical practice” by integrating the basic drug researches with the development of industrialization. The degree of safety, effectiveness, stability, and quality control of TCM preparations determines the effectiveness of medication, the cost and economic benefits of medicines. Researches on ideal dosage form design, administration way and preparation technology will give rise to the transformation of research findings from laboratory to industrialization. However, this transformation needs to constantly solve the problems in process, technology and quality based on the actual productive situation, and keep contact with the clinical medical practice, and modify and refine the quality of TCM preparations, so as to meet the clinical requirements. In addition, by researching on the key techniques and core problems of the modernization in TCM preparations, a series of bottleneck problems affecting the advancing of TCM preparations will be elimilated gradually, such as unclear material base of preparations, improper processing and incomplete quality evaluation, so that the dosage modernization, quality standardization and production industrialization will be achieved for lifting the overall capasity of China’s pharmaceutical industry, giving full play to the advantages and functions of the whole industry, and strenthening TCM core competitiveness in the globe.

四、中药药剂学常用术语
1.1.4 Commonly-Used Terms of TCM Pharmaceutics

1. 饮片、植物油脂和提取物 饮片系指药材经过炮制后可直接用于中医临床或制剂生产使用的处方药品。植物油脂和提取物系指从植物、动物中制得的挥发油、油脂、有效部位和有效成分。其中，提取物包括以水或醇为溶剂经提取制成的流浸膏、浸膏或干浸膏，含有一类或数类有效成分的有效部位和含量达到 90% 以上的单一有效成分。

(1) Pieces, Vegetable Lipids and Extracts Pieces refer to the processed medicinal materials which can be directly used in the clinics or preparation production. Vegetable lipids and extracts refer to the volatile oil, grease, effective parts and effective components made from plants and animals. Among them, the extracts include liquid extract, extract or dry extract, which are extracted in the solvent water or alcohol, with the effective parts, effective components or an effective component whose single useful content can reach 90%.

2. 药物与药品 凡用于预防、治疗和诊断疾病的物质称为药物，包括原料药与药品。药品一般是指原料药经过加工制成具有一定剂型，可直接应用的成品。

(2) **Medication and Medicine Products** Those substances used for the provention, treatment and diagnosis of diseases are named medication, including the originals and their products. Medicine products refer to the processed products with certain dosage forms and can be directly applied.

3. 剂型 根据药物的性质、用药目的和给药途径将原料药加工制成适合于预防、治疗和诊断疾病需要的不同给药形式称为药物剂型，简称剂型。它是药物施用于机体前的最后形式。如牛黄解毒片、复方丹参片、元胡止痛片等具有相同的药物应用形式"片剂"。目前常用的中药剂型有汤剂、散剂、丸剂、片剂等 40 余种。一个药物处方可以有多种剂型，如在藿香正气系列制剂中有藿香正气水、藿香正气口服液、藿香正气胶囊、藿香正气丸、藿香正气滴丸、藿香正气片、藿香正气颗粒剂等。

(3) Dosage Forms Dosage forms are different dosages which are prepared based on the drugs' properties, the treatment purposes and the administration routes for the purpose of prevention, treatment and diagnosis of diseases. They are called dosage forms for short. It is the last form of medicine before applying to the patients. For instance, Niuhuang Jiedu Tablets, Fufang Danshen Tablets and Yuanhu Zhitong Tablets are in the same application form "tablet". Nowerdays, there are over 40 TCM dosage forms, such as decoction, powder, pill, tablet, etc.. A formula can show itself in many forms. For example, concerning Huoxiang Zhengqi series, there are Huoxiang Zhengqi Tincture, Huoxiang Zhengqi Oral Liquid, Huoxiang Zhengqi Capsule, Huoxiang Zhengqi Pill, Huoxiang Zhengqi Drop Pill, Huoxiang Zhengqi Tablet, and Huoxiang Zhengqi Granule, etc..

案例导入 ¦ Case example

案例 1-1 藿香正气水

1-1 Huoxiang Zhengqi Tincture

处方： 苍术 160g 陈皮 160g 厚朴（姜制）160g 白芷 240g 茯苓 240g 大腹皮 240g 生半夏 160g 甘草浸膏 20g 广藿香油 1.6ml 紫苏叶油 0.8ml

Ingredients: Pericarpium Atractylodes Rhizoma 160g, Citri Reticulatae 160g, Magnoliae Officinalis Cortex (stir-baked with ginger juice) 160g, Angelicae Dahuricae Radix 240g, Poria 240g, Arecae Pericarpium 240g, Pinelliae Rhizoma 160g, Glycyrrhizae Extract 20g, Patchouli Oil 1.6ml, Perillae Folii Oil 0.8ml.

功能与主治： 解表化湿，理气和中。用于外感风寒、内伤湿滞或夏伤暑湿所致的感冒，症见头痛昏重、胸膈满闷、脘腹疼痛、呕吐泄泻；胃肠型感冒见上述证候者。

Functions and Indications: It is used to relieve the exterior symptems, resolve damp, regulate qi and stomach for the treatment of common cold caused by external wind-cold, internal damp stagnation or summer dampness, manifested as headache, dizziness, chest, stuffiness, fullness and stomachache vomiting, and diarrhoea; stomach flu with the symptoms described above.

制法： 以上十味，苍术、陈皮、厚朴、白芷分别用 60% 乙醇作溶剂，浸渍 24 小时后进行渗漉，前三味各收集初漉液 400ml，白芷收集初漉液 500ml，备用，继续渗漉，收集续漉液，浓缩后并入初漉液中。茯苓加水煮沸后，80℃ 温浸二次，第一次 3 小时，第二次 2 小时，取汁；生半夏用冷水浸泡，每 8 小时换水一次，泡至透心后，另加干姜 13.5g，加水煎煮二次，第一次 3 小时，第二次 2 小时；大腹皮加水煎煮 3 小时，甘草浸膏打碎后水煮化开；合并上述提取液，滤

过，滤液浓缩至适量。广藿香油、紫苏叶油用乙醇适量溶解。合并以上溶液，混匀，用乙醇与水适量调整乙醇含量，并使全量成2050ml，静置，滤过，灌装，即得。

Making Procedure: Macerate separately Atractylodis Rhizoma, Citri Reticulatae Pericarpium, Magnoliae Officinalis Cortex and Angelicae Dahuricae Radix for 24hours, using 60% ethanol as solvent. Percolate it, collect 400ml of the initial percolate of the former three drug each and 500ml from the first liquid of angelica dahurica. Collecingt the successive percolates, condensing, and combining them with the initial percolates respectively. Boiling Poria with water and macerating it at 80°C water twice, for, 3 hours and 2 hours respectively and collecting the decoctios; macerating raw Pinelliae Rhizoma with cold water, change water every 8 hours until it is soft thoroughly, then adding dried ginger 13.5g, decocing it with water twice for 3 hours and 2 hours respectively; decocting Arecae Pericarpium with water for 3 hours, pulverising Glycyrrhizae Extract and dissolving it by boiling water; then, putting all the above decoction together, getting it filtered, concentrated until proper amount left. Dissolving Patchouli Oil and Perillae Folii Oil in a right amount of ethanol. Placing the above solutions in a container to be mixed well; adjusting the ethanol content with ethanol and water, to make up the total amount to 2050ml, then, to have it stood still filtered and botting completion.

规格：每支装10ml。

Specifications: 10ml per vial.

用法与用量：口服，一次5~10ml，一日2次，用时摇匀。

Usage and Dosage: For oral administration, 5-10ml once, twice a day, shaking the vial fully before use.

注解：①原方始载于《太平惠民和剂局方》。原方由十一味药组成：大腹皮、白芷、紫苏、茯苓（去皮）各一两，半夏曲、白术、陈皮（去白）、厚朴（去粗皮，姜汁炙）、苦桔梗各二两，藿香（去土）三两，甘草（炙）二两半。

Notes: ① The original recipe was first recorded in *Taiping Huimin Heji Jufang*. It consists of 11 drugs: yi(one) liang for each of the Arecae Pericarpium, Angelicae Dahuricae Radix, Perilla and Poria (pilled); er(two) liang for each of the Pinellia tuber leaven, Atractylodis Macrocephalae Rhizoma, Citri Reticulatae Pericarpium(the white part removed), Magnoliae Officinalis Cortex(the thick skin removed and stir fried with ginger juice), bitter Platycodonis Radix, Patchouli (soil removed); san (three) liang, Glycyrrhizae Radix et Rhizoma Praeparata Cummelle er (two) liang ban (half).

新方十味，即原方去桔梗，并且将其中三味改用提取物以定量加入，即甘草浸膏、广藿香油、紫苏叶油。另外，白术换苍术；半夏曲用生半夏；引药去大枣。不仅对原处方做了修订，并由散剂（煮散）改为酊剂。

The present recipe contains ten drugs, i.e. Platycodon grandiflorum, is deselected from the old formula and fixed amount of abstrats of three of them are used, i.e. extractum Glycyrrhizae, Patchouli oil and Perilla leaf oil. Becides, Atractylodes macrocephala is replaced by Atractylodes Lancea, Pinellia tuber leaven was replaced by raw Pinellia ternate and the guiding drug jujube is removed, too. Not only the original prescription is revised, but also the powder (boiled powder) is changed into tincture.

②本方中以含挥发油的药味为多，原方剂为散剂水煎服。而改变剂型后若要使挥发油溶解，用作溶媒的醇就须提高到一定浓度（45%~50%），这样有利于有效成分的溶解，保证产品的疗效。

② In this prescription, more drugs contains volatile oil, and the originally it was decocted with water for the decoction. If the volatile oil is to be dissolved after the dosage form is changed, the alcohol used as the solvent must be increased to a concentration of 45% - 50%, which is conducive to the dissolution of effective ingredients and ensures the healing effectiveness.

③本品根据大腹皮、半夏、茯苓等药材中含生物碱、苷类、有机酸类等易溶于水的有效成分，选择水为提取溶媒，主要有效成分提取较完全；但用水作溶媒提取出的杂质较多，同时易生霉变质，故将乙醇渗漉液与水煎液混合，醇沉除杂，使不溶于乙醇的杂质，如黏液质、糊化淀粉、多糖等沉淀，到达分离精制的目的，保证了制剂的有效性和稳定性。

③ This product’s solvent is water for better effective abstracts based on the alkaloids, glycosides, organic acids and other effective ingredients of drugs soluble in water, such as Arecae Pericarpium, Pinelliae Rhizoma and Poria. However, there are impurities in the solution which apts to be deteriorated with molds. So, the ethanol percolate is added into the decoction, then such impurities as mucus, gelatnized starch and polysaccharides will be removed in the form of sedimentation and the solution is purified. The seperation makes refined solution. In this way, the effectiveness and stability of the preparation are guaranteed.

④制剂中乙醇含量高于 20% 时，即可防腐，故酊剂中无需加入防腐剂等辅料。

④ When the alcohol is higher than 20% in content, the preparation is antiseptic. So, tincture preparations do not need antiseptics.

⑤将藿香正气水改剂为藿香正气口服液，属于改剂型较为成功的案例，其制备方法与酊剂基本一致，只是最后成品中主要溶媒为水，这样避免了酊剂醇浓度较高，有一定刺激作用，对某些患者不太适合的缺点。成品中含橙皮苷、厚朴酚等酸性物质，在贮藏过程中容易发生水解而影响药液 pH 环境，进而导致树胶等高分子物质的析出和药物成分含量降低，影响产品澄明度和稳定性，故在灭菌灌封前加入氢氧化钠溶液，调节 pH 至 5.8~6.2，抑制酸性物质的水解和沉淀的产生，保证成品的稳定性和有效性。

⑤ It’s a successful case to change the dosage form of Huoxiang Zhengqi Shui into Huoxiang Zhengqi oral liquid, the preparation method is basically the same as that of the tincture, except that the main solvent in the final product is water, which avoids the disadvantages of certain stimulating effect and unsuitable feeling for some patients because of the high concentration of alcohol in the tincture. The product contains acid substances such as hesperidin and honokiol, which are likely to be hydrolyzed during storage and affect the pH value environment of the solution, further, the precipitation of high molecular substances like gum will appear and the drug ingredients will go down which will affect the clarity and stability of the product. Therefore, sodium hydroxide solution will be added before sterilization and filling, and the pH value will be adjusted to 5.8-6.2 to inhibit the hydrolysis and precipitation of acid substances, so as to ensure the stability and effectiveness of the finished product.

思考题：①简述藿香正气系列制剂的剂型选择依据。

②不同浓度的乙醇加入制剂中，分别有什么作用？

Questions: ① Please brief principles in dosage form selections in of Huoxiang Zhengqi preparation series.

② What are the effects of different concentrations of ethanol added to the preparations?

---

4. 制剂 根据《中华人民共和国药典》(以下简称《中国药典》) 药品标准等将药物加工制成具有一定规格，可直接用于临床的药物制品，称为制剂。如四物汤合剂、藿香正气口服液、一清颗粒等。制剂一般指某一个具体品种，有时可以是各种剂型、各种具体制剂的总称。同种剂型可包括多种制剂。制剂的生产一般在符合 GMP 要求的中药制药企业或医院制剂室中进行。

(4) Processing Preparation Based on the *Pharmacopoeia of the people’s Republic of China* (*Chinese Pharmacopoeia* for short) and drug standards, drugs are processed into medication products in certain specifications, and used in clinics, are called preparations, such as Siwutang Mixture, Huoxiang Zhengqi Oral liquid, Yiqing Granules, etc.. The preparation means a specific one or a general term for various dosage forms. The same dosage form may cover a variety of preparations. The production of preparations is generally carried out in the TCM pharmaceutical enterprises or hospital preparation rooms where the GMP standards are conformed to.

5. 调剂 按照医师处方专为某一患者配制，注明用法用量的药剂调配操作，称为调剂。此操作一般在医院药房的调剂室中进行。

(5) Dispensing According to the doctor's prescription, that the preparation is specially made for an individual patient and with the indications of the usage and dosage, is called dispensing. This operation is generally carried out in the dispensing room of the hospital pharmacy.

6. 成方制剂 系指以中药饮片为原料，在中医药理论指导下，经药品注册主管部门批准的处方和制法大量生产，有特有名称并标明功能主治、用法用量和规格的药品称为成方制剂。其中单味处方者称为单味制剂。成方制剂习称中成药。

(6) Prescription Preparation Those preparations, with Chinese herbal pieces as raw materials, under the guidance of TCM theories and the prescriptions and productive means approved by the drug registration authority, the preparation being produced in large scale, processing unique names and indication/functions, usage, dosage and specifications, are called prescription preparations. The prescription having one drug is called single-drug preparation. The prescription preparations is habitually called the Chinese patent medicine.

7. 新药 新药是指未曾在中国境内上市销售的药品。

(7) New Medication It refers to medications having not been marketed in China.

第二节 中药药剂学的发展简况
1.2 The Advancing of TCM Pharmaceutics

PPT

一、中药药剂学发展的历史回顾
1.2.1 A Historical Review of the Development of TCM Pharmaceutics

中药药剂学的发展是在漫长的中医药发展进程中，在古今成方及剂型的演变过程中逐渐形成和完善的。随着社会的进步，科学技术的发展和医药水平的提高，中药药剂的剂型理论、制备方法、加工技术以及临床应用等不断发展与完善。

The development of TCM Pharmaceutics is gradually formed and perfected along with the development of Chinese medicine and the evolution process of ancient and modern formulas as well. With the social progress, sci-tech development and the medicine ascendance, the formulation theories, preparation method, processing technology and clinical applications of TCM Pharmaceutics are developing as well.

中药药剂的起源可追溯至公元前2000多年，相传夏禹时期“仪狄造酒”，并有多种药物浸制而成的药酒。同时期龙山文化出土的文物证明，当时的酿酒技术已趋成熟。随酿酒而发现的曲

（酵母），具有健脾胃、助消化、消积导滞的功效，是一种早期应用的复合酶制剂，沿用至今。

The source of TCM Pharmaceutics can be traced back to over 2000 B.C. It is said that "Yidi created wine" in the period of Xia Yu, and there were many kinds of medicinal liquor made by soaking herbs in liquors. The cultural relics unearthed in Longshan Culture prove that the brewing technology at the same period was nearly mature. Yeast was found in the brewing, which is good for strengthening the spleen and stomach, helping digestion, eliminating food accumulation and removing stagnancy. It is a kind of compound enzyme preparation used in the early time and lasted till now.

相传早在公元前 1700 多年的商汤时期，宰相伊尹首创汤剂，并著有总结了方剂与制药技术的专著《汤液经》。时至今日，汤剂仍是中医用药的常用剂型。

It's said that as early as 1700 BC in the Shang Tang period, Prime Minister Yi Yin initiated the soup decoction and wrote the monograph *Tangye Jing* which summarized the prescriptions and pharmaceutical techniques. Up to now, decoction is still the commonly-used dosage form of TCM.

公元前 475 年我国进入战国时期。该时期是我国中医药理论的奠基时期。我国现存的第一部医药经典著作《黄帝内经》著于此时，其中提出了"君、臣、佐、使"的组方原则。而同时代的《汤液醪醴论》中则论述了汤液醪醴的制法和作用，并记载了汤、丸、散、膏、药酒等不同剂型。各种剂型均有较明确的制法、用法、用量与适应证，此实为中药药剂学的先导。

China entered the Warring States period in 475 BC when the TCM theories foundation was laid. Compiled in this period was the first extant medical classic *Huangdi Neijing, Canon of Medicine)* in which the formula principles of "monarch, minister, assistant and guide" were put forward. *Tangye Laoli Lun (On Decoction and Ferment)* compiled in the same period, discussed their preparations and functions and different dosage forms, such as decoction, pills, powders, plasters and medicinal liquors were recorded. Each dosage form was elaborated for the preparation, usages, dosages and indications, which is regarded as the forerunner of TCM Pharmaceutics.

公元前 221 年 ~ 公元 219 年的秦、汉时期，是我国药剂学理论与技术显著发展的时期。西汉马王堆汉墓出土文物《五十二病方》中用药除外敷和内服外，尚有药浴法、烟熏或蒸气熏法、药物熨法等记载。丸剂是最常用的药物剂型，其记载的制法及应用为：以酒制丸，内服；以油脂制丸；以醋制丸，外用于熨法；制成丸后，粉碎入酒吞服等。

The Qin-Han Dynasties (221 BC-219 AD), witnessed the remarkable progress of pharmaceutical theories and techniques. In addition to external application and internal use, the using methods of medicine, in the *Prescriptions of Fifty-two Diseases* unearthed from Mawangdui Tomb of the Western Han Dynasty, also were included the herbal bath, fumigation or steam fumigation, medicine ironing and so on. Pills were very popular dosage form, whose preparation and application recorded are: making pills with wine, taking them internally; making pills with grease; making pills with vinegar, using them externally for ironing; pills could be smashed and taken with wine.

东汉时期成书的《神农本草经》是现存最早的本草专著。该书论及了制药理论和制备法则，并强调应根据药物性质需要选择剂型。其序例指出："药性有宜丸者，宜散者，宜水煎者，宜酒渍者，宜煎膏者，亦有一物兼宜者，亦有不可入汤酒者，并随药性，不得违越。"

Shengnong Bencao Jing (Shennong Herbal Classic) compiled in the Eastern Han Dynasty, is the earliest extant monograph on materia medica. The book discusses the pharmaceutical theories and rules, also emphasizes that dosage forms should be selected according to the needs of drug properties. The preface points out: "The properties of herbs may decide whether they are suitable for making into pills, powders, decoction with water, condensed decoctions or soaking in wine. There are herbs proper for all

dosage forms, while others improper for decoction with water or wine.The properties of medicine should not be violated."

东汉末年，张仲景的《伤寒论》和《金匮要略》，记载了煎剂、丸剂、散剂、浸膏剂、软膏剂、酒剂、栓剂等十余种剂型及其制备方法。另外，书中首次记载用动物胶汁、炼蜜和淀粉糊作为丸剂的赋形剂，沿用至今，为我国中药药剂学的发展奠定了良好的基础。

At the end of the Eastern Han Dynasty, Zhang Zhongjing's *Shanghan Lun (Treatise on Febrile Diseases)* and *Jinkui Yaolue (Synopsis of Prescriptions of the Golden Chamber)* recorded more than ten dosage forms and their preparation methods, such as decoction, pill, powder, extract, ointment, medicinal liquor and suppository. In addition, it was recorded for the first time that animal glue juice, refined honey and starch paste were used as excipients of pills, which are still used nowadays. This lays a solid foundation for the development of TCM pharmaceutics.

晋代葛洪著《肘后备急方》八卷，记载了铅硬膏、蜡丸、锭剂、条剂、药膏剂、灸剂、熨剂、饼剂、尿道栓剂等多种剂型。并首次提出"成药剂"的概念，主张批量生产贮备，供急需之用。

In Ge Hong's eight volumes of *Zhouhou Beiji Fang*, (*Urgent Recipes at Hand*)of the Jin Dynasty (265AD-42OAD), recorded are such dosage forms as lead hard paster, wax pill, pastille, medicated roll, ointment, paste, mugwort stick, iron agent, cake agent, urethra suppository, etc.. The concept of "drug preparation" was put forward for the first time, and mass production and storage were advocated for urgent use.

梁代陶弘景在《本草经集注》中提出以治病的需要来确定剂型，指出："疾有宜服丸者，宜服散者，宜服汤者，宜服酒者，宜服膏煎者"。在该书序例中附有"合药分剂料理法则"，指出药物的产地和采治方法对其疗效有影响。《本草经集注》还考证了古今度量衡，并规定了汤、丸、散、膏、药酒的制作常规，实为近代制剂工艺规程的雏形。

In the Liang Dynasty, Tao Hongjing proposed in the *Bencaojing Jizhu* (*Notes on Herbal Classic*) that the dosage forms should be determined based on the disease's treatment. He pointed out that "Diseases may adapt to pills, powders, decoctions, wines, or soft extracts". In the preface, the book ranked "the arrangement rules of mixture and separation", pointing out that drug's growing place and the methods of collection and preparation would affect the curative effect. In addition, the ancient and then weights and measures were also verified in the notes of *Ben Cao Jing Ji Zhu*, and the production routine of decoction, pill, powder, ointment and medicinal wine was stipulated, having formed the prototype of modern preparation process.

公元659年即唐代显庆四年，唐朝政府组织编纂并颁布的《新修本草》是我国历史上第一部官修本草。其也是世界最早的一部全国性药典，它比欧洲1498年出版的地方性药典《佛洛伦斯药典》早800多年，比欧洲第一部全国性药典《法国药典》早1100多年，这也是我国作为文明古国的标志之一。唐代医药学家孙思邈的《备急千金要方》和《千金翼方》分别收载成方5300首和2000首，有汤剂、丸剂、散剂、膏剂、丹剂、灸剂等剂型。其中著名的成药有磁朱丸、紫雪、定志丸等，至今沿用不衰。《备急千金要方》设有制药总论专章，叙述了制药理论、工艺和质量问题，促进了中药药剂学的发展。稍后王焘所著的《外台秘要》收方6000余首，在每个病名的门下都附有处方、制备方法等。

In 659 AD, the fourth year of Xianqing Emperor of the Tang Dynasty, the government organized the compilation and promulgation of the *Xinxiu Bencao(Newly-revised Herbal Classic)*, which is the first officialy-revised Materia Medica in China. It is also the earliest state pharmacopoeia in the world, over 800 years earlier than the local Pharmacopoeia *"Florence Pharmacopoeia"* published in Europe in 1498, and more than 1100 years earlier than the first National Pharmacopoeia *"French Pharmacopoeia",* which

serves as one of the symbols of China as an ancient civilized nation. Sun Simiao, a medicine master in the Tang Dynasty, compiled *Beiji Qianjin Yaofang* (*Essential Prescriptions Worth a Thousand Gold for Urgencies*) and *Qianjin Yifang* (*A Supplement to the Essential Prescritions Worth a Thousand Gold*), in which were collected 5300 and 2000 prescriptions respectively, including decoction, pill, powder, plaster, pill, moxibustion and other dosage forms. Among them, the famous patent medicines are Cizhu pills, Zixue pills and Dingzhi pills, which are still in use. There is a special chapter on the pharmacy introduction in "*Beiji Qianjin Yaofang*" which describes the pharmaceutical theories, technology and quality problems, pushing TCM Pharmaceutics forward. Later, in Wang Tao's *Wai Tai Mi Yao* (*Essential Secrets from Outside the Metropolis*), he collected more than 6000 prescriptions, with prescriptions and preparation methods attached to each disease.

公元960~1367年的宋、元时期，中药成方制剂得到巨大发展，中药制剂初具规模。公元1080年由太医局颁布的《太平惠民和剂局方》，为我国历史上第一部由官方颁发的制剂规范，也是世界上最早的具有药典性质的药剂方典。该书共收载中药制剂788种，卷首有"和剂局方指南总论"，文中对"处方""合药""服饵""服药食忌"和"药石炮制"等均作专章讨论。书中收载的很多方剂和制法至今仍为传统中成药制备与应用时所沿用。该书可视为中药药剂发展史上的第一个里程碑。

During the Song and Yuan Dynasties (960-1367 AD), TCM preparations developed rapidly, and the scale of TCM Pharmaceutics began to take shape. In 1080, *Taiping Huimin Heji Jufang* (*Pacific Prescriptions Beneficial for People*) was issued by Royal Medicinal Bureau, which is the first official pharmaceutical standard in the Chinese history and the earliest pharmaceutics with Pharmacopoeia meanings in the world. The works contains 788 preparations, and the head chapter covers a general introduction to the guidelines of *He Ji Ju Fang*, in which special chapters are dedicated to "prescriptions", "combined drugs", "drug baits", "food taboo in drug application" and "processing of medicinal stones". Many prescriptions and methods in the book are still used in processing and applying TCM patent medicines. The book should be regarded as the first milestone in Chinese pharmaceutics history.

此外，当时的民间方书《小儿药证直诀》《金匮要略方论》《济生方》《普济本事方》亦收载了很多疗效确切的中药制剂，如抱龙丸、七味白术散、六味地黄丸等。

Moreover, the then folk prescriptions such as *Xiaoer Yaozheng Zhijue, Jinkui Yaolue Fanglun, Jisheng Fang, Puji Benshi Fang*, also contained many effective preparations, such as Baolong Pill, Qiwei Baizhu Powder, Liuwei Dihuang Pill, etc..

明、清时期（公元1369~1911年），中药成方及其剂型也有充实和提高。朱橚《普济方》收载成方61739首，对外用的膏药、丹药及药酒专篇介绍。李时珍《本草纲目》是对我国16世纪以前本草学的全面总结，其中载药1892种，附方剂13000余首，剂型近40种，其论述范围广泛、内容丰富，是对我国16世纪以前本草学的全面总结，对方剂学、药剂学等学科都有重大贡献。本草纲目巨帙远传海内外，影响深远。

During the Ming and Qing Dynasties (1369-1911 AD), prescriptions and dosage forms were enriched and upgraded. Zhu Yi's *Puji Fang* contains 61739 prescriptions, illustrating plasters, pills and medicinal liquor for external use. Li Shizhen's *Bencao Gangmu* (*Compendium of Materia Medica*) is a comprehensive summary of Materia Medica before the 16th century in China. It contains 1892 drugs, over 13000 prescriptions and nearly 40 dosage forms, with extensive and rich statements, contributing greatly to TCM Formulae, TCM Pharmaceutics and other disciplines. *Ben Cao Gang Mu* influences the world far and wide.

清代赵学敏《本草纲目拾遗》对民间草药作了广泛收集与整理，全书共载药物921种，新增

的就有716种之多，极大的丰富了我国药学宝库。另外，《证治准绳》中的二至丸、水陆二仙丹、《外科正宗》中的冰硼散、如意金黄散等一直沿用至今。而《理瀹骈文》则系统论述了中药外用膏剂的制备与应用。

Bencao Gangmu Shiyi compiled by Zhao Xuemin in the Qing Dynasty extensively collected and sorted out the folk herbal medicines. There are 921 drugs in the book, 716 being new, and enriching the drug treasure house. Further more, Erzhi Pill and Shuilu Erxian Pill in *Zhengzhi Zhunsheng* (*Standards of Syndrome and Treatment*), Bingpeng Powder and Ruyi Jinhuang Powder in the *Waike Zhengzong* (*Anthentic External Medicine*) are followed till now. The preparation and application of plaster for external use are systematically discussed in the book *Liyue Pianwen*.

鸦片战争以后，由于时局动荡、西方现代医学的涌入，中医药学发展一度受阻，但同时也在艰难中蕴发出了新的生机。

After the Opium War, TCM progress was once blocked due to then turbulence of the situation and the influx of modern western medicine, but at the same time, the new vitality was hidden and going to develop in the difficulties.

历代主要中药药剂学理论成就详见表1-1。

Theory Formation of TCM Pharmaceutics in history is shown in Table 1-1.

表1-1　历代主要中药药剂学理论成就

论著	时代	成就
《汤液经》	商汤时期	为我国最早的方剂与制药技术专著
《黄帝内经》	战国时期	我国现存的第一部医药经典著作，提出了“君、臣、佐、使”的组方原则
《神农本草经》	东汉时期	我国现存最早的本草专著，论及制药理论和制备法则，强调根据药物性质需要选择剂型
《肘后备急方》	晋代	葛洪著，首次提出“成药剂”的概念，主张批量生产贮备，供急需之用，并收载多种剂型，将成药、防疫药、兽用药剂分专章论述
《本草经集注》	梁代	陶弘景著，提出以治病的需要来确定剂型；规定了汤、丸、散、膏、药酒的制作常规，为近代制剂工艺规程的雏形
《新修本草》	唐显庆四年	又称《唐新修本草》或《唐本草》，我国由政府颁布的第一部药典，也是世界上最早的一部全国性药典
《太平惠民和剂局方》	宋、元时期	为我国历史上由国家颁发的第一部制剂规范

Table 1-1　Theory Formation of TCM Pharmaceutics in History

Book	Dynasty	Achievement
Tangye Jing	Shang Tang Period(16-11 century BC)	The earliest monograph on prescription and pharmaceutical technology
Huangdi Neijing	The Warring States Period (403-221BC)	The first medical classic extant in China, the principles of “monarch, minister, assistant and envoy”were raised
Shennong Bencao Jing	The Eastern Han Dynasty (25-22OAD)	The earliest monograph on materia medica extant in China, dealing with pharmaceutical theories and preparation rules, emphasizing the selection of dosage forms in light of drug properties
Zhouhou Beiji Fang	The Jin Dynasty (265-420 AD)	Written by Ge Hong,“patent medicine” was first put forward, advocating mass production and their storage for urgent use, a variety of dosage forms were collected. The patent medicine, epidemic prevention medicine and veterinary medicine were elaborated in separate chapters

(Continued)

Book	Dynasty	Achievement
Bencaojing Jizhu	The Liang Dynasty (502-557 AD)	Tao Hongjing proposed to determine the dosage form based on the diseases and stipulated the production routine of decoction, pill, powder, ointment and medicinal wine, which was the prototype of modern preparation processing
Xinxiu Bencao	Four years of Tang Emperor Xianqing(618-907 AD)	It is also known as "Tang Xin Xiu Ben Cao"(the Newly-Revised Materia Medica". The first Pharmacopoeia issued by the government in China, as well as in the world
Taiping Huimin Heji Jufang	the Song and Yuan Dynasties (960-1368)	The standards of drug preparation issued by the state in the history of China

二、新中国成立后中药药剂学的主要成就

1.2.2 The Major Achievements after the Founding of New China

中华人民共和国成立后，在党和政府的高度重视下，中医药事业有了前所未有的发展。中药制剂的研究、生产、流通和使用等方面也随之出现突破性进展。尤其是实施《药品管理法》《新药审批办法》和中成药 GMP 审核制度以来，我国创新中药的开发研究和中药制剂生产进入了一个新的发展时期，逐步走上了规范化、科学化和法制化轨道。同时，中药剂型理论的相关研究也取得了一定成果。归纳起来主要有以下几方面。

After the founding of the people's Republic of China, with the great concern of the party and the government, the traditional Chinese Medicine has developed unprecedentedly. The research, production, circulation and use of TCM preparations have also made breakthroughs. Especially, since the implementation of *Drug Administration Law, New Drug Examination and Approval Measures* and GMP audit system of Chinese patent medicine, the R&D of innovative Chinese medicine and the production of drug preparations have entered into a new advancing period, and gradually embarked on a standardized, scientific and legal track. At the same time, some outcomes have gained in the study of TCM dosage form theories. They are as follows:

1. 中药制剂的文献研究 为继承、发掘祖国医药宝库中传统中成药的处方和生产工艺，中国中医研究院中药研究所先后汇编出版了《全国中成药处方集》（1962 年）和《中药制剂手册》（1965 年），前书收载成方 6000 余首、中成药 2700 余种，后书收载制剂 555 种。国家医药管理局中成药情报中心站的《全国中成药产品目录》（一、二两部），收载中成药 9089 种，包括 43 种剂型。另有《中药制剂汇编》（1983 年）收载中药提取制剂达 4000 种、剂型 30 余种等。此外，《中华本草》《中药方剂大辞典》等传统中医药巨著也收载了大量中药成方制剂。

(1) Literature Study on Dosage Preparation The Institute of Chinese Materia Medica of the Chinese TCM Institute compiled and published the *National Formulary of Chinese patent medicine* (*1962*) and the *Manual of traditional Chinese medicine preparation* (*1965*). The former contains more than 6000 prescriptions, 2700-plus patent medicines, and the latter includes 555 preparations. There are 9089 Chinese patent medicines, including 43 dosage forms, in the *National catalog of Chinese patent medicines* (two parts, Ⅰ and Ⅱ) issued by the information Center of Chinese Patent Medicines of the State Administration of TCM. Further more, in the *Compilation of traditional Chinese medicine preparations* (1983) there are 4000 preparations extracted from drugs and more than 30 dosage forms.

Moreover, TCM masterpieces such as *Chinese Materia Medica* and *Dictionary of traditional Chinese medicine prescriptions* embrace a large number of TCM prescriptions.

2. 中药制剂的基础理论研究 对中药制剂的溶出度、生物利用度及配伍组方等基础理论的研究，对阐明中药制剂的生物有效性，正确选择药物剂型、合理拟定生产工艺、准确控制药品质量、有效监控临床用药具有指导作用；对提高中药药剂的生产技术水平，制备安全、有效、稳定且可控的产品具有重要意义。如银黄口服液与其片剂生物利用度比较研究表明，口服液黄芩苷、绿原酸血药峰浓度和血药达峰时间均优于片剂，生物利用度口服液也高于片剂。再如六神丸配伍组方研究表明，麝香、牛黄、蟾蜍的配合应用在抑制动物肉芽肿形成方面具有相乘的效果，且三者的用量以 3∶2∶2 为最佳；而雄黄、麝香、牛黄在强心方面具有协同作用。

(2)Foundmental Theory Study on TCM Preparation The studies on the theories of dissolution, bioavailability and compatibility of TCM preparations will play a guiding role in clarifying their biological effectiveness, correctly selecting the dosage forms, reasonably formulating the production process, accurately controlling drug quality and effectively supervizing the clinical use. It is of great significance for the better TCM Pharmaceutics production technology, and for making safe, effective, stable and controllable products. For example, the comparative study of bioavailability between Yinhuang Oral Liquid and its tablets showed that the concentration of baicalin and chlorogenic acid in the blood and the time of reaching the peak in the blood were both better than that of the tablets, and the bioavailability of the oral liquid was also higher than that of the tablets. Another example, the study on the compatibility of Liushen Pill shows that the cooperation of musk, bezoar and toad has a multiplier effect in inhibiting the formation of animal granuloma, and the best ratio of the three in the dosage is 3∶2∶2, while realgar, musk and bezoar have a synergistic effect in fortifying the heart.

3. 中药制剂的剂型改进与创新研究 在我国中药工业化发展的同时，对中成药传统剂型及其产品的科学化、新型化、方便化、高效化等方面进行了许多有益的探索，取得了一定的成绩。首先对有确切疗效的传统中药成方制剂进行革新改进，使得传统中成药能够缩小服用剂量、提高临床疗效、有利于工业生产等。如汤剂改制成颗粒剂（如五苓散颗粒）、口服液（如四逆汤口服液）、糖浆剂（如养阴清肺糖浆）、注射剂（如生脉注射液）等；丸剂改制成片剂（如银翘解毒片）、口服液（如杞菊地黄口服液）、酊剂（如藿香正气水）、滴丸剂（如苏冰滴丸）、气雾剂（如宽胸气雾剂）等。其次还创制出许多新剂型，为丰富临床用药、充分发挥药物疗效及方便药物应用等作出贡献。如天花粉粉针剂、康莱特静脉注射乳剂、鸦胆子油静脉注射乳剂、喜树碱静脉注射混悬剂、牡荆油微囊片、复方丹参膜剂、复方大黄止血海绵、宽胸气雾剂、小儿解热镇痛栓剂等。其中，清开灵注射液、参附注射液、双黄连粉针、速效救心丸、麝香保心丸、葛根芩连微丸及复方丹参滴丸等 37 个品种被国家中医药管理局定为中医医院急诊必备中成药。

(3) Researches on the Improvement and Innovation of Dosage Forms TCM industrialization is upgrading, concurrently, many beneficial explorations have been carried out on the traditional dosage forms for the scientific, new, convenient and efficient dosage forms and their results are inspiriting. First of all, TCM prescriptions with definite curative effect are modified for reducing the amount, increasing the curative effect and easy for production. For example, the decoction is changed into granule (like Wulingsan granules), oral liquid (like Sinitang oral liquid), syrup (like Yangyin Qingfei Syrup), injection (such as Shengmai Injection), etc.; the pill is changed into tablet (such as Yinqiao Jiedu Tablet), oral liquid (such as Qiju Dihuang Oral Liquid), tincture (such as Huoxiang Zhengqi Tincture), dropping pill (such as Subing Dropping pill), aerosol (such as Kuanxiong Aerosol) etc.. Secondly, a few new dosage forms have been created, which contribute to enriching clinical medication, giving full play to drug

efficacy and facilitating drug application, including Tianhuafen Powder injection, Kanglaite Intravenous Injection Emulsion, Brucea Javanica Oil Intravenous Injection Emulsion, Camptothecin Intravenous Injection Suspension, Vitex Oil Microcapsule Tablet, Fufang Danshen Membrane doses, Fufang Dahuang Hemostatic Sponge, Kuanxiong Aerosol, Xiaoer Jiere Zhentong Suppository, etc.. Among them, 37 varieties, such as Qingkailing Injection, Shenfu Injection, Shuanghuanglian Powder injection, Suxiao Jiuxin Pill, Shexiang Baoxin Pill, Gegen Qinlian Micropill and Fufang Danshen Dropping pill, have been approved as essential Chinese patent medicine for emergency treatment by the State Administration of TCM.

4. 中药制剂新辅料的研究 辅料在制剂的研究中占据重要的地位，不仅是原料药物制剂成型的物质基础，而且与制剂工艺过程的难易、药品的质量、给药途径、临床疗效，以及新剂型、新制剂的开发等方面密切相关。药用辅料与制剂理论、制剂技术与设备是构成药剂学不可缺少的组成部分。中药制剂使用辅料的特点是“药辅合一”，即在选用辅料时注重“辅料与药效相结合”。

(4) Researches on New Auxiliary Materials in TCM Preparations Auxiliary materials play an important role in the research of preparations. They are not only the material base for the formation of raw drug preparations, but have a lot to do with the easy or hard preparation processing, the preparation quality, the medication access, the clinical efficacy, as well as the development of new dosage forms and new preparations. Pharmaceutical excipients and preparation theory, technology and equipment are indispensable components of pharmaceutics. The feature of auxiliary materials used in TCM preparation shows “two-in-one unity”, i.e. the integration of excipients and healing effectiveness must be underscored.

目前，一些新辅料如天然大分子物质、纤维素衍生物、淀粉衍生物、合成/半合成油脂、磷脂、合成表面活性剂、乙烯/丙烯酸/可生物降解聚合物的应用，为中药缓释、控释、靶向制剂等各种给药系统的研究提供了必备的物质基础。

At present, some new auxiliary materials, such as natural macromolecular substances, cellulose derivatives, starch derivatives, synthetic / semi synthetic oils, phospholipids, synthetic surfactants, ethylene / acrylic acid / biodegradable polymers, have provided requisite material base for the researches on various drug delivery systems, such as modified-release, controlled-release and targeted preparations.

5. 中药制剂新技术与新设备的研究 创新的粉碎技术如超微粉碎、超低温粉碎等，提高了细胞的破壁率，增加药物的比表面积，提高了溶解速度和生物利用度；先进的提取分离技术如超临界流体萃取、微波萃取、动态循环阶段连续逆流提取、大孔树脂分离、膜分离、高速离心等提高了产品的纯度，降低了服用量；新兴的干燥技术如冷冻干燥、喷雾干燥、沸腾干燥、真空干燥等，效率高、速度快、干燥均匀、节约能源，且避免了高温对热敏物质的破坏，确保了产品质量的稳定和临床疗效。另外，薄膜包衣、环糊精包合、固体分散、微囊化、微乳化、缓控释、经皮给药、靶向给药，以及原位凝胶、纳米囊泡、脂质体等新型制剂技术及相关设备，有的已应用于生产，有的仍在研发。其中“超临界二氧化碳萃取中药有效成分产业化应用技术”“中药超微粉体关键技术的研究及产业化”等技术已获得突破，在产业中推广应用。

(5) Researches on New Technology and Equipments for TCM Preparations New Pulverizing techniques such as ultrafine pulverization and ultralow temperature pulverization enhance the cell wall broken rate, increase drug surface area, good for the dissolution rate and bioavailability; advanced extraction and separation technologies such as supercritical fluid extraction, microwave extraction, continuous countercurrent extraction in the dynamic cycle stage, macroporous resin separation, membrane separation, and high-speed centrifugation, etc. improve the purity of the products and reduce the dosage consumption; New drying technologies, such as freeze drying, spray drying, boiling drying, vacuum drying, etc. are efficient, speedy,

balanced dry and energy saving, and fending off the damage to heat sensitive materials, so, ensuring product quality, stability and clinical efficacy. Moreover, membrane coating, cyclodextrin inclusion, solid dispersion, microencapsulation, microemulsification, sustained-controlled release, transdermal delivery, targeting drug delivery, in situ gel, nano-sized vesicles, liposomes and other new preparation technologies and related equipments have been operated in production, and some are in the stage of R&D. Among them, "supercritical carbon dioxide extraction of drug effective ingredients industrializational application technology", "researches on industrialization of key technologies of drug ultra micro powder" and other technologies have gained breakthroughs, having been widely spread and applied in the industry.

快速搅拌制粒机、沸腾制粒机、喷雾干燥机、一步制粒机、粉末直接压片机、高速压片机、中药防黏冲压片机等国内外先进成套装备引进和应用，大幅提升了我国中药制药装备水平，加快了中药制剂工艺参数在线检测和自动化控制系统及其装备的产业化开发与应用，促进了中药制剂产业的技术升级。

Rapid mixing granulator, boiling granulator, spray dryer, one-step granulator, powder to tablets via direct compression machine, high-speed tablet pressure machine, drug anti sticking tablet machine and other advanced sets of equipments at home and abroad have been ushered in and applied, which have greatly expedited the level of pharmaceutical apparatus, accelerating the industrialization of TCM preparation process parameter online detection and automatic control system and equipment, and upgrading techniques of TCM preparation industry.

6. 中药制剂新质量标准体系的建立 随着现代分析技术与方法在中药制剂质量控制中的应用，现已逐步建立起中药制剂质量标准体系。中药及其制剂的质量可控性、有效性的技术保障不断提升，中药制剂质量标准内容渐趋科学规范合理。这在《中国药典》中得到了充分体现。中药制剂在不同剂型常规标准（如崩解时限、重量差异、澄清度、微粒细度等）、成分鉴别（包括理化鉴别、薄层色谱鉴别等）及含量控制（主药、毒剧药成分含量测定等）等项目和指标方面逐步完善的同时，《中国药典》还增订了安全卫生标准（如微生物、重金属、砷盐、农残等限度以及药品有效期）。如现行版《中国药典》明确规定了中药注射剂和儿童常用品种的重金属和有害元素限度标准，所有中药制剂必须标明有效期且最长不得超过 5 年等。薄层色谱法、气相色谱法、高效液相色谱法等现代检测技术和方法在中药制剂生产、研究中已普遍使用，液相色谱 - 质谱联用、分子鉴定、薄层 - 生物自显影技术等新方法也已采用。

(6) Establishment of New Quality Standard System for TCM Preparations Along With the application of modern analytical techniques and methods in the quality control of TCM preparations, the quality standard system of them have been gradually established. The technical guarantee for drugs' quality controllability and effectiveness and their preparations has kept ramping up and the quality standard clauses are progressively scientific, standardized and rational. This has been fully embodied in the *Chinese Pharmacopoeia*. TCM preparations have been improved step by step in routine standards of different dosage forms (such as disintegration time limit, weight variation, clarity, particle size, etc.), component identification (including physical and chemical identification, TLC identification, etc.) and composition control (main drug, content determination of toxicants, etc.). In the mean time, the safety and health standards (such as the limits of microorganisms, heavy metals, arsenic salts, agricultural residues, etc. as well as the expiry date of drugs are also updated in the *Chinese Pharmacopoeia*. For example, the current edition of the *Chinese Pharmacopoeia* clearly specifies the limit standards of heavy metals and harmful elements in TCM injections and children's medicine. and all TCM preparations must be marked with a validity period of less than 5 years. Thin layer chromatography, gas chromatography,

high performance liquid chromatography and other modern detection technologies and methods have been widely used in the production and researches of TCM preparations, and new methods such as liquid chromatography-mass spectrometry, molecular identification, thin layer biological self-development technology have also been adopted.

7. 中药制剂现代化产业体系的形成 经过多年的调整、改造和扩建，一大批符合 GMP 要求的创新中药制剂现代化产业体系已经形成。具有中医药特色的中药提取、纯化、浓缩、干燥、制粒、包衣等的新技术、新工艺、新方法、新设备正在中药制剂生产、研究中应用并普及。中成药工业生产的单元操作系统、物料与热量平衡、原材料与中间体质量控制以及中试放大等研究与应用已取得显著进展。上述诸多成果目前已成功转化为生产力，产生了巨大的社会和经济效益，同时对学科本身和中医药事业的发展亦有重大而深远的影响。然而，为促进中成药工业现代化进程，中药制剂系统工程的研究还需进一步加强。

(7) Formation of Modern Industrial System of TCM Preparations After many years's adjustment, transformation and expansion, a large number of modernization industry systems of preparations with innovation have been formed, which conform to GMP requirements. The new technologies, processes, methods and installations, with TCM features like extracting, purifying, concentrating, drying, granulating and coating, are applied and popularized in the production and researches of preparations. Remarkable progress has been made in the researches and applications of unit operating system, technique of balance between material and heat, quality control between raw materials and intermediates, and pilot scale-up in the production of Chinese patent medicine. At present, many of the above achievements have been successfully transformed into productive forces, which has produced huge social and economic benefits, and also has a significant and far-reaching impact on the development of the discipline itself and the TCM cause. However, to promote the modernization process of Chinese patent medicine industry, the researches on the TCM preparation system engineering should go on with even greater exertion.

第三节 药物剂型的分类

1.3 Classification of Drug Dosage Forms

PPT

药物剂型的种类繁多，为了便于学习、研究和应用，需要对剂型进行分类。目前剂型分类方法主要有以下几种。

There is a large variety of drug formulations. In order to facilitate the study, research and application, classification of dosage forms should be done. At present, the classification methods are mainly as follows.

一、按物态分类

1.3.1 Classification by Physical States

即根据药物物态的差异将药物剂型划分为固体、半固体、液体和气体等类型。固体剂型如散剂、颗粒剂（冲剂）、丸剂、片剂、胶剂等；半固体剂型如内服膏滋、外用膏剂、糊剂等；液体

剂型如汤剂、合剂（含口服液剂）、糖浆剂、酒剂、酊剂、露剂等；气体剂型如气雾剂、喷雾剂、烟剂等。相同物态的制备特点、用药起效时间和贮运有相似之处。例如固体剂型多需粉碎和混合；半固体剂型多需熔化和研匀；液体剂型多需提取和分离操作。用药起效时间以液体、气体剂型为最快，固体剂型较慢；固体制剂便于贮运，液体制剂易产生沉淀。

Based on the differences of drug states, drug dosage forms can be grouped into solid, semi-solid, liquid and gas forms, etc. Solid dosage forms--powders, granules, pills, tablets, glue, etc.; Semi-solid dosage forms--Gaozi(drug cream) for oral administration, ointments for external use, pastes, etc.; Liquid dosage forms-- decoction, mixture (including oral liquid), syrup, medicinal liquor, tincture, distillate, etc.; Gas dosage forms-aerosol, spray, fumicant and so on. The drugs with same physical state have similarities in the preparation specialties, effect starting time, perservation and carriage. For instance, solid dosage forms need to be crushed and mixed, semi-solid dosage forms, melted and ground, liquid dosage forms, extracted and separated. Liquid and gas dosage forms are the fastest to take effect, while solid dosage forms are slower. Solid dosage forms are apt to be stored and transported, and liquid dosage forms are apt to give rise to precipitates.

这种分类法在制备、贮藏和运输上较有意义，但是过于简单，缺少剂型间的内在联系，实用价值较低。

This classification method is not bad in preparation, storage and transportation, but it's too simple, lacking intrinsic links between dosage forms, so, its practical value is short.

二、按制备方法分类
1.3.2 Classification by Processing Methods

即将主要工序采用相同方法制备的剂型列为一类。例如浸出药剂是将用浸出方法制备的汤剂、合剂、酒剂、酊剂、流浸膏剂与浸膏剂等归纳为一类；无菌制剂是将用灭菌方法或无菌操作法制备的注射剂、滴眼剂等列为一类。

The dosage forms prepared by the same method in the main process are classified into one category. For example, the dosage forms by drug leaching form a group, containing decoction, mixture, medicinal liquors, tincture, fluid extract and extract; Aseptic preparation is for injections and eye drops which are prepared by sterilization methods or aseptic operation.

这种分类法有利于研究制备的共同规律，但归纳不全，而且某些剂型随着科学的发展会改变其制法，故同样具有一定的局限性。

This classification method is good for studying the common regularities of preparations, but with limitation, especially when the processing is in the changing.

三、按分散系统分类
1.3.3 Classification by Dispersing System

此法按剂型分散特性分类，便于应用物理化学原理说明各类剂型的特点，分类如下。

This method groups the dosage forms with dispersing features for the sake of describing each dosage in physical or chemistry laws. The groups are as follows:

1. 真溶液类剂型 如芳香水剂、溶液剂、醑剂、甘油剂及部分注射剂等。

(1) True Solution Dosage Form Such as aromatic water, solution, spirit, glyceritum and some

injections.

2. 胶体溶液类剂型 如胶浆剂、火棉胶剂、涂膜剂等。

(2) Colloidal Solution Dosage Form Such as mucilage, collodion, smeared film, etc..

3. 乳浊液类剂型 如乳剂、静脉乳剂、部分搽剂等。

(3) Emulsion Dosage Form Such as emulsion, intravenous emulsion, some liniments, etc..

4. 混悬液类剂型 如洗剂、混悬剂等。

(4) Suspension Dosage Form Such as lotion, suspension, etc..

5. 气体分散体剂型 如气雾剂等。

(5) Gas Dispersion Dosage Form Such as aerosol, etc..

6. 固体分散体剂型 如散剂、丸剂、片剂等。

(6) Solid Dispersion Dosage Form Such as powder, pill, tablet, etc..

这种分类法最大的缺点是不能反映用药部位与方法对剂型的要求，甚至一种剂型由于辅料和制法的不同而必须分到几个分散系统中去，因而无法保持剂型的完整性。例如注射剂中包括了溶液型、混悬型、乳浊型及粉针型等，合剂、软膏剂也存在类似情况。此外，中药汤剂可同时包含有真溶液、胶体溶液、乳浊液和混悬液。

It is the biggest disadvantage of this classification that it can't reflect the requirements of the dosage form for the application site and method, and even a dosage form must be divided into several dispersion systems due to the different auxiliary materials and preparation methods, so it can't maintain the integrity of the dosage form. For example, the injection form includes solution type, suspension type, opacification type and powder injection type. The mixture and ointment also have similar situation. In addition, decoction can simultaneously contain true solution, colloidal solution, emulsion and suspension.

四、按给药途径与方法分类

1.3.4 Classification by Medication Route and Administration

将采用同一种给药途径和方法的剂型列为一类，分类如下。

The same medication access and methods of dosage forms are in the same category, as follows:

（一）经胃肠道给药的剂型

(1) Dosage Forms of Gastrointestinal Administration

汤剂、合剂（口服液）、糖浆剂、煎膏剂、酒剂、流浸膏剂、散剂、颗粒剂（冲剂）、丸剂、片剂、胶囊剂等。经直肠给药的剂型有灌肠剂、栓剂等。

Decoction, mixture (oral liquid), syrup, decoction, medicinal liquor, fluid extract, powder, granule (granules), pill, tablet, capsule, etc.. The dosage forms of transrectal administration include enema, suppository, etc..

（二）不经胃肠道给药的剂型

(2) Dosage Forms of Non-gastrointestinal Administration

1. 注射给药 注射剂（包括肌内注射、静脉注射、皮下注射、皮内注射及脊椎腔注射等）。

① Administration by Injection Injection (including intramuscular injection, intravenous injection, subcutaneous injection, intradermal injection, spinal cavity injection, etc.).

2. 经皮肤给药 有软膏剂、膏药、橡胶膏剂、糊剂、搽剂、洗剂、涂膜剂、离子透入剂等。

② Transdermal Administration There are ointments, plasters, rubber plasters, pastes, liniments, lotions, smeared films, ion penetration agents, etc..

3. 经黏膜给药 有滴眼剂、滴鼻剂、含漱剂、舌下片、吹入剂、栓剂、膜剂及含化丸等。

③ Mucosal Routes of Drug Administration There are eye drops, nasal drops, gargarisms, sublingual tablets, blowing agents, suppositories, smeared films and containing pills.

4. 经呼吸道给药 有气雾剂、吸入剂、烟剂等。

④ Administration via Respiratory Tract There are aerosols, inhalants, and fumigants, etc..

这种分类方法与临床用药结合得比较紧密，并能反映给药途径与方法对剂型制备的特殊要求。缺点是往往一种剂型，由于给药途径或方法的不同，可能多次出现，使剂型分类复杂化，同时这种分类方法亦不能反映剂型的内在特性。

This classification is closely coupled with clinical medication, and able to show the special requirements of the ways and methods of administration for preparations. But its shortcoming lies on that one dosage form presents many times due to the different ways or methods of administration, which makes the classification complicated. Meanwhile, this classification can't reflect the inherent features of dosage forms.

上述各类分类方法各有特点与不足，实际工作中常采用综合分类法。

Each of above classifications has its own advantages and deficiencies. So, the comprehensive classification method is practically often used.

第四节 中药剂型选择的基本原则

1.4 The Essential Principles for the TCM Dosage Form Selection

PPT

剂型是药物使用的必备形式，药物剂型必须与给药途径相适应。虽然药物疗效主要取决于药物本身，但在一定条件下，剂型对药物疗效的发挥也可起到关键性作用，主要表现为对药物释放、吸收的影响。同一种药物，由于剂型种类不同，所选用的辅料、制备方法、工艺操作不同，往往会使药物的稳定性和药物起效时间、作用强度、作用部位、持续时间以及副作用等出现较大的差异，进而影响药物的治疗效果。因此剂型的选择是中药制剂研究与生产的重要内容之一。一般而言，剂型的选择应遵循以下基本原则。

The dosage form is a necessary form for medication, which must be matched with the route of administration. Although the curative effect mainly depends on the medicine itself, yet, under certain conditions, the dosage form can also play a crucial role in terms of drug release and absorption. One drug, in different dosage forms, may produce its different stability, effect starting time, intensity, location, duration and side effects due to different auxiliary ingredients, processing and techniques used in the dosage forms, as a result, the therapeutic effect goes down. Therefore, the choice of dosage forms is very important in the research and production of TCM preparational. In general, the selection of dosage forms should abide by the following principles.

一、根据防治疾病的需要选择剂型

1.4.1 To Select the Dosage Forms in Line with the Disease Prevention and Treatment

《本草经集注》载："疾有宜服丸者，宜服散者，宜服汤者，宜服酒者，宜服膏煎者"，即应当根据防治疾病的具体需要而选择不同的剂型。同一药物因剂型或给药方式的差异，会呈现不同的药理作用。如大承气汤在治疗肠梗阻等急腹症中，口服汤剂疗效良好，而注射剂则不能呈现促进肠套叠的还纳作用。枳实煎剂具行气宽中、消食化痰的作用；而若遇到休克病人，则应使用枳实注射剂，取其起效迅速、升压、抗休克的作用。另外，改变药物剂型有时候能起到扩大适应证、降低毒副作用的效果。如用洋金花单味药口服治疗慢性支气管炎时，虽疗效较明显但易出现口干、眩晕、视力模糊等副作用，采用复方洋金花栓剂治疗却能减轻或消除上述副作用。

In *Bencaojing Jizhu*, it is stated that "each illness may be proper for taking pills, or powders, or decoction, or medicinal liquors or soft extracts", meaning, different dosage forms should be selected according to the specific needs of disease prevention and treament. One drug may give rise to different pharmacological effects because of different dosage forms or administration ways. For example, Dachengqi Tang Decoction, in treating the acute abdominal problem, like intestinal obstruction, oral decoction creates good effectiveness, while injection can't promote intussusception. Zhishi Decoction is good for qi's flowing and chest loosening, digesting food and resolving phlegm. In case of patient in shock, Zhishi Injection will perform swiftly to gear up blood pressure and combat-shock. In addition, changing dosage forms may broaden indications and descend side effects. For example, in the treatment of chronic bronchitis by oral administration of single drug, Yangjinhua, the side effects such as dry mouth, vertigo and blurred vision easily occur although the curative effect is obvious, yet, the above side effects can be alleviated or eliminated by the compound Yangjinhua suppository.

不同给药途径的药物剂型，起效时间快慢不同。通常而言，由快到慢的给药途径排序为：静脉注射 > 吸入给药 > 肌内注射 > 皮下注射 > 直肠或舌下给药 > 口服给药（液体制剂）> 口服给药（固体制剂）> 经皮给药。药物的吸收、分布、代谢、排泄与疗效的发挥有着密切的关系，故应从防治疾病的角度选择剂型：急症用药宜选用发挥疗效迅速的剂型，如注射剂、气雾剂、滴丸、舌下片、合剂、保留灌肠剂等；慢性疾病用药宜选用作用缓和、持久的剂型，如丸剂、片剂、煎膏剂及长效缓释制剂等；皮肤疾患用药宜选用软膏剂、橡胶膏剂、外用膜剂、涂膜剂、洗剂、搽剂等；某些局部黏膜用药宜选用栓剂、膜剂、条剂、线剂、酊剂等。

Drug dosage forms with different administrations have different onset time. Generally, the sequence of administration from the fast to the slow is like this: intravenous injection > inhalation administration > intramuscular injection > subcutaneous injection > rectal or sublingual administration >oral administration (liquid preparation) > oral administration (solid preparation) > percutaneous administration. The absorption, distribution, metabolism and excretion of drug preparations immediately affect curative effect. Therefore, the dosage forms should be selected from the perspective of disease prevention and treatment: the dosage form serving for rapid curative effect should be selected for urgent cases, such as injection, aerosol, drop pill, sublingual tablet, mixture, retention enema, etc.; the dosage form with mild and lasting effect, such as pills, tablets, soft extracts, long-term sustained-release preparations, etc. for chronic diseases, i.e. ointment, rubber paste, external film, smeared films, lotion liniment etc. for skin diseases; suppository, film, strip, thread, tincture, etc. for some local mucosal areas.

案例导入 ¦ Case example

案例 1-2 复方丹参滴丸

1-2 Fufang Danshen Dripping Pills

处方：丹参适量　三七适量　冰片适量

Ingredients: Salvia Miltiorrhizae Radix et Rhizoma, Notoginseng Radix et Rhizoma, Borneolum Syntheticum, etc.

功能与主治：活血化瘀，理气止痛。用于气滞血瘀所致的胸痹，症见胸闷、心前区刺痛；冠心病心绞痛见上述证候者。

Functions and Indications: To activate blood, resolve stasis, regulate qi and relieve pain. It is used for the treatment of chest *bi* syndrome caused by qi stagnation and blood stasis, manifested by oppression in the chest, and stabbing pain in the precordium; angina pectoris in coronary heart disease with the symptoms mentioned above.

制法：以上三味，冰片研细；丹参、三七加水煎煮，煎液滤过，滤液浓缩，加入乙醇，静置使沉淀，取上清液，回收乙醇，浓缩成稠膏，备用。取聚乙二醇适量，加热使熔融，加入上述稠膏和冰片细粉，混匀，滴入冷却的液体石蜡中，制成滴丸，或包薄膜衣，即得。

Making Procedure: Cooking Salvia Miltiorrhiza Radix et Rhizoma and Notoginseng Radix et Rhizoma with water, having the decoction filtered and concentrated, adding some ethanol, placing it still for setting. Concentrating the supernatant to a thick extract, recycling the alcohol; Pulverising Borneolum Syntheticum into fine powder, heating to melt some polyethylene glycols. All above prepared materials are put together and mixed evenly. Then, dripping the mixture into cool liquid paraffin for drop pills, or being coated with film, to have film coated drop pills.

用法与用量：吞服或舌下含服。一次 10 丸，一日三次。28 天为一个疗程，或遵医嘱。

Usage and Dosage: For oral or sublingual administration, 10 pills one time, three times a day, twenty-eight days a course, or as advised by health professionals.

注解：①丹参、三七采用水提法，在于将丹参中水溶性的酚酸类成分和三七中皂苷全部提取出来，但出膏量较大，故采用乙醇沉淀，以除去蛋白质、淀粉和多糖等杂质，减少服用量。

Notes: ① Water abstration of Salvia Miltiorrhizae Radix et Rhizoma and Notoginseng Radix et Rhizoma is for fully abstracting water-soluble phenolic acids from Salvia Miltiorrhizae Radix et Rhizoma and saponins from Notoginseng Radix et Rhizoma, Ethanol precipitation is used to remove such impurities as protein, starch and polysaccharide and reduce the dose-taken since the amount of ointment is large.

②冰片研细，易分散在熔融混匀的聚乙二醇和丹参、三七提取物中；成品采用包薄膜衣，可防止冰片的升华和保证外观的美观；冰片的升华作用会导致滴丸形成花斑，应注意贮存温度。

② The Borneolum Syntheticum is finely ground for easily being dispersed in the polyethylene glycol and extracts of Salvia Miltiorrhizae Radix et Rhizoma and Notoginseng Radix et Rhizoma; the film-coated products are good at preventing Borneolum Syntheticum's sublimation and for pretty appearance of the pills; the sublimation of Borneolum Syntheticum might lead to the formation of blobs, so the storage temperature should be with caution.

③药物制成滴丸以后，药物在基质中的分散呈分子状态、胶体状态或微粉状结晶，为高度分散状态，而基质为水溶性（如聚乙二醇类），则可增加或改善药物的溶解性能，加快药物的溶出速度和吸收速度，提高药物的生物利用度。

③ After drugs having been made into dropping pills, the dispersion of the drugs in the base material is in the form of molecular state, colloidal state or micro powder crystal, highly dispersed, while the base material is water-soluble (such as polyethylene glycol), which can increase or improve the solubility of the drugs, speed up the dissolution and absorption of the drugs, and boost the bioavailability of the drugs.

④复方丹参滴丸溶化时间在3分钟以内，缓解心绞痛的时间在3~8分钟，可直接含化、吸收，不但能预防心血管疾病，还可用于心绞痛发作的急救。

④ The dissolution time of Fufang Danshen Dropping Pills is within 3 minutes, and the time to relieve angina is 3-8 minutes. It can be directly sucked and absorbed. Not only for preventing cardiovascular diseases, but also for emergency treatment of angina.

思考题：①复方丹参滴丸的成功研制，应用了哪些新技术或新方法？

②查阅有关复方丹参滴丸的研制与开发的过程，谈谈个人看法。

Questions: ① What new technology or methods have been adopted for the successful development of Fufang Dropping Pills?

② Consuling the process of R&D of Fufang Danshen Dropping Pills, then, talking about your personal viewpoints.

二、根据药物性质选择剂型

1.4.2 To Choose Dosage Form According to Drugs' Properties

中药制剂多为复方，所含成分极为复杂。在选择药物剂型前，必须认真进行组方药物的研究，重点研究活性成分的溶解性、稳定性和刺激性大小等，在符合临床用药要求的前提下，充分考虑所设计剂型对主要药物活性成分溶解性、稳定性、刺激性的影响，且每种剂型均有一定的载药范围，应根据处方剂型大小，结合其他因素综合考虑应制成何种剂型。

Most of TCM preparations are from compound prescriptions, consisting of extremely complicated ingredients. Before selecting dosage forms, prudent studied must be done for the solubility, stability and irritation of active ingredients. When the clinical medication requirements are met, the impact of the dosage form on solubility, stability, irritation of the main drug's active ingredients should be taken into full consideration. And further, each dosage form has its own capacity to drug loading. So, the dosage form should be decided based on the size of the prescription and other factors.

一般而言，含难溶性或在水中不稳定的成分的药物、主含挥发油或有异臭的药物不宜制成口服液等液体剂型。药物成分易被胃肠道破坏或不被其吸收，对胃肠道有刺激性，或因肝脏“首过作用”（或称“首关效应”“第一关卡效应”），而疗效显著降低的药物等均不宜设计为口服剂型。成分间易产生沉淀等配伍变化的组方，则不宜制成注射剂和口服液等液体剂型。如黄连的主要成分小檗碱，水中溶解度很小，肌内注射2~5ml（1mg/ml）很难达到有效抗菌浓度，且因为小檗碱季铵盐结构难以透过肠壁而吸收，因此治疗肠道感染，黄连素以口服给药剂型为佳；又如，黄连、黄柏中的小檗碱与大黄中的鞣质在水溶液中易生成鞣酸小檗碱沉淀，故含上述药材的处方不宜制成注射剂或口服液。药材富含糖类、胶类等活性成分者，其出膏率较高，浸膏吸湿性强，若制成硬胶囊剂则可能导致服用剂量大，制剂稳定性差。如八味丸治疗糖尿病用药材粉末有效，而水浸膏无效，与该丸中主要药味之一山茱萸所含的齐墩果酸、熊果酸在水中不能溶出有关。

Generally speaking, drugs containing insoluble or unstable ingredients in water, and drugs containing volatile oil or abnormal odor are improper to be processed into liquid dosage form like oral liquid, etc.. The drug ingredients easy to be impaired or not absorbed by the gastrointestinal tract, or irritating the gastrointestinal tract, or the effect steps down because of the "first-pass effect" of the liver, are not adequate in oral dosage forms. Those prescription's ingredients apt to set sediment should not be used in the forms of injection and oral liquid. For example, berberine, the main component part of Coptidis Rhizoma, is hard soluble in water. It's difficult to achieve an effective antibacterial concentration by intramuscular injection of 2-5ml (1mg/ml). Moreover, the quaternary ammonium salt structure of berberine is difficult to be absorbed through the intestinal wall, so it's better to choose Berberine oral administration for the treatment of intestinal infection. Another example, that the berberine in Rhizoma Coptidis, Rhizoma Cypresses and tannin in rhubarb are easy to form tannic acid berberine precipitation in aqueous solution, so the prescriptions containing the above medicinal materials are not adequate for making injection or oral solution. Other medicinal materials are rich in active ingredients like saccharides and glues, the extraction rate is high, and the extract with strong hygroscopicity. If they are made into hard capsules, the larger dose-taken may need and the preparation will not be stable in property. For example, Bawei Pill is effective for the treatment of diabetes, while water extract is ineffective because the oleanolic acid and ursolic acid included in Corni Fructus, one of the essential medicinal herbs of the pills, can't be dissolved in water.

三、根据原方不同剂型的生物药剂学和药代动力学特性选择剂型

1.4.3 Dosage Forms Selection Based on the Specialities of Biopharmaceutics and Pharmacokinetic in Different Dosage Forms of the Original Prescriptions

不同处方、不同药物、不同的有效成分应选择各自相适宜的剂型。若根据所选剂型要求制定的工艺路线不能使有效成分被最大限度地提取并保留于成品中，或制剂疗效差、不稳定，无法制定质量规格和标准，则所选剂型就不合理。为了客观地评价所确定剂型的合理性，要有资料证明所选剂型最优。因此，如果是改进剂型，药物应与原剂型药物作对比实验；如果是新研制的药物，应将该处方药物制成符合临床用药目的和药物理化性质的两种以上不同剂型的药剂，通过体内药代动力学（如测定血浆原型药浓度或尿中原型药排泄总量、代谢物尿排泄总量计算生物利用度）、药理效应法、体外溶出度法等的研究，反映药物不同剂型生物利用度的差异，从中优选出生物利用度较高的剂型。

Different formulations, different drugs and different effective ingredients should be teamed up with their own suitable dosage forms. The selected dosage form might be unreasonable, if the process route established according to the requirements of the selected dosage form fails to maximize the extraction and reserve of effective ingredients in the finished product, or the efficacy is poor and unstable, and the quality specifications and standards can't be formulated. In order to objectively evaluate the rationality of the determined dosage form, it's necessary to have data to prove that the selected dosage form is the best. Therefore, in the to-be-improved dosage form, the new drugs should be compared with those in the original dosage form; If it's a newly developed prescription, the drugs should be made into two or more different dosage forms which should reach the clinical purpose and physicochemical properties, By means of studies on pharmacokinetics *in vivo* (such as the determination of plasma prototype drug concentration or total excretion of prototype drug in urine, the calculation of bioavailability of total excretion of metabolites in urine), pharmacological effect method, *in vitro* dissolution method, etc., the

difference of bioavailability of different dosage forms of drugs is shown, and the dosage forms with higher bioavailability are selected.

有些药物溶液状态不稳定，需制成固体制剂。如天花粉用于中期妊娠引产疗效较好，其有效部位为蛋白质，对热很不稳定，其水溶液也不稳定，用丙酮分级沉淀制得具有一定分子量的蛋白质，经无菌分装、冷冻干燥制成粉针剂，临用前用新鲜灭菌注射用水配制。不仅制剂质量稳定，而且通过改变给药途径，提高了疗效、降低了毒副作用。

Some medicine solutions are unstable and need to be made into solid preparations. For example, Tianhuafen Powder has good effect on induced labour in mid-term pregnancy of which the effective part is protein, unstable to heat and water, so, the protein with certain molecular weight could be prepared by acetone precipitation. The powder injection was made by freezing-drying and kept in aseptic bottles, then prepare it with fresh sterile water before using it as injection. Now not only the quality of the preparation is stable, but also the therapeutic effect scale up and the side effects decline because of the administration alteration.

四、根据生产条件和“五方便”的要求选择剂型

1.4.4 Selecting Dosage Forms in Accordance with Production Conditions and “Five Conveniences”

药物剂型的选择在满足防治疾病需要和符合药物本身及其成分性质的前提下，应根据中药制药企业的技术水平和生产条件选择剂型。剂型不同，采用的工艺路线不同，对所需的技术、生产环境、设备、工人素质等都有不同的要求。若目前尚缺乏生产该剂型的符合药品生产质量管理规范（GMP）要求的车间，在临床用药、药物性质许可的前提下，可更换具备生产条件的其他剂型。当然，必要的厂房设施、仪器设备、制剂技术是确保剂型选择准确的重要条件。

Also the technical level and productive conditions of the pharmaceutical enterprises should be considered seriously in the selection of dosage forms with the prerequisite of the following：dosage forms meet the diseases’ prophylaxis and treament; conform to the drugs and their properties. Different dosage forms and different process routes require different technology, productive environment, equipments and workers’ quality. If the workshop can not meet the requirements of GMP to produce this dosage form, other dosage forms can be chosen to replace it when clinical medication and preparation nature can be reached. By all means, the necessary plant facilities, instruments and apparatuses, and technology are important to ensure the accurate selection of dosage forms.

剂型设计还应考虑“五方便”（服用、携带、生产、运输、贮藏方便）的要求，就携带、贮运而言，剂量小且质量稳定的固体制剂优于液体制剂。如汤剂味苦量大、服用不便，将部分汤剂处方改制成颗粒剂、口服液、胶囊剂等，既保持汤剂疗效好的特点，又易于服用。甘草主产于我国西北、东北及内蒙古一带，在制剂中用量很大，可以考虑在产地将甘草制成甘草浸膏，以便于运输。对于儿童用药还应尽量做到色美、味香、量宜、效高，并能多种途径给药，可考虑制成口服液、微型颗粒剂、滴鼻剂、微型保留灌肠剂、栓剂、注射剂等。

The “five conveniences” (taking, carrying, producing, transporting and storing conveniences) should also be considered in the dosage form design. In terms of carrying, storage and transportation, solid preparations with small dosage and stable quality are superior to liquid preparations. For example, the decoction is bitter in taste and large in amount, and inconvenient to take, some decoction prescriptions are to be changed into granules, or oral liquid, or capsules, etc., which will maintain not only the features

of decoctions' good effectiveness, but are easy to be taken. Glycyrrhizae Radix et Rhizoma grows in the northwest, northeast and Inner Mongolia of China. It is popularly used in most of preparations. So, it is good that Glycyrrhizae Radix et Rhizoma Licorice extract is to be prepared in the growing areas for the convenience of transportation. For children, it is better to make the medicine beautiful in color, fragrant in smell, and appropriate in quantity and good in effect. For them the oral liquid, micro granules, nasal drops, fine retention enema, suppository, injection, etc. are all handy forms.

第五节 中药药剂工作的依据

1.5 Basis of TCM Pharmaceutics Work

PPT

中药药剂的法定依据是指中药药剂工作中应遵循的国家药品标准及相关管理法规。我国目前药品所有执行标准均为国家注册标准。国家注册标准，是指原国家卫生部或药品监督管理局批准给申请人特定药品的标准，生产该药品的药品生产企业必须执行该注册标准。包括药典标准、新药转正标准（不断更新）、进口药品标准、《中华人民共和国卫生部中药成方制剂药品标准》（1998 年至今发布 20 册，收载中药成方制剂 4061 种）等。部颁标准、局颁标准的性质与作用同《中国药典》，都归属于国家药品标准，作为药物生产、供应、使用、监督等部门检验质量的法定依据，具有法律的约束力。

The legal basis of TCM Pharmaceutics is the national drug standards and the concerning regulations that should be followed in the work of Pharmaceutics of TCM. At present, all executive standards of drugs in China follow the State Registration Standards, which indicates that the specific medicine standards approved by the Ministry of Health P.R. China or the State Medicine Supervision and Administration (the manufacturing enterprises) should abide by the applicants in their implementation. They are *Pharmacopoeia Standard, New Drug Normalization Standard* (constantly updated), Imported Drug Standard, *Drug Standard of the Ministry of Health P.R. China·Composition Principles of Chinese Patent Drugs* (20 volumes have been published since 1998, and 4061 Chinese patent drugs collected), etc.. The properties and functions of the standards issued by the Ministry or the provincial Bureau are equal to those of *Chinese Pharmacopoeia*. They all belong to the national drug standards which are serving as legal binding force for the inspection departments of medicine production, supply, use, supervision and so on.

一、药典

1.5.1 Pharmacopoeia

（一）药典的性质与作用

(1) The Nature and Function of Pharmacopoeia

药典是一个国家记载药品质量、规格、标准的法典。由国家组织药典委员会编纂，并由政府颁布施行，具有法律的约束力。药典中收载疗效确切、毒副作用小、质量稳定的常用药物及其制剂，规定其质量标准、制备要求、鉴别、检查、含量测定、功能与主治及用法与用量等，作为药物生产、检验、供应与使用的依据。药典在一定程度上反映了该国家药物生产、医疗和科技的水

平，也体现了医药卫生工作的特点和服务方向。药典在保证人民用药有效、安全，促进药物研究和生产方面有重大作用。

Pharmacopoeia is a national code recording the drugs'quality, specifications and standards, compiled by the Chinese Pharmacopoeia Commission, promulgated and implemented by the government, with legal binding force. Pharmacopoeia contains common drugs and their preparations with definite curative effects, small toxic and side effects and stable quality, and their specific quality standards, preparation requirements, identification, inspection, content determination, functions and indications, usage and dosage, etc. Serving as the basis in drug production, inspection, supply and application. To certain extent, the Pharmacopoeia manifestes the level of medication production, medical therapies and science and technology of the country, and also shows the medicine/health features and service orientation. Pharmacopoeia plays an essential role in ensuring the effectiveness and medication safety and promotion of medicine research and production.

随着医药科学的发展，新药及新的试验方法亦不断出现，为使药典适应科技的发展，药典每隔几年修订一次。在修订出版新药典前往往发行该版的补充本，以使新的研究尽快地用于实践中。

With the advancing of medical science, new medication and new test methods keep emerging.To couple with the sci-tech progress, the Pharmacopoeia is revised every several years. Before the revision and publication of the new pharmacopoeia, the supplementary edition of it is often issued, for the sake of earlier usage of new researches in practice.

（二）中国药典

(2) Chinese Pharmacopoeia

1930 年国民党政府卫生署编纂了《中华药典》第一版，主要参考英、美国家药典编写而成，规定的药品标准不适合我国的实际情况。该药典出版后，直到中华人民共和国建立，20 年之久也未修订过。

The first edition of the *Chinese Pharmacopoeia* was compiled in 1930 by the health department of the then government, with consulting the Pharmacopoeia of the United Kingdom and the United States, of which the medication standards failed to match with the actual situation in China. The Pharmacopoeia had not been revised for 20 years until the establishment of the People's Republic of China.

中华人民共和国建立以来，《中国药典》至今已颁发了 11 版（1953 年版、1963 年版、1977 年版、1985 年版、1990 年版、1995 年版、2000 年版、2005 年版、2010 年版、2015 年版以及 2020 年版），每版药典在前版药典的基础上，在品种、标准和检测水平上有大幅度的增修和提高。

Since the founding of the People's Republic of China, nine editions of *Chinese Pharmacopoeia* have been issued up to now (1953 edition, 1963 edition, 1977 edition, 1985 edition, 1990 edition, 1995 edition, 2000 edition, 2005 edition, 2010 edition, 2015 edition and 2020 edition). On the basis of the previous edition, each new edition of Pharmacopoeia is largely revised and geared up in varieties, standards and detection level.

《中国药典》由凡例、正文、通用技术要求和索引组成。凡例是使用本药典的总说明，包括药典中各种计量单位、符号、术语等的含义及其在使用时的有关规定。正文是药典的主要内容，叙述本部药典收载的所有药物和制剂。通用技术要求叙述本部药典所采用的检验方法、制剂通则、药材炮制通则、对照品与对照药材及试药、试液、试纸等。索引设有中文、汉语拼音、拉丁名和拉丁学名索引，以便查阅。

The *Chinese Pharmacopoeia* is composed of general notices, text, general principle and index. Notices are the general description for the use of this Pharmacopoeia, covering various measurement units, symbols, special terms, etc. and relevant regulations in use. The text is the principal portion of the Pharmacopoeia, elaborating on all drugs and preparations embodied in it. The test methods, general principles of preparation, general principles of drug processing, reference materials and reference medicinal materials as well as test drug, test solution, test paper, etc. are all described in the general principle part. The index has the Chinese, Pinyin, Latin name and Latin scientific name index for easy reference.

（三）其他药典简介

(3) Briefing of the Other Pharmacopoeia

1. 美国药典（简称 U.S.P.） 由美国政府对药品质量标准和检定方法作出的技术规定，也是药品生产、使用、管理、检验的法律依据，对于在美国制造和销售的药物和相关产品而言，《美国药典》是唯一由美国食品药品监督管理局（FDA) 强制执行的法定标准，USP 标准在全球 130 多个国家得到认可和使用。USP 于 1820 年出版了第 1 版，1950 年以后每五年出一次修订版，自 2002 年开始，每年发布一版，并从 1980 年第 15 版 USP 起，将收载 USP 中所使用到的药用辅料标准的美国处方集并入 USP 中，前面内容为 USP，后面为 NF，在 NF 中还收载了 USP 尚未收入的新药和新制剂，目前 USP 最新版为 2013 年 12 月出版的第 37 版（USP37-NF32）。

① ***U.S. Pharmacopoeia (U.S.P. for short)*** The technical regulations made by the U.S. government on drug quality standards and inspection methods are the legal basis for drug production, use, management and inspection. The *U.S. Pharmacopoeia* is the only legal standards enforced by the U.S. Food and Drug Administration(FDA) for drugs and related products manufactured and sold in the United States. *USP* standards are recognized and used in more than 130 countries. USP was first published in 1820, having been modified every five years since 1950, and published one edition every year since 2002. Since the 15th edition of *USP* in 1980, the US prescription collection containing the standards of pharmaceutical excipients used in USP was moved into *USP*. The former content is *USP*, and the latter is *NF*. New drugs and new preparations that USP has not yet collected are also in *NF*. Currently, the latest version of *USP* is the 37th Edition (USP37-NF32) published in December 2013.

2. 欧洲药典（简称 E.P.） 由二十六国和欧共体协议编订，由欧洲药品质量委员会编辑出版。有英文和法文两种法定文本，其成员包括了欧盟在内的 37 个成员和 23 个观察员，《欧洲药典》于 1977 年出版第 1 版，1980~1996 年出版第 2 版，分 2 部 4 册。第一册是通则，包括各种分析方法、传统药物分析方法、制剂技术、试剂等；第二册为各论，分 3 册，共收载 133 种药物及制剂。第 3 版为合订本，于 1997 年出版，第 4 版于 2002 年 1 月生效。现行版为第 8 版。

② ***European Pharmacopoeia (E.P. for short)*** The *European Pharmacopoeia* (E.P.) is compiled by agreement between the 26 countries and the European Community and it's edited and published by the European Drug Quality Commission. There are two legal texts in English and French. There are 37 members and 23 observers from the European Union. The first edition of the *European Pharmacopoeia* was published in 1977, and the second edition, from 1980-1996, in two parts by four volumes. The first volume is about general principles, including analysis methods, traditional medication analysis methods, preparation technology, reagents, etc.; the second volume is on theories, within three volumes, having 133 drugs and preparations. The third edition is a combined one published in 1997 and the fourth edition came into force in January 2002. The current one is the eighth edition.

3. 日本药典（日本药局方，简称 J.P.） 首版于日本明治 19 年（公元 1886 年）出版，由日本药局方编集委员会编纂，由厚生省颁布执行，分两部出版，第一部主要收载原料药及基础制剂，第二部主要收载生药、家庭药制剂和制剂原料。

③ ***Japanese Pharmacopoeia (J.P. for short)*** The first edition of *Japanese Pharmacopoeia* was published in Meiji 19 (1886 A.D.), compiled by the Compilation Committee of Japan Drug Administration, and promulgated and implemented by the Ministry of Health, Labour and Welfare. There are two parts. The first part states active pharmaceutical ingredients (APIs) and basic preparations, and the second part contains crude drugs, family medicine preparations and preparing raw materials.

4. 国际药典（简称 Ph.Int.） 世界卫生组织（WHO）为了统一世界各国药品的质量标准和质量控制方法，于 1951 年正式出版了第一部《国际药典》(第 1 版)，1955 年出版了第二部，1959 年出版了补充版。由于各国的新药研究、剂型的发展，及以生物效应为主的制剂试验方法等的飞速发展，使得建立一个能指导各国药典体制的想法在能力和时间上皆缺乏可能性。因此各国根据各自的情况制定本国的药典。故于 1967 年发行《国际药典》(第 2 版）时就改名为《药品质量控制规格》，副名为《国际药典》(第 2 版)，突出药品质量管理标准的作用。1971 年又专门出版了补充版。第 3 版分 5 卷出版，1979 年出版了第一卷《一般分析方法》；1981 年出版了第二卷《质量规格》；1988 年出版了第三卷《质量规格》。第四卷（1994 年）为有关试验、方法的信息，以及药品原料、赋形剂的一般要求和质量说明等。第五卷（2003 年）为剂型通则、制剂各论，以及药品原料和质量标准等。《国际药典》对各国药典无法律约束力，仅供各国编纂药典时作为参考标准。

④ ***International Pharmacopoeia (Ph.Int for short)*** In order to unify the drug quality standards and quality control methods in the world, the World Health Organization (WHO) had the first edition of *International Pharmacopoeia* published in 1951, the second edition in 1955 and the supplementary edition in 1959. Thanks to the rapid ramp-up in new drug researches, dosage forms and test methods of preparations mainly based on biological effects in various countries, it is impossible for ability and time to set up a pharmacopoeia system to offer guidance to the world. Therefore, countries formulated their own Pharmacopoeia according to their own situation. So, the second edition of the *International Pharmacopoeia* issued in 1967, was renamed *Drug Quality Control Specifications* and the subname *The Second Edition of the International Pharmacopoeia,* highlighting the role of drug quality management standards. A supplementary edition was specially published in 1971, The third edition was assorted with five volumes, the first volume of *General Analysis Methods* was published in 1979, the second volume of *Quality Specifications* in 1981, and the third volume of *Quality Specifications* in 1988. The fourth volume (1994) accounted for the experiments and method, as well as the general requirements and quality for raw materials of medication and excipients. The fifth volume (2003) was about the generalrules of dosage forms, theories of preparations, as well as the medication raw materials and quality standards. The *International Pharmacopoeia* has no legal binding force on Pharmacopoeia of different countries. It only serves as reference in compiling Pharmacopoeia for countries.

二、局颁、部颁药品标准
1.5.2 Drug Standards Issued by Either the Administration or the Ministry

在原国家食品药品监督管理局（现国家药品监督管理局）成立前，由卫生部颁布的药品标准，称为《部颁药品标准》，包括中药材分册、中药成方制剂分册共 20 册，共收载品种 4052 种。由国家药品监督管理局（原国家食品药品监督管理局）颁布实施的药品标准，称为《局颁药品标准》。《部颁药品标准》《局颁药品标准》的性质与作用与《中国药典》类似，具有法律的约束力，都归属于国家药品标准，作为药物生产、供应、使用、监督等部门检验质量的法定依据。

Prior to the establishment of the China Food and Drug Administration (present the State Medical

Products Supervision and Administration), the drug standards issued by the Ministry of Health P.R. China was called the *Drug Standards issued by the Ministry*, consisting of volumes on TCM herbal substances and Chinese patent medicine, with a total of 20 volumes, and 4052 varieties. The drug standards promulgated and implemented by the National Medical Products Supervision and Administration (the former China Food and Drug Administration) are called *the Drug Standards issued by the Administration.* The character and function of the *Drug Standards issued by the Ministry* and the *Drug Standards issued by the Administration* are the same to those of the *Chinese Pharmacopoeia*, which are legally authentic and in scope of the national drug standards. They are the legal rules for the inspection quality of medication production, supply, use, supervision and other departments.

三、药品管理法规
1.5.3 Drug Administration Rules and Regulations

为对药品的研发、生产、流通、使用以及监督管理实行严格的法制化管理，我国颁布《中华人民共和国药品管理法》作为药事基本法，设立药品质量管理规范体系以及众多药事管理法律法规等，对保证公众用药安全性、有效性、科学性等具有重大意义。

In a bid to carry out a strict legal administration for medication R&D, production, circulation, application, supervision and management, China has promulgated the *Drug Administration Law of the People's Republic of China* as the basic law of drug affairs and set up a quality management standard system and many administration rules and regulations, which is of great significance to ensure the safety, effectiveness and scientificity for the public.

1. 中华人民共和国药品管理法 《中华人民共和国药品管理法》简称《药品管理法》，我国第一部《药品管理法》自 1985 年 7 月 1 日起施行。该法在加强药品监督管理、打击制售假劣药品行为、保证人民用药安全有效方面发挥了十分重要的作用。随着我国市场经济体制的推行和加入 WTO，对外开放的进一步扩大，于 2001 年 2 月 28 日首次修订《药品管理法》。2019 年 8 月 26 日第十三届全国人民代表大会常务委员会第十二次会议对《药品管理法》进行再次修订，并于 2019 年 12 月 1 日起施行。

(1) Drug Administration Law of the People's Republic of China The *Drug Administration Law of the People's Republic of China* is abbreviated as the *Drug Administration Law*. The first *Drug Administration Law* of China came into force on July 1, 1985. This law has played an essential role in bolstering drug supervision and management, cracking down on the manufacture and sale of fake and inferior drugs, and so safeguarding the medication safety and effectiveness. With the implementation of China's market economy system and accession to WTO, and the further expansion of opening up, the newly revised *Drug Administration Law* was first amended on February 28, 2001. Recently, the *Drug Administration Law* was revised at the 12th meeting of the Standing Committee of the 13th National People's Congress on August 26, 2019, and went into effect on December 1, 2019.

根据《药品管理法》，2002 年 9 月 15 日起又施行了《药品管理法实施条例》，并先后于 2016 年 2 月 6 日和 2019 年 3 月 18 日进行了相关修订。其特点是：全面体现了药品监督管理体制改革的精神和原则；进一步完善了行政执法手段，明确了权力和责任的关系；加大了对制售假劣药品等违法行为的处罚力度，完善了法律责任制度；增加了近十几年来在实践中探索出来的行之有效的最新药品监管制度；增加了人民群众普遍关心的热点问题，为更好地依法制药奠定了法律基础。

Following the *Drug Administration Law*, *the Regulations for the Implementation of the Drug*

Administration Law has been implemented since September 15, 2002. The relevant amendments were made on February 6, 2016 and March 18, 2019. Its particularities lie in fully presenting the spirit and principles of reforming the drug supervision and management system; further ameliorating the means of administrative law enforcement, and clarifying the relationship between authorities and responsibilities; amplifying the punishment for illegal acts such as manufacturing and selling fake and inferior drugs, and bettering the legal liability system; increasing the effective and new drug regulatory system explored in practice for years; adding hot issues of common concern to the people. And so, it lays a legal foundation for the better legal pharmacy.

2. 药品注册管理办法　药品注册是指国家药品监督管理局根据药品注册申请人的申请，依照法定程序，对拟上市销售的药品的安全性、有效性、质量可控性等进行系统评价，并决定是否同意其申请的审批过程。药品的注册管理办法是为了保证药品的安全、有效和质量可控，规范药品注册行为而制定的管理办法，在我国境内申请药物临床试验、药品生产和药品进口，以及进行药品审批、注册检验和监督管理，均适用本办法。

(2) Administration of Drug Registration　Drug registration refers to the examination and approval process in which the National Medical Products Administration in line with the legal procedure systematically evaluates the safety, effectiveness and quality controllability of the drugs to be marketed applicated by the drug registration applicant, and determines whether or not to say yes to the application. The administration of drug registration are formulated to guarantee the medication's safety, effectiveness and quality, and standardize medication registration doings. These measures are applicable to the application for medication clinical trials, production and drug imports within the territory of China, as well as drug approval, registration inspection and supervision.

药品注册申请分为：①新药申请；②已有国家标准的药品申请；③进口药品申请；④补充申请。

Drug registration applications cover those: ① new drug application; ② extant national standard drug application; ③ imported drug application; ④ supplementary application.

为了规范新药的研制，加强新药的审批管理，卫生部于 1985 年 7 月 1 日发布了《新药审批办法》。1992 年 9 月 1 日又发布了《有关中药部分的修订和补充规定》。1998 年我国组建国家药品监督管理局后，对《新药审批办法》进行了修订，并于 1999 年 5 月 1 日起施行。于 2002 年 12 月 1 日起我国施行了《药品注册管理办法》(试行)，其后原国家食品药品监督管理局又分别于 2005 年 5 月 1 日和 2007 年 10 月 1 日两次颁布施行了新的《药品注册管理办法》。目前，《药品注册管理办法》已由国家市场监督管理总局于 2020 年 1 月 15 日再次更新，自 2020 年 7 月 1 日起正式施行，原《药品注册管理办法》同时废止。

To standardize the advancement of new drugs and enhance the examination and approval of them, the Ministry of Health, Labour and Welfare issued the *Measures for Examination and Approval of New Drugs* on July 1, 1985. On September 1, 1992, the *Revised and Supplementary Provisions on Chinese Medicine* were issued. After the establishment of the National Medical Products Administration in 1998, the *Measures for the Approval of New Drugs* were revised and put into effect on May 1, 1999, and on December 1, 2002. The *Measures for the Administration of Drug Registration* (for Trial Implementation) were put into effect in China. Subsequently, the former National Medical Products Administration issued and implemented the new *Measures for the Administration of Drug Registration* on May 1, 2005 and October 1, 2007 respectively. Recently, the *Measures for the Administration of Drug Registration* have been renewed by the State Administration for Market Regulation on January 15, 2020, and came into force on July 1, 2020. The original *Measures for the Administration of Drug Registration* was abolished

simultaneously.

3. 药品生产质量管理规范（简称 GMP）《药品生产质量管理规范》系指在药品生产过程中，运用科学、合理、规范化的条件和方法保证生产优良药品的一整套科学管理方法。GMP 的实施，确保了制剂生产、管理的规范性。现行 GMP 的类型大致分为 3 类：一是国际性的 GMP，如 WTO 的 GMP，欧洲自由贸易联盟的 GMP、欧洲共同体的 GMP、东南亚国家联盟的 GMP 等；二是国家性的 GMP，如美国、日本、英国、法国、澳大利亚、中国的 GMP；三是制药行业性的 GMP，如美国制药联合会、日本制药协会、中国医药工业公司及中国药材公司制订的 GMP 等。

(3) Good Manufacturing Practice (GMP for short) *Drug Production Quality Management Standard* refers to a set of scientific management methods to ensure the production of good drugs by using scientific, reasonable and standardized conditions and methods in the process of drug production. The implementation of GMP ensures the standardization of preparation production and management. There are 3 types of current GMP: the first, international GMP, such as WTO GMP, European Free Trade Union (EFTA) GMP, European Community GMP, Association of South-East Nations (ASEAN) GMP, etc.; the second, national GMP, such as the United States, Japan, the United Kingdom, France, Australia and China; the third, GMP in the pharmaceutical industry, such as GMP formulated by the American Pharmaceutical Federation, Japan Pharmaceutical Association, China Pharmaceutical Industry Corporation and China pharmaceutical company.

GMP 是药品生产企业管理生产和质量的基本准则。早在 1963 年，美国 FDA 便制订了 GMP，并于 1964 年开始以法令形式正式实施，1976 年 FDA 又对 GMP 进行了修订。1975 年 WHO 修订发表了作为世界各国实行 GMP 的指导性文件。我国于 1988 年颁布实施 GMP，并于 1992 年重新修订，1998 年国家药品监督管理局组建后，又颁布了《药品生产质量管理规范》（1998 年修订版），2010 年再次对 GMP 进行修订，现行的 GMP 为 2011 年 3 月 1 日起施行的《药品生产质量管理规范（2010 年修订版）》。目前，我国现有中药制药企业皆已通过了 GMP 认证。

GMP is the essential standard for drug manufacturing enterprises to manage production and quality. As early as in 1963, the U.S. FDA formulated GMP, which was officially implemented in the form of laws and regulations in 1964. In 1976, FDA revised GMP again. In 1975, WHO revised and published the guidance document for GMP implementation in the world. China promulgated and implemented GMP in 1988, and revised it again in 1992. After the establishment of the National Medical Products Administration in 1998, the *Drug Production Quality Management Standard* (1998 Revision) was promulgated and the GMP was revised again in 2010. The current GMP is the GMP (2010 Revision) having been implemented since March 1, 2011. At present, China's existing pharmaceutical enterprises of traditional Chinese medicine have all obtained GMP certificates.

（傅超美　廖　婉）

岗位对接

重点小结

题库

第二章　中药调剂
Chapter 2　Traditional Chinese Medicine Prescription Filling

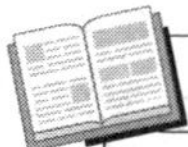

学习目标 | Learning Goals

知识要求：

1．**掌握**　处方的调配程序与注意事项。

2．**熟悉**　中药"斗谱"排列的一般原则，处方药、非处方药的基本概念；中药毒性药品种及用量；处方禁忌药。

3．**了解**　处方种类与格式；中药学的配伍变化与现代研究简况。

能力要求：

学会处方调配程序及注意事项，并能分清处方药与非处方药。

Knowledge requirements:

1. To master the formulation procedures and cautions.

2. To be familiar with the principles of traditional Chinese medicine ranking and the concept of prescription drugs and over-the-counter drugs, the type and quantity of the toxic drugs of traditional Chinese medicine and the prescription of contraindicated drugs.

3. To know the type and the form of prescriptions and compatibility changes of traditional Chinese medicine and the modern research.

Ability requirements:

Learn the formulation procedures and cautions and be able to distinguish between prescription drugs and over-the-counter drugs.

第一节　概述
2.1　Overview

PPT

中药调剂系指调剂人员根据医师处方，按照配方程序和原则，及时、准确地调配和发售药剂的操作技术。

Traditional Chinese medicine dispensing refers to the operative technique of the drug being dispensed and sold timely and accurately by the dispensers according to the prescription and the formulation procedures and principles.

中药调剂是中医药学的重要组成部分，其起源和发展有着悠久的历史。商代《汤液经法》《周礼》中始载汤剂的创制，标志了中药饮片调剂配方技术的初步形成。

Traditional Chinese medicine dispensing is an important part of traditional Chinese medicine. Its origin and development has a long history. Decoction first sets out in Shang Dynasty *Tang Ye Jing Fa* and *ZhouLi*, which marks that the pieces of Traditional Chinese Medicine dispensing technology has initially been formed.

第二节 处方

2.2 Prescription

PPT

一、处方的概念与种类

2.2.1 The Concept and Type of Prescription

（一）概念

(1) The Concept

处方系指由注册的执业医师和执业助理医师在诊疗活动中为患者开具的，由取得药学专业技术职务任职资格的药学专业技术人员审核、调配、核对，并作为患者用药凭证的医疗文书。

Prescription refers to medical documents prescribed by medical practitioners and assistant practitioners for patients in the clinical process, which is audited, dispensed and checked by pharmaceutical technical professionals and is used as a medical record of medication evidence.

（二）种类

(2) The Type

1. 法定处方 系指国家药品标准收载的处方，具有法律的约束力。

① **Official prescription** Refers to the prescription listed in the National Drug Standards, which is legally binding.

2. 协议处方 系指医院医师与药房根据临床需要，互相协商所制定的处方。

② **Agreed prescription** Refers to the prescription prescribed by hospital physician and pharmacy after interactive negotiation according to the clinical needs.

3. 医师处方 系指医师对患者治病用药的书面文件。包括药品名称、给药量、给药方式、给药天数及制备等内容。

③ **Physician prescription** Refers to the written document on the treatment and medication of the patient, including the drug name, dosage, method of administration and preparation, etc.

4. 经方、古方和时方 经方系指经典医学书籍中收载的处方。古方泛指古典医籍中记载的处方。时方系指从清代至今出现的处方。

④ **Classic prescription, ancient prescription and Shi prescription** Classic prescription refers to the prescription recorded in the classic medical books. Ancient prescription refers to the prescription recorded in the ancient Chinese medical books. Shi prescription refers to the prescriptions that have been kept since the Qing dynasty.

5. 单方、验方和秘方 单方一般系指较简单的处方，通常只有1~2味药。验方系指民间和医师积累的经验处方。秘方一般系指过去秘而不传的单方和验方。

⑤ **Single prescription, empirical prescription and secret prescription** Single prescription generally refers to a simple prescription, containing usually only 1 or 2 drugs. Empirical prescription refers to the prescription accumulated by folks and physicians. Secret prescription refers to the single prescription and empirical prescription that were kept as secrets.

二、医师处方的内容
2.2.2 Contents of A Doctor's Prescription

完整的医师处方包括以下各项。

A complete physician prescription includes:

1. 处方前记 包括医疗机构名称、处方编号、科别、处方日期、姓名、性别、年龄、临床诊断及可添加特殊要求的项目。

(1) The preface of prescription Including the name of the medical institution, prescription number, department, date, name, gender, age, clinical diagnosis and other particularly required items.

2. 处方正文 包括药品名称、规格、数量、用法用量。中成药还应当标明剂型，中药饮片处方的书写，一般应当按照"君、臣、佐、使"的顺序排列。

(2) The text of prescription Including drug name, specifications, quantity, dosage and administration. The prescription of Chinese patent medicine should clearly indicate its dosage form. The writing of decoction pieces should be arranged in the order of monarch, minister, assistant and guide generally.

3. 处方后记 包括医师签名，药品金额以及审核、调配、核发、发药药师签名或加盖专用签章。

(3) The post-script of prescription Including the signature of the physician, the price of the drug, the signature or the special seal of the pharmacist for auditing, dispensing and checking and delivering drug.

三、处方药与非处方药
2.2.3 Prescription Drugs and Over-The-Counter Drugs

1. 处方药 系指必须凭执业医师或执业助理医师处方才可调配、购买和使用的药品。

(1) Prescription drug Refers to the drug that must be dispensed, purchased and used according to the prescription prescribed by medical practitioners or assistant practitioners.

2. 非处方药 系指不需凭执业医师或执业助理医师处方即可自行判断、购买和使用的药品，又称为柜台发售药品（over the counter，OTC）。根据药品的安全性，非处方药分为甲、乙两类。非处方药有其专有标识，为椭圆形背景下的OTC三个英文字母，甲类非处方药专有标识为红色，乙类非处方药为绿色。

(2) Nonprescription drug Refer to the drug that can be purchased and used without a prescription

from a practicing physician or assistant practicing physician. It is also called over-the-counter drugs (OTC for short). The nonprescription drugs are divided into Class A drugs and Class B drugs according to the level of safety. OTC drugs have their own labels with the three letters of OTC in an oval backdrop. Class A is labeled red, while class B is labeled green.

第三节 中药处方的调配

2.3 Allocation of Traditional Chinese Medicine Prescriptions

PPT

一、处方的调配程序

2.3.1 Formulation Procedures

中药处方的调配程序为：审方→计价→调配→复核→发药。

Allocation of traditional Chinese medicine prescriptions procedures:
auditing → pricing → dispensing → reviewing → delivering drug.

（一）审方

(1) Auditing prescriptions

1. 审查项目 审方是调剂工作的关键环节，审方内容包括：

① **Auditing items** Auditing prescriptions is the key link of prescription filling.
The contents of auditing prescriptions include:

（1）处方医师、开方时间、患者姓名、年龄、性别。

a. Prescribers, date, the patient's name, age and gender.

（2）药名、剂量、规格、用法与用量等。

b. Drug name, dosage, specification, dosage and administration et al.

（3）方字迹是否清晰、配伍禁忌或超剂量的处方。

c. Is the handwriting of prescription clear? Is there incompatibility of drugs or overdosage?

2. 毒性药与配伍禁忌

② **Toxic drugs and incompatibility**

（1）毒性药 系指毒性剧烈，治疗量与中毒量接近，使用不当可致人中毒或死亡的药物。调剂人员应严格遵循毒性中药的剂量与用法规定。

a. Toxic drugs Refer to drugs with severe toxicity, whose therapeutic dose is close to the toxic dose. Toxic drugs can cause poisoning or death if used improperly. The dispensers should strictly follow the dosage and usage of toxic traditional Chinese medicine.

（2）配伍禁忌 中药配伍"七情"中相反和相恶，均使药物配伍后产生抑制和对抗作用。对于十八反、十九畏的药物，须避免盲目配合应用。

b. Incompatibility The antagonism and mutual inhibition of traditional Chinese medicine compatibility (seven relations) after compatibility. Blind compatibility of the drugs in eighteen antagonisms or nineteen counteractions should be avoided.

（3）妊娠禁忌 凡能影响胎儿生长发育、有致畸作用，甚至造成堕胎的中药为妊娠禁忌用药。

c. The contraindication in pregnancy Traditional Chinese medicines that can affect the growth of a fetus, have teratogenic effect, and even cause abortion are contraindicated for pregnancy.

3. 并开药物与脚注

③ Combination prescription and footnote

（1）并开药物 系指将处方中 2~3 种中药开在一起。

a. Combination prescription refers to that 2 or 3 kinds of traditional Chinese medicine are prescribed together.

（2）脚注 系指医师开处方时在某味药的上角或下角所加的简单要求。

b. Footnote refers to the simple requirement that the physician places on the upper or lower corner of a drug when prescribing.

（二）计价

(2) Pricing

药价的计算要按当地物价部门统一规定的办法和计价收费标准执行，不得任意改价或估价。

The calculation of drug prices should be carried out in accordance with the uniform measures and charge standard by the local pricing department. No arbitrarily changing or evaluating.

（三）调配

(3) Dispensing

配方时按处方药物顺序逐味称量，间隔摆放，多剂处方应先称取总量，然后按等量递减的方法进行称量分配。需特殊处理的药物应单独包装，并注明处理方法。

The medicinal materials in the prescription should be weighed in correspondence to the sequence of the prescription and separately placed. The total weight of multi-dose prescriptions should be weighed first, and then weighed and distributed according to the method of increment by equal quantity. The drug requiring special treatment should be separately packed and the treatment method should be indicated.

（四）复核

(4) Reviewing

复核具体要求如下：

The specific requirements for the review are as follows:

1. 注意调配的药味和称取的分量与处方是否相符。

① Pay attention to whether the categories and the weight of the dispensed drugs are in accordance with the prescription.

2. 饮片有无生虫、发霉及变质现象，有无以生代制、生制不分的处方应付错误，整药、籽药有无应捣未捣的情况。

② Pay attention to whether there are insects, mildew and deterioration of the prepared slices; whether there are mistakes of raw products instead of processed products on prescriptions; whether there are entire or seed drugs not mashed that is their due.

3. 需特殊处理的药物是否按要求单包并注明用法，贵重药、毒性药是否处理得当。

③ Pay attention to whether the drug requiring special treatment is separately packed and the treatment method is indicated as required; whether precious drugs and toxic drugs are processed appropriately.

（五）发药

(5) Delivering Drugs

发药时要注意：

The specific requirements for delivering drugs are as follows:

1. 认真核对取药凭证、姓名、剂数。

① Check the receipt, name and the number of doses carefully.

2. 向患者说明用法、用量、禁忌等。

② State the dosage, administration and contraindication et al.

3. 耐心回答病人提出的有关用药问题。

③ Answer the medication questions for the patients with patience.

二、中药“斗谱”的排列原则

2.3.2 The Principle of Traditional Chinese Medicine Ranking

“斗谱”一般排列原则如下：

The principle of“Dou Pu” ranking is as follows:

（一）按用药频率和质地排列

(1) Ranking by Medication Frequency and Textures

根据临床用药情况将饮片分为常用饮片、次常用饮片和不常用饮片。常用饮片装入药斗架的中层，不常用饮片装在上层，较常用饮片装在两者之间。

According to clinical medication, prepared slices of traditional Chinese medicine are divided into the most commonly used pieces, the second most commonly used pieces and the infrequently used pieces. The most commonly used pieces are placed in the middle layer of the drug hopper shelves, the infrequently used pieces are placed in the top layer, and the second commonly used pieces are placed in between.

（二）按方剂组成排列

(2) Ranking by Prescription Composition

同一方剂内药物宜装在同一药斗或临近药斗中，以方便调配。

To facilitate dispensing, the pieces of traditional Chinese medicine in the same prescription should be packed in the same drug hopper or the closer bucket.

（三）按入药部位排列

(3) Ranking by The Part of Medicinal Materials

如按根、茎、叶、花、果实、种子及动物药、矿物药等分类装入药斗。

The pieces of traditional Chinese medicine is placed in different drug hopper according to classification such as root, stem, leaf, flower, fruit, seed and animal medicine, mineral medicine.

（四）按药物性味功能排列

(4) Ranking by Nature and Flavor and Function of Drugs

性味功能相近的排列在一起。

The pieces of traditional Chinese medicine with the similar nature and flavor and function are arranged together.

第四节 中药饮片形式的沿革

2.4 History of The Forms for Pieces of Traditional Chinese Medicine

PPT

中药饮片分为传统中药饮片、新型中药饮片两大类。

The pieces of Traditional Chinese medicine are divided into two categories: Traditional pieces of traditional Chinese medicine and new pieces of traditional Chinese medicine.

一、传统中药饮片

2.4.1 Traditional Pieces of TCM

传统中药饮片有诸多不足，已不能适应当前中医药事业发展的需要。

Traditional pieces of TCM have many shortcomings, which have not been able to meet the needs of the development of traditional Chinese medicine.

二、新型中药饮片

2.4.2 New Pieces of TCM

（一）小包装中药饮片

(1) Small Package of Pieces of TCM

小包装中药饮片是将加工炮制后合格的中药饮片按设定的剂量单味定量包装，由配方药师直接数包调配而无需称量的一种新型中药饮片。特点：具有方便贮存保管、提高调剂效率、计量准确。

Small package of pieces of TCM are new pieces of TCM, which are packaged by qualified pieces of TCM according to the set dose, and then dispensed by the pharmacist according to quantity without weighing. Characteristics: convenience for storage, improving dispensing efficiency and accurate measurement.

（二）中药配方颗粒

(2) Traditional Chinese Medicine Particle Prescription

中药配方颗粒又称免煎中药，是根据各类药材的不同特性，参照传统煎煮法，利用现代工艺提取、浓缩、干燥、制粒等多道工序精制而成的单味中药产品。这种饮片形式既保持了原中药饮片的性味、归经和功效等特性，同时提高了有效成分和（或）组分含量，减少了用药剂量，使调剂更加科学准确，提高了调剂人员的工作效率，携带服用更方便。

Traditional Chinese medicine particle prescription also known as non-decoction Chinese medicine, which is a single traditional Chinese medicine product prepared by using modern technology such as extraction, concentrate, dry, granulation according to the different characteristics of each medicine, and referring to the traditional decoction method. Traditional Chinese medicine particle prescription not only maintains the characteristics of the original Chinese medicine decoction pieces, such as nature and flavor, channel tropism and efficacy, but also improves the content of the active ingredients and/or components,

岗位对接

重点小结

题库

reduces the dosage, makes the dispensing more scientific and accurate, improves the dispensing staff's work efficiency, and makes it more convenient to carry and take.

（三）超微中药

(3) Ultramicro Traditional Chinese Medicine

超微中药饮片加工成粒径为微米级的新型中药饮片。其特点是通过微粉化技术将药材粉碎至1~75μm，使中药细胞壁破碎，药材表面积增加，孔隙率增大，促进了药物成分的溶出。超微中药既保持了中药特性，又能随症加减、方便使用，也是现阶段比较理想的中药新型饮片。

Ultramicro pieces of TCM are processed into new micrometre-scale pieces of TCM. Its characteristic is to grind the medicinal materials to the size of 1-75μm by micronization technology, so that the cell wall of traditional Chinese medicine is broken, the surface area of the medicinal materials increases, the porosity increases, and the dissolution of active ingredients improves. Ultramicro traditional Chinese medicine not only maintains the characteristics of traditional Chinese medicine, but also can modify according to symptoms, be convenient to use. So it is ideal new pieces of TCM at present.

（张纯刚）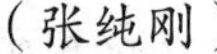

第三章　制药卫生
Chapter 3　Pharmaceutical Hygiene

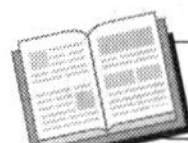

学习目标 | Learning Goals

知识要求：

1. **掌握**　常用灭菌方法和主要防腐剂的正确用法。

2. **熟悉**　制药卫生的意义和基本要求，预防药剂污染的主要环节。

3. **了解**　制药环境卫生的要求和管理、无菌操作和无菌检查。

能力要求：

学会微生物限度标准、各种灭菌方法的特点及应用要点、常用防腐剂的用法等，能应用于制剂实际生产中微生物的控制。

Knowledge requirements:

1. To master common sterilization methods and correct usage of main preservatives.

2. To be familiar with the significance and basic requirements of pharmaceutical hygiene, and the main contents of pharmaceutical pollution prevention.

3. To know the requirements and management of pharmaceutical environmental hygiene, aseptic manipulation and sterility inspection methods.

Ability requirements:

To be able to use various sterilization methods, preservatives and the standard of pharmaceutical hygiene.

第一节　概述
3.1　Overview

PPT

一、制药卫生的含义
3.1.1　Definition of Pharmaceutical Hygiene

制药卫生是药品生产管理的一项重要内容，涉及药品生产的全过程，是防止微生物污染的重要措施，可保证药品质量，是药品生产最基本的要求之一。

Pharmaceutical hygiene is an important part of pharmaceutical production management, which involves the entire process of pharmaceutical production. It is an important measure to ensure the quality of finished products and prevent microbial contamination, and is one of the most basic requirements for pharmaceutical production.

药品生产周期长，涉及因素复杂，存在微生物污染的机会，导致药品变质、腐败、疗效降低或失效，甚至可能产生对人体有害的物质，因此采取有效的制药卫生措施是确保药品质量的重要因素。

The production cycles of drugs are long and the factors involved are complicated. There are chances of being contaminated by microorganisms, which leads to deterioration, corruption, reduction or ineffectiveness of drugs, and may even produce harmful substances to the human body. Therefore, it is important factor to take effective pharmaceutical hygiene measures to ensure the quality of drugs.

二、中药的微生物限度标准

3.1.2 Microbial Limit Standards of TCM

现行版《中国药典》对中药提取物、饮片、中药制剂的微生物限度做了具体规定。制剂通则品种项下要求无菌的制剂、原辅料和用于手术、烧伤或严重创伤的局部给药制剂应符合无菌检查法规定。非无菌不含药材原粉的中药制剂的微生物限度标准见表 3-1。

The Chinese Pharmacopoeia in-use has specified the microbial limits of TCM extracts, decoction pieces, and TCM preparations. General rules of preparations of the variety requirements of sterile preparations, raw and auxiliary materials and preparations for local administration for surgery, burns or severe trauma should meet the requirements of the sterility inspection law. The non-sterile microbial limit standards of Chinese medicinal preparations without raw material, powder are shown in Table 3-1.

表 3-1 非无菌不含药材原粉的中药制剂的微生物限度标准

<table>
<tr><th colspan="2">给药途径</th><th>需氧菌总数（cfu/g、cfu/ml 或 cfu/10cm^2）</th><th>霉菌和酵母菌总数（cfu/g、cfu/ml 或 cfu/10cm^2）</th><th>控制菌</th></tr>
<tr><td rowspan="2">口服给药</td><td>固体制剂</td><td>10^3</td><td>10^2</td><td rowspan="2">不得检出大肠埃希菌（1g 或 1ml）；含药材原粉的化学药品制剂及含脏器提取物的制剂还不得检出沙门菌（10g 或 10ml）</td></tr>
<tr><td>液体制剂</td><td>10^2</td><td>10</td></tr>
<tr><td colspan="2">口腔黏膜给药制剂
齿龈给药制剂
鼻用制剂</td><td>10^2</td><td>10</td><td>不得检出大肠埃希菌、金黄色葡萄球菌、铜绿假单胞菌（1g、1ml 或 10cm^2）</td></tr>
<tr><td colspan="2">耳用制剂
皮肤给药制剂</td><td>10^2</td><td>10</td><td>不得检出金黄色葡萄球菌、铜绿假单胞菌（1g、1ml 或 10cm^2）</td></tr>
<tr><td colspan="2">阴道、尿道给药制剂</td><td>10^2</td><td>10</td><td>不得检出大肠埃希菌、金黄色葡萄球菌、铜绿假单胞菌、耐胆盐革兰阴性菌（1g 或 1ml）</td></tr>
<tr><td rowspan="2">直肠给药</td><td>固体制剂</td><td>10^3</td><td>10^2</td><td rowspan="2">不得检出金黄色葡萄球菌、铜绿假单胞菌（1g 或 1ml）</td></tr>
<tr><td>液体制剂</td><td>10^2</td><td>10^2</td></tr>
<tr><td colspan="2">其他局部给药制剂</td><td>10^2</td><td>10^2</td><td>不得检出金黄色葡萄球菌、铜绿假单胞菌（1g、1ml 或 10cm^2）</td></tr>
</table>

Table 3-1　Microbial limit standards for non-sterile traditional Chinese medicine preparations without medicinal raw powder

Route of Administration		TAMC (cfu/g, cfu/ml or cfu/10cm²)	TYMC (cfu/g, cfu/ml or cfu/10cm²)	Control bacteria
Oral administration	Solid preparations	10^3	10^2	No *E. coli.* (1g or 1ml) ; No *Salm.spp.*in preparation with raw medicinal powder and organic extraction (10g or 10ml)
	Liquid preparations	10^2	10	
Oral mucosal preparation Gingival administration preparation Nasal preparations		10^2	10	No *E. coli.*, *Sta.*, *Psa.* (1g, 1ml or 10cm²)
Ear preparations Dermal preparations		10^2	10	No *Sta.*, *Psa.* (1g, 1ml or 10cm²)
Vaginal and urethral administration preparations		10^2	10	No *E. coli.*, *Sta.*, *Psa.*, bile tolerant gram negative bacteria (1g or 1ml)
Rectal administration	Solid preparations	10^3	10^2	No *Sta.*, *Psa.*(1g or 1ml)
	Liquid preparations	10^2	10^2	
Other topical administration preparations		10^2	10^2	No *Sta.*, *Psa.* (1g, 1ml or 10cm²)

Note: TAMC: total aerobic microbial count; TYMC: total combined yeasts and mold count; *Sta.*: *Staphylococcus aureus*; *Psa.*: *Pseudomonas aeruginosa*; *E. coli*: *Escherichia coli*; *Salm.spp.*: *Salmonella* species.

非无菌含药材原粉的中药制剂的微生物限度标准见表 3-2。

Microbial limit standards for non-sterile traditional Chinese medicine preparations containing raw powder of medicinal material are shown in Table 3-2.

表 3-2　非无菌含药材原粉的中药制剂的微生物限度标准

给药途径		需氧菌总数（cfu/g、cfu/ml 或 cfu/10cm²）	霉菌和酵母菌总数（cfu/g、cfu/ml 或 cfu/10cm²）	控制菌
固体口服给药制剂	不含豆豉、神曲等发酵原粉	10^4 （丸剂 3×10^4）	10^2	不得检出大肠埃希菌（1g）；不得检出沙门菌（10g）；耐胆盐革兰阴性菌应小于 10^2（1g）
	含豆豉、神曲等发酵原粉	10^5	5×10^2	
液体口服给药制剂	不含豆豉、神曲等发酵原粉	5×10^2	10^2	不得检出大肠埃希菌（1ml）；不得检出沙门菌（10ml）；耐胆盐革兰阴性菌应小于 10（1ml）
	含豆豉、神曲等发酵原粉	10^3	10^2	
固体局部给药制剂	用于表皮或黏膜不完整	10^3	10^2	不得检出金黄色葡萄球菌、铜绿假单胞菌（1g 或 10cm²）；阴道、尿道给药制剂还不得检出白色念珠菌、梭菌（1g 或 10cm²）
	用于表皮或黏膜完整	10^4	10^2	

续表

给药途径		需氧菌总数（cfu/g、cfu/ml 或 cfu/10cm^2）	霉菌和酵母菌总数（cfu/g、cfu/ml 或 cfu/10cm^2）	控制菌
液体局部给药制剂	用于表皮或黏膜不完整	10^2	10^2	不得检出金黄色葡萄球菌、铜绿假单胞菌（1g 或 10cm^2）；阴道、尿道给药制剂还不得检出白色念珠菌、梭菌（1ml）
	用于表皮或黏膜完整	10^2	10^2	

Table 3-2 Microbial limit standards for non-sterile traditional Chinese medicine preparations containing raw powder of medicinal materials

Route of Administration		TAMC (cfu/g, cfu/ml or cfu/10cm^2)	TYMC (cfu/g, cfu/ml or cfu/10cm^2)	Control bacteria
Oral solid administration	Without fermented raw powder such as SSP and MMF	10^4 (pill 3×10^4)	10^2	No *E. coli*.（1g）; No *Salm. spp.*（10g）; bile tolerant gram negative bacteria<10^2（1g）
	With fermented raw powder such as SSP and MMF	10^5	5×10^2	
Oral liquid administration	Without fermented raw powder such as SSP and MMF	5×10^2	10^2	No *E. coli*.（1ml）; No *Salm. spp.*（10ml）; bile tolerant gram negative bacteria<10（1ml）
	With fermented raw powder such as SSP and MMF	10^3	10^2	
Topical administration solid preparations	For incomplete epidermis or mucosa	10^3	10^2	No *Sta.*, *Psa.*（1g or 10cm^2）; No candida albicans, clostridium in Vaginal and urethral preventive preparations（1g or 10cm^2）
	For complete epidermis or mucosa	10^4	10^2	
Topical administration liquid preparations	For incomplete epidermis or mucosa	10^2	10^2	No *Sta.*, *Psa.*（1g or 10cm^2）; No candida albicans, clostridium in Vaginal and urethral preventive preparations（1ml）
	For complete epidermis or mucosa	10^2	10^2	

Note: SSP: *semen sojae preparatum*; MMF: *massa medicate fermentata*; TAMC: total aerobic microbial count; TYMC: total combined yeasts and mold count; *Sta.*: *Staphylococcus aureus*; *Psa.*: *Pseudomonas aeruginosa*; *E. coli*: *Escherichia coli*; *Salm.spp.*: *Salmonella* species.

中药提取物、中药饮片、非无菌的药用原料及辅料微生物限度标准见表 3-3。

Microbial limit standards for traditional Chinese medicine extracts, decoction pieces and non-sterile medicinal raw materials and excipients owe shown in Table 3-3.

表 3-3 中药提取物、中药饮片非无菌的药用原料及辅料微生物限度标准

	需氧菌总数（cfu/g、cfu/ml 或 cfu/10cm^2）	霉菌和酵母菌总数（cfu/g、cfu/ml 或 cfu/10cm^2）	控制菌
中药提取物	10^3	10^2	限度未做统一规定
中药饮片	限度未做统一规定	限度未做统一规定	不得检出沙门菌（10g）；耐胆盐革兰阴性菌应小于 10^4（1g）
药用原料与辅料	10^3	10^2	限度未做统一规定

Table 3-3 Microbial limit standards for traditional Chinese medicine extracts, decoction pieces and non-sterile medicinal raw materials and excipients

	TAMC (cfu/g, cfu/ml or cfu/10cm^2)	TYMC (cfu/g, cfu/ml or cfu/10cm^2)	Control bacteria
Traditional Chinese medicine extracts	10^3	10^2	Limits are not uniform
Decoction pieces	Limits are not uniform	Limits are not uniform	No *Salm.spp.* (10g); bile tolerant gram negative bacteria<10^4 (1g)
Medicinal raw materials and excipients	10^3	10^2	Limits are not uniform

霉变、长螨者，以不合格论。

Those which have mildew or mites are regarded as unqualified.

三、预防中药制剂污染的措施

3.1.3 The Methods of Preventing Herbal Preparation Contamination

（一）原辅料的处理

(1) Processing of Raw Materials and Excipients

中药制剂原料带有大量微生物、虫卵及杂质，投料前对原材料进行洁净处理，可以避免或减少微生物污染。

The raw materials of TCM preparations contain many microorganisms, insect eggs and impurities. So the raw materials are cleaned before feeding to avoid or reduce microbial pollution.

中药材可通过筛选、剪切、刮削、剔除、刷擦、碾串及泡洗方法，达到规定净度的质量标准。常用洗药机、干式表皮清洗机、带式磁选机、机械化净选机组等。

TCM materials can be picked, cut, scraped, eliminated, brushed, purified through grinding, and soak-washed to meet the required quality standards. Commonly medicine washing machine, belt magnetic separator and so on are used.

中药材前处理生产操作，必须与其他制剂生产严格分开，炮制操作应有良好的通风、除烟、除尘、降温设施。

The pretreatment production operation of Chinese medicinal materials must be strictly separated from the production of other preparations, and the processing operation should have good ventilation, smoke removal, dust removal, and cooling facilities.

防止中药材在贮藏过程中污染，采用干燥养护技术、气调养护技术、射线辐射杀虫养护技术、包装防霉养护技术、气幕防潮养护技术等。

Dry maintenance technology, air conditioning maintenance technology, radiative insecticidal method, air curtain moisture-proof maintenance technology can be used to prevent pollution of TCM materials during storage.

中药制剂制备过程中使用的辅料，都应符合相应的质量标准，使用前应严格按照标准进行选择并做适当处理。

The excipients often used in the manufacture of TCM preparations should meet the corresponding quality standards, and be selected, handled properly before use.

（二）生产过程的控制

(2) Control of the Production Process

生产过程中，防止微生物污染，可采用阶段性生产方式；分隔区域内生产不同品种药品；空气洁净级别不同区域应有压差控制；密闭系统生产；干燥设备的进风应有空气过滤器，排风应有防止空气倒流装置；液体制剂的部分工序应当在规定时间内完成；按剂型特点规定贮存期和贮存条件。

During the production process, staged production methods can be used to prevent microbial pollution; different types of drugs are produced in separate areas; pressure difference control should exist in areas with different air cleanliness level; production should be finished in closed system; The air inlet of the drying equipment should have an air filter, and the air exhaust should have a device to prevent air flow back, and part of the process of liquid preparation should be completed within the specified time. preparation, filtration, potting, sterilization of liquid preparation should be completed within the required time; based on the characteristics of different dosage forms, preparations should be stored under different condition with various shelf lives.

案例导入 ¦ Case example

案例 3-1　川芎饮片的炮制

3-1　Processing of *Ligusticum Chuanxiong Hort*

功能主治：活血行气，祛风止痛。用于胸痹心痛，胸胁刺痛，跌扑肿痛，月经不调，头痛，风湿痹痛。

Functions and indications: To Promote blood circulation, dispel wind and relieve pain. It is used for chest pain, chest rib pain, tingling pain, irregular menstruation, headache, rheumatic pain.

制法：原料药→预处理→净制加工→软化处理→水分检查→切片→干燥→精制

Making Procedure: Raw medicinal material → Pretreatment → clean Processing → Softening → Moisture measurement → Slicing → Drying → Purifying

用法用量：3~10g。

Dosage: 3-10g.

注解：①预处理过程是指对川芎表皮的清洗；②净制过程是通过筛选除去药材中的泥沙、石块等杂质；③精制则是通过筛选除去碎末。

Notes: The pretreatment process refers to the cleaning of the epidermis of *Ligusticum chuanxiong*; The clean process is to remove impurities such as sand, stones, etc.; Purifying removes debris through sieves.

第二节　制药环境的卫生管理

3.2 Management of the Pharmaceutical Environment

PPT

一、中药制药环境的基本要求

3.2.1 The Basic Requirements of the Pharmaceutical Environment

《中华人民共和国药品管理法》《中华人民共和国药品管理法实施办法》《药品生产质量管理

规范》等法规对药品生产企业的环境、布局、厂房和设施等方面提出了基本要求。

The Drug Administration Law of the People's Republic of China, the Rules for the Implementation of the Drug Administration Law of the People's Republic of China, and the Good Manufacturing Practice, etc. set forth basic requirements for the environment, layout, factory buildings and facilities of pharmaceutical manufacturers.

（一）厂区环境

(1) Plant Environment

厂房所处的环境应当能够最大限度的降低物料或产品遭受污染的风险。

The environment of the factory should be able to minimize the contamination risk of materials or products.

（二）厂房设计与设施要求

(2) Plant Design and Facility Requirements

生产、行政、生活和辅助区总体布局应当合理，不得相互妨碍。中药材前处理工序，应当进行粉尘扩散和水蒸气控制，避免污染；应当设置表面平整光洁的净选台。提取、浓缩、收膏工序宜采用密闭系统进行操作，并在线清洁。中药注射剂浓配前的精制工序应至少在D级洁净区内完成。非创伤面外用中药制剂及其他特殊的中药制剂可在非洁净厂房内生产，但必须有效的控制与管理。

The overall layout of production, administration, living and auxiliary areas should be reasonable and should not interfere with each other. In the pre-treatment process of TCM materials, dust diffusion and water vapor management should be controlled to avoid pollution and cross-contamination; the clean benches with smooth surface should be set up. The extraction, concentration, and decoction collection processes should be operated with closed system and cleaned online. The exquisite process before the concentration of TCM injections should be completed at least in the D-class clean zone. Non-traumatic external TCM preparations and other special TCM preparations can be produced in non-clean workshops, but must be effectively controlled and managed.

二、洁净室的净化标准

3.2.2 Purification Standards of Lean Room

利用空气洁净技术，能使洁净室达到一定洁净度。洁净室可分为四个级别（表3-4）。

The use of air cleaning technology can make clean room reach a certain degree of cleanliness. Clean rooms can be divided into four levels (Table 3-4).

A级：高风险操作区。

Class A: High-risk operating area.

B级：无菌配制和灌装等高风险操作A级洁净区所处的背景区域。

Class B: Background area where Class A clean area is located for high-risk operations such as aseptic preparation and filling.

C级和D级：无菌药品生产过程中重要程度较低操作步骤的洁净区。

Class C and D: Clean area with less important operational steps in the production of sterile medicines.

表 3-4 各级别空气悬浮粒子的标准

洁净级别	悬浮粒子最大允许数 /m³			
	静态		动态	
	≥ 0.5μm	≥ 5.0μm	≥ 0.5μm	≥ 5.0μm
A 级	3520	20	3520	20
B 级	3520	29	352000	2900
C 级	352000	2900	3520000	29000
D 级	3520000	29000	不作规定	不作规定

Table 3-4 Standards for All Levels of Airborne Particles

Cleanliness levels	Maximum allowable number of airborne particles /m³			
	Static state		Dynamic state	
	≥ 0.5μm	≥ 5.0μm	≥ 0.5μm	≥ 5.0μm
A Class	3520	20	3520	20
B Class	3520	29	352000	2900
C Class	352000	2900	3520000	29000
D Class	3520000	29000	No rule	No rule

洁净室室温为 18~26℃，相对湿度为 40%~60%。洁净室必须保持正压，以防止低级洁净室的空气逆流至高级洁净室中。生产车间按洁净度等级的高低依次排列，并有相应的压差。

The clean room's temperature is 18 to 26℃, and the RH is 40% to 60%. The clean room must maintain positive pressure to prevent the air in the lower clean room from flowing back into the higher clean room. The production plants are arranged in order according to the degree of cleanliness, and there is a corresponding pressure difference.

三、空气洁净技术与应用
3.2.3 Air Clean Technology and Application

空气洁净技术是指创造洁净空气环境的各种技术的总称。目前，常用的空气洁净技术是非层流型洁净技术和层流洁净技术。非层流洁净技术是用高度净化的空气将操作室内的尘粒加以稀释的空气净化方式，气流形式是乱流。层流洁净技术是用高度净化的气流作载体，将操作室内的尘粒以平行层流状态排出的空气净化方式，气流形式是层流。

The air clean technology involves various technologies that create a clean air environment. The commonly used air cleaning technologies are non-laminar and laminar flow cleaning technology.

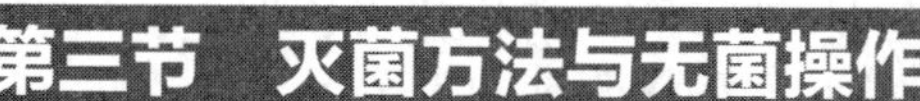

第三节　灭菌方法与无菌操作

灭菌方法的操作包括：灭菌：用物理或化学方法将所有致病和非致病的微生物、细菌的芽孢全部杀死的操作；防腐：用物理或化学方法防止和抑制微生物生长繁殖的操作；消毒：用物理或化学方法将病原微生物杀死的操作。

一、灭菌方法

（一）物理灭菌法

1. 干热灭菌法　利用火焰或干热空气进行灭菌的方法。加热使蛋白质变性或凝固，破坏核酸，酶失活，微生物死亡。

（1）火焰灭菌法　用火焰直接灼烧达到灭菌目的。适宜于耐火材质的物品与用具的灭菌。

（2）干热空气灭菌法　利用高温干热空气达到灭菌的方法。在高温烘箱或干热灭菌柜中进行。干热空气灭菌法采用的温度一般比湿热灭菌法高，一般规定：160~170℃ 灭菌 2 小时以上，170~180℃ 灭菌 1 小时以上或 250℃ 灭菌 45 分钟以上。适宜于耐高温的玻璃、金属制品以及不允许湿气穿透的油脂类材料和耐高温的粉末材料等。不适宜于大部分药品及橡胶、塑料制品的灭菌。

2. 湿热灭菌法　利用饱和水蒸气或沸水灭菌的方法。湿热潜热大，穿透力强，容易使蛋白质变性或凝固，灭菌效果可靠。

（1）热压灭菌法　利用高压饱和水蒸气杀灭微生物的方法。是药品生产中使用最广泛、效果最可靠的灭菌方法。适宜于耐热压灭菌的药品、玻璃容器等。

热压灭菌温度、压力、时间要求：115℃，表压力 68.6kPa，绝对压力 166.7kPa，40 分钟；121.5℃，表压力 98.0kPa，绝对压力 196.1kPa，30 分钟；126.5℃，表压力 137.2kPa，绝对压力 235.3kPa，15 分钟。

（2）煮沸灭菌法　利用沸水加热灭菌的方法。煮沸时间 30~60 分钟。

（3）流通蒸汽灭菌法　常压下使用 100℃ 流通蒸气加热灭菌的方法。灭菌时间 30~60 分钟。一般作为不耐热无菌产品的辅助灭菌手段。

（4）低温间歇灭菌法　将待灭菌物品于 60~80℃ 加热 1 小时，杀灭其中细菌繁殖体，然后在室温或 37℃ 恒温箱中放置 24 小时，待芽孢继续发育成为繁殖体，再进行加热灭菌。按此法反复操作 3 次以上，直至杀灭全部细菌繁殖体和芽孢。该法适用于必须加热灭菌但又不耐较高温度的药品。

（5）影响湿热灭菌的因素（Factors that affect moist-heat sterilization）

①微生物的种类和数量　微生物种类和发育阶段不同，其耐热、耐压性有很大差异。耐热耐压次序为芽孢 > 繁殖体 > 衰老体。灭菌物品中微生物数量越少，灭菌时间越短。

②蒸汽性质　饱和蒸汽热含量高，穿透力强，灭菌效力高；湿饱和蒸汽，热含量低，穿透力差；过热蒸汽类似干热空气，穿透力弱。

③制剂中介质的性质　制剂中含有营养物质，能增强微生物抗热性。一般情况下微生物在不同环境下的耐热次序为中性 > 碱性 > 酸性。

④灭菌温度与时间　灭菌温度与灭菌时间成反比。

3. 紫外灭菌法　用紫外线灭菌的方法。灭菌紫外线波长 200~300nm，其中最强的是 254nm。

紫外线可促使核酸蛋白变性，同时照射空气后产生微量臭氧，共同发挥杀菌作用。该法广泛用于空气灭菌与表面灭菌。

4. 微波灭菌法 利用频率在300MHz~300kMHz之间的高频电磁波产生热灭菌的方法。能穿透到介质的深部，使其加热表里一致。适用于水性药液、饮片及固体制剂的灭菌。

5. 辐射灭菌法 利用放射源辐射的γ射线灭菌的方法。穿透力强、灭菌效率高，对灭菌物料温度影响小，适用于不耐热药物制剂的灭菌，尤其适用于已包装药品的灭菌。但是设备费用高，有时会降低某些药物的药效。

6. 滤过除菌法 采用无菌滤器过滤，去除介质中微生物，达到除菌目的的方法。主要用于不耐热的低黏度药物溶液和相关气体物质的除菌。除菌滤膜孔径一般不超过0.22μm。

（二）化学灭菌法

化学灭菌法是使用化学药品直接作用于微生物进行灭菌的方法。原理：使病原体蛋白质变性而死亡；与细胞的酶系统结合，影响其代谢；降低细菌的表面张力，增加菌体浆膜的通透性，使细胞破裂或溶解。

1. 气体灭菌法 使用化学药品形成气体或蒸气达到灭菌目的的方法。适用于环境消毒，不耐热医用设备器具的消毒。

（1）环氧乙烷灭菌法 穿透力强，灭菌谱宽，对多数物品呈惰性，无损害。但是易燃易爆，对皮肤和眼黏膜有损害，吸入产生毒性。

（2）甲醛蒸气熏蒸法灭菌法 杀菌效力大，穿透力差，主要用于空气杀菌。

（3）其他蒸气熏蒸灭菌法 丙二醇、乳酸、三甘醇、过氧醋酸等均可以蒸气熏蒸形式用于室内灭菌。

2. 药液法 化学药品作为溶液灭菌剂以喷雾、涂抹或浸泡的方法达到消毒的目的。多数化学灭菌剂不能杀死芽孢，主要用于其他灭菌法的辅助灭菌措施，适用于皮肤、无菌器具等消毒。

（1）醇类 乙醇、异丙醇、氯丁醇等。使菌体蛋白变性杀死细菌繁殖体，不能杀死芽孢。

（2）酚类 苯酚、甲酚、氯甲酚等。

（3）氧化剂 过氧乙酸、过氧化氢、臭氧等。

（4）表面活性剂 洁尔灭、新洁尔灭等季铵盐类阳离子表面活性剂。

（5）其他 部分含氯化合物、含碘化合物、酸类化合物和酯类化合物等也具有杀菌消毒功效。

案例导入

案例3-2 六味地黄丸

处方： 熟地黄120g 酒茱萸60g 牡丹皮45g 山药60g 茯苓45g 泽泻45g

制法： 以上六味，牡丹皮用水蒸气蒸馏法提取挥发性成分；药渣与酒萸肉20g、熟地黄、茯苓、泽泻加水煎煮二次，每次2小时，煎液滤过，滤液合并，浓缩成稠膏；山药与剩余酒萸肉粉碎成细粉，过筛，混匀，与上述稠膏和牡丹皮挥发性成分混匀，制丸，干燥，打光，即得。

功能主治： 滋阴补肾。用于肾阴亏损，头晕耳鸣，腰膝酸软，骨蒸潮热，盗汗遗精，消渴。

用法用量： 口服。一次8丸，一日3次。

注解： ①稠膏是由煎煮液浓缩而成，即已高温灭菌，因此在制丸前无需其他灭菌措施；

②山药与酒茱萸细粉应灭菌后方可制丸；

③本浓缩丸应采用低温灭菌法（如微波灭菌法、辐射灭菌法等）灭菌。

思考题： 本品制备中药粉可采用哪种灭菌方法？

二、无菌操作法

无菌控制条件下制备无菌制剂的操作方法，制备过程中须保持无菌度。

（一）无菌操作室的灭菌

操作室的灭菌多采用除菌和灭菌相结合的方式：操作室内空气的灭菌采用过滤介质除菌、气体灭菌、紫外线灭菌等；用具、地面、墙壁采用加热灭菌和液体灭菌等方法。

（二）无菌操作

操作人员应按操作规程更衣和洗手，各洁净区的着装与洁净度级别相适应。大量无菌制剂的生产在无菌操作室内进行，小规模生产主要在层流洁净工作台、无菌操作柜进行。

（三）无菌检查

无菌检查应在环境洁净度 B 级背景下的局部 A 级洁净度的单向流空气区域内或隔离系统中进行，全过程应严格遵守无菌操作，可按照现行版《中国药典》中“无菌检查法”项下具体规定和方法检查。

三、F 与 F_0 值在灭菌中的意义与应用

为了保证最终产品的无菌效果，目前多采用 F 与 F_0 作为验证灭菌可靠性的参数。

（一）微生物致死时间曲线与 D 值

研究表明，灭菌时微生物的死亡速度属于一级或近似一级动力学过程，符合下列方程：

$$\lg N_t = \lg N_0 - \frac{kt}{2.303} \tag{3-1}$$

式中，N_0 为原始微生物数，N_t 为 t 时残存的微生物数，k 为灭菌速度常数。微生物残存数的对数 lgN_t 对时间 t 作图，可得一条直线，斜率为 $-k/2.303$。式（3-1）也可改写为：

$$t = \frac{2.303}{k}(\lg N_0 - \lg N_t) \tag{3-2}$$

D 值为，在一定灭菌温度下被灭菌物品中杀灭微生物 90% 或残存 10% 所需的时间。

$$D = t = \frac{2.303}{k}(\lg 100 - \lg 10) = \frac{2.303}{k} \tag{3-3}$$

D 值也可以看作被灭菌的物品中微生物数降低一个数量级或一个对数值所需的时间。

D 值越大表明微生物耐热性越强。微生物种类、环境、灭菌条件不同，D 值也不同。

（二）Z 值

Z 值是衡量温度对 D 值影响的参数。它是在一定温度条件下对特定的微生物灭菌时，降低一个 $\lg D$ 所需升高的温度数。

$$Z = \frac{T_1 - T_2}{\lg D_2 - \lg D_1} \tag{3-4}$$

式中，D_2 为温度 T_2 的 D 值，D_1 为温度 T_1 的 D 值，将式（3-4）重排，得：

$$\frac{D_2}{D_1} = 10^{\frac{T_1 - T_2}{Z}} \tag{3-5}$$

设 Z=10℃，T_1=110℃，T_2=121℃，则 D_2=0.079D_1。即 110℃灭菌 1 分钟与 121℃灭菌 0.079 分钟，灭菌效果相当。

Z 值越大表明微生物对灭菌温度变化的“敏感性”越弱，通过升高灭菌温度来加速杀死微生物的效果越不明显。

（三）F 与 F_0 值

1. F 值　在一定灭菌温度 T，给定 Z 值所产生的灭菌效果，与参比温度 T_0 给定 Z 值所产生的灭菌效果相同所相当的时间。

$$F=\int_0^T 10^{\frac{T_1-T_2}{Z}}$$

$$\text{或 } F=\Delta t\sum 10^{\frac{T-T_0}{Z}} \tag{3-6}$$

式中，Δt 为测量被灭菌物品温度的时间间隔，通常为 0.5~1 分钟或更小。T 为每个 Δt 测得的被灭菌物品的温度。

F 值还可以看作 D 值与微生物降低值的乘积，即：

$$F=D_{\mathrm{T}}(\lg N_0-\lg N_t) \tag{3-7}$$

式中，N_t 为灭菌后预期达到的微生物残存数，一般认为 N_t 为 10^{-6} 即认为达到可靠的灭菌效果，故：

$$F=D_{\mathrm{T}}(\lg N_0-\lg 10^{-6}) \tag{3-8}$$

式中，F 值是在一定温度下，杀死容器内全部微生物所需时间。

2. F_0 值　对于湿热灭菌，参比温度为 121℃，参比微生物选择嗜热脂肪芽孢杆菌，Z 值为 10℃，此时得到的 F 值称为 F_0 值。用公式表示为：

$$F_0=\Delta t\sum 10^{\frac{T-121}{10}} \tag{3-9}$$

式中，F_0 值是一定灭菌温度（T），Z 值为 10℃产生的灭菌效果，与 121℃时 Z=10℃产生的灭菌效力相同时所相当的时间。即 F_0 是将被灭菌物品在灭菌过程中不同灭菌温度下的灭菌时间折算成与 121℃灭菌等效的灭菌时间。

目前灭菌设备带有自动计算 F_0 值程序，可根据实际灭菌过程计算。

由于 F_0 值综合考虑了温度与时间对灭菌效果的影响，而且以“标准状态”作为参照，较科学、准确地对灭菌程序进行设计和验证。保证灭菌效果，应尽量减少被灭菌物中的初始菌数，同时增加 50% 的 F_0 值，如规定 F_0 为 8 分钟，实际操作可控制为 12 分钟。

第四节　防腐与防虫

3.4 Anti-Corrosion and Pest Control

PPT

中药制剂的防腐与防虫是保证制剂质量的重要环节。

The antiseptic and insect control of Chinese medicine preparations is an important link to ensure the quality of the preparations.

一、防腐与防虫措施
3.4.1　Anti-Corrosion and Pest Control Measures

防腐，实际药品生产过程中不能完全杜绝微生物的污染，制剂中存在的少量微生物会在适宜条件下滋长和繁殖，导致霉败变质。所以有针对性的选择应用防腐剂，是中药制剂防腐的有效手段之一。

Microbial contamination cannot be completely eliminated in the actual pharmaceutical production process, and a small amount of microorganisms present in the preparation will grow and multiply under appropriate conditions, which will lead to mildew and deterioration. Therefore, the targeted selection and application of preservatives is an effective method for the preservation of TMC preparations.

防虫，主要防止仓库害虫的危害。由于中药及中药制剂的特点，若加工制备不当、保管不善，较其他制剂更容易被害虫感染，导致虫害。

Pest control prevents the damage of warehouse pests. Due to the characteristics of TMC and its preparations, if they are improperly prepared and stored, it is likely to be infected by pests than other preparations.

二、防腐剂
3.4.2　Preservatives

防腐剂是防止药物制剂由于微生物污染而产生变质的添加剂。优良的防腐剂要求：用量小，对人体无害、无刺激性，无不良气味；水中溶解度能达到有效抑菌浓度；抑菌谱广，对大多数微生物抑制作用较强；理化性质稳定，不与制剂中的其他成分起反应，不易受温度和 pH 影响，可长期贮存。

Preservatives are additives that prevent the deterioration of pharmaceutical preparations due to microbial contamination. Excellent preservative requirements: small dosage, harmless to human, no irritation, no bad odor; water solubility can reach effective bacteriostatic concentration; wide antimicrobial spectrum, strong inhibitory effect on most microorganisms; stable physical and chemical properties, no reactions with other ingredients in the preparation, no effect of temperature and pH, and long-time storage.

1. 苯甲酸与苯甲酸钠　苯甲酸未解离分子发挥防腐作用，酸性溶液（pH4）中抑菌效果最好。一般用量为 0.1%~0.25%。

(1) Benzoic acid and sodium benzoate　The un-ionized molecules in benzoic acid play the preservative role, and the antibacterial effect is best in acid solution (pH4). The general dosage is 0.1%-0.25%.

2. 对羟基苯甲酸酯类（尼泊金类）　对羟基苯甲酸酯类有甲酯、乙酯、丙酯和丁酯。酸性溶液中作用最强，在微碱性环境由于酚羟基解离、酯水解，导致作用减弱。该类抑菌剂的效力随着烷基碳数增加而增加，而溶解度递减。故该类抑菌剂常合并使用，协同作用效果更佳。一般用量为 0.01%~0.25%。

(2) Parabens　Parabens are methyl, ethyl, propyl and butyl. The effect is the strongest in acidic solution, and the effect is weakened in the slightly alkaline environment due to dissociation of phenolic

hydroxyl groups and hydrolysis of the ester. The effectiveness of parabens increases with the number of alkyl carbons, while the solubility decreases. Therefore, the synergistic effect of this preservative is better. The general dosage is 0.01%-0.25%.

聚山梨酯、PEG 等与本类防腐剂产生络合作用，增加该类防腐剂水中溶解度，但减弱其抑菌效力，应避免合用。

Polysorbate, PEG, etc. produce complexation with parabens, with complex compound increasing the solubility of parabens in water, but weakening its antibacterial effect, so they should not be used in combination.

3. 山梨酸及其盐 对霉菌和细菌均有较强抑菌作用，其未解离分子发挥防腐作用，常用浓度 0.15%~0.25%。其钾盐的溶解度大于山梨酸。

(3) Sorbic acid and its salts It has strong bacteriostatic effects on molds and bacteria, and its un-ionized molecules play the preservative role, and the common concentration is 0.15%-0.25%. Its potassium salt is more soluble than sorbic acid.

4. 三氯叔丁醇 常用浓度 0.25%~0.5%，一般用于微酸性注射液或滴眼液中，本品有局麻作用。

(4) Chlorobutanol The common concentration is 0.25%-0.5%, and it is used in slightly acidic injections or eye drops. Chlorobutanol has a local anesthetic effect.

5. 酚类及其衍生物 常作注射剂的抑菌剂。苯酚有效抑菌浓度一般为 0.5%，低温及碱性溶液中抑菌效力较强，与甘油、油类或醇类共存时抑菌效力降低。甲酚用量为 0.25%~0.3%，抑菌效力比苯酚强 3 倍，毒性及腐蚀性比苯酚小，不易溶于水。

(5) Phenols and their derivatives They are often used as preservatives for injections. The effective concentration of phenol is 0.5%. The bacteriostatic effect is strong in low temperature and alkaline solutions, and is reduced when coexisting with glycerol, oils or alcohols. The dosage of cresol is 0.25%-0.3%, the bacteriostatic effect is 3 times stronger than that of phenol, the toxicity and corrosivity are less than that of phenol, but it is not easily soluble in water.

岗位对接

6. 季铵盐类 常用洁尔灭、新洁尔灭和杜灭芬，用量约 0.01%，具有杀菌和防腐作用。洁尔灭、新洁尔灭一般用于外用溶液，杜灭芬可作口含消毒液。本类化合物在 pH<5 时作用减弱，遇阴离子表面活性剂时失效。

(6) Quaternary ammonium Jieermie, Xinjieermie and Dumiefen are commonly used. The dosage is about 0.01%. Jieermie and Xinjieermie are used for external solution. Dumiefen is used as oral disinfectant. Benzene compounds effect weaken at pH <5 and fail when meeting anionic surfactants.

重点小结

7. 苯甲醇 常用浓度为 1%~3%，适用于偏碱性注射液，有局部止痛作用。

(7) Benzyl alcohol The concentration is 1%~3%. It is suitable for alkaline injections. It has local analgesic effect.

题库

8. 有机汞类 常用硝酸苯汞和硫柳汞。

(8) Organic mercury Phenylmercury nitrate and thimerosal are commonly used.

9. 其他 20% 以上乙醇以及 30% 以上的甘油溶液具有防腐作用。部分植物挥发油也有防腐作用。

(9) Other More than 20% ethanol and more than 30% glycerol solution have antiseptic effect. Some plant volatile oils also have antiseptic effects.

（柯 瑾）

第四章　粉碎、筛析、混合与制粒

Chapter 4　Pulverization, Sieving, Mixing and Granulation

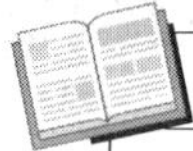

学习目标 | Learning Goals

知识要求：

1. **掌握**　药物粉碎、筛析、混合与制粒的目的和原理及常用方法。

2. **熟悉**　粉体学基本特征；粉碎、筛析、混合与制粒常用机械的性能与使用方法。

3. **了解**　粉体学在药剂中的应用。

能力要求：

学会不同物料应用不同原理的设备进行粉碎、筛析、混合、制粒操作，会运用粉体的特性来提高制剂的质量，提高药物的疗效。

Knowledge requirements:

1. **To master** the purpose, principle and common methods of pulverization, sieving, mixing and granulation of drugs.

2. **To be familiar with** essential features of micromeritics, mechanical properties and usage of machines for pulverization, sieving, mixing and granulation.

3. **To know** the application of micromeritics in pharmaceutics.

Ability requirements:

Learn to pulverize, sieve, mix and granulate different materials with various devices, to improve the quality of preparations and the efficacy of drugs depending on the characteristics of powder.

第一节 粉碎

4.1 Pulverization

一、粉碎的含义与目的

4.1.1 Definition and Purpose of Pulverization

粉碎是借助机械力或其他方法将大块的固体物料碎裂成所需粒度的操作过程。粉碎的目的在于：①增加药物的表面积，促进药物的溶解和吸收，利于有效成分的浸出或溶出；②便于调剂操作；③为制备多种液体和固体剂型奠定基础。

Pulverization is the process of breaking large pieces of solid material into desired size by mechanical force or other means. The purpose of crushing is: ① to increase the superficial area of the drug, to promote the dissolution and absorption of the drug, in favor of extraction or dissolution of the effective ingredients; ② to facilitate dispensing; ③ Lay the foundation of Preparing a variety of liquid and dosage forms.

二、常用的粉碎方法

4.1.2 Methods of Pulverization

（一）干法粉碎

(1) Dry Grinding

干法粉碎是指药物经适当方法干燥后，药物中的水分降低到一定限度（一般少于 5%）再进行粉碎的方法，适合绝大多数中药材的粉碎。

Dry pulverization refers to a method in which, after the drug has been dried by an appropriate method, the moisture in a drug is reduced to a certain limit (usually less than 5%) and then pulverized, which is suitable for pulverization of most Chinese medicinal materials.

1. 单独粉碎 将一味中药单独粉碎，便于应用于各种复方制剂中。通常需要单独粉碎的中药包括：贵重中药（如牛黄、羚羊角、西洋参、麝香等，可避免损失）；毒性或刺激性强的中药（如红粉、轻粉、蟾酥、斑蝥等，主要目的是避免损失和对其他药品的污染）；氧化性与还原性强的中药（如雄黄、火硝、硫黄等，主要目的是避免混合粉碎时发生爆炸）；以及质地坚硬，不便与其他药混合粉碎的中药（如磁石、代赭石等）。

① Pulverize separately The traditional Chinese medicine will be crushed separately, which is convenient to be used in various compound preparation.

Some Traditional Chinese Medicines usually need pulverizing separately, which include: valuable drugs (e.g. bezoar, antelope horn, ginseng, musk, etc.); toxic or irritating drugs (e.g. venenum bufonis, cantharides, etc. the main purpose is avoid loss and pollution to other drugs to avoid explosion); strongly oxidizing and reducing drugs; (e.g. realgar, sulphur etc.) and hard materials that are not get mixed with other materials (e.g. Magnetitum, reddle, etc.).

2. 混合粉碎 即将处方中全部或部分药材混合在一起进行粉碎，可使粉碎与混合操作同时进行，并克服单独粉碎中的困难。复方制剂多数药材采用此法粉碎。根据药物的性质和粉碎方式的不同，有时需采用特殊的粉碎方法。介绍如下：

② **Mixed pulverization** All or part of the medicinal materials in the prescription is mixed together for pulverization, so that the pulverization and mixing operations can be performed simultaneously, and the difficulty in separate pulverization can be overcome. Most medicinal materials of compound preparations are crushed by this method. Depending on the nature of the medicine and the method of crushing, special crushing methods are needed. The introduction is as follows:

（1）串料粉碎 对于含大量糖分、树脂、树胶、黏液质的药材，其黏性大，吸湿性强，粉碎困难。可先将处方中其他中药粉碎成粗粉，再将黏性药材陆续掺入，逐步粉碎至所需粒度。需要串料粉碎的中药，有乳香、没药、黄精、玉竹、熟地、山茱萸、肉苁蓉、枸杞、麦冬等。

a. Pulverization by mixing adhesive materials For the medicinal materials containing a lot of sugar, resin, gum, mucus, with strong viscosity, and hygroscopicity. The other traditional Chinese medicines in the prescription can be first crushed into coarse powder, and then the viscous herbs are added, gradually crushed to the required particle size. There are frankincense, myrrh, Polygonatum, Fragrant Solomonseal Rhizome, Rehmannia Glutinosa etc.

（2）串油粉碎 含大量油脂性成分的药材，如桃仁、苦杏仁、酸枣仁、火麻仁等，虽易于粉碎，先过筛困难。可先将处方中其他中药粉碎成粗粉，再陆续掺入此类药材，逐步粉碎成所需粒度；或先将油脂类中药研成糊状再与其他药物粗粉混合粉碎至所需粒度。

b. Pulverization by mixing greasy materials The medicinal materials containing a large number of fatty ingredients, such as Peach kernel, Bitter Apricot Seed, Spina date seed, etc., with sieving difficult. Other traditional Chinese medicines in the prescription can be first crushed into coarse powder, and then this kind of medicinal materials were joining, gradually crushed into the required particle size. Or grind the oily Chinese medicine into a paste first, and then mix with other medicine coarse powder crushed to the required particle size.

（3）蒸罐粉碎 先将处方中其他中药粉碎成粗粉，再将粗粉与用适当方法蒸制过的动物类或其他中药混合，经干燥，再粉碎至所需粒度。需蒸罐粉碎的中药主要是动物的皮、肉、筋、骨及部分需蒸制的植物药，如乌鸡、鹿胎、制何首乌、酒黄芩、熟地、酒黄精、红参等。

c. Steamed before pulverization Some traditional Chinese medicine are steamed with an appropriate method at first, then mixed with the coarse powder and be crushed to the required particle size. These materials are mainly animal skins, meat, tendons, bones, and some plant medicines that need steaming, such as Pullus Cum Osse Nigro, Deer fetus, Polygonum multiflorum, Radix Ginseng Rubra etc.

（二）湿法粉碎

(2) Wet Pulverization

湿法粉碎是指往药物中加入适量水或其他液体并与之一起研磨粉碎的方法（又称加液研磨法）。通常选用液体是以药物遇其不膨胀、两者不起变化、不妨碍药效为原则。粉碎过程中，液体分子很容易渗入药物颗粒的内部，有效削减其分子间内聚力，从利于粉碎；对于毒剧性、刺激性强的药物，此法可避免粉尘飞扬。具体如下：

Wet grinding is the process of adding an appropriate amount of water or other liquid to grind together, which is applicable to some toxic, irritating drugs and also can avoid dust flying (Also named liquid-adding pulverization).The principle of liquid selection is that drugs doesn't swell and change, don't hinder the efficacy of drugs. During the pulverization process, water or other liquid molecules infiltrate into the cracks inside the drug, effectively reducing the cohesion between the molecules, thereby facilitating the pulverization of the drug.

1. 水飞法 利用粗细粉末在水中悬浮性的不同，将不溶于水的药物反复研磨至所需粒度的粉碎方法。具体操作：将药物事先打成碎块，放入研钵中，加适量水后研磨。研磨过程有细粉漂浮在水面或混悬在水中，将水液倾出，余下药物再加水反复研磨，重复操作直至全部研细。倾出的混悬液全部合并，沉淀得到湿粉，干燥，即得极细粉。中药矿物类、贝壳类，如朱砂、珍珠、炉甘石等，常用“水飞法”粉碎。但水溶性的矿物类药不能采用水飞法，如芒硝、硼砂等。现在多用球磨机代替传统低效率的手工研磨，既保证了药粉细度又提高生产效率，但耗时仍较长，需持续转动60~80小时。

① **Elutriation** A method of grinding the insoluble drug repeatedly to the required particle size by using the suspension difference of fine and coarse powder in large amounts of water. Fine powder floats or suspends in the water, the rest of the medicine is milled with water repeatedly. Pour out all suspension and precipitation to get wet fine powder. Minerals, shellfish, such as Cinnabar, Pearl, Calamine, are commonly pulverized with elutriation method. Now the ball mill is used instead of the traditional low-efficiency manual grinding. However, it still takes a long time and requires continuous rotation of 60~80h.

2. 加液研磨法 指在粉碎的药物中加入少量液体后研磨至所需粒度的方法。比如粉碎冰片、薄荷脑时通常加入少量的乙醇或水；粉碎麝香时常加入少量水，俗称为“打潮”，尤其剩下异常坚硬的麝香渣时，“打潮”更易研碎。中药传统粉碎方法中对冰片和麝香的粉碎有个原则，即“轻研冰片，重研麝香”。

② **liquid-adding pulverization** A process of adding a small amount of liquid to a crushed drug and grinding it to a desired size. For example, Borneol, Menthol and Musk are usually crushed by this way. When crushing musk, a small amount of water is often added, commonly known as “tide” , especially when the abnormal and hard musk residue is left, “tide” is easier to grind. There is a principle for the crushing of borneol and musk in the traditional grinding method of traditional Chinese medicine, it’s often to grind Borneo lightly and musk heavily. Based on experience, it is often to grind borneol lightly and musk heavily.

案例导入 ¦ Case example

案例 4-1 “水飞”朱砂

4-1 “Water Fly” Cinnabar

制法：取原药材，用磁铁吸去铁屑，置乳钵中，加入适量清水研磨成糊状，再加多量清水搅拌，静置，倾取上层混悬液。沉淀再如上法，反复操作多次，直至手捻细腻无亮星为止，弃去杂质，混悬液合并，静置后倾去上层清水，沉淀60℃以下烘干，过200目筛。

Making Procedure: Take the original medicinal materials, use magnet to absorb the iron filings, put them in the mortar, add some water to grind them into paste, then add more water to mix them, stand still, pour the upper suspension. Precipitate again as above method, repeat the operation for many times until it become fine powder.Discard the impurities, combine the suspension, after standing, dump the upper water, precipitate it to dry below 60°C, and pass the 200 mesh-sieve.

注解：朱砂经“水飞”后，能除去杂质，降低毒性，增加纯净度，粒度达到极细，便于制剂，故无论内服外敷，朱砂均宜用极细粉。

Notes: After elutriation, cinnabar can remove impurities, reduce toxicity, increase purity, and achieve extremely fine particle size, which is convenient for preparation.

（三）低温粉碎

(3) Cryogenic Grinding

即将物料冷却后或在冷却条件下进行粉碎的方法。低温下有些药材黏性与延展性降低，脆性增加易于粉碎。其特点为：①适用于在常温下难以粉碎、软化点低、熔点低、热可塑性物料，如树胶、树脂、干浸膏等；②富含糖分，具一定黏性的药物；③一定程度保留挥发性成分；④可获得更细的粉末。

Often, some materials (e.g gum, resin, dry extract) with high viscosity and low ductility, and elastic and heat-sensitive materials cannot be finely ground. In cryogenic grinding, nitrogen or carbon dioxide is used to lower the temperature of these materials to their precise embrittlement point, prior to grinding. This process has proven to be a cost- and energy-efficient compliment to traditional size-reduction methods.

（四）超微粉碎

(4) Superfine Grinding

超微粉碎，又称超细粉碎。系指采用适当的设备将药物粉碎至粒径为 75μm 以下的粉碎技术。超微粉碎后的粒径达到微米级，显著增加了药物的表面积，植物药材细胞破壁率达 95% 以上。但设备耗能较大。有利于增大药物成分的释放或溶出，提高难溶性药物的生物利用度，为混悬型注射剂、滴眼剂等制备创造了条件。

Superfine grinding means a comminution technique by which materials are pulverized to a particle size of less than 75μm. The surface area and bioavailability of the drug increase significantly in this way. To the benefit of the preparation of suspension injections and eyedrops.

超微粉体又称超细粉体，分为微米级、亚微米级以及纳米级。粉体粒径为 1~100nm 的称为纳米粉体；粒径为 0.1~1μm 的称为亚微米粉体；粒径大于 1μm 的称为微米粉体。

Ultra fine powder is divided into micron level, submicron level and Nano level. The powder with a particle size of 1-100nm is called Nano powder; the particle size with a particle size of 0.1-1 μ m is called submicron powder; the particle size with a particle size greater than 1 μ m is called micron powder.

三、粉碎原则

4.1.3 Principle of Pulverization

在中药粉碎过程中，应遵循以下原则：①粉碎前后应保持药物的组成和药理作用不变；②根据应用目的和药物剂型控制适当的粉碎程度；③粉碎过程中应及时过筛，以免部分药物过度粉碎，且可提高效率；④中药较难粉碎部分如叶脉、纤维、油脂等应以适当方法处理，不随意丢弃；⑤粉碎过程注意安全防护，尤其对于毒性、刺激性大的药物。

In the process of crushing, the following principles should be followed: ① The composition and pharmacological action of the drug should be kept unchanged before and after grinding. ② According to the application purpose and drug dosage form to choose the appropriate degree of crushing. ③ There should be a timely screening in the process of crushing. ④ Some parts of Chinese medicine is difficult to crush, such as veins, fibers, grease, etc. should be treated with appropriate methods rather than randomly discarded. ⑤ Pay attention to safety protection during crushing, especially for toxic and irritating drugs.

四、粉碎设备
4.1.4 Equipment of Pulverization

目前粉碎的设备有很多，主要通过研磨、撞击、挤压、劈裂等作用实现对物料的粉碎。常用的粉碎设备有以下几种。

At present, there are many crushing equipments, mainly through grinding, impact, extrusion, splitting and other functions to achieve the crushing of materials. Commonly used crushing equipment are as follows.

（一）常规粉碎设备
(1) Conventional Crushing Equipment

1. 柴田式粉碎机 亦称万能粉碎机，在各类粉碎机中粉碎能力最大，撞击伴以劈裂、撕裂与研磨而粉碎，是中药厂普遍应用的粉碎机，如图 4-1 所示。该机的特点是细粉率高，可得到 120 目（七号筛）的细粉，广泛适用于黏软性、纤维性及坚硬的中药的粉碎，但对油性过多的药料不适用。

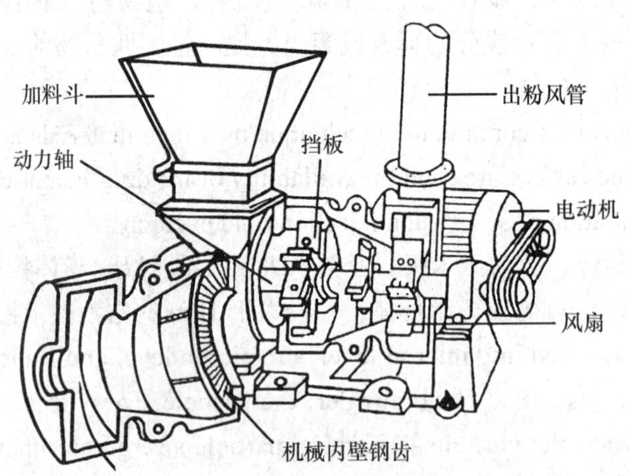

图 4-1 柴田式粉碎机示意图

Figure 4-1 Shibata-type Mill

1. 加料斗 Feed inlet 2. 动力轴 Power shaft 3. 挡板 Board 4. 出粉风管 Outlet 5. 电动机 Electric motor 6. 风扇 Air fan 7. 机械内壁钢齿 Steel tooth

① **Shibata-type mill** Shibata-type mill is also known as universal pulverizer. It has the largest crushing capacity among all kinds of pulverizer as shown in Figure 4-1. The impact is accompanied by splitting, avulsion and grinding. The machine can get 120 mesh of fine powder, widely used for the crushing of sticky, fibrous and hard traditional Chinese medicine, but not for oily materials.

2. 万能磨粉机 是一种应用较广的粉碎机，药材被撞击伴撕裂、研磨而粉碎。如图 4-2 所示。万能磨粉机适宜粉碎各种干燥的非组织性药物（如中草药的根、茎、叶和皮等）及结晶性药物和干浸膏的粉碎，但粉碎过程会发热，因此不适宜粉碎含有大量挥发性成分、黏性强或软化点低且遇热发黏的药物。

② **Hammer mill** Size reduction by impact can be carried out using a hammer mill. Hammer mills consist of a series of four or more hammers, hinged on a central shaft which is enclosed within a rigid metal case, as shown in Figure 4-2. During milling the hammers swing out radially from the rotating central shaft. Particles are retained within the mill by a screen that allows only adequately comminuted

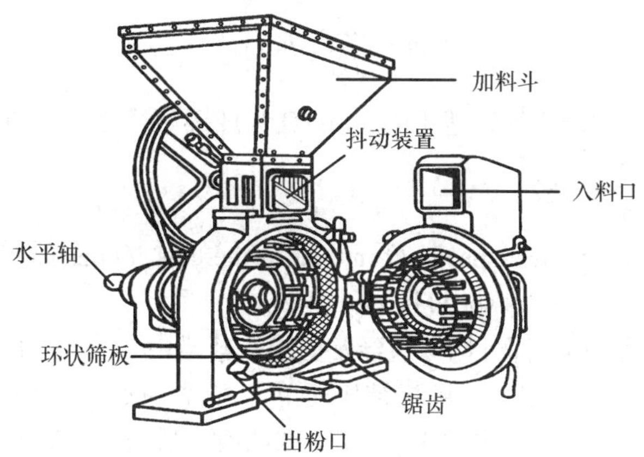

图 4-2 万能磨粉机示意图

Figure 4-2 Hammer Mill

1. 水平轴 horizontal shaft 2. 环状筛板 Annular sieve plate 3. 加料斗 Feed hopper 4. 抖动装置 Shaking device 5. 入料口 Feed inlet 6. 锯齿 Hammers 7. 出粉口 Outlet

particles to pass through. Heat will be generated during crushing, so volatile components, or products with strong viscosity are not appropriate to comminution in this way.

3. 球磨机 广泛应用于干法粉碎，以撞击和研磨作用为主的粉碎机械，如图 4-3 所示。 为了有效的粉碎物料，球磨机必须有一定的转速，使圆球从最高的位置以最大的速度下落。这一转速的极限值称为临界转速，它与球罐的直径有关，可由下式求出：

③ Ball mill A ball mill is an example of crushing method which produces size reduction by both impact and attrition of particles, as shown in Figure 4-3. In order to effectively crush the material, the ball mill must have a certain speed, so that the ball fall to the base of the drum from the highest position with the maximum speed, a cascading action is produced.The limit value of this speed is called the critical speed and related to the diameter of the drum.

$$n_{临(\text{critical})} = \frac{42.3}{\sqrt{D}}\ (\text{r/min}) \tag{4-1}$$

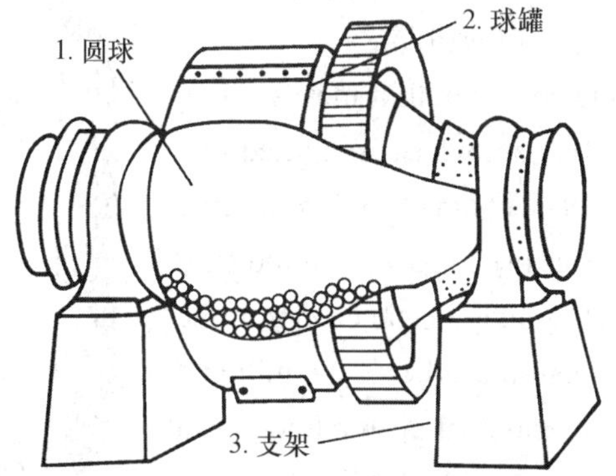

图 4-3 球磨机示意图

Figure 4-3 Ball Mill

1. 圆球 2. 球罐 3. 支架

1. Ball 2. Spherical tank 3.Support

$$n = \frac{32}{\sqrt{D}} \text{ (r/min)} \tag{4-2}$$

式中，$n_{临}$为球罐每分钟的临界转速（r/min）；D 为球罐直径（m）。在实际工作中，一般采用临界转速的 75%，即$n = \frac{32}{\sqrt{D}}$（转 / 分钟）。

Where, $n_{clinical}$ means the clinical speed per minute of the tank, D means diameter of sphere tank. In practice, generally 75% of the clinical speed is used (4-2).

由于操作时圆球不断磨损，部分圆球须经常更换。球罐中装填圆球的数目不宜太多，一般圆球体积仅占球罐容积的 30%~35%。球磨机结构简单、密封，操作时粉尘不会飞扬，适用于粉碎结晶性药物（如明矾、朱砂、硫酸铜等）、树脂（如松香、乳香）、树胶（如桃胶、阿拉伯胶等）及其他植物药材浸提物（如儿茶）。对具有很大吸湿性的浸膏（如大黄浸膏等）可防止吸潮；对具有挥发性的药物（如麝香等）、贵重药物（如羚羊角、鹿茸等）以及与铁易起作用的药物均可用瓷质球磨机进行粉碎。还可用在无菌条件下，进行无菌药粉的粉碎和混合。球磨机除可广泛应用于干法粉碎外，亦可用于湿法粉碎。如用球磨机水飞制备的炉甘石、朱砂等粉末可达到七号筛的细度，比干法制备的粉末润滑，且可节省人力。

Ball mills consist of a hollow cylinder mounted such that it can be rotated on its horizontal longitudinal axis.The cylinder contains balls that occupy 30–35% of the total volume, the ball size being dependent on feed and mill size.The factor of greatest importance in the operation of the ball mill is the speed of rotation. The ball mill is suitable for crushing crystalline medicine, resin, gum, some medicinal materials extract (e.g.Catechu), Volatile drugs, valuable drugs etc.It can also be used to crush and mix aseptic powder under aseptic conditions. Ball mill can be widely used in both dry and wet grinding for impalpable powder.

（二）超微粉碎设备

(2) Superfine Grinding Equipment

1. 流能磨 如图 4-4 所示，系利用高速流体（空气、蒸汽或惰性气体）使药物的颗粒之间以及颗粒与室壁之间发生碰撞、冲击、研磨而产生强烈的粉碎作用，适于脆性及坚硬的矿物药料，但药料应预粉碎，可得到 5μm 以下的均匀的粉体。粉碎过程中，由于气流在粉碎室中膨胀时的冷却效应，被粉碎物料温度不会升高，因此本法适应于抗生素、酶、低熔点及其他对热敏感药物的粉碎。

① **Fluid energy mill** Fluid energy mill, it means strong comminution made by a fluid, usually air, which is injected as a high-pressure jet through nozzles at the bottom of the loop (Figure 4-4). The high velocity of the air gives rise to zones of turbulence into which solid particles are fed.The high kinetic energy of the air causes the particles to impact with the sides of the mill and with other particles with sufficient momentum for fracture to occur, and with no temperature rise. Therefore, this method is suitable for antibiotics, enzymes, low melting point and other heat-sensitive drugs.

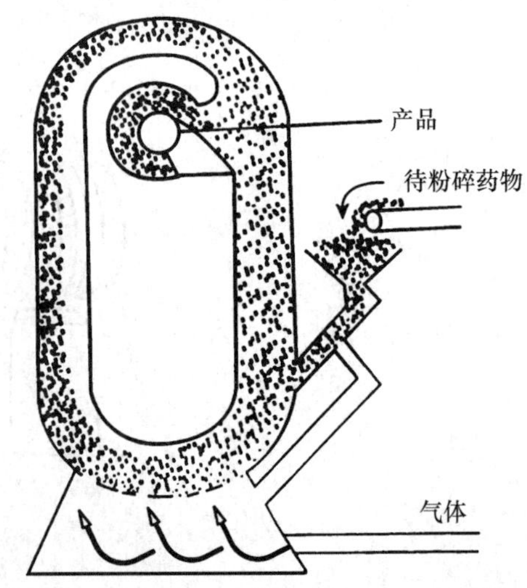

图 4-4 流能磨示意图

Figure 4-4 Fluid Energy Mill

1. 产品 Classifier removes fine particles and air 2. 待粉碎药物 Solids inlet 3. 气体 Air inlet jet

2. 振动磨 如图 4-5 所示，系利用研磨介质（球形、柱形或棒形）在振动磨筒体内做高速振动产生撞击、摩擦等作用，得到超细粉末的一种粉碎设备。可以通过改变研

磨介质的数量，调节振动的幅度，以适应不同物料，获得不同细度的微粉。也可在无菌条件下进行无菌粉末的粉碎和混合。

② **Vibration mill** An alternative to hammer milling which produces size reduction is vibration milling (Figure 4-5).

During milling the whole tank is vibrated and size reduction occurs by repeated impact and friction. Comminuted particles fall through a screen at the base of the mill, a cascading action is produced. The efficiency and crusher time of vibratory milling is greater than ball mill.

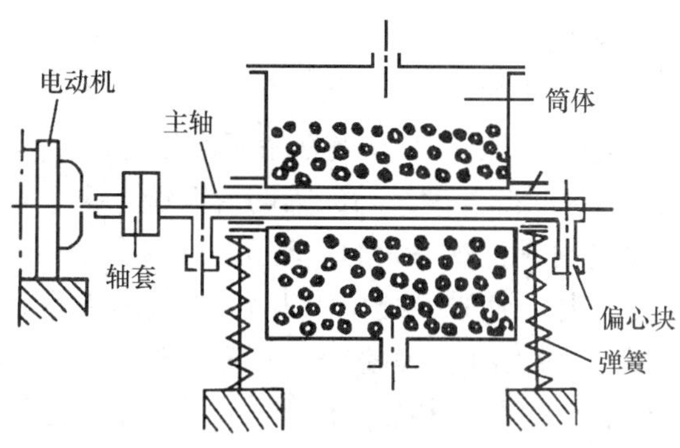

图 4-5 振动磨示意图

Figure 4-5 Vibration Mill

1. 电动机 Drive motor 2. 轴套 Axle sleeve 3. 主轴 Principal axis 4. 筒体 Tank 5. 偏心块 Out of balance weight 6. 弹簧 Spring mounting

振动磨可以干法或湿法作业。在工业上应用时一般是连续操作，即物料连续进入筒体并自筒体排出。振动磨与球磨机相比，其粉碎比更高（可达 300~400 目）；粉碎时间短；可连续粉碎；可以通过改变粉碎的条件（如研磨介质的数量、振动时间）得到超细粉末。

The vibration mill can be operated in dry or wet methods. In industrial applications, it is generally a continuous operation, that is, materials continuously enter the cylinder and are discharged from the cylinder. Compared with the ball mill, the vibration mill has a higher crushing ratio (up to 300-400 mesh); the crushing time is short; it can be crushed continuously; the ultrafine powder can be obtained by changing the crushing conditions (such as the number of grinding media, vibration time).

第二节 筛析

PPT

英文翻译

筛析是固体粉末的分离技术。筛即过筛，是指粉碎后的药料粉末通过网孔性的工具，使粗粉与细粉分离的操作；析即离析，是指粉碎后的药粉借空气或液体（水）流动或旋转的力，使粗（重）粉与细（轻）粉分离的操作。

一、筛析的目的

筛析的目的：①将粉碎好的药粉或颗粒按不同的粒度范围分为不同等级，供制备各种剂型的需要；②对药粉同时起混合作用，保证物料组成的均一性；③及时将符合细度的药粉筛出，可避免过度粉碎，减少耗能，提高效率。

二、药筛和粉末的分等

1. 药筛的种类 药筛系指按药典规定，全国统一用于药剂生产的筛，或称标准药筛。在实际生产中，也常使用工业用筛，这类筛的选用，应与药筛标准相近，且不影响药剂质量。

药筛可分为两类：编织筛与冲眼筛。编织筛的筛网由铜丝、铁丝等金属丝或尼龙丝、绢丝等非金属丝编织而成，也有采用马鬃或竹丝编织的。其孔径可编得极细小，但筛线易于移位变形，故常将金属丝线于交叉处压扁固定。细粉一般用编织筛或空气离析等方法筛析。冲眼筛系在金属板上冲压出圆形或多角形的筛孔，常用于高速粉碎过筛联动的机械上及丸剂生产中分档。

2. 药筛的规格 《中国药典》一部所用的药筛，选用国家标准的 R40/3 系列，共规定了 9 种筛号，一号筛的筛孔内径最大，依次减小，九号筛的筛孔内径最小。具体规定见表 4-1。

表 4-1 《中国药典》筛号、筛目、筛孔内径对照表

筛号	筛孔内径平均值（μm）	筛目（孔 /2.54cm)
一号筛	2000 ± 70	10
二号筛	850 ± 29	24
三号筛	355 ± 13	50
四号筛	250 ± 9.9	65
五号筛	180 ± 7.6	80
六号筛	150 ± 6.6	100
七号筛	125 ± 5.8	120
八号筛	90 ± 4.6	150
九号筛	75 ± 4.1	200

目前制药工业上，习惯以目数来表示筛号及粉末的粗细，多以每英寸（2.54cm）长度有多少孔来表示。例如每英寸有 200 孔的筛号称为 200 目筛，筛号数越大，粉末越细。凡能通过 200 目筛的粉末称为 200 目粉。

3. 粉末的分等 粉碎后的粉末必须经过筛选才能得到粒度比较均匀的粉末，以满足制剂生产和临床需求。筛选方法是以适当筛号的药筛过筛，所有粒径小于筛孔的粒子都能通过筛网，比如通过一号筛的粉末，是指不仅仅是近于 2mm 直径的粉粒，包括所有能通过二号至九号筛甚至更细的粉粒。富含纤维的药材在粉碎后，有的粉碎呈棒状，其直径小于筛孔，而长度则超过筛孔直径，有可能在筛析时这类粉粒仍可通过筛网，存在于筛过的粉末中。为了更好控制粉末的均匀度，需用两种孔径的药筛对粉末的细度进行规定。现行版《中国药典》一部规定了六种粉末规格，具体见表 4-2。

表 4-2 粉末的分等标准

等级	分等标准
最粗粉	能全部通过一号筛，但混有能通过三号筛不超过 20% 的粉末
粗粉	能全部通过二号筛，但混有能通过四号筛不超过 40% 的粉末
中粉	能全部通过四号筛，但混有能通过五号筛不超过 60% 的粉末
细粉	能全部通过五号筛，并含能通过六号筛不少于 95% 的粉末
最细粉	能全部通过六号筛，并含能通过七号筛不少于 95% 的粉末
极细粉	能全部通过八号筛，并含能通过九号筛不少于 95% 的粉末

三、影响过筛的因素

1. 药粉性质 它是影响过筛效率的主要因素，黏性小、流动性好的粉体较易过筛。药粉中含水量过高时应充分干燥后再过筛。易吸潮的药粉应及时过筛或在干燥环境中过筛。富含油脂的药粉易结成团块，很难通过筛网，可采用串油法使易于过筛外，也可先进行脱脂使能顺利过筛。若含油脂不多时，先将其冷却再过筛，可减轻黏着现象。

2. 振动速度 药粉在静止情况下由于受相互摩擦及表面能的影响，易形成粉块不通过筛孔，因此过筛时需不断振动。当施加外力振动时，各种力的平衡受到破坏，小于筛孔的粉末才能通过。粉末在筛网上的运动速度不宜过快，粉末才可落入筛孔；但速度也不宜过慢，否则效率降低。

3. 粉末量 药筛内放入粉末不宜太多，让粉末有足够的余地在较大范围内移动而便于过筛。但也不宜太少，否则影响过筛效率。

四、过筛和离析的设备

（一）过筛器械与应用

过筛器械种类繁多，应根据对粉末粗细的要求、粉末的性质及数量来适当选用。在药厂成批生产中，多采用粉碎、筛粉、空气离析、集尘联动装置，以提高粉碎与过筛效率，保证产品质量。在小批量生产及实验室中，常用手摇筛、振动筛粉机、悬挂式偏重筛粉机以及电磁簸动筛粉机。

1. 手摇筛 系由不锈钢丝、铜丝、尼龙丝等编织的筛网，固定在圆形或长方形的竹圈或金属圈上。按照筛号大小依次叠成套（亦称套筛），最粗号在顶上，其上面加盖，最细号在底下，套在接受器上，用手摇动过筛。此筛适用于少量药物粉末、毒性、刺激性或质地轻的药物粉末的过筛，可以避免细粉飞扬。如图 4-6 所示。

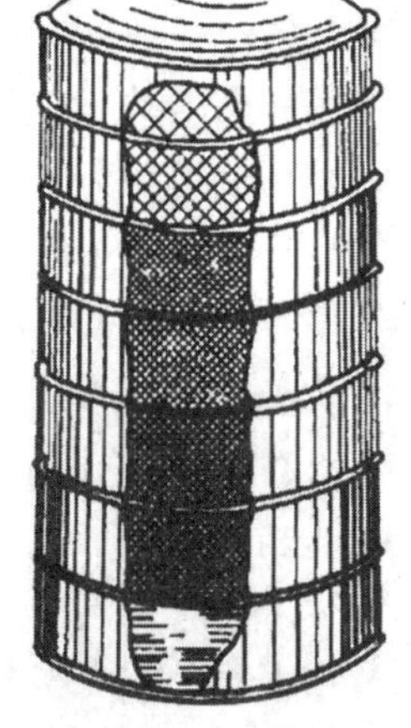

图 4-6 手摇筛

2. 振动筛粉机 如图 4-7 所示。又称筛箱，系指由电机带动偏心轮对连杆产生往复平动和振动而筛选粉末的装置。适用于无黏性的植物药、化学药物、毒性药、刺激性药及易风化或易潮解的药物粉末过筛。过筛完毕后，需静置适当时间，使细粉下沉再开启。圆形振动筛又称为旋转式振动筛粉机，能够连续进行筛分操作，具有分离效率高、占地少、重量轻等优点，目前中药生产企业较多使用。

3. 悬挂式偏重筛粉机 系指筛粉机挂于弓形铁架上，铁架上装有偏重轮，当偏重轮转动时，不平衡惯性使药筛产生簸动，如图 4-8 所示，此种筛构造简单，效率高，但不能连续工作，粗粉积多时，需将粗粉取出，再开动机器添加药粉，是间歇性操作，适用于矿物药、化学药或无显著黏性的中药粉末过筛。

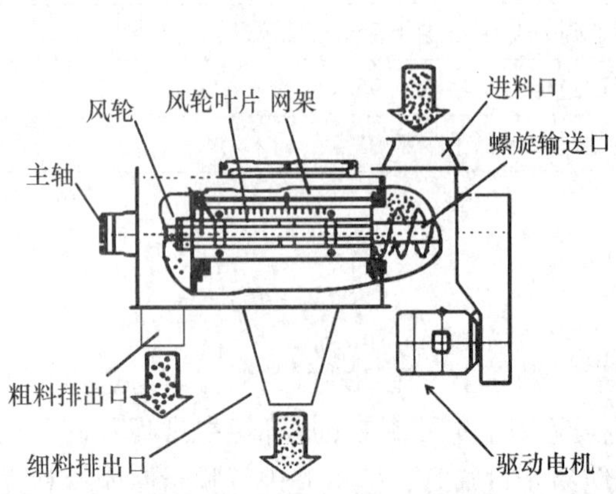

图 4-7 振动筛粉机示意图

主轴 Principal axis 风轮 wind wheel 风轮叶片 Rotor blades
网架 net rack 进料口 feed inlet 螺旋输送口 screw port
驱动电机 Drive motor 细料排出口 Fine outlet
粗料排出口 coarse outlet

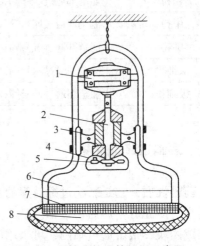

图 4-8 悬挂式偏重筛粉机示意图

1. 电动机 Motor 2. 主轴 Principal axis
3. 轴座 Axle bed 4. 保护罩 Protect cover
5. 偏重轮 Wheel 6. 加粉口 Drug inlet
7. 筛子 Sieve 8. 接收器 Receiver

4. 电磁簸动筛粉机 电磁簸动筛粉机是一种利用较高频率（高达每秒 200 次以上）与较小幅度（其振动幅度在 3mm 以内）往复振荡的筛分装置，如图 4-9 所示。由于振幅小，频率高，药粉易于通过筛网，适用于筛分黏性较强的药粉，如含油或树脂的药粉。

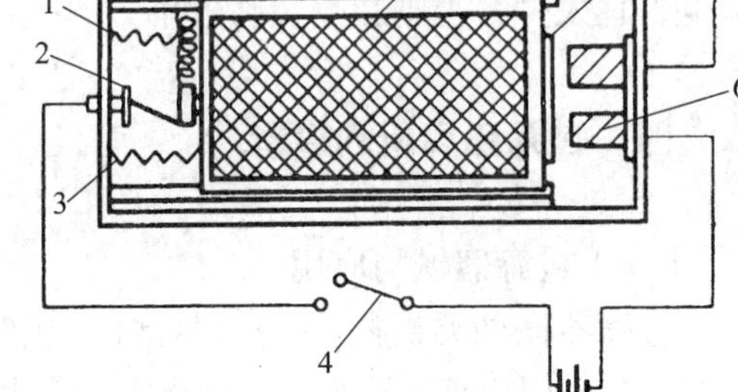

图 4-9 电磁簸动筛粉机

1、3. 弹簧 spring 2. 控制器 controller 4. 开关 switch
5. 电源 power 6. 电磁铁 electromagnet 7. 衔铁 armature
8. 筛网 sieve

（二）离析器械与应用

中药粉碎时经常用到的粉碎机，如万能粉碎机等装有风扇。随着粉碎过程的进行，一定细度的药粉会被风扇吹出机外，使粗、细粉靠风力得以分离，经粉碎机粉碎的细粉被风扇吹出后，再用旋风分离器将药粉从气流中分离，最后用袋滤器将残余气流中的极细粉再分离出来。常用的离析器械包括如下两种：

1. **旋风分离器** 是利用离心力来分离气体中细粉的设备。如图 4-10 所示，含细粉气体以很大的速度进入旋风分离器，沿器壁成螺旋运动。细粉受到离心力作用被抛向器壁，逐渐被撞击沉降下来，落入出粉口。旋风分离器构造简单、分离效率为 70%~90%。操作时注意气体的流量不应太小。

2. 袋滤器 袋滤器在制药工业中应用较广，是进一步分离气体与细粉的装置。其构造如图 4-11 所示。滤袋是用棉织或毛织品制成的圆袋，以列管形式平行排列而成，当含有极细粉的气体进入后，空气可透过滤袋，极细粉被截留在袋中。袋滤器的网眼密集，能截留直径小于 1μm 的药物细粉，截留效率可高达 94%~99%。但缺点是滤布磨损和被堵塞较快，不适用于高温潮湿的气流。如使用棉织品，其气流温度不超过 65℃；用毛织品截留微粒效果好，但不宜超过 60℃。目前，国内中药厂常将粉碎机和旋风分离器与袋滤器串联组合起来，成为药物粉碎、分离的整体设备。

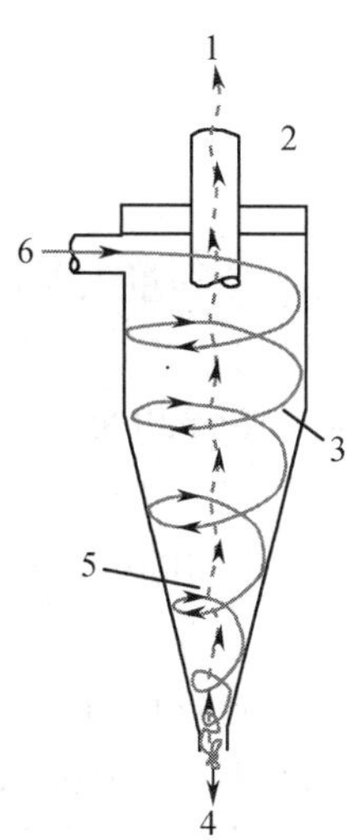

图 4-10 旋风分离器原理图

1. 出气口 fluid outlet 2. 涡漩导向器 Vortex finder
3. 粒子与流体的外涡漩 Outer vortex of particles and fluid
4. 粒子出口 Particle outlet 5. 流体的内涡漩 Inner vortex of fluid
6. 悬浮粒子 Particles in suspension

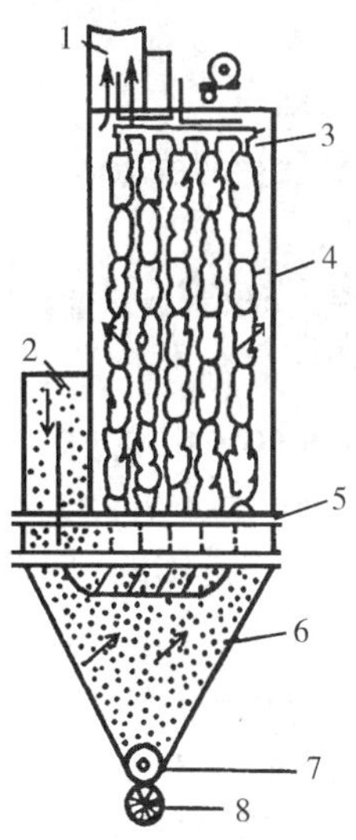

图 4-11 袋滤器示意图

1. 排气管 Filter outlet 2. 气体入口 Air inlet 3. 框架 Chamber
4. 滤袋 Filter bag 5. 分配花板 Filter head plate
6. 气室 Air chamber 7. 螺旋输送器 Spiral conveyor
8. 闸门 Gate

第三节 混合

4.3 Mixing

一、混合的含义与目的

4.3.1 Definition and Purpose of Mixing

混合是指将两种或两种以上的固体粉末相互均匀分散的过程或操作。

Mixing may be defined as a unit operation that aims to treat two or more components, each unit (particle, molecule, etc.) of the components lies as nearly as possible in contact with a unit of each of the other components.

混合的目的是使多组分含量均匀一致。混合操作对制剂的外观及内在质量都影响重大。如在片剂生产中，混合不好会出现色斑、崩解时限不合格等现象，且影响药效。特别是治疗窗窄的小剂量药物，主药含量不均匀对制剂疗效带来影响，甚至带来危险。因此，混合操作是保证制剂产品质量的主要措施之一。

Whenever a product contains more than one component, a mixing or blending stage will be required in the manufacturing process in assuring the quality of pharmaceutical products. Especially for small dose drugs with narrow therapeutic window, the uneven content of main drug will affect the efficacy of the preparation and even bring danger.

二、混合方法
4.3.2 Mixing Method

1. 搅拌混合 适合于少量药物的配制，可以反复搅拌使之混合。药物量大时该法不易混匀，实际生产常用搅拌混合机。

(1) Stirring mixture Stirring mixture is suitable for the preparation of small amounts of medicine. Agitator mixer is common in practical production.

2. 研磨混合 将药物的粉末在容器中研磨混合，适用于结晶体药物的混合，不适于吸湿性和爆炸性成分的混合。

(2) Grind mixture The medicine powder is ground and mixed in the container, suitable for the mixture of crystalline medicine, not for the mixture of hygroscopic and explosive components.

3. 过筛混合 指通过适宜孔径的筛网使药物达到混合均匀的方法。但对于密度相差悬殊的组分来说，过筛以后须加以搅拌才能混合均匀。一般用于不含细料的粉末，如散剂的大生产，常用 3 号筛过筛 1~2 次，将药粉混匀。

(3) Sieving mixture Sieving mixture means mixing drugs through a sieve of suitable size, But for components with very different densities, they must be stirred after sieving to mix them evenly. Generally used for fine powder，for example in the preparation of powder, drugs usually sieve by No. 3 screening once or twice to be mixed uniformity.

三、混合机械
4.3.3 Mixer

1. 容器固定型混合机 是指容器不会进行旋转等运动，物料靠容器内叶片、螺带或气流的搅拌作用进行混合的设备。

(1) Container fixed mixer Refers to the equipment that the container will not rotate and other materials, and the materials are mixed by the stirring action of the blades, spiral belts or airflow in the container.

（1）搅拌槽型混合机 主要结构为混合槽，槽上有盖，均由不锈钢制成。槽内装有“~”形的搅拌浆，在电动机的带动下，搅拌浆绕水平轴转动，用以混合粉末。该机器除适用于各种药粉混合以外，还可用于颗粒剂、片剂、丸剂制软材，亦用于软膏剂基质的混合。如图 4-12 所示。

① *Ribbon mixer* The ribbon mixer can be used for either solid-solid or liquid-solid mixing, also can be used for preparation of granule, tablet and pill, even the mixture of ointment matrix Figure 4-12.

（2）双螺旋锥形混合机 是一种新型混合装置。对于大多数粉粒状物料都能满足混合要求。由锥形容器和内装的螺旋桨、摆动臂和传动部件等组成，如图 4-13 所示。螺旋推进器在容器内既有自转又有公转。该机特点是：混合速度快，混合度高，混合量比较大也能达到均匀混合，而且动力消耗较其他混合机少。

② *Conical-Screw Mixer* The mixer provides a very mild shearing action and was used for solid-solid blending and liquid-solid blending in wet granulating. The screw shaft rotates around the periphery of the cone and the screw turns such that the pitch transfers the material from the bottom of the mixer to the top. The big advantage of such units is that when filled to any height, the same mixing action is

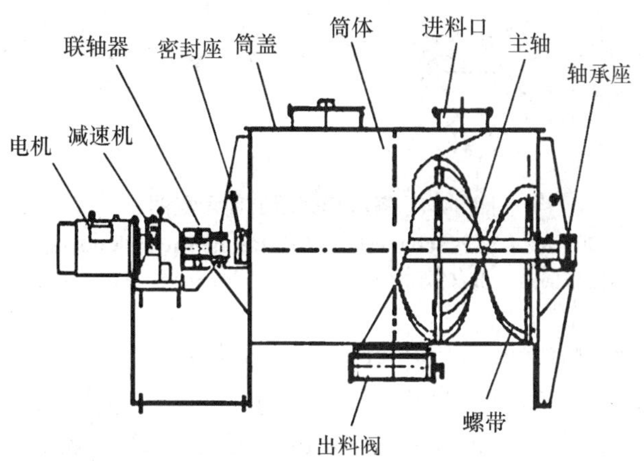

图 4-12 槽型混合机示意图

Figure 4-12 Ribbon Mixer

电机 motor 减速机 reducer 联轴器 Shaft coupling 密封座 Seal holder 筒盖 Packing gland
筒体 Mixer 进料口 Feed inlet 主轴 Drive shaft 轴承座 Bearing block

obtained, and the power consumption is less than other mixers (Figure 4-13).

2. 容器旋转型混合机 其特点：①分批操作，适宜多品种小批量生产。②适用于轻度混合，尤其是比重相近的细粉粉末。③对于黏附性、凝结性的粉体必须在机内设置强制搅拌叶或挡板，或加入钢球。④可用带夹套的容器进行加热或冷却操作。

(2) Conical-screw mixer Its characteristics: ① Batch operation, suitable for production of small batches of many varieties. ② Suitable for mild mixing, especially fine powder with similar specific gravity. ③ For the adhesive and coagulating powder, a forced stirring blade or baffle must be set in the machine, or a steel ball should be added. ④ The container with jacket can be used for heating or cooling operation.

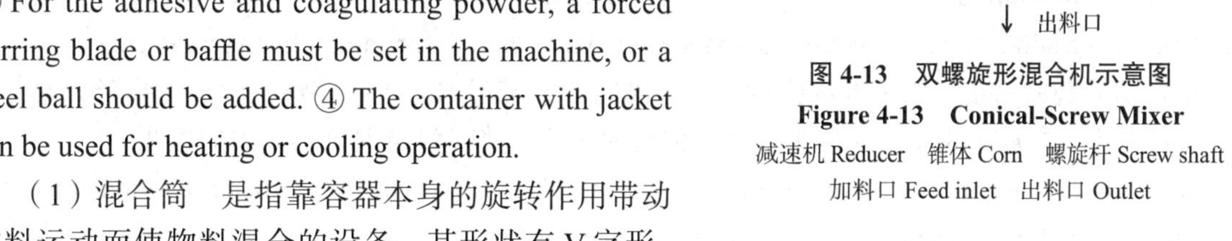

图 4-13 双螺旋形混合机示意图

Figure 4-13 Conical-Screw Mixer

减速机 Reducer 锥体 Corn 螺旋杆 Screw shaft
加料口 Feed inlet 出料口 Outlet

（1）混合筒 是指靠容器本身的旋转作用带动物料运动而使物料混合的设备，其形状有 V 字形、双圆锥形及正方体形等。如图 4-14 所示，混合筒的转速应控制在一定范围，如转速太快，则使粉末由于离心力作用而紧贴筒壁，降低混合效果。

① The first general class of mixers are those which create particle movement by rotation of the entire mixer shell or body. A schematic of the three types listed below.Blender speed may also be a key to mixing efficiency (Figure 4-14).

（2）三维混合机 滚筒同时具有转动、平移和摆动三种运动方式，设备可以各个方向进行扭动。在医药生物工程中，这种混合机是效能最高的混合机。对湿度、柔软度、密度不同的粉末的混合，都可达到最佳效果。如图 4-15 所示。

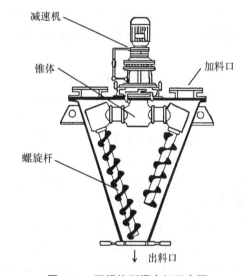

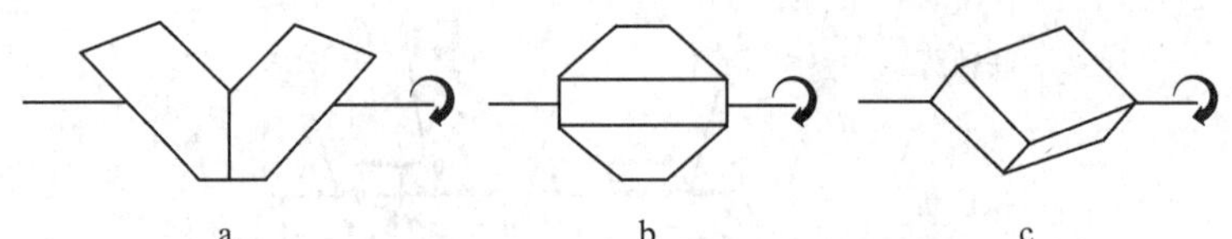

图 4-14 各种形式混合筒示意图

Figure 4-14 Schematics of Rotating Shell Blenders

a. V 型 V-shaped blender b. 双圆锥型 double-cone blender c. 正立方体型 cube-blender

② *3D Motion Mixer* Mixing container is suspended on the ends of driving, and driven shafts through two joints, which are crossing and vertical to each other in the space. When driving shaft is driven to rotate, joint makes the container perform composite motions, including horizontal moving, rotation and turning in the space. By which, materials also performs 3-dimensional motion inside the container. Several kinds of materials inside the container flow, diffuse, penetrate each other and finally form uniform status (Figure 4-15).

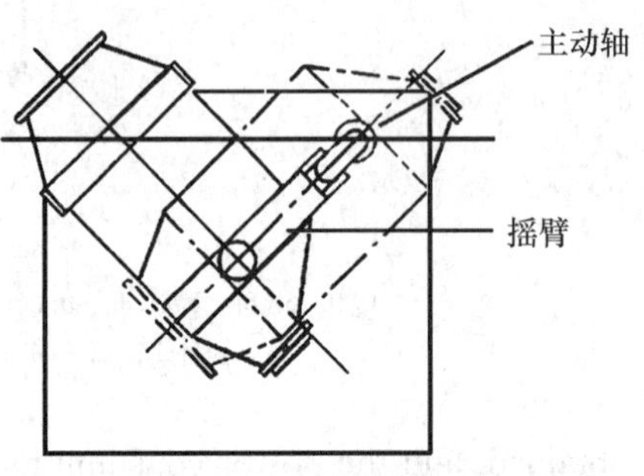

图 4-15 三维混合机示意图

Figure 4-15 Three-dimensional Motion Mixer

主动轴 Driving shaft 摇臂 Rocker arm

四、影响混合的因素
4.3.4 Factors Affecting Mixing

1. 各组分药物比例量 组分药物比例量相差悬殊，不易混合均匀。特别粒径相差越大，比例量对混合程度影响越大。此时应采用“等量递增法”混合，即将量小组分与等量量大组分，同时置于混合器中混匀，再加入与混合物等量的量大组分稀释均匀，如此倍量增加至加完全部的量大组分为止，混匀，过筛。

(1) Proportion of each component When there is a large difference in the proportion of drugs, the “equal increment method” shall be adopted for mixing, that means equal volume components mix at the same time. Then add a large amount of components equal to the mixture and dilute them evenly.

2. 各组分药物密度 组分药物密度相差悬殊时，较难混匀。一般应将密度小（质轻）者先放入混合容器中，再放入密度大（质重）者，混合时间应适当，注意混合操作中的检测。

(2) Drug density of each component It is difficult to mix the mixture when the density of the components is different. Generally, those with low density (light weight) should be put into the mixing container first, and then those with high density (heavy quality).

3. 各组分药物色泽 组分药物的色泽相差悬殊时，可采用“打底套色法”来解决。具体方法是：量少的，色深的药粉先放入研钵中（在此之前先用量大的药粉预饱和研钵内表面）作为基础，即“打底”；再将量多的、色浅的药粉逐渐分次加入研钵中，研磨至均匀，颜色变浅，即“套色”。

(3) Drug color of each component When the color of the component drug is very different, It is often to put dark powder first into the mortar (Pre-saturated mortar inner surface with power of larger amounts) as the basis, then a large amount of light colored powder gradually into the mortar several times.

4. 各组分药物的粉体性质 组分药物的粒子形态、粒度分布、含水量、黏附性等粉体性质均会影响混合的均匀性。若组分药物粒度分布相差悬殊，一般先将粒径大者放入混合容器中，再放

入粒径小者；若处方中有液体组分，可用处方中其他组分吸收该液体，常用稀释剂有碳酸钙、蔗糖、葡萄糖等；当混合组分因彼此间摩擦带电阻碍混合时，常可加入少量表面活性剂以提高表面导电性或在较高湿度下（>40%）下混合，亦可加入润滑剂（如硬脂酸镁）作抗静电剂。

(4) Powder properties of each component The particle morphology, particle size distribution, water content, adhesion and other powder properties of the component drugs will affect the mixture uniformity. If the particle size distribution of the drug components is very different, generally, the large particle size is first put into the mixing container, and then the small particle size; If there is a liquid component in the prescription, other components in the prescription can be used to absorb the liquid. Common diluents include calcium carbonate, sucrose, glucose, etc. When mixed components are prevented from mixing by friction charges between them, a small amount of surfactant can be added to improve the surface conductivity or to mix at a higher humidity (>40%). A lubricant (such as magnesium stearate) can also be added as an antistatic agent.

案例导入 ¦ Case example

案例 4-2　益元散

4-2　Yiyuan San

处方： 滑石 30g　甘草 5g　朱砂 1.5g

Ingredients： Talc 30g; Liquorice 5g; Cinnabar 1.5g

功能与主治： 消暑利湿。用于感受暑湿、身热心烦、口渴喜饮、小便赤短等症。

Functions and indications: To relieve heat and dampness, to remove body heat and upset, thirsty and fond of drinking, red short urination.

制法： 以上三味，滑石、甘草粉碎成细粉；朱砂飞成极细粉，与上述粉末配研过筛，混匀，即得。

Making Procedure： The above three flavors, talcum and licorice are crushed into fine powder; cinnabar is grinded to extremely fine powder, which is obtained by grinding, sieving and mixing with the above powder.

用法与用量： 调服或煎服，一次 6g，一日 1~2 次。

Usage and dosage: Taking decoction, 6g once, 1-2 times per day.

注解： 益元散方中朱砂质重色深，量少且有毒，而滑石粉色浅、量大，宜采用打底套色法混合。

第四节　制粒

4.4　Granulation

一、制粒的含义与目的

4.4.1　The Meaning and Purpose of Granulation

制粒是指往粉末状的药料中加入适宜的润湿剂和黏合剂，经加工制成具有一定大小的颗粒状物体的操作。制得的颗粒可以直接作为颗粒剂，也可以作为胶囊剂、片剂生产中的中间体。

Granulation refers to the operation of adding suitable wetting agent or adhesive to the powder and making granule of certain size. Granules are used as an intermediate in tablet or capsule manufacture.

制粒的目的：①较细粉而言，颗粒可改善物料的流动性；②防止多组分药物的分层离析；③防止生产中粉尘的飞扬和在器壁上的黏附；④在片剂生产中可改善压力的传递。

Purpose of granulation includes:

• To prevent segregation of the ingredients of the powder mix.
• To improve the flow properties of the mix.
• To improve the compaction characteristics of the mix.
• To prevent flying upward and sticking on the machine of the powder mix.

二、制粒的方法与设备
4.4.2 Methods and Equipment of Granulation

（一）湿法制粒
(1) Wet Granulators

1. 挤出制粒 在药粉中加入适量黏合剂制成软材后，用强制挤压的方式使其通过具有一定孔径的筛网或孔板而制粒的方法。这类制粒设备有摇摆挤压式、旋转挤压式、螺旋挤压式等（图 4-16）。

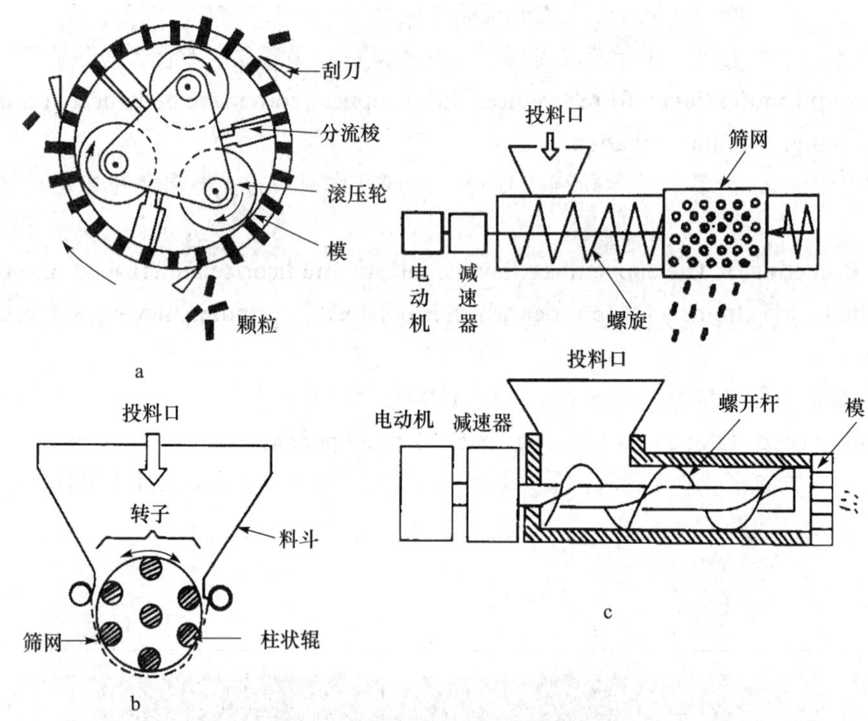

图 4-16 挤压式制粒机示意图

Figure 4-16 Schematic Representation of Production Extruders

a. 环模式辊压制粒机 Ring type roller granulator b. 摇摆式制粒机 Oscillating granulator c. 螺旋挤压制粒机 Screw-feed extruders

a：刮刀 Blade 分流梭 Spreader 滚压轮 Rolling wheel 模 Rolling die 颗粒 Granule

b：投料口 Feeder nose 转子 Rotor 筛网 Sieve screen 料斗 Feed container 柱状辊 Cylindrical roller

c：电动机 Motor 减速器 Reducer 投料口 Feeder nose 筛网 Sieve screen 螺开杆 Screw pole 螺旋杆 Screw rod 模 Rolling die

① **Extrusion/spheronization**　Extrusion/spheronization is a multi-step process used to make uniformly sized spherical particles.it is primarily used as a method to produce multi-particulates for controlled drug release applications. The main steps of the process are dry mixing of ingredients, wet massing, extrusion and spheronization (Figure 4-16).

2. 高速搅拌制粒　又称快速搅拌制粒（图 4-17），是将药粉、药用辅料加入容器中，通过高速旋转的搅拌桨的搅拌作用和制粒刀的切割作用，完成混合并制成颗粒的方法。主要由容器、搅拌桨、切割刀组成。通过调整搅拌桨和切割刀的转速可控制粒度的大小。

② **High-speed mixer/granulator**　The machines have a mixing bowl containing an agitating valve which revolves in the horizontal plane and a breaker blade which revolves in vertical plane. The advantage of this method is that powder blending, wet massing and granulation are all performed in a few minutes in the same piece of equipment (Figure 4-17).

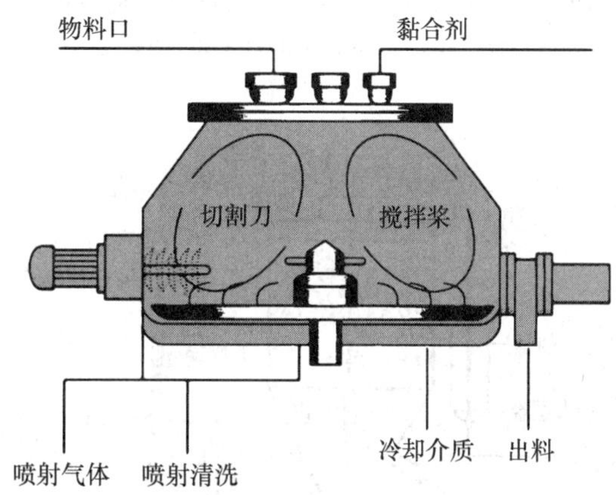

图 4-17　高速搅拌制粒

Figure 4-17　High-Speed Mixer/Granulator

物料口 Feeder nose　黏合剂 Adhensive　切割刀 Chopper　搅拌浆 Mixing shaft
喷射气体 Injection gas　喷射清洗 Spray wash　冷却介质 Cooling medium　出料 Outlet

3. 流化喷雾制粒　是指利用气流使药粉（或辅料）呈悬浮流化状态，再喷入黏合剂（或中药流浸膏）液体，使粉末聚结成粒的方法。设备如图 4-18 所示。由于将混合、制粒、干燥等操作在一台设备内完成，又称一步制粒或沸腾制粒。

③ **Fluidized-bed granulators**　Fluidized-bed granulators have a similar design and operation to fluidized-bed driers, i.e. the powder particles are fluidized in a stream of air, but in addition granulation fluid is sprayed from a nozzle onto the bed of powders. All the granulation processes which include mixing, granulation, drying are performed in one unit, saving labor costs, transfer losses and time (Figure 4-18).

该法得到的颗粒粒度均匀，外形圆整，流动性较好，适用于对湿和热敏感的药物制粒，也适用于小丸或颗粒等固体剂型的薄膜包衣或缓释控释的包衣。缺点是动力消耗大，药物粉末飞扬，极细粉易损失。

The particle size obtained by this method is uniform, round in shape and good in fluidity. The disadvantages is that the equipment is initially expensive, there are numerous apparatus, process and product parameters which affect the quality of the final granule.

4. 喷雾干燥制粒　是将药物浓缩液送至喷嘴后与压缩空气混合形成雾滴喷入干燥室中，在热气流的作用下雾滴很快被干燥成球状颗粒，干燥室温度一般为 120℃ 左右。装置如图 4-19 所示。

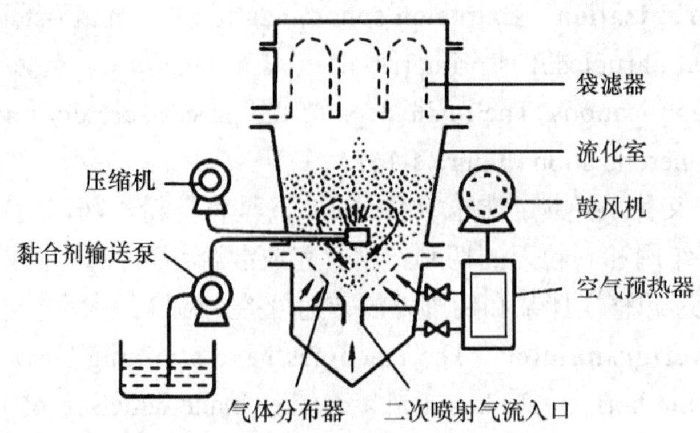

图 4-18 流化床制粒

Figure 4-18 Fluidized-Bed Granulators

压缩机 Compressor 黏合剂输送泵 Adhesive transfer pump 袋滤器 Exhaust filter 流化室 Product container 鼓风机 Air blower 空气预热器 Air pre-heater 气体分布器 Gas distributor 二次喷射气流入口 Secondary air inlet

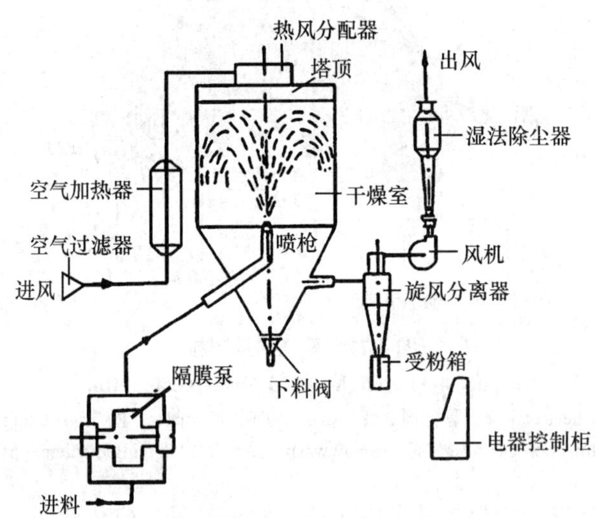

图 4-19 喷雾干燥制粒

Figure 4-19 Spray Driers

空气加热器 Air-heater 空气过滤器 Air filter 进风 Air inlet 进料 Feedstock 热风分配器 Hot air distributor 塔顶 Top of equipment 干燥室 Drying chamber 喷枪 Spray nozzle 下料阀 Discharge valve 出风 Air outlet 湿法除尘器 Dust washer 风机 Air blower 旋风分离器 Cyclone separator 受粉箱 Discharge port 电器控制柜 Electric appliances control

喷雾干燥制粒干燥速度较快，制得的颗粒溶解性、分散性和流动性都较好，适合中药全浸膏片浓缩液直接制粒，还适用于微粉辅料、热敏性物料及微囊、抗生素等的生产制备。

④ **Spray driers** Granular product is made from a solution or a suspension, which may be of drug alone, a single excipient or a complete formulation.

The primary advantages of the process are the short drying time and the minimal exposure of the product to heat due to the short residence time in the drying chamber. This means that little deterioration of heat-sensitive materials takes place in this equipment (Figure 4-19).

5. 滚转制粒 是将浸膏或半浸膏细粉与适宜的辅料混匀，置包衣锅或适宜的容器中转动，在滚转中将润湿剂乙醇或水呈雾状喷入，使药粉润湿黏合成粒，继续滚转至颗粒干燥。此法适用于中药浸膏粉、半浸膏粉及黏性较强的药物细粉制粒，类似泛丸的过程，多用于小丸粒制备。

⑤ **Spheronizers/pelletizers** For some applications it may be desirable to have a dense, spherical pellet of the type difficult to produce with the equipment described above. Such pellets are used for controlled drug release products following coating with a suitable polymer coat and filling into hard gelatin capsules.

The process is carried out by putting the extract or semi-extract with appropriate auxiliary materials in the coated pot or appropriate container for rotation. Ethanol or water is sprayed in a mist form in the roll, so that the powder wets and binds to form particles, and continue to roll until the particles dry.

（二）干法制粒

(2) Dry Granulators

干法制粒是靠压缩力使粒子间产生结合力，无须加热与干燥的步骤，原理为重压成粒的物理过程。其优点是使药物避免受湿、热的影响，可以缩短工时。常用滚压法和重压法制备。

Dry granulation converts primary powder particles into granules using the application of compressing force without the intermediate use of a liquid, meanwhile, it avoids heat combinations and drying steps which may degrade the product. Two pieces of equipment are necessary for dry granulation: first, a machine for compressing the dry powders into compacts or flakes and second, a mill for breaking up these intermediate products into granules.

1. 滚压法制粒 将药物粉末和辅料混匀后，使之通过转速相同的 2 个滚动圆筒间的缝隙压成所需硬度的薄片，然后通过颗粒机破碎制成一定大小的颗粒的方法。目前国内已有滚压、碾碎、整粒的整体设备。如国产干挤制粒机。

① **Roller compaction** Roller compaction is an alternative gentler method, the powder mix being squeezed between two counter-rotating rollers to form a compressed sheet, then the sheet is broken immediately into flakes by using gentler treatment like oscillating granulator.

2. 重压法制粒 又称压片制粒法。将药物与辅料混匀后，通过压片机压成大片，然后再破碎成所需大小的颗粒。生产过程分进料、重压和粉碎三步。

岗位对接

干法制粒还存在一些问题，很多药物和辅料并无可压缩性，难以重压制粒，粉碎制成颗粒时极易产生较多细粉及需要特殊的生产设备，在实际生产中，除干浸膏直接粉碎成颗粒应用较多外，其他只有少部分产品使用此法。

重点小结

② **Slugging** Slugging also known as tablet granulation method. After mixing the medicine with the auxiliary materials, it is compressed into large pieces by a tablet machine, and then broken into granules of the desired size. The production process is divided into three steps: feeding, pressing and crushing.

题库

There are still some problems with dry granulation, many drugs and auxiliary materials are not compressible, it is difficult to press granulation, and it is easy to produce more fine powder when crushed into granules and requires special production equipment. Except that the paste is directly crushed into granules, there are many applications, and only a few products use this method.

（王　芳）

第五章　散剂
Chapter 5　Powders

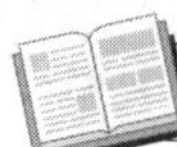

学习目标 | Learning Goals

知识要求：

1. **掌握**　各类散剂的制法。
2. **熟悉**　散剂的含义、特点与质量检查。
3. **了解**　散剂的分类。

能力要求：

学会各类散剂的制备与质量检测方法，能制备不同类型的散剂，并检查和评价散剂的产品质量。

Knowledge Requirements:

1. **To master** the preparations of powders.
2. **To be familiar with** the definition, characteristics and quality inspection of powders.
3. **To know** the classification of powders.

Ability Requirements:

To be able to prepare the powders and grasp their quality-test for the quality evalustion /control.

第一节　概述
5.1　Overview

PPT

一、散剂的含义
5.1.1　The Definition of Powders

散剂系指饮片或提取物经粉碎、均匀混合制成的干燥粉末状剂型。

A powder is a dosage form, referring to a dry powder made of even mixture of smashed herbs or herbal extracts.

散剂在《黄帝内经》《伤寒杂病论》等古典医籍中均有收载，元代王海藏《汤液本草 · 东垣用药心法》有"散者散也，去急病用之"的论述。散剂可直接用水送服，也可在皮肤、口腔、咽

喉等局部敷用，迄今仍为常用固体剂型。

Powders are recorded in *Huang Di Nei Jing* (Canon of Yellow Emperor) and *Shang Han Za Bing Lun*.

In the Yuan Dynasty, the book named *(Dongyuan Medication Thoughts. Materia Medica of Decoction*) written by Wang Haizang stated "Powders are loose and scattering, using in urgent cases". The powder can be taken with water, or applied on the skin, in the mouth, throat, etc.. It is a commonly-used solid dosage form.

二、散剂的特点
5.1.2 The Characteristics of Powders

散剂具备以下特点：①粉末比表面积大，易分散、奏效迅速；②制法简单，剂量易于调节；③对疮面有一定的机械性保护作用；④运输、携带、贮藏较方便。由于药物粉末的比表面积较大，使药物易吸潮变质，且药物刺激性和相关化学活性也相应增加，故剂量较大、易吸湿或易氧化、刺激性大、腐蚀性强、含挥发性成分较多的药物不宜制成散剂。

Powders have the following characteristics:

① The powder has a larger specific surface, is easy to disperse, and works in short time;

② Powders' making is simple, and the dose is easy to be adjusted;

③ It has a certain mechanical protective effect on the sore surface;

④ It is handy to be transported, carried and stored.

Due to the larger specific surface, of the powder, the drug is prone to absorb damp and go bad, the drug irritant and relevent chemical activities also increase accordingly. Therefore, those drugs with large doses moisture-absobent, quick oxidation, or with strong irritants, strong corrosiveness and containing much volatile components should not be made into powders.

三、散剂的分类
5.1.3 The Classification of Powders

按给药途径，散剂可分为：口服散剂与局部用散剂。按处方药物组成，散剂可分为：单味药散剂与复方散剂。按分装剂量，散剂可分为：单剂量包装的散剂与多剂量包装的散剂。按药物性质，散剂可分为：含毒性药散剂、含低共熔混合物散剂、含液体成分散剂等。

Concerning the administration ways, powders can be divided into orally-taken powders and powders for topical use. Concerning the prescription drugs, powders can be: single drug powder and compound ones. Concerning the packing dose, powders can be single dose or multidose. According to the nature of the drug, powders can be toxic powders, eutectic powders, and liquid-containing dispersants.

PPT

第二节 散剂的制备

5.2 Preparation of Powders

一、一般散剂的制备

5.2.1 Preparation of General Powders

一般散剂的制备工艺流程如图 5-1 所示。

Preparation process of general powders as shown in Figure 5-1.

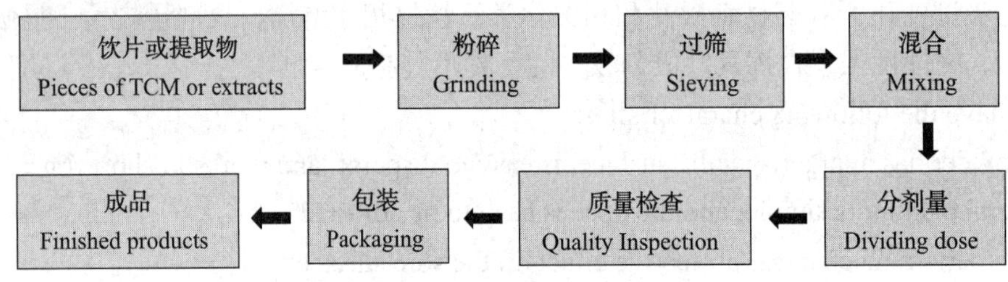

图 5-1 一般散剂的制备工艺流程

Figure 5-1 Preparation Process of General Powders

1. 粉碎与过筛 饮片或提取物均应根据药物的性质及临床用药要求选择适宜的方法和设备粉碎成一定粒度并过筛备用。药物的粉碎与过筛方法、常用器械详见本书第四章。

(1) Grinding and Sieving The decoction pieces or extracts should be ground into fine particles and sieved according to the properties of drugs and clinical requirements. For the methods of drug-grinding and sieving and commonly-used tools, see Chapter 4 of this book.

2. 混合 混合是散剂制备的关键操作。散剂应当含量均匀、色泽一致。混合的主要方法有研磨混合法、搅拌混合法和过筛混合法。混合方法选用和混合器械详见本书第四章。

(2) Mixing Mixing is a key operation of preparing powders. The powder should be uniform in content and color. The mixing methods mainly consist of abrasive mixing, stirring mixing and sieve mixing. The selection of mixing methods and mixing instruments are detailed in Chapter 4 of this book.

3. 分剂量 分剂量系指将混合均匀的散剂按照所需剂量分成相等份数的操作。散剂常用的分剂量方法包括：

(3) Dose-Dividing Dividing dose refers to the operation of dividing a fully-mixed powder into equal portions based on the prescription requirement.

The methods of dividing doses of powders are as follows:

重量法：按规定剂量用天平或戥秤逐包称量。该法剂量准确，但操作效率低且难以机械化，适于含毒药物或贵重细料药物的散剂。

Weighing:In line with the prescriptive dosage, weighing them bag by bag with scales. This method has accurate dose, but low in speed, and inconvenient to usher in machines. So, this method is proper for powders with toxic ingredients or valuable drugs.

容量法：用容量药匙或散剂自动分装机等进行分剂量。该法分量差异可控，效率高且可机械

化生产。

Volumetric method: In this method a volumetric spoon or automatic dispensing machines are used for dosing, which can control the slim weight differences, The efficacy is high and proper for mechanized production.

4. 包装与贮藏 散剂比表面积大，粉末易吸湿、结块、挥发性成分易挥损甚至变色、分解等，从而影响用药安全，故散剂生产环境的相对湿度应控制在临界相对湿度以下，并选择透湿性较小的包装材料与贮藏条件延缓散剂的吸湿，常用的包装材料包括蜡纸、玻璃瓶、塑料瓶、铝塑袋等。

(4) Packing and Storage Powders, because of the large specific surface, are apt to agglomerate and absorb moisture, and their volatile components are easy to be impaired and even discolored or decomposition, which will affect the therapeutic safety. Therefore, the production environmental relative humidity should be controlled below the critical relative humidity, and the packaging materials with little moisture-penetrability and profitable storage conditions to delay the damp-absorption should be used. The commonly-used packaging materials include wax paper, glass bottles, plastic bottles, aluminum bag, etc..

散剂可单剂量包（分）装，多剂量包装者应附分剂量的用具。含有毒性药的口服散剂应单剂量包装。

The powders can be packed in single-dose packages (divided); powder of multidoses packaging should be with dosing tools. Toxic drugs should be packed in single dose.

除另有规定外，散剂应密闭贮存，含挥发性原料药物或易吸潮原料药物的散剂应密封贮存。

Unless otherwise specified, powders should be preserved in well closed containers, powders containing volatile or hygroscopic drugs should be preserved in sealing containers.

案例导入 ¦ Case example

案例 5-1 冰硼散

5-1 Bingpeng San

处方：冰片 50g 硼砂（煅）500g 朱砂 60g 玄明粉 500g

Ingredients: Borneolum Syntheticum 50g; Borax(calcined)500g; Cinnabaris 60g; Natrii Sulfas Exsiccatus 500g.

功能与主治：清热解毒，消肿止痛。用于热毒蕴结所致的咽喉疼痛、牙龈肿痛、口舌生疮。

Functions and indications: Heat-clearing and detoxicating, detumescence and pain- relieving. Used for the treament of sore throat, swollen gingiva, sore mouth and tongue caused by accumulated heat-toxin.

制法：朱砂水飞成极细粉，硼砂粉碎成细粉，将冰片研细，与上述粉末及玄明粉配研，过筛，混匀，即得。

Making Procedure: To grid Levigate Cinnabaris into ultra fine powder, and pulverize Borax into fine powders. Grid Borneolum Syntheticum and then mix the three, sieve the mixture again. It is down.

用法与用量：吹敷患处，每次少量，一日数次。

Usage and dosage: Apply small dose of the powder to the affected area, several times a day.

注解：（1）玄明粉为芒硝经纯化后，风化失去结晶水而得，较芒硝作用缓和。外用治疮肿丹毒，咽肿口疮。

（2）硼砂煅制后失去结晶水又名煅月石。

（3）冰片即龙脑，外用能消肿止痛。冰片系挥发性药物，故在散剂制备时最后加入，同时密

封贮藏以防成分损失。

（4）本品为粉红色粉末；气芳香，味辛凉。本品含朱砂，不可多服；孕妇及肝肾功能不全者禁用；破伤出血者不可外敷。

Notes:

① Natrii Sulfas Exsiccatus comes from purified mirabilite, weathered and crystal water lost, whose effect is more mitigating than mirabilite. Use it externally for the treatment of sores erysipelas, pharyngeal swelling and mouth sores.

② Borax is also known as calcined moonstone, after its crystal water loss by calcining.

③ Borneolum Syntheticum is also called camphol, externally use of it can reduce swelling and pain. Borneolum Syntheticum is a volatile drug, that's why it should be added in at the end of the preparation and sealed up when stored aside in case of component loss.

④ This product is a pink powder with aromatic smell and pungent-cool flavor. Since it contains cinnabais, do not take it in excess; Pregnant women and patients who have hepatic and renal dysfunctions are prohibited from having it. Do not apply to bleeding wounds.

思考题：方中朱砂质重、色深、有毒、量少，为提高混合效率，应遵循哪些混合原则？

Questions: The Cinnabaris is heavy in quantity, dark in color, light in weight, and with toxics, so, what mixing principles should be followed to improve mixing efficiency?

二、特殊散剂的制备
5.2.2 Preparation of Special Powders

1. 含毒性药物的散剂 此类药物剂量小，有效剂量与中毒剂量接近，为使用药剂量准确，通常在毒剧药物或含毒性成分中药饮片粉末中添加适量的稀释剂采用等量递增法混合制成稀释散使用。根据药物的稀释比例，稀释散通常又称为倍散，例如 1 份药物与 9 份稀释剂混匀制成的散剂成为十倍散。药物稀释比例应根据用药剂量确定，一般剂量在 0.01~0.1g 者可制成十倍散，剂量在 0.01g 以下则多制成百倍或千倍散。稀释剂应是惰性粉末，常用乳糖、淀粉、糊精、硫酸钙等，而以乳糖为最佳。

(1) Powders Containing toxic drugs The toxic drugs is small in dose and the healing effectiveness is close to the intoxication. In order to get the accurate dose mostly, it should be carried out that proper diluents are added into the powders which contain toxic components or toxic herbs by equivalent increment method, so as to get a dilute powder.According to the dilution ratio of the drugs, the diluted powder is also named multiple-powder. For example, one portion drug and nine portions diluents mixed together are named tenfold powder. The dilution ratio of drugs should be determined according to the dose. The general dose of 0.01-0.1g can be made into tenfold powders, while the dose below 0.01g can be made into hundredfold or thousandfold powders. Diluents should be inert powders, such as lactose, starch, dextrin, calcium sulfate, etc. of which lactose is the best.

倍散配制过程中，为便于观察混合是否均匀及区别倍散的浓度，常添加食用色素胭脂红、苋菜红、靛蓝等着色剂。着色剂一般多稀释成低浓度贮备粉使用，且应在第一次稀释药物时加入。

In the preparation of severalfold powders, to better the observation of the uniform, and the concentration of severalfold powders, food colorants, such as rouge red, amaranth, indigo and other colorants.should be added. Colorants are generally diluted into a lower concentration powder and used at

the first diluent.

案例导入 ¦ Case example

案例 5-2 九分散

5-2 Jiufen San

处方： 马钱子粉 250g 麻黄 250g 乳香（制）250g 没药（制）250g

Ingredients: Powder of Strychni Semen Pulveratum 250g; Ephedrae Herba 250g; Olibanum (processed) 250g; Myrrha (processed) 250g

功能与主治： 活血散瘀，消肿止痛。用于跌打损伤、瘀血肿痛。

Functions and Indications: To activate blood and dissipate stasis, disperse swelling, and relieve pain. Used for traumatic injuries, swelling pain due to blood stasis.

制法： 麻黄、乳香、没药粉碎成细粉；马钱子粉与上述粉末配研，过筛，混匀，即得。

Making Procedure: To Pulverize Ephedrae Herba, Olibanum and Myrrha to fine powders, triturate with Strychni Semen Pulveratum, sieve and mix well, done.

用法与用量： 口服，一次 2.5g，一日 1 次，饭后服用；外用，创伤青肿未破者以酒调敷患处。本品含毒性药，不可多服，孕妇禁用；小儿及体弱者遵医嘱服用，破伤出血者不可外敷。

Usage and Dosage: Taken orally, 2.5g one time, once a day, after meals.External use: for topical administration, mix it with wine and apply it for swollen bruises on intact skin. This product contains toxic drugs, which cannot be used in excess, pregnant women are prohibited from using it; children and the weak should ask the doctor's advice, do not apply to bleeding wound areas.

注解：（1）本品为黄褐色至深黄褐色的粉末，遇热或重压易黏结；气微香，味微苦。

（2）马钱子粉的制法：取制马钱子，粉碎成细粉，测定士的宁、马钱子碱含量后，加适量淀粉，使士的宁含量为 0.78%~0.82%，马钱子碱含量不低于 0.50%。

（3）乳香、没药为树脂类药物，其生品气味辛烈，对胃刺激性较强，醋制后可缓和其刺激性，矫臭矫味，便于粉碎，同时能增强活血生肌、收敛生肌等功效。

Notes:

① The powder is tawny or dark tawny, in color, easy to be bonded by heat or heavy pressure; It is slightly fragrant and slightly bitter in taste.

② The preparation of Strychni Semen Pulveratum is as follows: Crush Strychni Semen into fine powder, measure the contents of strychnine and vauqueline, and add appropriate amount of starch, with strychnine content 0.78%-0.82%, and vauqueline content not less than 0.50%.

③ Raw Olibanum and Myrrha are resinous drugs with strong smell and strong stimulation to the stomach. But it is processed with vinegar the stimulation will ease off, and the odor and taste, are improved, so as to facilitate being crushed, and also the functions of activating blood circulation and generating muscles, are fortified.

思考题 ¦ Questions:

（1）乳香、没药可采用什么粉碎方法？

① What are the grinding methods respectively for Olibanum(processed) and Myrrha(processed)？

（2）为什么以炮制的马钱子粉入药？

② Why is the preperation added with processed Strychni Semen Pulveratum powder?

2. 含低共熔混合物的散剂 当两种或两种以上的药物混合时出现润湿或液化的现象称为低共熔现象，如薄荷脑与樟脑、薄荷脑与冰片、樟脑与水杨酸苯酯等。

(2) Powders containing eutectic mixture That the phenomenon of wetting or liquefaction appears while two or more drugs are mixed is named eutectic phenomenon, such as mixing menthol and camphor, menthol and borneol, camphor and phenyl salicylate, etc..

制备此类散剂通常有两种方法：①先形成低共熔物，再与其他固体粉末混匀；②分别以固体粉末稀释低共熔组分，再缓缓混合均匀。在选择方法时应考虑形成低共熔混合物对药效的影响以及处方中其他固体药物的剂量，若药物形成低共熔物后药效增强，则宜先形成低共熔物再与方中其他药物混合，反之亦然。处方中若含有挥发油或其他可与低共熔混合物相溶的液体时，可以将低共熔混合物溶解于其中，再采用喷雾法加入到其他固体成分中并混合均匀。

There are two preparations for those powders:

① Forming eutectic mixtures first, and then get it mixed with other solid powders;

② Diluting the eutectic components respectively with solid powders, and then mix them slowly and evenly. The influence of eutectic mixture on healing efficacy and the amount of other solid drugs in the prescription should be considered in the selection of method. If the healing efficacy can be enhanced after the formation of eutectic mixtures, it's advisable to form eutectic mixtures before mixing with other drugs in the prescription, and vice versa. If the prescription contains volatile oil or other liquid that can be dissolved with the eutectic mixtures, the eutectic mixtures can be dissolved in it, and then it is added to other solid components by spray and mixed evenly.

3. 含液体药物的散剂 当处方中含有挥发油、酊剂、流浸膏剂、药物煎液等液体药物时，应根据液体药物性质、剂量及方中其他固体粉末的多少而采用不同的处理方法：①液体组分量较小，可利用处方中其他固体组分吸收后研匀；②液体组分量较大，处方中固体组分不能完全吸收，可另加适量的稀释剂如磷酸钙、淀粉、糖粉、乳糖等辅料吸收；③液体组分含量过大且有效成分为非挥发性时，可加热蒸去大部分水分后再以其他固体粉末吸收，或加入固体粉末或稀释剂后，低温干燥，研匀过筛。④液体组分量过多、有效成分为热敏性药物且方中其他固体药物组分不能完全将其吸收时，需加入其他适宜辅料如乳糖、淀粉、蔗糖等吸收至不湿润为度。

(3) **Liquid-containing powders** The prescription may contain volatile oil, tincture, liquid extract, drug decoction and other liquid drugs, Various preparations should be chosen based on the properties of the liquid drugs, doses and the amount of other solid powders in the formulae:

① When liquid component is lesser in content the other solid components in the prescription can absorb it and they can be ground together evenly.

② When liquid component is more in content, which can not be completely absorbed an appropriate amount of diluents, such as calcium phosphate, starch, sugar powders, lactose and other excipients are to be added;

③ If the liquid component is too much and the effective components are non-volatile, the liquid component can be dried by heating or steaming, before being absorbed by other solid powders, or after adding solid powders or diluents, it is dried at low temperature, ground and sieved evenly.

④ When the amount of liquid components is too more, effective components are heat sensitive and the other solid drug components in the prescription can not completely absorb it, then, the other suitable excipients such as lactose, starch, sucrose will be added properly.

案例导入 | Case example

案例 5-3 蛇胆川贝散

5-3 Shedan Chuanbei Powder

处方：蛇胆汁 100g 川贝母 600g

Ingredients: Serpentis Fel 100g; Fritillariae Cirrhosae Bulbus 600g

功能与主治：清肺，止咳，除痰。用于肺热咳嗽，痰多。

Functions and indications: Clearing away heat from the lung, relieving cough and dispelling sputum. It is used for the treatment of cough due to lung heat with profuse sputum.

制法：川贝母粉碎成细粉，与蛇胆汁混匀，干燥，粉碎，过筛，即得。

Making Procedure: Fritillariae Cirrhosae Bulbus is pulverized into fine powder, mixed thoroughly with Serpentis Fel, dried, crushed, sifted, and done.

用法与用量：口服，一次 0.3~0.6g，一日 2~3 次。

Usage and dosage: Taken orally. 0.3-0.6g one time, 2-3 times a day.

注解：本品为浅黄色至浅棕黄色的粉末；味甘、微苦。蛇胆汁中含有较多的水分，用川贝母细粉吸收后干燥，有利于加速干燥，且药物分散均匀。

Notes: This product is a pale yellow to pale brown yellow powder; with sweet flavor, and slightly bitterness. Serpentis Fel contains more water, which can be absorbed by powder of Fritillariae Cirrhosae Bulbus, for dryness, This is conducive for the powder's faster drying, and evenly scattering.

4. 眼用散剂 眼用散剂是由提取物、饮片制成的用于眼部发挥治疗作用的无菌散剂。其制法与一般散剂相似，但应注意：①配制眼用散剂的药物多经水飞或流能磨粉碎成能通过 200 目筛的极细粉；②配制用具应灭菌，配制操作应在清洁、避菌环境下进行；③成品应经灭菌、遮光、密封，置阴凉处保存。

案例导入

(4) Ophthalmic powders Ophthamal powder is a kind of aspetic powder made of extracts and decoction pieces for the treatment of eye ailments. The preparation method is similer to the general powders but the following should be noted: ① In the preparation drugs mostly are refined with water or fluid-energy mills into the ultra fine powders, which should get through 200 mesh sieve; ② The tools of preparation are sterilized, and the operations should be in a clean and germfree environment; ③ The finished product should be sterilized, shaded, sealed, and stored in a cool place.

第三节 散剂的质量要求与检查

5.3 Quality Requirements and Inspections of Powders

PPT

一、散剂的质量要求

5.3.1 Quality Requirements of Powders

1. 粒度 除另有规定外，一般口服散剂应为细粉；用于儿科及外用散剂应为最细粉；用于烧伤或严重创伤的外用散剂通过六号筛的粉末重量不得少于95%；眼用散剂应为极细粉。

(1) Particle size Unless otherwise specified, general oral powders should be fine powders, while for pediatrics and topical use they should be very fine powders. No less than 95% weight of the powders used for topical burns or severe trauma should pass through sieve No.6 Ophthalmic powders should be ultra fine powder.

2. 外观均匀度 散剂一般应干燥、疏松、混合均匀、色泽一致。

(2) Uniformity of appearance Powders should be dry, loose, well-mixed and uniform in appearance and colour.

3. 水分 除另有规定外，散剂含水分不得超过9.0%。

(3) Determination of water Unless otherwise specified, Powders' water-containing should not exceed 9.0%.

4. 装量差异 单剂量包装的散剂，其每袋（瓶）内容物重量，与标示量相比，超出限度的不得多于2袋（瓶），并不得有1袋（瓶）超出限度1倍。

(4) Dose content uniformity For a single-dose powder, the weight of content in each bag (bottle) should not exceed the limit by more than 2 bags (bottles) and not exceed the limit by 1 bag (bottle) twice as much as the indicated weight.

5. 无菌 眼用散剂及用于烧伤或严重创伤的局部用散剂应无菌。

微生物限度、装量、药物的鉴别与含量等均应符合相应要求。

(5) Sterility The powders should be sterile for eyes, topical burns or severe trauma.They should meet the corresponding requirements in microbial limit, dosage, drug identification and content.

岗位对接

二、散剂的质量检查项目

5.3.2 Inspection Items of Powder Quality

重点小结

粒度、外观均匀度、水分、装量差异（单剂量包装的散剂）、装量（多剂量包装散剂）、无菌（用于烧伤、严重创伤或临床必需无菌的局部用散剂）、微生物限度检查等应符合现行版《中国药典》质量要求。

题库

Inspection items, such as particle size, uniformity of appearance, moisture content, content uniformity (powders packaged in single-dose), Filling (multi-dose packaged powders), sterility (powders used for burns, severe trauma or topical application), and microbial limit inspection, etc., all should be conformed to the quality standards of the current edition of *Chinese Pharmacopoeia.*

（廖 婉 傅超美）

第六章　浸提、分离与纯化、浓缩与干燥
Chapter 6　Extraction, Separation and Purification, Concentration and Drying

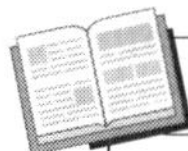

学习目标 | Learning Goals

知识要求：

1. 掌握　浸提过程及其影响因素；常用的浸提、分离、纯化方法；影响药液浓缩效率的因素与常用浓缩方法；影响干燥的因素与常用干燥方法及注意事项。

2. 熟悉　中药浸提、分离、纯化的目的；常用的浸提溶剂。

3. 了解　常用浸提辅助剂；中药成分与疗效的关系；常用的浸提、浓缩、干燥设备。

能力要求：

能根据药物的种类和性质，选用相应的方法进行提取、分离纯化、浓缩干燥。

Knowledge requirements:

1. To master the extraction process and its influencing factors; commonly used methods for extraction, separation, and purification; factors affecting the concentration efficiency and common methods for concentration; and factors affecting drying and common methods and precautions for drying.

2. To be familiar with the purposes of extraction, separation, and purification of traditional Chinese medicine (TCM); and commonly used extraction solvents.

3. To know the commonly used auxiliary adjuvants; the relationship between the composition of TCM and curative effect; and the commonly used equipments for extraction, concentration, and drying.

Ability requirements:

To be able to extract, separate and purify, concentrate and drying the TCM according to the character of material.

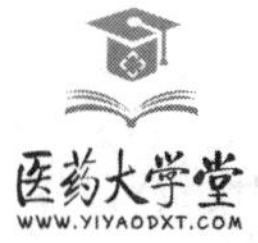

第一节　概述

6.1 Overview

PPT

中药制剂与西药制剂最大的差别在于中药制剂的原料是中药饮片或中药提取物。采用适宜的方法和技术将中药饮片或复方的药效物质最大限度地提取出来，以保证中药制剂特有的功能与主治，是中药制剂的关键。

The largest difference between TCM preparation and chemical medicine preparation is the nature of material. The raw material of TCM preparation is decoction piece or extract. Using appropriate method and technique to extract effective substance from TCM decoction piece maximally is the key point for TCM preparation, which ensures the unique functions and curative effects of TCM preparation.

一、浸提、分离与纯化的目的

6.1.1 Purposes of Extraction, Separation and Purification

中药制剂的疗效，很大程度上取决于浸提、分离、纯化等方法的选择是否恰当，工艺设计是否科学、合理。提取、分离纯化的目的在于：最大程度浸提出有效成分或有效部位；最低限度浸出无效甚至有害物质；减少服用量；增强制剂稳定性；提高疗效；适于工业化规模生产。

The efficacy of TCM preparation, largely depends on the appropriate selection of methods for extraction, separation, and purification. The purposes of extraction, separation and purification include obtaining the active ingredients or effective part maximumly; lowering the content of invalid or harmful substances; reducing the amount of consumption; enhancing the stability of the preparation; improving efficacy; and matching industrial-scale production.

中医治病的特点是复方用药，发挥多成分、多途径、多环节、多靶点的综合作用和整体效应。在拟定提取纯化工艺时，应在尽可能满足临床疗效的基础上，根据处方中各组成药物的性质、拟制备的剂型，结合生产设备、技术条件、经济的合理性等，选择和确定最佳提取纯化工艺。

The characters of TCM preparation are compound medication and integrated effect achieved by multi-components acting on multi targets and pathways.

For extraction and purification process setting, the best extraction purification process should be selected to fulfill TCM clinical efficacy. In addition, factors such as the nature of the composition of the drug, formulation, production equipment, technical condition, and economic rationality should be considered.

二、浓缩与干燥的目的

6.1.2 Purposes of Concentration and Drying

浓缩是中药制剂原料成型前处理的重要单元操作。其目的在于将不挥发或挥发性物质与在同一温度下具有挥发性的溶剂（如乙醇或水）分离至某种程度，得到具有一定密度的浓缩液。

Concentration is an important step before preparation. The purpose is to separate non-volatile

or volatile substances from solvents (such as ethanol or water) to a certain extend and to obtain a concentrated liquid with certain density.

干燥是中药制剂原料成型前处理的另一重要操作单元。在药剂生产中，新鲜药材除水，原辅料除湿，以及颗粒剂、片剂等剂型的制备过程中都会用到干燥。干燥的好坏，将直接影响中药制剂的内在质量。

Drying is another important step before preparation. In pharmaceutical production, drying is frequently involved in various processes including removing water from fresh herb and raw material, and preparation of granule and tablet. Drying could directly affect the inherent quality of TCM preparation.

三、中药成分与疗效

6.1.3 Composition and Efficacy of TCM

中药中所含的成分十分复杂，概括起来可分为四类，即有效成分（包括有效部位）、辅助成分、无效成分和组织成分。

Composition of TCM is very complex, and it can be classified into four categories, namely effective composition (including effective part), auxiliary composition, invalid composition and tissue composition.

1. 有效成分 有效成分是指起主要药效的物质。一般指化学上的单体化合物，含量达到 90% 以上，能用分子式和结构式表示，并具有一定的理化性质，如乌头碱、麻黄碱、青蒿素等。一种中药往往含有千百个有效成分，而一个有效成分又有多方面的药理作用。

(1) Effective composition The effective composition refers to the substance with curative effect. Generally, it refers to a chemical compound with purity up to 90%, which can be described with molecular formula and structure, such as aconitine, ephedrine, and artemisinin. A TCM often contains hundreds of effective compositions, and an effective substance may possess many pharmacological effects.

有效部位是指当一味中药或复方提取物中的一类或几类有效成分的含量达到总提取物的 50% 以上的具有药理活性的混合体。中药提取时往往得到的是有效部位，如总生物碱、总皂苷、总黄酮、挥发油等。应用有效部位在药理和临床上能够代表或部分代表原中药或复方的疗效，有利于发挥其综合效能，符合中医用药的特点。

Effective part refers to a bioactive mixture contain one or several effective compositions with content up to 50% of the total extract of TCM. Effective part is the most common form of TCM extraction, and it can be total alkaloid, total saponin, total flavonoid, and volatile oil. The effective part can represent or partially represent TCM for clinical treatment, which exerts efficacy comprehensively and has the similar function with TCM.

2. 辅助成分 辅助成分系指本身无特殊疗效，但能增强或缓和有效成分作用的物质，或指有利于有效成分的浸出或增强制剂稳定性的物质。如大黄中所含的鞣质能缓和大黄的泻下作用。

(2) Auxiliary composition Auxiliary composition has no special therapeutic effect, but could enhance or alleviate the effect of the active composition, or improve extraction efficiency and enhance the stability of preparation. For example, tannin in rhubarb can reduce the diarrhea effect of rhubarb.

3. 无效成分 无效成分系指无生物活性，不起药效的物质，有的甚至会影响浸出效能，制剂的稳定性，外观和药效等。例如蛋白质、鞣质、脂肪、树脂、淀粉、黏液质、果胶等。

(3) Invalid composition Inactive composition is non-bioactive substance, and some of them may

even affect extraction efficiency, formulation stability, appearance and efficacy. Such as protein, tannin, fat, resin, starch, mucus, and pectin.

4. 组织物质 组织物质系指一些构成中药细胞或其他的不溶性物质，如纤维素、栓皮、石细胞等。

(4) Tissue composition Tissue composition refers to cell of material or the insoluble component of TCM, such as cellulose, cork, and stone cell.

第二节 浸提

6.2 Extraction

PPT

浸提系指采用适当的溶剂和方法将中药所含的有效成分或有效部位提取出来的操作。

Extraction refers to an operation using appropriate solvent and method to extract the effective component or effective parts of TCM.

一、浸提过程

6.2.1 Extraction Process

一般可分为浸润、渗透、解吸、溶解、扩散等几个相互联系的阶段。

Generally, it can be divided into several correlated stages, such as infiltration, permeation, desorption, dissolution, and diffusion.

1. 浸润与渗透阶段 浸提溶剂与饮片接触混合后，使饮片表面湿润，并进一步渗透进细胞组织中，这一过程为浸润与渗透阶段。

(1) Infiltration and permeation stage Soak the TCM decoction piece with extraction solvent, and make solvent penetrate into the tissue.

2. 解吸与溶解阶段 需解除中药中各种成分之间或与细胞壁之间的亲和力，才能使各种成分转入溶剂中，这种作用称为解吸。浸提溶剂进入细胞组织后与解吸后的各种成分接触，使部分有效成分以分子、离子或胶体粒子等形式或状态转入溶剂，这是溶解阶段。

(2) Desorption and dissolution stage Desorption means to remove the affinity between the various components of TCM and cell wall, which makes extraction easier. For dissolution, the extraction solvent enters the cell and contacts with various components after desorbing, so that effective component can transferred into solvent in the forms of molecular, ionic, or colloidal particle.

3. 扩散阶段 浸出溶剂溶解大量药物成分后形成的浓溶液具有较高的渗透压，从而形成扩散点，不停地向周围扩散其溶解的成分以达到渗透压平衡。

(3) Diffusion stage The concentrated solution contains a lot of component and thus has high osmotic pressure, leading to component diffusion continuously to achieve osmotic pressure balance.

在浸出过程中，有两种类型的扩散方式，一种是在静止的条件下，完全由于溶质分子浓度不同而扩散；另一种为对流扩散，即在扩散过程中由于流体的运动而加速扩散。

During the extraction, two diffusion ways are involved. One is diffusion under completely static

condition, which realized by the concentration gradient of solute. Another one is convection diffusion in which the diffusion is accelerated by the movement of fluid.

二、影响浸提的因素
6.2.2 Factors Affecting Extraction

浸出溶剂，浸出方法，中药的性质如粒度、表面状态，浸提的温度、压力，浓度差，pH 值以及新技术的应用等因素，均能影响提取效率。

The factors affecting extraction include extraction solvent, extraction method, properties of TCM (such as particle size and surface state), temperature, pressure, concentration difference, pH value and the application of new technology.

1. 中药粒度 中药粒度主要影响渗透与扩散两个阶段。通常饮片粉碎越细，浸出效果越好。但过细的粉末反而妨碍浸出过程。

(1) Particle size The particle size of TCM mainly affects permeation and diffusion. In most of cases, the smaller particle size is, the better extraction efficacy achieved. But the tiny powder could hinder the extraction.

2. 浸提温度 浸提温度升高，可促进成分的溶解与扩散，提高浸出效果。但温度不宜过高。

(2) Extraction temperature Increasing extraction temperature can improve the dissolution and diffusion speed of TCM component, and thus receives a better extraction effect. But the temperature should not be too high.

3. 中药成分 有效成分通常为小分子化合物，扩散较快，在最初的浸出液中占比例高，随着扩散的进行，高分子杂质溶出逐渐增多。因此，浸提次数不宜过多，一般 2~3 次即可。

(3) Component of TCM The effective component of TCM is usually small molecule compound, which spread faster and occupy a higher proportion in the initial extraction solution. With the progress of diffusion, the polymer impurity dissolution would be increase. Therefore, the frequency of extraction should not be too much, and usually 2-3 times are appropriate.

4. 浸提时间 浸出量与浸提时间成正比，浸提时间越长，浸出的物质越多，当扩散达到平衡后，浸出不再受时间影响，应更换新的溶剂。

(4) Extraction time The longer the extraction time is, the more extract will be obtained. When the diffusion reaches equilibrium, the extraction is no longer affected by time, and solvents should be replaced.

5. 浓度差 浓度差是指中药组织内的溶液与组织外部周围溶液的浓度差值，它是扩散作用的主要动力。浸提过程中，适当应用和扩大浸出过程的浓度差，将有利于提高浸提效率。

(5) Concentration difference It refers to the concentration difference between the out-layer solution and the solution around the tissue of TCM, and it is the main driving force for diffusion. In the process of extraction, the proper expansion of the concentration difference could improve extraction efficiency.

6. 浸提压力 加压可加速溶剂对质地坚硬的中药的浸润与渗透过程，缩短浸提时间。但当中药组织内已充满溶剂之后，加压对扩散速度没有影响。对组织松软的中药，容易浸润的中药，加压对浸出影响不明显。

(6) Extraction pressure The pressure increasement can accelerate speed of infiltration especially

for the hard material of the TCM, and shorten the extraction time. However, the pressure has no effect on the diffusion rate when the tissue of the TCM is filled with solvent. For soft and easy infiltrated TCM material, the effect of pressure on extraction is tiny.

7. 溶剂 pH 值 在中药浸提过程中，调节适当的pH值，有助于中药中某些弱酸、弱碱性有效成分在溶剂中的解吸和溶解。

(7) pH value of solvent Appropriate pH value of solvent would increase desorption and dissolution efficiency of some weak alkaloid and organic acid.

8. 新技术 近年来新技术的不断推广，不仅可加快浸提过程，提高浸提效果，而且有助于提高制剂质量，如超声波提取法、微波加热提取法、超临界流体提取法等。

(8) New technology In recent years, the continuous promotion of new technology can not only accelerate the extraction speed, improve the extraction efficiency, but also help to improve the quality of the preparation, such as ultrasonic extraction, microwave heating and supercritical fluid extraction.

三、常用浸提溶剂
6.2.3 Commonly Used Extraction Solvent

优良的溶剂应能最大限度地溶解和浸出有效成分，最低限度地浸出无效成分和有害物质；不与中药成分发生化学变化，不影响其稳定性和药效；本身性质稳定，比热小，安全无毒，价廉易得，可回收利用。

Excellent solvent should be able to maximize the dissolution and extraction of active composition, minimize the extraction of ineffective and harmful compositions, bring no chemical change to the TCM composition, and cause no effect on stability and efficacy. It also should be non-toxic, cheap, and recyclable.

1. 水 水价廉易得、极性大、溶解范围广，能浸出生物碱盐类、苷、有机酸盐、鞣质、蛋白质、树胶、色素、多糖类（果胶、黏液质、菊糖、淀粉等），以及酶和少量的挥发油等。缺点是浸出选择性差，容易浸出大量无效成分，易霉变且能引起一些有效成分的水解，浸提液滤过、纯化困难等。

(1) Water The advantages of water used as solvent include low price, easy to obtain, high polarity, and wide dissolution range. It can extract alkaloid salt, glycoside, organic acid salt, tannin, protein, gum, pigment, polysaccharide (pectin, mucus, inulin, starch, etc.), enzyme, and a small amount of volatile oil. The shortcomings are poor selectivity leading to extraction of ineffective component and high risks for mold and hydrolyzation of effective component is difficult to filter and purify the solution.

2. 乙醇 乙醇能与水以任意比例混溶。其最大优点是可通过调节乙醇的浓度，选择性地浸提中药中某些有效成分或有效部位。一般乙醇含量在90%以上时，适于浸提挥发油、有机酸、树脂、叶绿素等；乙醇含量在50%~70%时，适于浸提生物碱、苷类等；乙醇含量在50%以下时，适于浸提苦味质、蒽醌苷类等化合物；乙醇含量大于40%时，能延缓许多药物的水解，如酯类、苷类等成分，增加制剂的稳定性；乙醇含量达20%以上时具有防腐作用。

(2) Ethanol Ethanol and water can be mixed with each other at any proportion. The greatest advantage for ethanol as solvent is that it can selectively extract effective component or effective part of TCM by adjusting the concentration of ethanol. Ethanol above 90% is suitable for the extraction of volatile oil, organic acid, resin, and chlorophyll. 50%-70% ethanol is suitable for the extraction of alkaloid and glycoside. Ethanol below 50% is suitable for the extraction of bitter taste component, anthraquinone glycoside. Ethanol above 40% could delay the hydrolyzation of many drugs, such as ester, glycoside and other component, and increase the stability of the preparation. Ethanol above 20% has antiseptic effect.

3. 亲脂性有机溶剂 亲脂性的有机溶剂，如乙醚、丙酮、三氯甲烷、石油醚等，很少用于中药提取，一般仅用于某些有效成分的纯化，使用这类溶剂，最终产品必须进行溶剂残留量的限度测定。

(3) Lipophilic organic solvent Lipophilic organic solvent, such as ethyl ether, acetone, trichloromethane and petroleum ether, are seldom used for the extraction of TCM. Generally, they are only used for the purification of some effective components. The residual of these solvents must be determined for the final product.

四、浸提辅助剂
6.2.4 Extraction Auxiliary

浸提辅助剂系指能提高浸提效能，增加成分的溶解度、制剂的稳定性以及去除或减少杂质，提高制剂的质量而特加的物质。常用的浸提辅助剂有酸、碱及表面活性剂等。

Auxiliary agent can improve the extraction efficiency, increase the stability of the composition and preparation, reduce impurity, and improve the quality of the preparation. The commonly used extraction auxiliaries are acid, alkali and surfactant.

1. 酸 加酸的主要目的是促进生物碱的浸出；提高部分生物碱的稳定性；使有机酸游离，便于用有机溶剂浸提；除去酸不溶性杂质等。常用的酸有硫酸、盐酸、醋酸、酒石酸、枸橼酸等。

案例导入

(1) Acid The purposes of adding acid is to promote the extraction of alkaloid, improve the stability of alkaloid, free organic acid, to easy to extract with organic solvent and remove acid insoluble impurity. The commonly used acids are sulfuric acid, hydrochloric acid, acetic acid, tartaric acid, and citric acid.

2. 碱 碱性水溶液可溶解内酯、蒽醌及其苷、香豆素、有机酸、某些酚性成分，但同时碱性水溶液亦能溶解树脂、某些蛋白质等杂质。常用的碱为氨水、碳酸钙、氢氧化钙、碳酸钠和石灰等。

(2) Alkali Alkaline solution can dissolve lactone, anthraquinone and its glycoside, coumarin, organic acid, and phenolic component. But alkaline water solution can also dissolve impurity such as resin and protein. The commonly used alkalis are ammonia, calcium carbonate, calcium hydroxide, sodium carbonate, and lime.

3. 表面活性剂 选用适宜的表面活性剂可增强中药的浸润性，如阳离子型表面活性剂的盐酸盐等，用于生物碱的提取；非离子型表面活性剂一般不影响药物的有效成分，毒性较小或无毒性，故常选用。

(3) Surfactant Surfactant can enhance the wettability of TCM. Cationic surfactant hydrochloride is used for the extraction of alkaloid. Nonionic surfactant generally does not affect the effective component of TCM, and it is frequently used due to its low or non-toxicity.

五、常用浸提方法与设备
6.2.5 Commonly Used Extraction Method and Equipment

常用的浸提方法主要有煎煮法、浸渍法、渗漉法、回流法、水蒸气蒸馏法等。近年来，超临界流体提取法、超声波提取法、微波提取法、半仿生提取法等新技术也应用于中药制剂提取的研

究中。

The commonly used extraction methods include decoction, impregnation, percolation, reflux, and water distillation. In recent years, supercritical fluid extraction, ultrasonic extraction, microwave extraction, semi bionic extraction and other new technologies have also been applied.

1. 煎煮法 是用水作溶剂，加热煮沸浸提中药有效成分的常用提取方法。

(1) Decoction Decoction is a common method using boiling water to extract effective component of TCM.

（1）操作方法 即将中药饮片或粗粉置煎煮器中，加水浸泡适宜时间，加热至沸，保持微沸一定时间，滤过，滤液保存，药渣再依法煎煮，合并各次煎出液，即得。

常用设备有敞口倾斜式夹层锅，圆柱形不锈钢钢罐、多能提取罐等。

① Operation Raw material should be soaked for a suitable time. Then, heat to boiling, keep boiling for a time, filter, decoct the residue of raw material again according to requirement, and combine the filtrate at last. Common equipment include open inclined mezzanine pot, cylindrical stainless steel tank, multi-function extraction tank.

（2）应用特点 煎煮法经济、简单、易行，符合中医传统用药习惯。适用于有效成分能溶于水，且对湿、热较稳定的中药。浸提成分谱广，还可杀酶保苷，杀死微生物。但一些不耐热及挥发性成分易被破坏或挥发损失；提取物杂质较多，煎出液易霉败变质，应及时处理。

② Character This method is economical, simple and easy to use, which is in accordance with traditional application form of TCM. It is suitable for extraction of water soluble and hydrothermal stable component. It can also inactivate enzyme in material to prevent hydrolyzation of glycoside and kill microorganism. However, some thermal unstable and volatile components can be easily destroyed or volatilized. In addition, the decocting liquid is easy to become moldy, and thus should be treated in time.

2. 浸渍法 浸渍法是用定量的溶剂，在一定的温度下，浸泡中药的提取方法。

(2) Impregnation Impregnation refers to extracting TCM at a certain temperature with a quantitative solvent.

（1）浸渍法的类型 浸渍法按提取温度和浸渍次数可分为：冷浸渍法、热浸渍法、重浸渍法。冷浸渍法又称常温浸渍法。热浸渍法需水浴或蒸汽加热至 40~60℃ 浸渍。重浸渍法即多次浸渍法。

① *Types of impregnation* Impregnation can be divided into cold impregnation, hot impregnation, and repeated impregnation according to the extraction temperature and the times. The cold impregnation method is also known as the normal temperature impregnation. The hot impregnation process requires water bath or steam heating to 40-60℃. The repeated impregnation refers to extract the material for several times.

常用设备有圆柱形不锈钢罐、搪瓷罐等。

The commonly used equipments include cylindrical stainless steel can and enamel can.

（2）应用特点 浸渍法适用于黏性药物、无组织结构中药、新鲜及易膨胀的中药、价格低廉的芳香性中药。不适于贵重中药、毒性中药及制备高浓度的制剂。

② *Character* This method is suitable for extraction of adhesive, unstructured, fresh and low cost, and aromatic TCM. It is not suitable for the extraction of valuable and toxic TCM, and for the production of highly concentrated TCM preparation.

3. 渗漉法 渗漉法是将中药粗粉置渗漉器内，溶剂连续地从渗漉器的上部加入，渗漉提取液

不断地从其下部流出的提取方法。

(3) Percolation Transfer TCM powder into percolator, add solvent continuously from the upper percolator, and make solvent dropping continuously from the lower part of the percolator.

（1）渗漉法的类型 渗漉法根据操作方法的不同，可分为单渗漉法、重渗漉法、加压渗漉法、逆流渗漉法。

① *Types of percolation* It can be divided into four ways, including single time percolation, repeated percolation, pressurize percolation, and countercurrent percolation.

1）单渗漉法 其操作流程为：粉碎→润湿→装筒→排气→浸渍→渗漉。

a. Operation process for Single time percolation:

Crushing → wetting → canister-fulling → exhausting → impregnating → percolating.

案例导入 | Case example

案例 6-1 大黄流浸膏

6-1 Rhei Radix et Rhizoma Liquid Extract

处方： 大黄（最粗粉）1000g 60% 乙醇 适量

Prescription: Rhei Radix et Rhizoma (coarse powder) 1000g; 60% ethanol (defined amount)

功能与主治： 用于便秘及食欲不振。

Functions and indications: For constipation and inappetence syndrome.

制法： 取大黄（最粗粉）1000g，用 60% 乙醇作溶剂，浸渍 24 小时后，以 1 ~3ml/min 的速度缓缓渗漉，收集初漉液 850ml，另器保存，继续渗漉，至渗漉液色淡为止，收集续漉液，浓缩至稠膏状，加入初漉液，混匀，用 60% 乙醇稀释至 1000ml，静置，待澄清，滤过，即得。

Making Procedure: Macerate 1000g of the coarse powder of Rhei Radix et Rhizoma in 60% ethanol for 24h and percolate slowly at a speed of 1-3ml per minute. Reserve 850ml of the initial percolate and continue to percolate until the percolate becomes pale in color reserve the succersive percolate. Concentrate the successive percolate to a thick extract, mix well the initial percolate and dilute with 60% ethanol to produce a volume of 1000ml. Allow to stand until the fluid become clear and filter.

用法与用量： 口服，一次 0.5~1ml，一日 1~3ml。

Usage and Dosage: For oral administration; 0.5-1ml liquid per time, 1-3ml liquid a day.

注解： ①大黄饮片粉碎为最粗粉进行渗漉，粒度较适宜，过细易堵塞，吸附性增强，浸出效果差；过粗不易压紧，粉柱增高，减少粉粒与溶剂的接触面，浸出效果差，溶剂耗量大。

Notes: ① The material must be coarse powder. Fine powder may block the outlet of percolator, and reduce extract efficacy. Over coarse powder leads to the increased height of percolator and amount of solvent, and decreased contact surface area between powder and solvent, which reduce extract efficacy.

②药粉在装渗漉筒前应先用浸提溶剂润湿。填装时，先在渗漉器底部装假底并铺垫适宜滤材，将已润湿的药粉，分层均匀装入，松紧一致，再从上部添加溶剂，同时打开下部渗漉液出口排除空气。装筒后，添加溶剂至浸没药粉表面数厘米，浸渍 24~48 小时，使溶剂充分渗透扩散。

② The powder should be wetted before loading. For loading, install percolate bottom and adequate filter material for the percolator, fill the wet powder evenly, then add the solvent from the top of the percolator, and meanwhile open the bottom outlet of percolator to exclude air. After loading, add the solvent until liquid level is a few centimeters higher than the powder level. Then percolate for 24-48h until the solvent percolate sufficiently.

③渗漉速度应适当，一般 1000g 中药的渗漉速度，每分钟以 1~3ml 为宜。

③ The percolating speed should be appropriate. Usually the proper speed is 1-3ml per minute for the percolation of 1000g crude drug.

思考题：采用渗漉法进行大黄流浸膏制备的关键技术包括哪些？

Questions: What are the key techniques for the preparation of Rhubarb liquid extract by percolation method?

2）重渗漉法　重渗漉法是将多个渗漉筒串联排列，渗漉液重复用作新药粉的溶剂，进行多次渗漉以提高渗漉液浓度的方法。

b. Repeated percolation　Re-percolation method is to reuse percolation solvent to percolate new powder in percolator series so as to improve the concentration of extract.

（2）应用特点　渗漉法属于动态浸出，溶剂的利用率高，有效成分浸出完全。适用于贵重中药、毒性中药及高浓度制剂及有效成分含量较低中药的提取。通常采用不同浓度的乙醇或白酒作为溶剂。

② *Character*　Percolation belongs to the dynamic extraction, and it has the advantages of solvent saving and complete extraction of effective component. It is suitable for the extraction of toxic TCM, high concentration preparation, and TCM with low content effective component. Alcohol or liquor of different concentrations are usually used as solvents.

案例导入

4. 回流法　回流法是用乙醇等挥发性有机溶剂提取中药成分，其中挥发性溶剂馏出后又被冷凝，重复流回浸出器中浸提中药，循环直至有效成分提取完全的方法。

(4) Reflux　Reflux is to extract the component of TCM with volatile organic solvent such as ethanol by evaporation and condensation. In this circulation, solvent can be reused and the effective component is extracted completely.

（1）回流法的类型　可分为回流热浸法及回流冷浸法。回流热浸法溶剂只能循环使用，不能更新，通常需更换溶剂 2~3 次，溶剂用量较多。回流冷浸法溶剂既可循环使用，又能不断更新，故溶剂用量较回流热浸法、渗漉法少，浸提更完全。

① *Types of reflux*　It can be divided into hot reflux and cold immersion reflux. For hot reflux, heated solvent can be recyclable but cannot be replaced with in a circulation. It usually needs replacing the solvent for 2-3 times, and a large amount of solvent is necessary. For cold immersion reflux, solvent can not only be recycled but also be replaced constantly, which brings higher extraction efficacy and lower solvent consumption.

（2）应用特点　回流法需连续加热，浸提液在蒸发锅中受热时间较长，不适用于易被热破坏的中药成分的浸提。

② *Character*　For hot reflux, continuous heating is needed for a few hours, and it is not suitable for the extraction of thermal instable component of TCM.

5. 水蒸气蒸馏法　水蒸气蒸馏法是指将含有挥发性成分的中药与水共蒸馏，使挥发性成分随水蒸气一并馏出，并经冷凝分取挥发性成分的一种提取方法。

(5) Steam distillation　Steam distillation refers to distill TCM which contain volatile component by water steam, and condense to make steam and volatile component separated.

（1）水蒸气蒸馏法的类型　水蒸气蒸馏法可分为：共水蒸馏法（即直接加热法）、通水蒸气蒸馏法及水上蒸馏法三种。为提高馏出液的纯度或浓度，一般需进行重蒸馏，收集重蒸馏液。但蒸馏次数不宜过多。一般使用多功能提取罐进行水蒸气蒸馏提取。

① *Types of steam distillation* Steam distillation can be divided into three types: water and material co-distillation (direct heating), direct steam distillation and water distillation. In order to improve the purity or concentration of the distillate, distillation is usually repeated, collect the distillate. But the frequency of distillation should not be too high. Generally, multi-function extraction tank is used for steam distillation extraction

（2）应用特点 水蒸气蒸馏法适用于具有挥发性，能随水蒸气蒸馏而不被破坏，与水不发生反应，难溶或不溶于水的化学成分的提取、分离，如挥发油。

案例导入

② *Character* This method is suitable for the extraction and the separation of volatile component, which cannot be damaged by steam distillation or do not react with water, and is insoluble in water.

6. 超临界流体提取法 超临界流体提取法是利用超临界状态下的流体为萃取剂提取中药有效成分的方法。作为一种高效、清洁的新型提取、分离手段，其优点有：①提取速度快，效率高；②提取温度低，无氧，中药成分不易分解；③可选择性地提取中药成分；④工艺简单，溶剂可循环利用。适合于挥发性较强的成分、热敏性物质和脂溶性成分的提取分离。可用作超临界流体的气体很多，二氧化碳应用最广。其缺点为一次性设备投资过大，应用范围较窄。

(6) Supercritical fluid extraction Supercritical fluid extraction (SFE) is a method to extract the effective component of TCM by using the fluid under supercritical state as the extractant. As a new method of extraction and separation, it has the characters of: ① The extraction speed is fast and the efficiency is high; ② The extraction temperature is low, anaerobic, which would help the stabilization of effective composition of TCM; ③ Selective extraction; ④ The process is simple and the solvent can be recycled. So, this method is suitable for the extraction and separation of volatile component, heat sensitive substance and fat-soluble component. A large amount of carbon dioxide gas can be consumed, and it is the most widely used supercritical fluid. Its disadvantage is that the investment on equipment is relatively high.

7. 其他提取法

(7) Others extraction methods

（1）超声波提取法 系指利用超声波通过增大溶剂分子的运动速度及穿透力以提取中药有效成分的方法。

① *Ultrasonic extraction method* This method refers to extract effective component of TCM by ultrasonic wave that could increase the velocity and penetration ability of solvent molecule.

（2）微波提取法 系指利用微波（频率在 0.3~300GHz 之间，波长在 1mm~1m 之间的电磁波）强烈的热效应进行提取的一种方法。

② *Microwave extraction method* A method of extracting effective component of TCM by strong thermal effect of microwave (frequency between 0.3-300GHz, wavelength between 1mm and 1m).

第三节 分离与纯化

6.3 Separation and Purification

一、分离

6.3.1 Separation

中药品种多，来源复杂，提取液是多种成分的混合物，既含有效成分，又含无效杂质，需对中药提取液进行分离，常用分离方法有：沉降分离法、离心分离法和滤过分离法。

TCM extract is a mixture which contains both active and ineffective components. It is necessary to purify extract of TCM. The common methods of separation include sedimentation, centrifugation and filtration.

1. 沉降分离法 沉降分离法是利用固体与液体介质密度相差悬殊，在静止状态下，液体中的固体微粒靠自身重力自然沉降而与液体分离。该方法简便易行，但耗时长、药渣沉淀吸附药液多。适于固体杂质含量高的水提液或水提醇沉（醇提水沉）液的粗分离；对料液中固体物含量少、粒子细而轻，料液易腐败变质者不宜使用。

(1) Sedimentation Sedimentation is to separate solid particle from liquid by its own natural gravity, which is realized by density difference between solid particle and liquid in a quiescent state. The method is simple and easy to control, but it takes a long time. So, it is suitable for the primary separation of water extract with high content of solid impurity, and the separation technique such as water extraction and alcohol precipitation (or alcohol extraction and water precipitation). It is not suitable for the separation of liquid with low content of solid, fine and light solid particle and perishable material.

2. 离心分离法 离心分离法是借助离心机的高速旋转，使料液中的固体与液体，或两种密度不同且不相混溶的液体产生大小不同的离心力而分离的方法。适用于含不溶性微粒的粒径很小或黏度很大的滤浆，或密度不同的不相混溶的液体。离心分离法能有效地防止中药提取液中有效成分的损失，最大限度的保存药物的活性成分，缩短工艺流程，降低成本。

(2) Centrifugation Centrifugation is to separate solid particle from liquid by centrifugal force, which is realized by centrifugal high-speed rotation. It is suitable for the separation of insoluble particle with small particle size, high viscosity liquid, and immiscible liquid. This method can reduce the loss of the active component, procedure, and cost.

常用离心机主要有：沉降式离心机、管式离心机、蝶片式离心机、滤过式离心机、三足式离心机、卧式刮刀离心机、活塞推料离心机等。

Commonly used centrifuges are: sedimentation centrifuge, tube centrifuge, disk centrifuge, filtration centrifuge, three-legged centrifuge, horizontal scraper centrifuge, and piston push centrifuge.

3. 滤过分离法 滤过分离法是指混悬液（滤浆）通过多孔的介质（滤材）时固体微粒被截流，液体经介质孔道流出达到固液分离的方法。

(3) Filtration Filtration refers to the process whereby fluid pass through a filter or a filtering medium.

（1）滤过机制 通常有两种，一种是过筛作用，料液中大于滤器孔隙的微粒全部被截留在滤过介质的表面，如薄膜滤过；另一种是深层滤过，微粒截留在滤器的深层，如砂滤棒、垂熔玻璃

漏斗等称为深层滤器。

① *Filtration mechanism* Usually two mechanisms are involved. One is sifting, particle larger than the pore of the filter is retained in the filtration media surface, such as membrane filtration. Another mechanism is deep filtration that the particle is trapped in the deep layer of filter, such as sand filter rod and glass filter.

（2）影响滤过速度的因素 影响滤过速度的因素主要有：滤渣层两侧的压力差、滤器的面积、滤材和滤饼毛细管半径、毛细管长度、料液黏度等。

② *Factors affecting filtration speed* The main factors affecting the filtration speed are: pressure difference on both sides of the filter residue layer, the filter area, filter media and filter capillary radius, capillary length, liquid viscosity and so on.

常用的助滤剂有活性炭、滑石粉、硅藻土、滤纸浆等，常用量为 0.2%~2%。

Commonly used filter aid includes activated carbon, talc, diatomaceous earth, and filter pulp, and the commonly used amounts of these filter aids are in the range of 0.2% to 2%.

（3）滤过方法与设备

③ *Filtering methods and equipments*

1）普通滤过

A. Common filtration

①常压滤过 常用玻璃漏斗、搪瓷漏斗、金属夹层保温漏斗。此类滤器常用滤纸或脱脂棉作滤过介质。一般适于小量药液的滤过。

a. Atmospheric pressure filtration Glass funnel, enamel funnel, metal sandwich insulation funnel are commonly used equipments. For filters medium, filter paper or cotton are widely adopted. This method is generally suitable for a small amount of liquid filtration.

②减压滤过 常用布氏漏斗、垂熔玻璃滤器（包括漏斗、滤球、滤棒）。布氏漏斗滤过多用于非黏稠性料液和含不可压缩性滤渣的料液，在注射剂生产中，常用于滤除活性炭。垂熔玻璃滤器常用于注射剂、口服液、滴眼液的精滤。

b. Vacuum filtration Buchner funnel, vertical melting glass filter (including funnel, filter ball, filter rod) are commonly used equipments. Buchner funnel filtration is suitable for separation of non-viscous liquid and incompressible residue. Vertical melting glass filter is commonly used for the production of injection, oral solution, and eye drop.

③加压滤过 常用压滤器和板框压滤机。板框压滤机适用于黏度较低、含渣较少的液体作密闭滤过，醇沉液、合剂配液多用板框滤过。常用板框压滤机。适用于黏度较低、含渣较少的液体加压密闭滤过，多用于醇沉液、合剂配液滤过，其效率高，滤过质量好，滤液损耗小。

c. Pressure filtration Pressure filter and frame pressure filter are commonly used equipments. Frame pressure filter is suitable for filtration of lower viscosity liquid. It has characters of high efficiency, good filtration quality and low filtrate loss.

2）薄膜滤过 薄膜滤过是利用对组分有选择透过性的薄膜，实现混合物组分分离的一种方法。按薄膜所能截留的微粒最小粒径，薄膜滤过可分为微孔滤过、超滤、反渗透。

B. Membrane filtration Membrane filtration is a method of separating mixture using a selectively permeable membrane. According to the minimum size of the particle, particle can be retained by the membrane. Membrane filtrations can be divided into microporous filtration, ultrafiltration, and reverse osmosis.

①微孔滤膜滤过 微滤所用微孔滤膜，孔径为 0.03 ~10μm，主要滤除直径≥ 50nm 的细菌和

悬浮颗粒。生产中主要用于精滤。微滤的特点：微孔滤膜的孔径高度均匀，孔隙率高，滤速快；滤膜质地薄，对料液的滤过阻力小，滤速快，吸附损失小；滤过时无介质脱落，对药液不污染；但易堵塞，故料液必须先经预处理。

a. Microporous membrane filtration Membrane for microfiltration has a pore size of 0.03 ~ 10μm, which is used to filter the bacteria and suspended particle with diameter ⩾ 50nm. Microfiltration characteristics: well-distributed pore size, high porosity, fast filtration; thin membrane texture, low filtration resistance to the liquid, low adsorption loss; no pollute to the liquid. However, liquid must be pre-treated to prevent blocking of membrane.

②超滤　超滤所采用的非对称结构的多孔超滤膜孔径为1~20nm，主要滤除直径为5~100nm的颗粒，故为纳米数量级（$nm=10^{-9}m$）选择性滤过的技术，是以压力差为推动力的膜分离过程。超滤常用于药物、注射剂的精制，不能用于高压消毒灭菌制剂的除菌；可用于蛋白质、酶、核酸、多糖类药物的超滤浓缩；蛋白质和酶类制剂的超滤脱盐；不同分子量的生化药物的分级分离和纯化。

b. Ultrafiltration Ultrafiltration membrane has a pore size of 1-20nm, which is used to remove particle of 5-100 nm. It can be used for ultrafiltration of protein, enzyme, nucleic acid and polysaccharide.

二、纯化
6.3.2 Purification

纯化是采用适当的方法和设备除去中药提取液中杂质的操作。常用的纯化方法有：水提醇沉法、醇提水沉法、超滤法、盐析法、酸碱法、澄清剂法、透析法、萃取法等。

The aim of purification is to remove impurity in TCM extract. Commonly used purification methods are: water extraction and alcohol precipitation, alcohol extraction and water sedimentation method, ultrafiltration, salting out, acid-base method, adding clarifier, dialysis, and extraction.

1. 水提醇沉法　水提醇沉法是先以水为溶剂提取中药有效成分，再用不同浓度的乙醇沉淀去除提取液中杂质的方法。广泛用于中药水提液的纯化，以降低制剂的服用量，或增加制剂的稳定性和澄清度。该法也可用于制备具有生理活性的多糖和糖蛋白。

(1) Water extraction and alcohol precipitation Water extraction and alcohol precipitation method is to use water as the solvent to extract active ingredients of Chinese medicine, and then add different concentrations of ethanol to remove impurity in the water extract. This method is widely used in the purification of TCM extract to reduce the amount of preparation, or increase the stability and clarity of preparation. The method can also be used to prepare physiologically active polysaccharide and glycoprotein.

（1）基本原理　根据中药成分在水和乙醇中的溶解性不同：通过水和不同浓度的乙醇交替处理，可保留生物碱盐类、苷类、氨基酸、有机酸等有效成分；去除蛋白质、糊化淀粉、黏液质、油脂、脂溶性色素、树脂、树胶、部分糖类等杂质

① *The basic principle* According to the different solubility of components of TCM in water and ethanol, the active components such as alkaloids salts, glycosides, amino acids and organic acids can be preserved by alternately treating water and different concentrations of ethanol. The protein, gelatinized starch and mucus, grease, fat-soluble pigment, resins, gum, some sugar and other impurity can be removed.

（2）操作要点　该纯化方法是将中药饮片先用水提取，再将提取液浓缩至约每毫升相当于原

中药 1~2g，冷却，加入适量乙醇，静置，冷藏适当时间，分离去除沉淀，回收乙醇，最后制成澄清的液体。具体操作时应注意以下问题。

② *Operation points* Extract the TCM slice with water first, then concentrate the extract solution to about 1 milliliter equivalent to 1-2g of TCM, cool, add an appropriate amount of ethanol, allow to stand and refrigerate for a suitable time, separate and remove the sediment, recover the ethanol, and finally become a clear liquid. The specific operation should pay attention to the following questions.

1）药液浓缩 水提取液应经浓缩后再加乙醇处理。

Liquid concentrate: Water extract should be concentrated and then add ethanol.

2）加醇的方式 分次醇沉或以梯度递增方式逐步提高乙醇浓度的方法进行醇沉。

The way to add alcohol: Alcohol precipitation or stepwise increase the concentration of ethanol to ethanol precipitation.

3）醇沉浓度的计算 每次需达到某种含醇量，应通过计算求得。

Calculation of alcohol sediment concentration:

$$C_{实}\ (C_{ture}) = C_{测}\ (C_{test}) + (20 - t) \times 0.4 \tag{6-1}$$

式中，$C_{实}$为乙醇的实际浓度（%）；$C_{测}$为乙醇计测得的浓度（%）；t 为测定时乙醇本身的温度。

C_{ture} is the alcohol actual concentration (%), C_{test} is measuring concentration (%), t is the temperature of the ethanol at the time of measurement.

4）密闭冷藏与处理 药液加至所需含醇量后，将容器口盖严，以防乙醇挥发。待含醇药液慢慢降至室温时，再移至冷库中，于 5~10℃ 下静置 12~24 小时，充分静置冷藏后，先虹吸上清液，可顺利滤过，下层稠液再慢慢抽滤。

Closed refrigeration and treatment: After the liquid is added to the desired alcohol content, the container is covered tightly to prevent ethanol volatilization. When the alcohol-containing liquid is slowly cooled to room temperature, it is moved to a cold storage room and allowed to stand at 5-10℃ for 12-24h. After fully standing for cold storage, the supernatant is siphoned first and filtered smoothly. Filter slowly again.

2. 醇提水沉法 先以适当浓度的乙醇提取中药成分，再加适量的水，以除去水不溶性成分。其基本原理与操作要点同水提醇沉法。适于提取药效物质为醇溶性或在醇水中均有较好溶解性的中药，可避免中药中大量淀粉、蛋白质、黏液质等高分子杂质的浸出；水处理又可较方便地将醇提液中的树脂、油脂、色素等杂质沉淀除去。应特别注意，如果药效成分在水中难溶或不溶，则不可采用水沉处理。

(2) Alcohol extraction and water sedimentation method First, use appropriate concentration of ethanol to extract TCM component, then add a suitable amount of water to remove water-insoluble ingredient. The basic principle and operation point are same with those of water extraction alcohol precipitation method. It is suitable for the extraction of alcohol-soluble active substance. It can avoid the extraction of a large number of high molecular impurities such as starch, protein and mucus in traditional Chinese medicine, and it is convenient for water treatment to remove the impurities such as resin, oil and pigment from alcohol extraction solution. Special attention shall be paid to the insoluble or insoluble components, which shall not be treated by water sedimentation.

3. 盐析法 盐析法是指在药物溶液中加入大量的无机盐，使某些高分子物质的溶解度降低沉淀析出，而与其他成分分离的方法。主要适用于蛋白质的分离纯化。此外，也常用于提高中药蒸馏液中挥发油的含量及蒸馏液中微量挥发油的分离。

(3) Salting out Salting-out method refers to adding a large amount of inorganic salt into the solution to reduce the solubility of some high-molecular substances and precipitate from solution. It is mainly used for protein purification. In addition, it is also commonly used to improve the content of volatile oil in TCM distillate and the separation of trace volatile oil in distillate.

盐析常用中性盐有：氯化钠、硫酸钠、硫酸镁、硫酸铵等。

Commonly used neutral salts are: sodium chloride, sodium sulfate, magnesium sulfate, ammonium sulfate and so on.

案例导入

4. 酸碱法 酸碱法是针对单体成分的溶解度与酸碱度有关的性质，在溶液中加入适量酸或碱，调节pH值至一定范围，使单体成分溶解或析出，以达到分离目的的方法。

(4) Acid-base method Adding appropriate amount of acid or alkali solution to adjust the pH to a certain range, which makes component dissolved or precipitated to achieve separation.

5. 大孔树脂吸附法 大孔树脂吸附法是利用其多孔结构和选择性吸附功能将中药提取液中的有效成分或有效部位吸附，再经洗脱回收，以除去杂质的一种纯化方法。大孔树脂由聚合单体和交联剂、致孔剂、分散剂等添加剂经聚合反应制备而成，是吸附树脂的一种。

(5) Macroporous resin adsorption Macroporous resin could selectively adsorb active component in TCM, which can be used to remove impurity in an extract. It is made by polymerization monomer and crosslinking agent, and other additives.

案例导入 | Case example

案例 6-2　三七总皂苷

6-2 Notoginseng Total Saponins

制法： 取三七粉碎成粗粉，用70%乙醇提取，滤过，滤液减压浓缩，滤过，过苯乙烯型非极性或弱极性共聚体大孔吸附树脂柱，用水洗涤，水洗液弃去，以80%的乙醇洗脱，洗脱液减压浓缩，脱色，精制，减压浓缩至浸膏，干燥，即得。

Method: Crash notoginseng into coarse powder and extract with 70% ethanol, and concentrate the extract under reduced pressure. Use macroporous resin to purify notoginseng total saponin by gradient elution with water and 80% ethanol separately. Discard the water eluent and concentrate the 80% ethanol eluent under reduced pressure to obtain dry matter.

注解： ①大孔吸附树脂作为一种分离手段，在中药皂苷类成分的分离、纯化研究中应用十分广泛。大孔树脂型号很多，性能用途各异，必须根据中药功能主治，分析可能的有效成分或有效部位的性质，根据"相似相溶"原则，筛选恰当型号的大孔树脂。

Notes: ① As a separation method, macroporous resin is widely used in the separation and purification of saponins in TCM, According to the principle of "similar compatibility", select appropriate type macroporous resin according to the character of active component or effective part.

②大孔吸附树脂的操作要点包括中药提取液的预处理，树脂型号及用量的选择，洗脱剂的种类及用量选择等。

② The key points of macroporous adsorption resin operation include pretreatment of Chinese medicine extract, selection of resin model and dosage, type and dosage of eluent, etc.

③乙醇提取液中含大量的脂溶性色素，可用1%的活性炭除去后，再进行大孔树脂的纯化。以饱和吸附量、洗脱率为指标考察5种大孔树脂D101、AB-8、HPD300、HPD400、HPD500对三七总皂苷的吸附和洗脱，结果5种树脂的饱和吸附量无明显差异；在静态洗脱中，D101型树

脂吸附的总皂苷较易洗脱，洗脱率达 88.12%，故选择 D101 型大孔树脂。

③ The adsorption and elution of Panax notoginseng saponin from five macroporous resins D101, AB-8, HPD300, HPD400 and HPD500 were investigated with saturated adsorption capacity and elution rate. The results showed that there was no significant difference in the saturated adsorption capacity among five resins. In the static elution, D101-type resin adsorption of total saponin is easier to elute, and elution rate is 88.12%. So D101-type macroporous resin was selected.

④在树脂纯化过程中，洗脱剂的浓度、用量、流速等是影响树脂纯化的重要参数，另外，树脂柱径高比、树脂柱的使用次数以及再生，都会影响树脂的分离纯化效果。

④ In the process of resin purification, the concentration, amount and flow rate of the eluent are important parameters affecting the purification of the resin. In addition, the resin column diameter-height ratio, the number of resin column used and the regeneration will affect the separation and purification of the resin.

⑤由于大孔吸附树脂含有微量苯、甲苯、二甲苯、二乙烯苯等有机溶剂，可能残留在产品中，因此现行版《中国药典》对三七总皂苷树脂残留溶剂的限度制订了标准。

⑤ Macroporous resin contains a trace of benzene, toluene, xylene, divinylbenzene and other organic solvents. So, a resin solvent limit was set in the current version of *Chinese Pharmacopoeia*.

思考题：如何评价大孔吸附树脂的安全性？

Questions: How to evaluate the safety of macroporous resin?

第四节 浓缩

6.4 Concentration

PPT

浓缩是采用适当的技术和方法，使溶液中部分溶剂气化或被分离移除，以提高溶液的浓度或使溶液达到饱和而析出溶质的过程。浓缩可分为蒸发浓缩、反渗透浓缩和超滤浓缩。目前在中药的浓缩过程中大多采用蒸发浓缩，即在沸腾状态下进行的传热传质过程，包括常压浓缩、减压浓缩、薄膜浓缩和多效浓缩等不同方式，应根据中药提取液的性质和蒸发浓缩的要求选择适宜的浓缩方法和设备。

Concentration refers to increase the density of the extract by removing solvent with appropriate technique and method. Concentration can be divided into evaporative concentration, reverse osmosis concentration and ultrafiltration concentration. At present, evaporation concentration is most adopted for the production of TCM, which is carried out in a boiling state to achieve massive transfer, including atmospheric concentration, vacuum concentration, film concentration and multi-effect concentration. Appropriate method and equipment should be selected according to the character of extract and requirement of concentration.

一、影响浓缩效率的因素
6.4.1 Factors Affecting the Efficiency of Concentration

1. 传热温度差（Δt_m）的影响 分子运动学说指出，气化是分子通过获得足够热能而使其振动能力超过分子间的内聚力而产生，故浓缩过程中必须不断给料液供热。

(1) Effect of temperature difference (Δt_m) Molecular kinematic theory points out that gasification is the result of molecule vibration when getting enough heat. So, the heat must be continuously supplied to the liquid during the concentration process.

提高 Δt_m 的方法：①提高加热蒸气的压力，但易导致热敏成分的破坏；②降低溶液沸点，可借助减压方法适当降低冷凝器中的二次蒸气压力，也可及时移去蒸发器中的二次蒸气。

Increase Δt_m method:

① Increase the pressure of the heated steam, but easily lead to the destruction of thermal unstable component.

② Reduce the boiling point of the solution.

注：①真空度不宜过高，否则会增加能量消耗，且溶液易因沸点降低而黏度增加，使传热系数降低；②加热温度一般恒定，溶剂蒸发后，溶液的浓度增加而沸点升高，导致 Δt_m 减小；③由于静压的影响，液层底部的沸点高于液面，Δt_m 变小，可通过控制液面的深度而改善。

Note: ① The degree of vacuum should not be too high.

② Heating temperature is generally constant. After the solvent evaporation, the solution concentration and boiling point are increased, resulting in Δt_m decrement.

③ Due to static pressure, the boiling point of bottom liquid layer is higher than that of the upper liquid layer. Thus, the depth of the liquid should be controlled to increase Δt_m.

2. 传热系数（K）的影响 一般而言，增大传热系数是提高蒸发浓缩效率的主要因素。可通过定期除垢，改进蒸发器结构，建立良好的溶液循环流动，排除加热管内不凝性气体等方法增大传热系数，以提高蒸发效率。

(2) Effect of heat transfer coefficient (K) In general, increasing the heat transfer coefficient is the main factor to increase the efficiency of evaporation and concentration. To improve the evaporation efficiency, regular removing dirt, improving the evaporator structure, establishing a good solution circulation, excluding the heating pipe non-condensable gas are necessary.

二、浓缩方法与设备
6.4.2 Concentration Method and Equipment

1. 常压浓缩 常压浓缩是指液体在一个大气压下蒸发的方法。该法耗时较长，易导致某些成分破坏。适用于对热较稳定的药液的浓缩。常用设备包括敞口倾倒式夹层蒸发锅、常压蒸馏装置等。

(1) Atmospheric pressure concentration Atmospheric pressure concentration refers to concentrate the liquid under normal atmosphere pressure. This method takes a long time, and easily leads to the component destruction. Common equipments include open-dumping mezzanine evaporation pot and atmospheric distillation unit.

2. 减压浓缩 减压浓缩是在密闭的容器内，抽真空降低内部压力，形成负压，使料液的沸点

降低的方法。

(2) Concentration under reduced pressure This operation is carried out in a closed container. By lowering the internal pressure, the liquid boiling point is reduced.

减压浓缩的特点为：①沸点降低，能防止或减少热敏性物质的分解；②增大传热温度差，提高蒸发效率；③能不断地排除溶剂蒸汽，有利于蒸发；④可利用低压蒸汽或废气作加热源；⑤缺点是耗能大，气化潜热增大，比常压浓缩消耗的热蒸汽量多。减压浓缩适用于含热敏成分药液的浓缩及需回收溶剂的药液的浓缩。

This method is characterized by:

① Reducing the boiling point, preventing or reducing the decomposition of heat-sensitive substances.

② Increasing the heat transfer temperature difference and increasing the evaporation efficiency.

③ Continuously excluding solvent vapor and facilitating evaporation.

④ Utilizing low-pressure steam or exhaust gas as heating sources.

⑤ Its disadvantage is the relatively high energy consumption.

This method is suitable for pharmaceutical solutions which contain thermosensitive components and those require solvent recovery.

减压浓缩装置，又称减压蒸馏装置。料液需回收溶剂时多采用此种减压蒸馏装置。对于以水为溶剂提取的药液，目前许多药厂使用真空浓缩罐进行浓缩。

Concentration under reduced pressure is suitable for the concentration of the liquid containing the thermosensitive component. At present, many pharmaceutical factories use vacuum concentration tank to concentrate the liquid medicine extracted with water as solvent.

3. 多效浓缩 将第一效蒸发器汽化的二次蒸汽作为热源通入第二效蒸发器的加热室作加热用，以此类推，依次进行多个串接，则称为多效浓缩。多效浓缩器是节能型浓缩器，节约热蒸汽和冷凝水，应用较多的是二效或三效浓缩，如三效浓缩罐，但是因药液受热时间长，不适于热敏性药物，另外该设备生产强度较低，设备复杂，清洗困难。

(3) Multi-effect concentration Multi-effect concentrator is an energy-saving equipment, saving hot steam and condensate water. It is not suitable for the evaporation of heat-sensitive drug due to long time heating, while the equipment is complex and difficult to clean.

4. 薄膜浓缩 薄膜浓缩是使料液沿加热壁呈薄膜状快速流动，同时与剧烈沸腾时所产生的大量泡沫相结合，达到增加料液的气化面积，提高蒸发浓缩效率的方法。其特点是蒸发速度快，受热时间短；不受液体静压和温度过热的影响，成分不易被破坏；可在常压或减压下连续操作；溶剂可回收重复使用；缺点是蒸发速度与热量供应平衡较难掌握，易造成料液变稠后黏附于加热面，影响蒸发。

(4) Thin film concentration Film concentration is to make the liquid flow rapidly along the heating wall in a thin film-like state, and mix with a large amount of foam generated by boiling, which could increase the gasification area and improve efficiency of concentration.

Its characteristics are fast evaporation speed, short heating time, avoiding hydrostatic pressure and overheating, the component are not easy to be destroyed. It can be continuously operated under atmospheric or reduced pressure, and solvent can be recycled for reuse. The disadvantage is the evaporation rate and heat supply balance are difficult to achieve, and easily lead to material thickening after adhesion to the heating surface and thus affect evaporation.

薄膜浓缩常用设备主要分为升膜式蒸发器、降膜式蒸发器、刮板式薄膜蒸发器和离心式薄膜

蒸发器四种。

Thin film concentration equipments commonly used include rising film evaporator, falling film evaporator, scraping film evaporator and centrifugal film evaporator.

第五节 干燥

6.5 Drying

PPT

干燥是利用热能或其他方式除去固体物质或膏状物中所含的水分或其他溶剂，获得干燥物的操作。其目的在于提高药物的稳定性、便于进一步加工处理，保证中药的内在质量。

Drying refers to an operation by using heat or other methods to remove water or other solvents contained in paste or solid matter and to get dry matter. The purpose of drying is to improve the stability of the drug, to facilitate further processing, and to ensure the inherent quality of TCM.

一、干燥的基本原理

6.5.1 The Principle of Drying

1. 物料中所含水分的性质

(1) The property of water

（1）结晶水　结晶水是化学结合水，一般用风化方法去除，在药剂学中不视为干燥过程。

① *Crystal water*　Crystal water is chemical bound water. It can be removed by weathering which is not considered as a drying process in pharmaceutics.

（2）结合水与非结合水　结合水指存在于细小毛细管中的水分和渗透到物料细胞中的水分。非结合水是指存在于物料表面的润湿水分、粗大毛细管中的水分和物料孔隙中的水分。

② *Bound water and unbound water*　Bound water refers to the water in small capillary and moisture penetrated in the cell of material. Unbound water refers to the wet water presented in the surface, wide-bore capillary, and the pore of material.

（3）平衡水分与自由水分　物料与一定温度、湿度的空气相接触时，将会发生排除水分或吸收水分的过程，直到物料表面所产生的蒸气压与空气中的水蒸气分压相等为止，物料中的水分与空气处于动态平衡状态，此时物料中所含的水分称为该空气状态下物料的平衡水分。

③ *Balance of water and free water*　When material encounter air with a certain temperature and humidity, the process of water exclusion or water absorption will occur, until the vapor pressure of the material surface is equal to the partial pressure of water vapor in the air. At this moment, the water in material and air are in a dynamic equilibrium state, and the water in material is called the equilibrium water under defined air state.

物料中所含的总水分为自由水与平衡水之和，在干燥过程中可除去自由水（包括全部非结合水和部分结合水），不能除去平衡水。

Total water in the material is the sum of the free water and the balance water, free water can be removed (including all unbound water and part of bound water), and the equilibrium water cannot be

removed during the drying process.

干燥效率不仅与物料中所含水分的性质有关，而且还取决于干燥速率。

Drying efficiency is not only related to the property of the water in material but also to the drying rate.

2. 干燥速率与干燥速率曲线 干燥速率是指在单位时间内，在单位干燥面积上被干燥物料中水分的汽化量。可用式（6-2）表示。

(2) Drying rate and drying rate curve Drying rate refers to the amount of vaporized water in the dried material per unit area of drying in the unit time. It can be expressed as the following formula (6-2):

$$U = \mathrm{d}w/(S \cdot \mathrm{d}t) \tag{6-2}$$

式中，U 为干燥速率 [$\mathrm{kg/(m^2 \cdot s)}$]；$S$ 为干燥面积（$\mathrm{m^2}$）；w 为汽化水分量（kg）；t 为干燥时间（s）。

U refers to the drying rate [$\mathrm{kg/(m^2 \cdot s)}$], S refers to drying area ($\mathrm{m^2}$), w refers to the water content of vaporization (kg), t refers to drying time.

当湿物料与干燥介质接触时，物料表面的水分开始汽化，并向周围介质传递。干燥过程是被汽化的水分连续进行内部扩散和表面汽化的过程，因此干燥速率取决于内部扩散速率和表面汽化速率，可以用干燥速率曲线来说明。干燥过程明显地分成两个阶段，等速阶段和降速阶段。在等速阶段，干燥速率与物料湿含量无关。在降速阶段，干燥速率近似地与物料湿含量成正比。

When wet materials encounter the drying medium, water on the surface of the material begins to vaporize, and transfer to the surrounding medium. Drying is a combination of the internal diffusion and the external vaporization of vaporized water. Therefore, drying rate depends on the rate of internal diffusion and the rate of external vaporization, and it can be described by drying rate curves. The drying process is obviously divided into two phases: the constant velocity phase and deceleration phase. In the constant velocity phase, the drying rate has no relationship with the water content of materials. However, in the deceleration phase, the drying rate is proportional to the water content of the material approximately.

二、影响干燥的因素

6.5.2 Factors Affecting Drying

1. 影响干燥的等速和降速阶段的因素

(1) Factors affecting drying constant velocity and deceleration phases

（1）等速阶段 在等速阶段，凡能影响表面汽化速率的因素都可以影响等速阶段的干燥。例如：干燥介质的种类、性质、温度、湿度、流速、固体物料层的厚度、颗粒的大小、空气和固体物料间的相互运动方式等。

① *Constant velocity stage* During the constant velocity phase, factors which can affect the rate of external vaporization also can affect the rate of constant drying phase. For example: the type of drying medium, the property, temperature, humidity, velocity, the thickness of solid material layer, the size of the particle, the way of the mutual movement between the air and the solid material etc.

（2）降速阶段 在降速阶段，干燥速率主要与内部扩散有关。因此，物料的厚度、干燥的温度等可影响降速阶段的干燥。

② *Deceleration phase* In the deceleration phase, the drying rate is mainly concerned with the internal diffusion. Therefore, the thickness of the material, the drying temperature can affect the deceleration phase of drying.

2. 影响干燥的具体因素

(2) Specific factors affecting drying

（1）被干燥物料的性质　系最主要的因素。湿物料的形状、大小及料层的厚薄、水分的结合方式都会影响干燥速率。一般说来，物料呈结晶状、颗粒状、堆积薄者，较粉末状及膏状、堆积厚者干燥速率快。

① *The property of material*　It is the main factor. Shape of wet material, size and thickness of material layer, the combined way of water can affect the drying rate. Generally, the drying rates for crystalline, granular, and thin stacking materials are faster than the those of the materials in the form of powder, paste, and thick stacking.

（2）干燥介质的温度、湿度与流速　在适当范围内，提高空气的温度，可加快蒸发速度，有利于干燥。但应根据物料的性质选择适宜的干燥温度，以防止某些热敏性成分被破坏。

② *The temperature, humidity and velocity of drying medium*　Within an appropriate range, increasing the temperature of air can accelerate the evaporation rate and benefits drying. However, suitable drying temperature should be selected according to the property of the material, to prevent the destruction of heat-sensitive ingredient.

空气的相对湿度越低，干燥速率越大。降低有限空间的相对湿度可提高干燥效率。

The lower the relative humidity of the air is, the greater the rate of drying is. Reducing the relative humidity in limited space can improve drying efficiency.

空气的流速越大，干燥速率越快。空气的流速加快，可减小气膜厚度，降低表面汽化阻力，提高等速阶段的干燥速率，但空气流速对内部扩散无影响，故对降速阶段的干燥速率影响较小。

The greater the flow rate of air is, the faster the drying rate is. Accelerating the flow rate of air can reduce the thickness of gas film, lower the resistance of external vaporization and increase the drying rate of the constant phase. But the air flow rate has no effect on the internal diffusion, and thus it has a limited effect on the drying rate in deceleration phase.

（3）干燥速度与干燥方式　当干燥速度过快时，物料表面的蒸发速度大大超过内部液体扩散到物料表面的速度，致使表面粉粒黏着，甚至熔化结壳，从而阻碍了内部水分的扩散和蒸发，形成假干燥现象，此问题常见于静态干燥中。动态干燥法颗粒处于跳动、悬浮状态，可大大增强其暴露面积，有利于提高干燥速率，但必须及时给足够的热能，以满足蒸发和降低干燥空间相对湿度的需要。

③ *Drying rate and drying method*　When drying is too fast, the rate of evaporation on the surface of material greatly exceeds the spreading rate of internal liquid to the material surface, resulting in adhesion of surface powder, or even melting to crust. This phenomenon hinders the diffusion and evaporation of internal water and forms a fake dryness, and it is commonly happened in static drying. Granule in dynamic drying is in a state of beating and suspension, which can greatly enhance its exposure area and improve the drying rate. Enough heat must be given promptly to meet the needs of evaporation and to reduce the relative humidity of the drying space.

（4）压力　压力与蒸发量成反比。减压是改善蒸发，加快干燥的有效措施。真空干燥能降低干燥温度，加快蒸发速度，提高干燥效率，产品疏松易碎，质量稳定。

④ *Pressure*　Evaporation is inversely proportional to the pressure. Reducing pressure is a measure to improve evaporation and accelerate drying. Vacuum drying can reduce the drying temperature, speed up the evaporation rate, improve drying efficiency, and make the product loose, friable and stable.

三、干燥方法与设备

6.5.3 Drying Methods and Equipments

在制药工业中，由于被干燥物料的形状是多种多样的，物料的性质各不相同，对干燥产品的要求各有差异，生产规模及生产能力各不相同。因此，采用的干燥方法与设备也是多种多样的。

In the pharmaceutical industry, the shape and property of the material, the requirement for dried product, and the production and production capacity are different. Therefore, drying method and equipment are varied.

1. 常压干燥 常压干燥是在常压下利用热的干燥气流通过湿物料的表面使水分汽化进行干燥的方法。

(1) Ambient pressure drying Ambient pressure drying refers to a drying method that makes hot drying air flow pass the wet material to remove the surface water of wet material.

（1）烘干干燥 烘干法是在常压下，将湿物料摊放在烘盘内，利用热的干燥气流使湿物料水分汽化进行干燥的一种方法。适用于对热稳定的药物。由于物料处于静止状态，所以干燥速度较慢，干燥时间长，易引起成分的破坏，干燥品较难粉碎。常用的设备有烘箱和烘房。

① *Baking drying* Baking drying is a method that makes wet material spread in the baking dish, and vaporizes the water in wet material by hot and dry air flow under atmospheric pressure. It is suitable for drugs stable to heat. Due to the stationary state of material, this method becomes slow and lasts a long drying time, leading to destruction of component and dry material hard. Drying oven and drying room are used commonly.

（2）鼓式干燥 鼓式干燥是将湿物料涂布在热的金属转鼓上，利用热传导方法使物料得到干燥的一种方法。适于浓缩药液及黏稠液体的干燥；可连续生产，根据需要调节药液浓度、受热时间（鼓的转速）和温度（蒸汽）；对热敏性药物液体可在减压情况下使用；干燥物料呈薄片状，易于粉碎。常用于中药浸膏的干燥和膜剂的制备。设备分单鼓式和双鼓式两种。

② *Drum-drying* Drum drying refers to plastering wet material on the hot metal drum and using heat conduction to obtain dry material. It is suitable for the drying of concentrated liquid and viscous liquid, and it can be used continuously by adjusting the liquid concentration, heating time (rotational speed of the drum) and temperature (steam). Heat-sensitive drug can be dried under the reduced pressure, and the dried material is flaky and easy to crush. This method is commonly used in the drying of TCM extract and in the preparation of film former. The equipments can be divided into sub-single drum and double drum.

（3）带式干燥 带式干燥是将湿物料平铺在传送带上，利用干热气流或红外线、微波等加热干燥物料的一种方法。在制药生产中，某些易结块和变硬的物料，中药饮片，颗粒剂、茶剂的干燥灭菌等多采用带式干燥设备。带式干燥设备可分为单带式、复带式和翻带式等。

③ *Belt-drying* Belt drying refers to spreading wet material tile on the conveyor belt and heating by dry and hot air, infrared, or microwave. In the drug production, belt drying is frequently used for drying and sterilization of easy caking and hardening material, TCM pieces, granule, and tea. Belt drying equipments can be divided into single-belt, double-belts and turning- belt.

2. 减压干燥 减压干燥又称真空干燥。它是在密闭的容器中抽去空气减压而进行干燥的一种方法。其特点是干燥的温度低，速度快；减少了物料与空气的接触机会，避免物料被污染或氧化变质；产品呈松脆的海绵状，易于粉碎。适于稠膏及热敏性或高温下易氧化，或排出的气体有使

用价值、有毒害、有燃烧性的物料的干燥。

(2) Depression drying Depression drying is also known as vacuum drying. It is used under the reduced pressure by exhausting air in a closed vessel. It is characterized by low drying temperature and high speed, which reduce the contact chance between material and air, and avoid contamination or oxidation deterioration of material. The product is crunchy and cavernous and easy to crush. It is suitable for the drying of thick paste, drug with heat-sensitive or easily oxidized characters, or the material releasing valuable gas, poison or combustible.

案例导入

3. 流化干燥

(3) Fluidized drying

（1）沸腾干燥法　它是利用从流化床底部吹入的热气流使湿颗粒悬浮，呈流化态，如“沸腾状”，热气流在悬浮的颗粒间通过，在动态下进行热交换，带走水分，达到干燥的一种方法，适于湿粒性物料的干燥。特点是气流阻力较小，物料磨损较轻，热利用率较高；干燥速度快，产品质量好。

① *Boiling drying* Boiling drying refers to making wet granule suspend in a fluidized state or a boiling state by the hot air blown from the bottom of the fluidized bed. The hot gas stream gets through the suspended particle with heat-exchanged, taking up water, to reach a purpose of drying. It is suitable for drying of wet grained material. Its characteristics are as follows: a smaller flow resistance, lighter wear, high efficiency of heating, fast drying rate, and good product quality.

目前在制药工业生产中应用较多的为负压卧式沸腾干燥装置。

Currently, negative pressure horizontal boiling drying device is used frequently in pharmaceutical industry.

（2）喷雾干燥法　喷雾干燥是用于液态物料干燥的流态化技术，是将液态物料浓缩至适宜的密度后，使之雾化成细小雾滴，与一定流速的热气流进行热交换，使水分迅速蒸发，物料干燥成粉末状或颗粒状的方法。

② *Spray drying* Spray drying is a fluidized technique used for the drying of liquid material. The liquid material is concentrated to a suitable density and atomized into fine droplet, and heat is exchanged between droplet and hot stream with certain flow rate, which makes water evaporation rapidly to obtain powder or granular.

喷雾干燥法的特点：药液瞬间干燥；受热时间短、温度低，操作流程管道化，符合 GMP 要求；产品质量好，多为疏松的细颗粒或细粉，溶解性能好，可保持原来的色香味。适用于液体物料，特别是含热敏性成分的液体物料的直接干燥，干燥后的制品可制得 180 目以上的极细粉，且含水量≤ 5%；对改善某些制剂的溶出速度具有良好的作用。

The characteristics of spray drying: instant drying; short heating time, low temperature, pipelined operation, meeting GMP requirements. Product has good quality, good solubility, original color and flavor, and form of loose particle or fine powder. This method is suitable for the drying of liquid material, especially for the direct drying of liquid material with heat-sensitive component. The dried product can generate very fine powder of 180 mesh or more, and the water content of the product is less than 5%. This method could improve the dissolution rate for certain preparation.

4. 冷冻干燥　冷冻干燥是将被干燥液体物料冷冻成固体，在低温减压条件下利用冰的升华性能，使物料低温脱水而达到干燥目的的一种方法，故又称升华干燥。

(4) Freeze-drying Freeze-drying refers to freezing the liquid material to be solid and dehydrating under the reduced pressure and low temperature condition to obtain dry material, which is based on the sublimation property of ice. So, it is also known as sublimation drying.

制品的冷冻干燥过程主要包括预冻、升华和干燥等阶段。药液在冻干前，需经滤过等预处理。

冷冻干燥的特点：物料在高真空和低温条件下干燥，成品多孔疏松，易溶解；含水量低，一般为1%~5%，有利于药品长期贮存；设备投资大，生产成本高。适于极不耐热物料的干燥，如血浆、血清、抗生素等。

The freeze-drying process mainly includes pre-freezing, sublimation and drying stages. Before lyophilization, liquid must be filtrated. The characteristics of freeze-drying: material is dried under the conditions of high vacuum and low temperature; finished product is porous and loose and can be dissolved easily; product has low water content, generally 1% to 5%, which is conducive to long-term storage. However, equipment investment is huge, and production cost is high. This drying method is suitable for the drying of extremely heat-sensitive material, such as plasma, serum and antibiotic.

5. 红外线干燥 红外线干燥是利用红外线辐射器产生的电磁波被含水物料吸收后，直接转变为热能，使物料中水分汽化而干燥的一种方法，属于辐射干燥。其特点是干燥速率快，热效率较高，适用于热敏性药物的干燥，特别适宜于熔点低、吸湿性强的药物，以及某些物体表层（如橡胶硬膏）的干燥。成品质量好，但电耗大。红外线干燥的设备常用振动式远红外干燥机。

(5) Infrared drying Infrared drying is another method to evaporate the water of material to achieve the purpose of drying. It belongs to radial drying. In this method, electromagnetic wave produced by infrared radiation machine is absorbed by water-bearing materials and then transferred into heat energy. This drying method is characterized by its fast-drying rate and high thermal efficiency, and it is suitable for the drying of heat-sensitive drug, especially suitable for those with low melting point, strong moisture absorbability as well as certain object whose surface (such as rubber plaster) is dry. Finished product has good quality, but drying procedure has large power consumption. Vibratory far infrared dryer is usually used for infrared drying.

岗位对接

6. 微波干燥 微波是一种高频波，制药工业上微波加热干燥只用915MHz和2450MHz两个频率，后者在一定条件下兼有灭菌作用。微波干燥的特点为：物料内外加热均匀，热效高，干燥时间短，对药物成分破坏少，且兼有杀虫及灭菌作用。适用于中药饮片、散剂、水丸、蜜丸、袋泡茶等制剂与物料的干燥。

重点小结

(6) Microwave drying Microwave is a high-frequency wave. In pharmaceutical industry, the microwave heating drying only uses two frequencies, 915MHz and 2450MHz. The latter one also has sterilization under certain condition. The characteristics of microwave drying: the internal and external parts of material are heated uniformly, it has high thermal efficiency, the drying time is short, and it causes less damage to the pharmaceutical ingredients and has insecticidal and sterile functions. This method is used for the drying material of TCM, powder, watered pill, honeyed pill and tea bag.

题库

（付　强）

第七章　浸出药剂
Chapter 7　Extractions

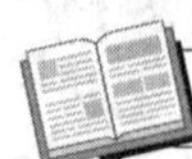

学习目标 | Learning Goals

知识要求：

1. 掌握　汤剂、中药合剂、糖浆剂、煎膏剂、酒剂、酊剂、流浸膏、浸膏剂、茶剂的含义、制法及注意事项。

2. 熟悉　浸出药剂的含义、特点及剂型种类；各种剂型的特点、质量检查及控制方法。

3. 了解　汤剂研究及剂改的进展；煎膏"返砂"的原因及解决途径；液体类浸出药剂的生霉发酵、浑浊、沉淀、水解的原因及解决途径。

能力要求：

学会各类浸出药剂的制备与质量检测方法，能制备不同类型的浸出药剂，并检查和评价浸出药剂的产品质量。

Knowledge requirements:

1. To master the definitions, preparations and precautions of decoctions, mixtures, syrups, concentrated decoctions, medicinal wines, tinctures, fluid extracts, extracts and medicinal teas.

2. To be familiar with the definition, characteristics and classifications of extractions; characteristics of various dosage forms and the quality inspection and control.

3. To know the research and development of decoction in dosage form innovations; the reasons for sugar recrystallization of concentrated decoctions and the corresponding solutions; the reasons and solutions for mould and fermentation, opacitas, sedimentation and hydrolysis.

Ability requirements:

To be able to manufacture and inspect various types of extract preparations; be able to manufacture extract preparations and inspect them, evaluate the product qualities.

第一节 概述
7.1 Overview

一、浸出药剂的含义
7.1.1 The Definition of Extractions

浸出药剂系指采用适宜的溶剂和方法提取饮片中有效部位（成分）而制得的供内服或外用的一类制剂。

Extractions are made by appropriate extraction methods to extract the active fractions or ingredients from prepared slices of TCM in suitable solvents. It can be used by oral or external.

浸出药剂常以水和不同浓度的乙醇为溶剂。以水为溶剂时，多用煎煮法制备；采用其他非水溶剂时，可选用渗漉法、浸渍法、回流提取法等方法制备。

Water and ethanol of different concentration are usually used as solvent. When water is used as solvent, decocting method is applied; when other nonaqueous solvent is used, percolation, impregnation and reflux can be chosen.

二、浸出药剂的特点
7.1.2 The Characteristics of Extractions

（一）优点
(1) Advantages

1. 体现方药多种成分的综合疗效与特点　浸出药剂具有方药各种成分的综合疗效，符合中医药理论。该类药剂与相应的单体相比，有些不仅疗效好，还能呈现单体化合物未起到的疗效。如麻黄浸出药剂，具有止咳平喘、发汗作用，而麻黄碱却只有止咳平喘作用。

① Embody the comprehensive functions and characteristics of TCM in the formula. It complies with the TCM theory that the extract preparations contain the comprehensive function of all the ingredients in the formula. Compared with corresponding monomers, extractions are not only better in effect but also present some efficacy that monomers don't have. For instance, extract of Ephedra sinica can relieve asthma and cough, as well as promote perspiration, while purified ephedrine can only relive asthma and cough.

2. 可以增强疗效，降低毒性　合理配伍的中药复方制剂，多种成分相辅相成或相互制约，可以增强疗效，降低毒性。例如四逆汤，强心升压效应优于方中各单味药，且能避免单味附子引起的异位心律失常，这也体现了“附子无干姜不热，得甘草则性缓”的传统论述。又如洋地黄叶中的洋地黄毒苷与鞣质结合存在，用乙醇提取制成酊剂，进入体内经分解、释放、起效，其作用缓和且毒性小，但精制成洋地黄毒苷单体后，作用强烈，毒性大且药效维持时间短。

② Appropriate formulation of TCM can not only enhance the effect but also reduce the toxicity. Take Sini Tang for example, not only the efficacy of heart-strengthening and pressure-boosting is more superior to any other single herb, but also avoid ectopic arrhythmia due to single application of Radix

Aconiti Lateralis Praeparata. This phenomenon reflects the traditional narrative "Radix Aconiti Lateralis Praeparata is not hot without Rhizoma Zingiberis and the hastiness of Radix Aconiti Lateralis Praeparata can be made rate with Radis Glycyrrhizae". Another example is Digotoxin from the Digitalis Fclia combined with tannin and after extracted by ethanol and prepared into tincture. The function is moderate and the toxicity is reduced after dissolution and release *in vivo*. However, if the digotoxin monomer is purified, both the effect and toxicity are increased, and the duration of treatment effect is much shorter.

3. 减少服用量 浸出药剂由于去除了部分无效成分和组织物质，相应地提高了有效成分的浓度，故与原方相比，减少了服用量，便于服用。

③ Reduce the dosage. Since part of the invalid components and tissues are removed in the extractions, the concentration of the active ingredients are increased. So compared with the original formula, the dosage is reduced and the administration is more convenient.

4. 部分药剂可作为其他剂型的原料 浸出药剂在提取过程中，除药酒、酊剂等可直接由提取液制备得到外，部分提取液需经浓缩成流浸膏、浸膏等作为原料，供进一步制备其他药剂。

④ Some preparations are used as raw materials for other dosage forms. Medicinal wines, tinctures can be prepared directly from the extract solution. Part of the extract solution need to be concentrated into fluid extracts, extracts, etc. as raw materials for furth preparation of other dosage forms.

（二）缺点

(2) Disadvantages

1. 稳定性差 浸出药剂多以水为溶剂，且常含有胶体物质、酶类，易产生陈化、成分酶解或滋生微生物，导致沉淀、变质；浸膏剂因水溶性成分多，易吸潮结块。含醇浸出药剂易因乙醇挥发而出现浑浊或沉淀。

① **Poor stability** Water is mostly used as the extracting solvent. The extractions usually contain colloids and enzymes, so it is inclined to precipitate or deteriorate due to aging, enzymatic hydrolysis or microbe proliferation. On the other hand, too many water-soluble ingredients in extracts tend to absorb moisture and cake. Ethanol containing extractions tend to present with opacitas or sediment because of the ethanol volatilization.

2. 运输不方便 浸出药剂多是液体，储存运输不如固体制剂方便。

② **Inconvenience in transportation** Compared with the solid preparations, it is not convenient to store and transport because most of extracts are liquid.

三、浸出药剂的分类

7.1.3 The Classification of Extractions

浸出药剂按照浸出过程和成品情况大致可分为以下几类。

According to the production process and the end item, extractions can be classified as follows:

1. 水浸出剂型 系指在一定的加热条件下，用水为溶剂浸出饮片中有效部位（成分），其成品为含水的制剂，如汤剂、合剂、口服液等。

(1) Water extracts By certain heating conditions, water is used to extract the active fractions (or ingredients) from prepared slices of Chinese crude drugs.The products contain water, such as decoctions, mixtures and oral solutions.

2. 含醇浸出剂型 系指在一定的条件下，用适宜浓度乙醇或酒为溶剂浸出饮片中有效部位（成分），制得的含醇制剂，如药酒、酊剂、流浸膏等。有些流浸膏虽然是用水浸出饮片中有效部

位（成分），但成品中仍加有适量乙醇。

(2) Ethanol-containing extracts It refers to extracts containing ethanol that are acquired by extracting the active fractions (or ingredients) from prepared slices of Chinese crude drugs with ethanol of suitable concentration or spirit, such as medicinal wines, tinctures, fluid extracts, etc. Some fluid extracts are extracted with water, but still added with proper ethanol.

3. 含糖浸出剂型 系指在水或含醇浸出制剂的基础上，按一定方法处理，加入适量蔗糖（或蜂蜜）或其他辅料制成。如煎膏剂、糖浆剂等。

(3) Sugar-containing extracts This type of extracts is prepared by adding some sucrose (or honey) or other excipients on the basis of the water or ethanol extracts in a certain way,, such as concentrated decoctions and syrups.

4. 无菌浸出剂型 系指用适宜的溶剂浸出饮片中有效部位（成分），经适当纯化处理，最终制成的无菌制剂，如中药注射剂等。

(4) Sterile extracts This type of extracts is made by extracting the active fractions (or ingredients) from the prepared slices of Chinese crude drugs with suitable solvents and then purifying, such as injections of TCM.

5. 其他浸出药剂 除上述剂型外，还有以浸出提取物为原料制备的颗粒剂、片剂、胶囊剂、浓缩丸剂、软膏剂、栓剂、气雾剂等。

(5) Other extracts Besides the dosage forms above, there still are granules, tablets, capsules, concentrated pills, ointments, suppositories and aerosols which are prepared from extracts.

第二节　汤剂

7.2　Decoctions

PPT

一、汤剂的含义

7.2.1　The Definition of Decoctions

汤剂又称“汤液”，系指将处方饮片或粗颗粒加水煎煮或用沸水浸泡，去渣取汁制成的液体剂型。其中以中药粗颗粒制备的汤液又称“煮散”。以沸水浸泡药物，服用时间和剂量不定或宜冷饮者，又称“饮”。汤剂主要供内服，也可供洗浴、熏蒸、含漱等外用。

Decoctions, also known as “soup”, are liquid dosage forms that are prepared by decocting the prepared slices or granules in water, removing the residues and taking the juice. Among them, those made by decocting coarse granules are also called “decocted powders”, while those macerated with boiling water and taken at random time and dose, or better to be taken coldly are also called “drink”. Decoctions are mainly for oral administration, and also for gargling, fuming or steaming and bathing.

二、汤剂的特点

7.2.2　The Characteristics of Decoctions

汤剂是中药应用最早、最广泛的一种剂型，具有以下特点：

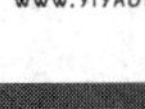

Decoctions are one of the oldest and most widely used dosage forms. The characteristics as follows:

（一）优点

(1) Advantages

1. 以水为溶剂，制法简单，吸收、奏效较为迅速，目前仍为中医临床广泛应用的剂型。

① Water is used as solvent. Because of the easy preparation, rapid absorption and effect, decoctions are still widely used dosage forms in clinical currently.

2. 组方灵活，适应中医临床辨证施治，随证加减用药的需要。

② The formula is flexible, complying with syndrome differentiation and treatment for TCM clinical practice. It can be modified according to symptoms.

3. 中药复方多种活性成分组成的复合分散体系（药物以离子、分子或液滴、不溶性固体微粒等多种形式存在于汤液中）充分发挥复方综合疗效。

③ The compound dispersing system consisted of multiple active ingredients in the formula (ionic, molecular or insoluble liquid drops or particles) can fully exert the comprehensive effects of the formula.

（二）缺点

(2) Disadvantages

1. 挥发性、脂溶性和难溶性成分的提取率或保留率低，可能影响疗效。

① It is hard to conserve volatile and insoluble ingredients, which may influence the treatment effects.

2. 味苦量大，病人依从性较差，特别是儿童难以服用。

② Bitter in taste and large in volume leads to poor compliance for patients, especially for children.

3. 需临用新制，多有不便。

③ It is not convenient for emergent or severe illnesses

4. 久置易发霉变质。

④ It tend to be moldy and decayed after prolonged storage.

三、汤剂的制备与影响质量的因素

7.2.3 Preparation of Decoctions and Factors That Influence the Quality of Decoctions

（一）汤剂的制备

(1) Preparation of Decoctions

1. 汤剂的制法 汤剂一般采用煎煮法制备。工艺过程如图 7-1 所示。

① **Preparation methods of decoctions** Decocting method is often used for decoctions. The procedures are shown in flow Figure 7-1.

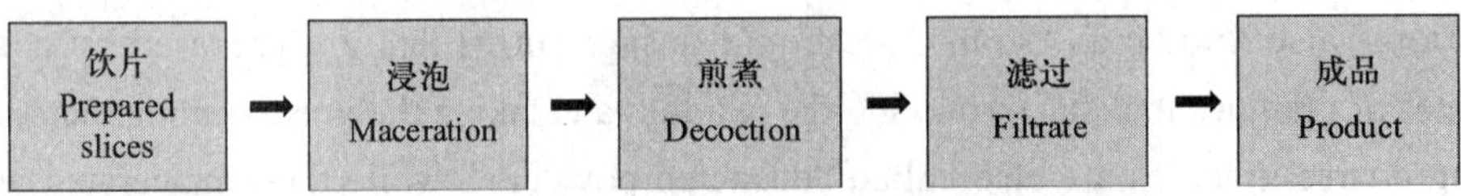

图 7-1 汤剂制备工艺流程

Figure 7-1 Preparation Process Flow of Decoctions

取中药饮片或粗颗粒，置于适宜的容器中，加适量的水浸泡适当时间，加热至沸，保持微沸一定时间，分离煎出液，药渣再煎煮 1~2 次，各次煎出液混合，即为汤剂。

Macerate the prepared slices in suitable container with water for a while, and then heat to boil for a certain period of time and separate extracts. The drug residues should be decocted once or twice more.

Combine all the filtrates to make decoctions.

2. 影响汤剂质量的因素 饮片质量、煎提条件等多个环节均与汤剂质量有关，应从严把握。汤剂内在质量首先在于饮片质量，应使用优质饮片，同时必须符合处方特定炮制要求。煎药器皿传统多用砂锅或陶器（瓦罐），也可选用搪瓷煎器、不锈钢或铝锅，医院煎药目前多已采用电热或蒸汽加热自动煎药机。铜铁器性质活泼，易与中药成分发生反应，忌用。煎煮用水最好采用软化水或纯化水，加水量头煎一般为中药饮片量的6~10倍，或没过药面2~5cm，二煎加水量适当减少。煎煮火候应沸前武火，沸后文火。汤剂煎煮时间通常头煎45~60分钟，二煎20~30分钟。一般煎煮2~3次。具体应视处方饮片性质、药量多少以及设备与工艺条件确定。煎煮最佳条件的控制，以有利有效成分溶出，防止有效成分损失，操作方便，汤液体积适中为原则。

② **Factors that affect the quality of decoctions** The quality of decoctions is associated with many factors, such as quality of prepared slices and decocting parameters, which should be strictly controlled. Fundamentally, the quality of decoctions is related to the quality of the prepared slices, the superior prepared slices should be used and processed according to specific requirements. Marmites or earthenware (crockeries) are frequently used for decocting in the past; ceramics, stainless steel or aluminum pots also can be chosen; in hospitals, automatic decocting machines powered by electricity or steam are widely used nowadays. Both ironware and copperware are forbidden to use, because it tend to react with TCM compositions due to their active chemical properties. Demineralized water or purified water is optimal in decoction. The amount of water is commonly 6 to 10 times of the weight of the prepared slices, or immersing the prepared slices by 2 to 5 cm for the first time and properly decreased for the second time. High heat should be used before ebullition and gentle heat after ebullition. The first time of decocting is 45 to 60 minutes and 20 to 30 minutes for the second time. Prepared slices are usually decocted for 2 to 3 times. The particular parameters depend on the properties and amounts of prepared slices, apparatuses and process conditions. The optimization of decocting conditions should be chosen by the principle which is beneficial to the dissolution of active ingredients, prevented the loss of active ingredients and prepared conveniently and proper volumes.

（二）特殊中药的处理

(2) Disposition of Special Materials

汤剂制备时，方中某些中药不宜或不能同时入煎，需要进行特殊的处理。

During the preparation of decoctions, some materials are not suitable or not able to be decocted together which need to special procedures.

（1）先煎 是将中药先于其他药材煎煮一定时间的操作。①矿物药、贝壳类、角甲类等，因质地坚硬，有效成分难以煎出，如寒水石、赤石脂、牡蛎、鳖甲、水牛角等，可先煎30分钟。②有毒中药，如乌头、附子、雪上一枝蒿、商陆等，要先煎1~2小时，以降低毒性，增加疗效。附子久煎不仅降低毒性，还可释放出钙离子，协同消旋去甲基乌头碱的强心作用。③有些中药先煎才有效，如石斛、天竺黄、藏青果、火麻仁等。石斛所含内酯类生物碱，只有久煎后的水解产物才有效。

① *Decocted earlier* Some materials are decocted for a certain time before the others. A.Minerals, seashells, horns and carapaces are hard in property and it is difficult for effective ingredients to get dissolved form them. For example, Gypsum Ru brum, Halloysitum Rubrum, ostrea gigas Thunberg, Carapax Amydae , Cornu Bubali can be decocted 30 minutes before other materials. B.Toxic medicinal materials, such as Radix Aconiti Carmichaeli, Radix aconite Lateralis Praeparata、Radix Aconiti Brachypodi Seu Penduli, Radix Aconiti Brachypodi Seu Penduli should be decocted 1 to 2hours to

reduce the toxicity and enhance the effects. Prolonged decoction of Radix aconite Lateralis Praeparata can not only reduce the toxicity, but also release ion calcium, which synergizes the cardiotonic function of demethylaconitine. C.Some medicinal materials can only be active after decocted for a long time, such as Dendrobii Caulis、Bambusae Concretio Silicea、Fructus Terminaliae Chebulae Immaturi、Cannabis Semen. The Lactone alkaloids in Dendrobii Caulis can only be active after hydrolysis caused by prolonged decoction.

（2）后下　①气味芳香，含有挥发性成分的中药，如薄荷、藿香、沉香、青蒿、细辛等，应在中药汤剂煎好前 5~10min 入煎，防止挥发性成分挥散损失。②不宜久煎的中药，如钩藤、杏仁、大黄、番泻叶等，后下可防止所含成分水解，药效降低。③含有共存酶的中药，如黄芩等，在沸后入煎，可以灭酶保苷，提高疗效。

② *Decocted later*　A.Aromatic herbs containing volatile ingredients, such as Menthae Haplocalycis Herba, Pogostemonis Herba, Aquilariae Lignum Resinatum, Artemisiae Annuae Herba, Asari Radix et Rhizoma, should be added 5 to 10 minutes before the decoction is done, in order to reduce the loss of volatile ingredients. B.Some herbs can't stand prolonged decoction, such as Uncariae Ramulus Cum Uncis, Armeniacae Semen Amarum, Rhei Radix Et Rhizoma, Sennae Folium. Later decoction can prevent the effective ingredients from hydrolysis and reduction of function. C. Medicinal materials containing coexisting enzymes, such as Scutellariae Radix, are added after boiling, in order to kill enzymes to reserve glycosides and enhance the effects.

（3）包煎　是将中药用滤过介质包裹后入煎的操作。①颗粒细小的花粉类中药，如松花粉、蒲黄；种子类，如葶苈子、菟丝子、苏子；中药细粉，如六一散、黛蛤散等。因其比表面积大，易浮于水面或沉入锅底，需用纱布包裹后与其他中药同煎。②含淀粉、黏液质较多的中药，如车前子、浮小麦、秫米等在煎煮过程中易粘锅底焦糊，并可导致汤剂黏度增加，不利于有效成分溶出和滤过，故需包煎。③附绒毛的中药，如旋覆花等，包煎可防止绒毛脱落进入汤剂刺激咽喉。

③ *Wrapped decoction*　It refers to the procedure that the herbs are decocted with the filtration materials wrapped outside. A.Pollens of small volumes, such as Pini Pollen, Typhae Pollen; seeds, such as Descurainiae Semen, Lepidii Semen, Cuscutae Semen, Perillae Fructus; fine powders of traditional Chinese medicine, such as Liuyi San, Daige San. Because of its large specific surface area, it tends to float on the surface or sink to the bottom, therefore it is necessary to be wrapped with gauze and decocted with other herbs. B. Materials that are abundant in starch or mucin, such as Plantaginis Semen, Fructus Tritici Levis, Fructus Setariae, are inclined to stick to the bottom of the decocting pots and get charred, making the decoction too viscous for extraction and filtration. C.For materials covered with floss, such as Inulae Flos, wrapped decoction can prevent the floss from entering the decoction and irritating the throat.

（4）另煎兑入　是将单味中药单独煎煮，煎出液兑入汤剂共服的操作。贵重中药，为防止其他药渣吸附导致成分损失，可单独煎煮取汁，兑入煎好的汤剂中一起服用。如人参、西洋参、鹿茸等。

④ *Decocting separately*　It refers to the procedure that a single herb is decocted separately, then mix the decoction together for administration. Precious materials, such as Ginseng Radix Et Rhizoma、Panacis Quinquefolii Radix、Cervi Cornu Pantotrichum, to keep the other residue from absorbing the effective ingredients, can be decocted alone and mixed with the prepared decoction for administration.

（5）榨汁　一些需取鲜汁的中药，可直接榨取汁液兑入煎好的汤剂中。如鲜生地、生藕、梨、韭菜、鲜姜、鲜白茅根等。竹沥直接兑入汤剂服用即可。

⑤ *Juicing*　A few single herb which need to take fresh juice, can be squeezed and mixed with the prepared decoctions. such as Rehmanniae Radix, Nelumbinis Rhizomatis Rhizoma, Fructus Pyri, Allii Tuberosi Folium, Zingiberis Rhizoma Recens, Imperatae Rhizoma. Succus Bambusae can be directly mixed with decoctions to use.

（6）烊化 胶类及一些易溶性中药可用开水溶化后兑入。如阿胶、龟甲胶、鹿角胶、鸡血藤膏、蜂蜜、饴糖等，若与其他中药共煎，不但使煎液黏度增大，其本身也易被药渣吸附损失。芒硝、玄明粉等亦可溶化后兑入。

⑥ *Melting* Glues and some soluble materials can be dissolved with hot water and mixed, such as Asini Corii Colla, Testudinis Carapacis et Plastri Colla, Cervi Cornus Colla, Spatholobi Caulis Colla, Mel, cerealose. If those are decocted with other materials, the decoction can be very viscous and they themselves are tend to be absorbed by the residues. Soluble minerals such as Natrii Sulfas, Natrii Sulfas Exsiccatus can also be added after dissolution.

（7）冲服 一些难溶于水的贵重药可制成极细粉兑入汤剂或用汤剂冲服。如牛黄、三七、麝香、羚羊角、朱砂等。

⑦ *Administered after dissovled* Some insolubly precious materials can be pulverized to impalpable powder and added into or mixed with decoction to take, such as Bovis Calculus, Notoginseng Radix et Rhizoma, Moschus, Saigae Tataricae Cornu, Cinnabaris.

除上述影响汤剂质量的因素外，对于汤剂疗效的发挥，还与服药方法、剂量、时间、服药时的饮食情况等因素有关。

Besides the mentioned factors above, the effect of decoctions is also related to the method of take herbs in treatment, dosage, time and the diet of administration

四、煎煮过程对药效的影响

7.2.4 Effects on the Efficacy of the Decoction Process

中药汤剂多为复方，复杂的成分群在煎煮时会发生一系列的物理化学变化，如成分增溶而增效，成分挥发或沉淀而减效，产生新的化合物等。

Decoctions are mostly the compound prescription. A series of physical and chemical changes are taken place during decocting, such as the solubilization leading to synergism, volatilization or precipitation lead to reduce the, or generating new compounds, etc.

1. 成分增溶而增效 复方合煎时，成分间可因增溶而增加某些难溶成分的提取率。如对当归承气汤的研究发现，增加当归的用量，汤液中磷脂的含量增加，大黄总蒽醌的溶出率也随之增加；麻黄、金银花与当归配伍，麻黄碱和绿原酸的溶出率也随当归用量的增加而增加，比无当归组增加 80%~100%。

(1) Synergism due to solubilization of ingredients When decocted together, the extraction rate of some insoluble ingredients can be enhanced due to solubilization. For example, it was reported that in Danggui Chengqi Decoction, the content of phospholipid in the decoction increased with the increasing of Angelicae Sinensis Radix, and so was the dissolution rate of the total anthraquinones from Rhei Radix et Rhizoma. When it comes to the compatibility of Ephedrae Herba, Lonicerae Japonicae Flos and Angelicae Sinensis Radix, the dissolution rate of ephedrine and chlorogenic acid increased with the increasing of Angelicae Sinensis Radix by 80% to 100% compared with the group without Angelicae Sinensis Radix.

2. 成分挥发或沉淀、药渣吸附而减效 挥发性成分在煎煮过程中挥散，受热时间越长损失越大。如柴胡桂枝汤中的桂皮醛煎出量仅为原中药的 5% 以下，而回流提取可达 54%；有些成分间

还可形成不溶性的沉淀而被滤除，如小檗碱和甘草酸、黄芩苷、鞣质等能产生沉淀；黄芩苷与麻黄生物碱也能生成沉淀。群药共煎，药渣吸附有效成分造成损失。贵重药应单煎或原药粉兑入。

(2) Effect reduction due to volatilization or precipitation of ingredients, or the absorption of residues Volatile ingredients are lost during decocting; the longer they are heated, the more they get lost. For example, the extraction rate of cinnaldehydum in Chaihu Guizhi Decoction was only 5% of the original material, while extracted with reflux method, the extraction rate could reach as high as 54%. Some reactions of ingredients may generate insoluble sediments and be filtrated. For example, the reactions between berberine and glycyrrhizic acid, baicalin, tannin produce sediment; the reaction between baicalin and ephedrine also produce sediment. In addition, when decocted all together, the residue may absorb the effective ingredients and cause loss. Therefore, precious medicinal materials should be singularly decocted or added as pulverized powders.

3. 产生新的化合物 汤剂在煎煮过程中，复方成分自身或成分间可发生相互作用，产生新的化合物。如麻黄汤中的麻黄碱和桂皮醛、氰基苯甲醛等成分生成新的化合物；生脉饮方中群药合煎，原来微量的人参皂苷 Rg_3、Rh_1、Rh_2 的含量高出单味人参煎剂含量的 54.83%、52.40%、113.64%。

(3) Generating new compounds During decocting, there may be reactions in the compounds themselves or among other compounds to generate new compounds. For example, the reaction between ephedrine and cinnaldehydum, cyanobenzaldehyde produced new compounds. When decocted together, the trace of ginsenoside Rg3, Rh1 and Rh2 were higher than those of singular decoction of Ginseng Radix Et Rhizoma by respectively 54.83%、52.40% and 113.64%.

另外，混煎可以增加某些成分的稳定性，从而提高疗效。如柴胡皂苷 D 在酸性环境中不稳定，若在方中配有龙骨、牡蛎等制酸物质，可增加柴胡皂苷 D 的稳定性，增加其在汤剂中的含量。

In addition, combined decoction can enhance the stability of some ingredients, hence rise the treatment effect. For example, Saikosaponin D is unstable in acid circumstances, but if combined with antiacid substances such as Os Draconis, Ostreae Concha, the stability of Saikosaponin D can be enhanced and the content of it in the decoction can be increased.

总之，煎煮过程是一个极复杂的过程，方药单煎合并不能完全等效于群药合煎。

In brief, the process of decoction is extremely complicated; the mix of decoctions of every single herb in the formula cannot completely equals the combined decoction.

案例导入 ¦ Case example

案例 7-1 大承气汤

7-1 Dachengqi Tang

处方：大黄（酒洗）12g 厚朴（去皮，炙）24g 枳实（炙）12g 芒硝 9g

Ingredients: Rhei Radix et Rhizoma(wine washed)12g; Magnoliae Officmalis Cortex (peeled and processed)24g; Aurantii Fructus Immaturus(processed)12g; Natvii Sulfas 9g

功能与主治：峻下热结。用于阳明腑实证，大便不通，频转矢气，脘腹痞满，腹痛拒按，按之则硬，甚或潮热谵语，手足濈然汗出，舌苔黄燥起刺，或焦黑燥裂，脉沉实。

Functions and indications: Dramatically purgation of heat accumulation. Used for excessive syndrome of Yangming organs, presenting with constipation, frequent fart, stuffy and full sensation in stomach, abdominal pain refusing to press, stiffness under pressing of abdomen, even with tidal fever,

paroxysmal perspiration in feet and hands, yellow and dry and pricking tongue coating or scorched black and dry and pricking tongue coating, sunken and solid pulse.

热结旁流证，下利清水，色纯青，其气臭秽，脐腹疼痛，按之坚硬有块，口舌干燥，脉滑实。

Diarrhea with retention, presenting with watery and stinky stool, black in its color, abdominal pain, hard with mass under pressure, dry mouth and tongue, smooth and solid pulse.

制法：取厚朴和枳实，加水2000ml，浸泡30分钟，加热至沸，保持微沸30分钟，加入大黄，保持微沸10分钟，滤过去渣，加入芒硝溶化后，即得。

Making Procedure: Macerate Magnoliae Officmalis Cortex and Aurantii Fructus Immaturus with 2000ml of water for 30 minutes, decoct for 30 minutes, add Rhei Radix et Rhizoma to decoct for another 10 minutes, filtrate, add Natrii Sulfas into the decoction.

用法与用量：顿服，通便后停用。

Usage and dosage: take at one draught, quit on defecation.

注解：①大黄泻下作用的成分为大黄总蒽醌苷类，对热不稳定，后下。

②芒硝可溶于水中，直接加入汤剂溶解即可。

Notes: ① The purgative ingredients in Rhei Radix et Rhizoma are the total anthraquinones, unstable to heat and should be decocted afterwards.

② Natvii Sulfas is soluble in water, therefore it can be added directly into the decoction.

思考题 ¦ Questions:

①中药在使用前为什么要进行相应的炮制？

① why should the herbs be processed correspondingly before use?

②中药制剂大生产煎煮时，一些特殊处理的饮片应如何处理？

② In mass production, how to handle some special slices?

第三节 中药合剂（含口服液）
7.3 Chinese Medicinal Mixture (Oral Liquid Included)

PPT

一、中药合剂的含义
7.3.1 The Definition of Chinese Medicinal Mixture

中药合剂系指饮片用水或其他溶剂，采用适宜的方法提取制成的口服液体制剂，单剂量包装者又称“口服液”。合剂一般采用煎煮法、渗漉法来制备，必要时酌加防腐剂和矫味剂，含糖量不得高于20%。

Mixtures are liquid preparations intended for oral administration, prepared by extracting the prepared slices with water or other solvents in appropriate ways (the single dose packed mixtures are also known as “oral solutions”. Mixtures are generally manufactured by decoction or percolation method. Preservatives and flavoring agents are added if necessary. The content of sugar should be no more than 20%.

二、中药合剂的特点

7.3.2 The Characteristics of Chinese Medicinal Mixture

中药合剂与口服液是在汤剂的基础上改进和发展起来的中药剂型，中药合剂一般选用疗效可靠、应用广泛的方剂制备，其特点是：

（一）优点

(1) Advantages

1. 能浸出饮片中的多种有效成分，保证制剂的综合疗效。

① Since multiple effective ingredients in the prepared slices can be extracted, the comprehensive effect of the formula can be ensured.

2. 与汤剂一样，吸收快，奏效迅速。

② As the decoctions, mixtures can be rapidly absorbed and exert the function.

3. 克服了汤剂临用煎煮的麻烦，使用方便。

③ The inconvenience of decoctions that have to be prepared right before clinical use has been eliminated, and therefore mixtures are quite handy.

4. 经过浓缩，服用量减小，且可加入矫味剂，外观和口感都较易接受。

④ The condensation procedure reduces the administration volume, and the flavoring agents are added to improve the appearances and tastes of mixtures.

5. 成品中多加入适宜的防腐剂，并经灭菌处理，密封包装，质量稳定。

⑤ Proper preservatives are usually added into the end products, plus sterilization and tight package, so mixtures are stable in quality.

6. 若单剂量包装（口服液）则携带、保存和服用更方便、准确。

⑥ If packed into single dose container (oral liquids), they are more convenient and accurate in transportation, storage and administration.

（二）缺点

(2) Disadvantages

1. 不能随证加减。

① The formula of mixtures cannot be modified with different patterns.

2. 合剂为水性液体制剂，属于复合分散系统，具有不稳定性，常有沉淀析出。

② Mixtures are aqueous liquid preparation, belong to composite dispersion system. Therefore, they are unstable to produce sediment.

3. 浓缩受热时间长，有效成分可能被破坏。

③ After a long period of heating in condensation, the effective ingredients may be destroyed.

4. 生产工艺较复杂，生产设备、工艺条件要求较高。

④ The procedures included in mixture manufacture are complicated, and the requirements for the equipment and conditions of production is high.

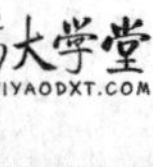

三、中药合剂的制法

7.3.3 Preparation of Chinese Medicinal Mixture

中药合剂制备工艺流程如图 7-2 所示：

The producing flow chart of Chinese medicinal mixtures are shown in Figure 7-2.

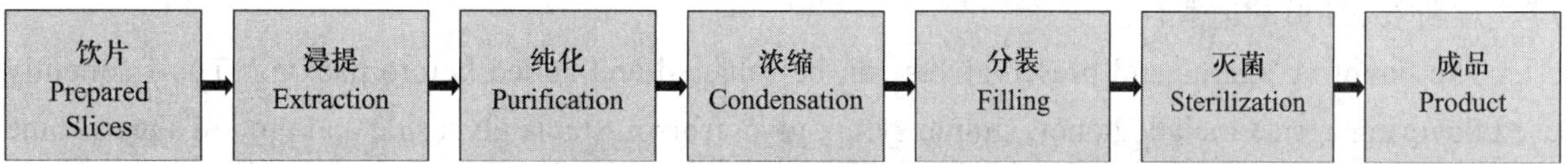

图 7-2 中药合剂的制备工艺流程

Figure 7-2 Preparation Process of Chinese Medicinal Mixtures

（一）浸提

(1) Extraction

一般采用煎煮法，因合剂投料较多，生产上多用具有一定规模的多功能提取罐，煎煮时间较长。含挥发性成分药材用“双提法”，或超临界流体提取收集挥发性成分，药渣与其他药材一起煎煮。热敏性成分多采用渗漉法，减压浓缩。

Decoction method is often applied. On account of the large volumes of the medicinal materials and the long period of processing, multi-functional extraction tanks are frequently used in mass production. “Double extraction method” is usually used for volatile herbs, or supercritical fluid extraction method is first used to collect the volatile ingredients then the residues are decocted with other herbs. The thermosensitive ingredients are extracted with percolation method and condensed with decompression method.

（二）纯化

(2) Purification

现行版《中国药典》规定，中药合剂贮藏期间只允许有少量轻摇易散的沉淀。为减少沉淀量，多需要纯化处理。可将煎出液放置，热处理冷藏，滤出不溶物；或用乙醇沉淀部分杂质，但需注意因沉淀包裹或吸附造成的成分损失；也可用超滤、离心、絮凝（甲壳素、明胶单宁、果汁澄清剂等）、酶解等方法进行净化。无论采用哪种纯化方法，都应注意对有效成分的影响。

According to the requirements of the current edition of *Chinese Pharmacopoeia,* mixtures should be clear, only a small amount of precipitates easily dispersed on shaking allowed. To minus precipitation, purification is possibly needed, in which the decoction is heated and kept in cold storage, and the insoluble is filtrated. Or part of impurity can be precipitated with ethanol (attention should be paid to the loss caused by the enveloping or absorption of precipitates). Ultrafiltration, centrifugation, flocculation (using chitsan, gelatin tannin or juice clarifiers), or enzymolysis methods can also be applied in purification. No matter which method is used, the influence on the effective ingredients should never be ignored.

（三）浓缩

(3) Condensation

净化后的提取液进行浓缩，浓缩程度一般以每日用量在 30~60ml 之间为宜，若太浓，分装困难；若太稀，服用量太大。煎出液经乙醇处理的应先回收乙醇，热敏性成分浓缩时应采用减压浓缩。

The purified extracts should then be condensed, the degree of which is about 30 to 60ml of administration volume per day. If it is too thick, it will cause trouble in packing; if it is too thin, the administration volume will be excessively large. Ethanol should be recovered for ethanol processed extracts, and decompression condensation should be used in the condensation of thermosensitive ingredients.

（四）配液

(4) Dosing

分装前可合理选加矫味剂和防腐剂。常用的矫味剂有蜂蜜、单糖浆、甘草甜素、甜菊苷、蛋

白糖等，也可加入天然香料；常用的防腐剂有山梨酸、苯甲酸、对羟基苯甲酸酯类，使用防腐剂应注意药液 pH 值的适宜性。

The flavoring agents and preservatives can be selected and added before packing. The frequently used flavoring agents include honey, simple syrup, glycyrrhizin, stevia glycoside and protein sugar; some natural perfumes can also be used. And the frequently used preservatives include sorbic acid, benzoic acid and parahydroxybenzoate esters. Attention should be paid to the suitability of pH values of the extracts for preservatives.

加入矫味剂和防腐剂后，搅匀，可按注射液制备工艺要求进行粗滤、精滤后，即得。处方中如含有酊剂、醑剂、流浸膏，应以细流缓缓加入药液中，随加随搅拌，使析出物细腻，分散均匀。配液时可根据需要加入适量的乙醇。

After the flavoring agents and preservatives are added, the mixture should be stirred to even, then rough filtration and refined filtration should be taken first according to the requirement of the preparation for injections. If tinctures, spirits or fluid extracts are involved in the formula, they should be slowly added into the extracts in a thin flow; stir while adding to make the educts silky and evenly dispersed. Suitable amount of ethanol can be added if necessary.

（五）分装

(5) Filling

配液好的药液应及时灌装于无菌洁净的干燥容器中，单剂量包装或多剂量包装。

The mixed liquid should be timely filled into sterile dry containers, in the form of single dose or multiple dose.

（六）灭菌

(6) Sterilization

一般采用煮沸法和流通蒸汽法进行灭菌。亦可在严格避菌条件下，灌装后不经灭菌，直接包装。

Generally boiling method and free flowing steam method are used in sterilization. Under strict aseptic condition, mixtures after filling can be packaged without sterilization.

中药合剂制备时还应注意：①制备过程严格避菌操作，减少污染，尽可能缩短时间；②标签应标明“服时摇匀”；③成品应贮存于阴凉干燥处。

There are some other precautions during preparation of Chinese medicinal mixtures: ① Strict aseptic manipulation is recommended in preparation, in order to reduce pollution and shorten the time as much as possible. ② The term “shaking before use” should be labeled. ③ The end products should be kept in cool and dry places.

四、中药合剂的质量要求与检查

7.3.4 Quality Requirements and Inspections of Chinese Medicinal Mixture

（一）合剂的质量要求

(1) The Quality Requirements of Mixtures

除另有规定外，合剂应澄清。在贮存期间不得有发霉、酸败、异物、变色、产生气体或其他变质现象，允许有少量摇之易散的沉淀。药液的 pH 值、相对密度以及装量、微生物限度均应符合规定要求。

Unless otherwise specified, mixtures should be clear without mold, rancidity, foreign substances, discoloration, gas generation or other degenerative phenomenon during storage. A little precipitates easily

dispersed by shaking can be allowed. The pH values and relative density, as well as packing volumes and microbial limit of mixtures should comply with the requirements.

（二）合剂的质量检查

(2) Inspection Items of Mixture Quality

1. pH 值 照现行版《中国药典》中的测定法测定。

① **PH value** should be inspected according to Determination of pH Value in the current edition of *Chinese Pharmacopoeia*.

2. 相对密度 照现行版《中国药典》中相对密度测定法测定。

② **Relative density** should be inspected according to Determination of Relative Density in the current edition of *Chinese Pharmacopoeia*.

3. 装量 取单剂量灌装的合剂供试品 5 支，将内容物分别倒入经标化的量入式量筒中，在室温下检视，每支装量与标示量相比较，少于标示量的不得多于 1 支，并不得少于标示量的 95%。

③ **Packing volumes** take 5 single dose mixtures, pore the inclusion into standardized measuring cylinder and inspect at room temperature. Compared with the labeled volume, the actual volumes that are less than the labeled volume should be no more than one, and no less than 95%of the labeled quality.

多剂量灌装的合剂，照现行版《中国药典》最低限度检测法检查。

Multiple dose mixtures should be inspected according to the requirements of Minimum Fill in current edition of *Chinese Pharmacopoeia*.

4. 微生物限度 照现行版《中国药典》微生物限度检测法检查。

④ **Microbial limit** should be inspected according to Microbial Examination in the appendix of the current edition of *Chinese Pharmacopoeia*.

案例导入 ¦ Case example

案例 7-2 小建中合剂

7-2 Xiaojianzhong Heji (Xiaojianzhong Mixture)

处方：桂枝 111g 白芍 222g 炙甘草 74g 生姜 111g 大枣 111g 饴糖 370g 苯甲酸钠 3g 蒸馏水适量

Ingredients: Cinnamomi Ramulus 111g; Paeoniae Radix Alba 222g; Glycyrrhizae Radix et Rhizoma Praeparata cum Melle 74g; Zingiberis Rhizoma Recens 111g; Jujubae Fructus 111g; Maltose 370g; Sodium benzoate 3g.

功能与主治：温中补虚，缓急止痛，用于脾胃虚寒，脘腹疼痛，喜温喜按，嘈杂吞酸，食少，胃及十二指肠溃疡见上述证候者。

Functions and indications: To warm the middle energizer, tonify deficiency, relax spasm and relive pain. Used for the pattern of spleen and stomach deficiency cold, manifested as pain in the epigastrium and abdomen, preference for warmth and pressing, stomach upset, acid reflus, and reduced food intake; gastric ulcer and duodenal ulcer with the symptoms described above.

制法：以上五味，桂枝蒸馏提取挥发油，蒸馏后的水液另器收集；药渣与炙甘草、大枣加水煎煮二次，每次 2 小时，合并煎液，滤过，滤液与蒸馏后的水溶液合并，浓缩至约 560ml，白芍、生姜用稀乙醇作溶剂，浸渍 24 小时后进行渗漉，收集渗漉液，回收乙醇后与上述药液合并，静置，滤过，另加饴糖 370g，再浓缩至近 1000ml，加入苯甲酸钠 3g 与桂枝挥发油，加水至 1000ml，搅匀，即得。

Making Procedure: Distill volatile oil from Cinnarnorni Ramulus and collect the aqueous solution in a separate container. Decoct the drug residue, Glycyrrhizae Radix et Rhizoma Praeparata Cum Melle and Jujubae Fructus with water twice, 2hours for each time, combine the decoctions and filter. Combine the filtrates with the above aqueous solution and concentrate to about 560ml. macerate Paeoniae Radix Alba and Zingiberis Rhizoma Recens for 24hours and percolate, using dilute ethanol as solvent. Collect the percolate, recover ethanol and mix with the above concentrated decoction. Allow to stand, filter, add 370g of maltose and concentrate to about 1000ml. add 3g of sodium benzoate, the volatile oil and a quantity of water to a volume of 1000ml and stir well.

用法与用量： 口服，一次 20~30ml，一日 3 次，用时摇匀。

Usage and dosage: For oral administration, 20-30ml per time, three times a day. Shake well before use.

注解： 对于处方中的饮片，要根据所含成分的性质和溶解能力，分别选择最佳溶剂和适宜的方法进行提取。提取液浓缩或回收乙醇，一般采用减压的方式。在最终的合剂中可以添加矫味剂和防腐剂。

Notes: The optimal solvents and extraction methods should be respectively chosen according to the properties and dissolution capacities of the effective ingredients in the prepared slices in the formula. Decompression method is commonly used to condense the liquid or recover the ethanol. Flavoring agents and preservatives can be added into the ultimate mixture.

思考题： 方中加入饴糖和苯甲酸钠的目的是什么？

Question: what are the purpose of adding the maltose and sodium benzoate?

第四节　糖浆剂

7.4 Syrups

PPT

一、糖浆剂的含义

7.4.1 The Definition of Syrups

糖浆剂是指含有饮片提取物的浓蔗糖水溶液，一般含糖量不得低于 45%（g/ml）。糖浆剂供内服。

Syrups are concentrated sucrose solutions which contain herbal extract. The sucrose concentration is no less than 45 %(g/ml). Syrups are intended to oral administration.

二、糖浆剂的特点

7.4.2 The Characteristics of Syrups

糖浆剂具有味甜量小、服用方便、吸收较快的特点，因含有糖和芳香性物质，口感较好，尤其适合于儿童用药；因含糖等营养物质，在制备和贮存过程中极易被微生物污染，制剂中需加入防腐剂；含糖量多，不适于糖尿病患者服用。

Syrups have the characteristics of sweet tastes and small volumes, easy to take and fast absorption.

Syrups taste good for there are sucrose and aromatic materials in syrups, especially for pediatric administration. With nutritional materials such as sucrose, syrups are liable to get contaminated by microbes during storage, so preservatives should be added. With much sucrose in syrups, they are not for diabetics.

三、糖浆剂的分类
7.4.3 The Classification of Syrups

根据糖浆剂的组成及用途可以分为以下几类：

According to the compositions and administration purposes, syrups can be divided into the following kinds:

1. 单糖浆 蔗糖的近饱和水溶液，其浓度为 85.0%（g/ml）或 64.71%（g/g）。不含任何药物，可用作矫味剂、助悬剂、黏合剂等。

(1) Simple syrups. Referring to the almost saturated aqueous solution of sucrose, with the concentration 85.0 %(g/ml) or 64.71 %(g/g), without any drug substance, used as the flavoring agent, suspending agent and adhesive.

2. 芳香糖浆 含芳香性物质或果汁的浓蔗糖水溶液。不作药用，主要用作矫味剂。如橙皮糖浆。

(2) Aromatic syrups. Referring to the strong aqueous solution of sucrose containing aromatic substances or juice, such as orange syrup, used as a flavoring agent not a medicine.

3. 药用糖浆 含有饮片或中药提取物的浓蔗糖水溶液，用于治疗。如复方百部止咳糖浆具有清肺止咳作用，五味子糖浆具有益气补肾、镇静安神作用。

(3) Medicinal syrups. Referring to the strong aqueous solution of sucrose containing extracts of prepared slices, used for clinical treatment, such as Compound Baibu Zhike Syrup, which has a function of long clearance and cough suppression and Wuweizi Syrup, which can replenish qi, engender fluid, tonify the kidney and calm the heart.

四、糖浆剂的制法
7.4.4 Preparation of Syrups

中药糖浆剂的制备工艺过程见图 7-3。

The procedure of preparation Chinese medicinal syrups is shown in Figure 7-3.

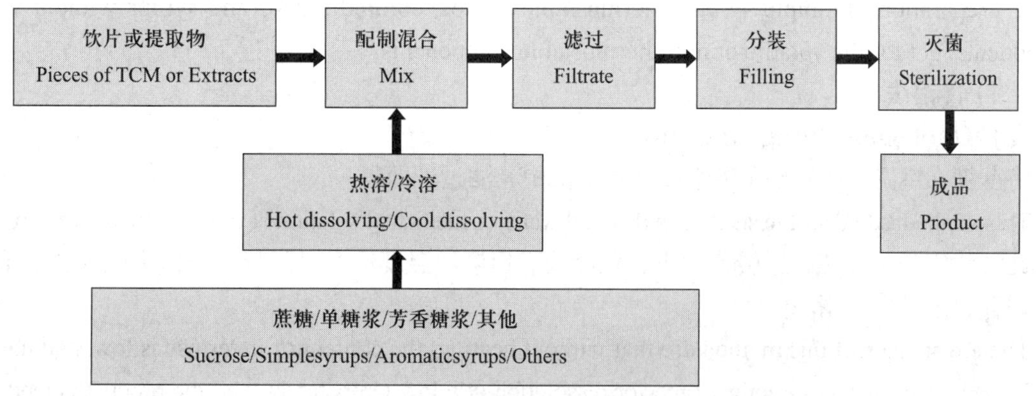

图 7-3 中药糖浆剂的制备工艺流程

Figure 7-3 Preparation Process of Chinese Medicinal Syrups

浸提、纯化、浓缩内容详见“中药合剂”相应项下。根据配制过程中蔗糖的加入方式，可分为溶解法和混合法，溶解法又包括热溶法和冷溶法。所用蔗糖应符合现行版《中国药典》规定。

For more details of extraction, purification and condensation, please refer to the contents under *Chinese Medicinal Mixtures*. According to different ways by which sucrose is added, preparation process of syrups are divided into dissolving method and blending method, and dissolving method further includes hot dissolving method and cool dissolving method. The sucrose used in preparation should be complied with the requirements of the current edition of *Chinese Pharmacopeia*.

（一）热溶法

(1) Hot Dissolving Method

将蔗糖加到沸腾的蒸馏水（或饮片浓煎液）中溶解，加入可溶性药物，搅拌溶解后，趁热滤过，自滤器上加蒸馏水至全量即得。若趁热滤过仍有困难者，可用滤纸浆、滑石粉等助滤剂，以吸附杂质，提高澄清度。

Dissolve sucrose in boiling distilled water (or condensed extracts of preparation slices), add soluble drug substances, stir to dissolve, filter while it is still hot, and add distilled water from the filter to the required volume. Filter aids such as filter paper pulp or talcum powder can be added if filtration is difficult, in order to absorb impurities and enhance the clarity.

加热溶解时间不宜太长（一般沸后 5 分钟即可），温度也不宜超过 100℃，避免蔗糖转化（蔗糖在加热或酸性条件下易水解成一分子果糖和一分子葡萄糖，果糖和葡萄糖 1∶1 的混合物也叫转化糖）。果糖受热易转化成有色物质，制品颜色加深，微生物在单糖中也容易滋生。

Heat time should not be too long, (commonly around 5 minutes after boiling), and the temperature should not be over 100℃ to avoid the inversion of sucrose (in the condition of heating or acid circumstances, one sucrose molecule is inclined to be hydrolyzed into one fructose molecule and one glucose molecule, the mixture of which is also called invert sugar). The fructose is easily converted into colored substances by heat, which leads to darken the color of the product. Meanwhile, microbes are liable to grow in monosaccharides.

此法优点是蔗糖溶解速度快，药液流动性好，容易滤过；加热可使糖中的蛋白质变性凝固，便于去除；可杀灭微生物，利于保存。适于单糖浆、不含挥发性成分的糖浆、热稳定性药物的糖浆剂及有色糖浆剂。但对挥发性、不耐热的药物不适合。

The advantages of this method are that sucrose can be rapidly dissolved. The liquid has good fluidity and is easily filtered. The proteins in sucrose can be denatured and concreted by heating, for easy removal. Microbes can be killed during heating, so it is beneficial to preserve. This method is intended for the preparation of simple syrups, thermostable syrups, colored syrups and syrups without volatile components, not for the volatile or non-thermostable components.

（二）冷溶法

(2) Cool Dissolving Method

将蔗糖在室温下溶解于蒸馏水或药物溶液中，滤过，即得。

This method is to dissolve sucrose in distilled water or medicinal solution at room temperature, then filter.

此法优点是不加热，含转化糖少，色泽浅。但溶解温度低，时间长，易污染微生物，不利于成品保存，故较少应用。

The advantages of this method are that without heating, the content of invertose is low, and the color is light. However, it takes a longer time for dissolution at a low temperature, and the product is tend to get contaminated by microbes, which is not good for preservation and storage, so it is used relatively more rarely.

适用于单糖浆和不宜加热的糖浆剂，如含挥发性成分、热敏性成分的药物。

This method is intended for the preparation of simple syrups and non-thermostable syrups, such as syrups containing volatile or thermosensitive components.

（三）混合法

(3) Blending Method

将药物与计算量的单糖浆直接混合或溶解制备糖浆剂的方法。根据药物的性质可分为以下几种情况：

This method is to directly blend or dissolve drug substances with calculated amount of simple syrup, depending on the properties of the drug substances, blending method are used as follows:

1. 水溶性固体药物 水中溶解度大的，先用少量蒸馏水制成浓溶液；水中溶解度小的，加适宜的辅助剂使溶解后与单糖浆混合。

① **The drug substances are soluble solid** If the solubility is high in water, strong solutions can be prepared first with small amount of distilled water; if the solubility is low in water, suitable auxiliary substances can be added first to dissolve then mixed with the simple syrup.

2. 药物为液体 水性液体可直接与单糖浆混匀；含乙醇液体与单糖浆混合时易产生浑浊，可加入适量的甘油，或加助滤剂滤过至澄清；若为挥发油，可先溶于少量的乙醇或应用增溶剂，溶解后与单糖浆混合。

② **The drug substances are liquid** Aqueous liquid can be mixed directly with the simple syrup; liquid containing ethanol tend to precipitate on mixing, therefore suitable amount of glycerin or filtrate aids can be added then filtrate until the liquid is clear; if the liquid is volatile oil, it can be dissolved with small amount of ethanol or solubilizer, and then mixed with the simple syrup after dissolution.

3. 饮片 应先提取、精制后加入单糖浆中；干浸膏先粉碎成细粉，加少量的甘油或其他稀释剂，在研钵中研匀后与单糖浆混合。

③ **Prepared slices** Prepared slices should be extracted and refined before add into the simple syrup. Dry extracts should be pulverized to fine powder first, then add small amount of glycerin or other dilutes, mix well, and mix with the simple syrup in the mortar.

中药糖浆剂一般从饮片开始，经提取、净化、浓缩至适当浓度，将浓缩液与糖或单糖浆、防腐剂、矫味剂等混合均匀，加水到全量，静置 24 小时，滤过即得。配制时应在清洁避菌的环境中进行，并应及时灌装于灭菌的洁净干燥容器中。

The preparation of Chinese medicinal syrups starts generally from the prepared slices, through extraction, purification and appropriate condensation, then the concentrates are mixed with sucrose or simple syrup, preservatives, flavoring agents, add water to the required volume, allow to stand for 24hours and filtrate. The mixing procedure should be carried out in clean and sterile environments, and be promptly irrigated into sterilized clean and dry containers.

五、糖浆剂的质量要求与检查及质量问题讨论

7.4.5 Discussion on Quality Control of Syrups

（一）糖浆剂的质量要求

(1) Quality Requirements for Syrup

除另有规定外，制剂应澄清。在贮存期间不得有发霉、酸败、产生气体或其他变质现象，允许有少量摇之即散的沉淀。

Unless otherwise specified, syrups should be clear. There are no mold rancidity, or generating gases or other metamorphism during storage. Small amount of precipitates easily dispersed on shaking is allowed.

糖浆剂含蔗糖量应不低于 45%（g/ml）。其他应符合现行版《中国药典》附录的相关规定。

The sucrose content in syrups should be no less than 45% (g/ml). Other aspects of syrups should comply with the corresponding requirements of the current version of *Chinese pharmacopeia*.

（二）糖浆剂的质量检查

(2) Quality Inspections of Syrup

1. pH 值 照现行版《中国药典》中 pH 值测定法测定。

① **pH value** Should be inspected according to Determination of pH Value in the current edition of *Chinese Pharmacopoeia*.

2. 相对密度 照现行版《中国药典》中相对密度测定法测定。

② **Relative density** Should be inspected according to Determination of Relative Density in the current edition of *Chinese Pharmacopoeia*.

3. 装量 取单剂量灌装的糖浆剂供试品 5 支，将内容物分别倒入经标化的量入式量筒中，在室温下检视，每支装量与标示量相比较，少于标示量的不得多于 1 支，并不得少于标示量的 95%。

③ **Packing volumes** Take 5 containers, pour the contents into a previously calibrated graduated cylinder as completely as possible. Measure the volume of the contents in each cylinder at room temperature. Not more than 1 of the volume should be less than labelled quantity, and none should be less than 95% of labelled quantity.

多剂量灌装的糖浆剂，照现行版《中国药典》中最低装量检测法检查。

Multi-dose syrups should comply with the test of Minimum Fill required by the current version of *Chinese pharmacopoeia*.

4. 微生物限度 照现行版《中国药典》中微生物限度检测法检查。

④ **Microbial limit** Should be inspected according to Microbial Examination in the current edition of *Chinese Pharmacopoeia*.

（三）糖浆剂质量问题讨论

(3) Discussion on the Quality of Syrup

糖浆剂存在的主要问题是长霉发酵和产生沉淀两大问题。

There are two main problems of syrups: mildew and fermentation, schlammbildung.

1. 长霉发酵 糖浆剂被微生物污染后长霉发酵，引起糖浆变质霉败。生产单位应从生产工艺管理、糖和原料的处理、配料、滤过和包装材料等各工序加强防范微生物污染的措施。另外，制剂中适当添加防腐剂（见本章中药合剂）。加防腐剂时一定要注意到糖浆 pH 值对防腐剂防腐效能的影响。

① **Mildew and fermentation** Syrups contaminated by microbes tend to mildew and ferment, which causes syrups to metamorphic mould. To prevent this phenomenon, the manufacturer should reinforce prevention against microbial pollution from every section of production, such as management of preparation process, disposition of sucrose and other raw materials, mixing, filtering and filling. In addition, suitable preservatives can be added into the preparations (referring to *Chinese medicinal mixture* in this chapter). Attention must be paid to the influence of pH value to the capacity of preservatives.

2. 沉淀问题 沉淀的来源主要有以下几方面：①药材中微小颗粒或杂质，净化处理不够；②药液中的高分子化合物陈化聚集沉降；③有些成分温度高时溶解，冷却到室温即沉淀析出；

④糖浆剂的 pH 值变化，某些物质溶解度降低而沉降；⑤所用糖含有较多杂质，是由滤过不彻底导致的。

② **Precipitation problems** The sources of sediment mainly include the following aspects: A.Tiny particles or impurities from prepared slices not completely eliminated. B. Aging, aggregation and sedimentation of polymeric compounds in the decoction. C.Solubility variation of some components ranging from high temperature to room temperature. D.Solubility decreasing of some components due to alteration of pH value. E.Too many impurities from sucrose, caused by incomplete filtration.

对于糖浆剂中的沉淀，应视具体情况采取相应的净化措施或添加适当的附加剂尽量减少沉淀出现。对于因热溶冷沉出现的沉淀，往往不认为是无效物质，因而现行版《中国药典》关于糖浆剂的质量标准中允许有少量轻摇即散的沉淀。

For the sediments in syrups, corresponding purification or suitable additives should be used depending on particular situation to reduce the precipitation as much as possible. Sediments due to alteration of temperature are not regarded as useless, that's why in the current edition of *Chinese Pharmacopeia* small amount of precipitates easily dispersed on shaking is allowed.

案例导入 ¦ Case example

案例 7-3 健脾糖浆

7-3 Jianpi Syrup

处方：党参 51.3g 炒白术 76.9g 陈皮 51.3g 枳实（炒）51.3g 炒山楂 38.5g 炒麦芽 51.3g 蔗糖 650g 苯甲酸 3g 蒸馏水适量

Ingredients: Codonopsis Radix 51.3g; Atractylodis Macrocephlae Rhizoma (stir-baked) 76.9g; Citri Reticulatae Pericarpium 51.3g; Aurantii Fructus Immaturus (stir-baked) 51.3g; Crataegi Fructus (stir-baked) 38.5g; Hordei Fructus Germinatus (stir-baked) 51.3g; sucrose 650g; Benzoic Acid 3g.

功能与主治：健脾开胃。用于脾胃虚弱，脘腹胀痛，食少便溏。

Functions and indications: To fortify the spleen and increase the appetite. Used for pattern of spleen-stomach weakness, manifested as distension and fullness in the epigastrium and abdomen, poor appetite and sloppy stool.

制法：以上六味，将陈皮提取挥发油，药渣与其余党参等五味加水煎煮三次，每次 1.5 小时，滤过，合并滤液，浓缩至 450ml。另取蔗糖 650g 加水适量煮沸，滤过，与浓缩液合并，加入苯甲酸钠 3g，混匀，放冷，加入陈皮挥发油，加水至 1000ml，混匀，即得。

Making Procedure: Extract the essential oil in Citri Reticulatae Pericarpium, decoct the residue and the other five ingredients with water for three times, 1.5hours for each time, filter, combine the filtrate and concentrate to 450ml. Weigh 650g of sucrose, add a quantity of water, and heat to boil, filter, combine with the concentrative liquid, add 3g of sodium benzoate, mix well and cool, add the essential oil of Citri Reticulatae Pericarpium, dilute with water to 1000ml, mix well.

用法与用量：口服，一次 10~15ml，一日 2 次。

Usage and dosage: For oral administration, 10-15ml per time, twice a day.

注解：本制剂采用混合法制备。浓缩时尽量采用减压浓缩，以减少成分受热破坏。

Notes: This preparation was manufactured with the blending method. Decompression concentration is recommended to lower the ingredient loss in heating.

思考题：①提取挥发油的方法有几种？

②用苯甲酸钠做防腐剂，制剂的 pH 值应在什么范围内？

Questions: ① How many methods are there to extract the volatile oil?

② If sodium benzoate is used as the preservative, what is the range of the pH value?

第五节　煎膏剂（膏滋）

7.5　Concentrated Decoctions

PPT

一、煎膏剂的含义

7.5.1　The Definition of Concentrated Decoctions

煎膏剂系指饮片用水煎煮，取煎煮液浓缩，加炼蜜或糖（或转化糖）制成的半流体制剂。煎膏剂以滋补为主，兼有缓慢的治疗作用，故又名膏滋。多用于慢性疾病，如益母草膏、养阴清肺膏等。

Concentrated decoctions are semi-fluid preparations which are prepared by decoction and concentrated, then adding honey or sugar (or invert sugar). Concentrated decoctions are mainly regarded to be tonifying with chronic treatment, so they are also called “tonifying extracts”, used for chronic diseases, such as Yimucao concentrated decoction, Yangyin Qingfei concentrated decoction.

二、煎膏剂的特点

7.5.2　The Characteristics of Concentrated Decoctions

（一）优点

(1)　Advantages

1. 药物浓度高，有良好的保存性。

① High concentration of components and fine storability.

2. 体积小，便于服用。

② Easily to take with small volume.

3. 含有蜂蜜、蔗糖而味美适口，病者乐于服用，如枇杷蛇胆川贝膏。

③ The patients are willing to take because of good taste by containing honey or sucrose,, such as Pipa Shedan Chuanbei concentrated decoction.

（二）缺点

(2)　Disadvantages

经过长时间的加热浓缩，成分易挥发或破坏。因而热敏性药物及挥发性成分为主的饮片不宜制成煎膏剂。

Heated for a long time during condensation, the effective components tend to be volatilized or destroyed. So thermosensitive materials or prepared slices mainly containing volatile components are not for concentrated decoctions.

三、煎膏剂的制法

7.5.3 Preparation of Concentrated Decoctions

煎膏剂用煎煮法提取，其一般工艺流程见图 7-4。

Decoction method is usually used for extraction. The preparation process is shown in Figure 7-4.

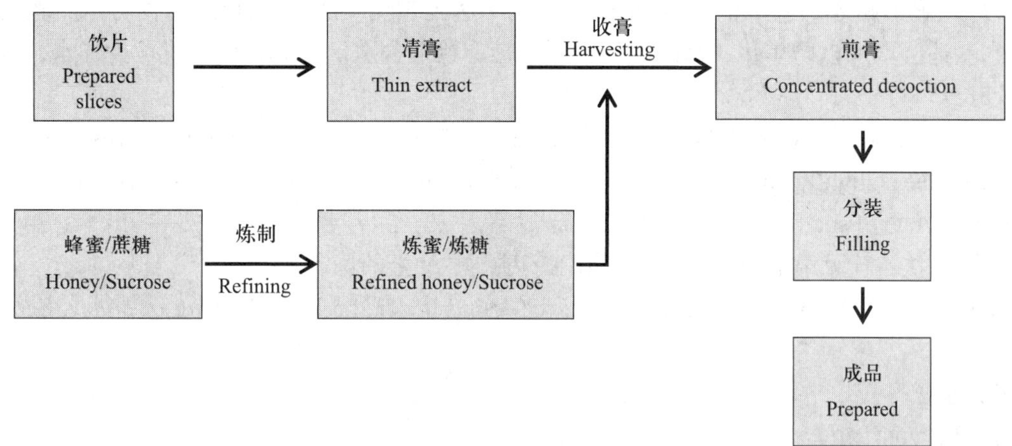

图 7-4 煎膏剂制备工艺流程图

Figure 7-4 Preparation Process of Soft Extract

（一）煎煮

(1) Decocting

根据处方饮片的性质，加水煎煮 2~3 次，每次 2~3h，滤过，合并滤液，静置，滤过。

Based on the properties of the prepared slices in the formula, decoct for 2-3 times, 2-3hours for each time, filter, combine the filtrate, leave to stand and filter again.

处方中若含胶类，如阿胶、鹿角胶等，除发挥治疗作用外，还有助于药液增稠收膏，应烊化后在收膏时加入。贵重细料药可粉碎成细粉待收膏后加入。

Colloidal materials in the formula, such as Colla Corii Asini and Colla Cornus Cervi help to increase the density of the extract, as well as their curative actions, so they should be added during harvest after dissolved. Precious materials with small quantity should be ground to fine powder and added after harvest.

（二）浓缩

(2) Condensing

将滤液浓缩至规定的相对密度，或趁热蘸取浓缩液滴于桑皮纸上，以液滴周围无渗出水迹为度。即得“清膏”。浓缩过程应注意防止焦糊。

Condense the filtrate to the required relative density, or to the degree that no water trace would be found after dripping a drop of the condensed extract onto a piece of mulberry paper. At this moment, the condensed extract is called thin extract. Scorches should be prohibited during condensation.

（三）炼糖（炼蜜）

(3) Refining Sucrose/Honey

煎膏剂中的蔗糖和蜂蜜必须炼制之后加入。炼糖（炼蜜）的目的在于除去杂质，杀灭微生物，减少水分，防止“返砂”（“返砂”是指煎膏剂贮藏过程中析出糖晶的现象。其可能原因是煎膏剂中总糖量过高或炼糖的转化率过低或过高所致。炼糖的目的之一在于使蔗糖部分转化成转化糖）。

Honey and sucrose should be refined before added. The aims are that eliminating impurities, killing microbes, reducing water content and preventing *sugar crystallization.* (*Sucrose crystallization* is a phenomenon of appearance of sucrose crystal during storage. Reasons for this phenomenon may be excessiveness of the total sugar or excessively high or low rate of conversion. One of the aims of refining sucrose is to partially convert sucrose to invert sugar.)

炼糖的方法：取蔗糖适量，加入糖量 50% 的水和 0.1% 酒石酸，加热溶解，保持微沸，炼至“滴水成珠，脆不黏牙，色泽金黄”，使糖的转化率达到 40%~50%，即得。冰糖含水量较小，炼制时加水量适当增加以防焦化，炼制时间相对较短。饴糖含水量较大，炼制时可少加水，炼制时间相对较长。

The way to refine sucrose: Add 50% of water and 0.1% of tartaric acid into the sucrose, dissolve by heating, keep them slightly boiling, until *droplets turns spheroid, color turns golden, crisp not sticky*, and the conversion rate of sucrose reaches 40%-50%.

炼蜜的方法：详见第十四章“丸剂”第三节项下“蜂蜜的炼制”。

The way to refine honey: More details can be found under the item *Refining of honey*, Section 3, Chapter 14.

（四）收膏

(4) Harvesting

除另有规定外，取清膏，于 100℃ 以下加入不超过清膏 3 倍量的炼糖或炼蜜。收膏时煎膏剂的相对密度一般为 1.4 左右。亦可采用经验方法判断：①沸腾时膏滋表面出现“龟背纹”，用细棒或膏滋板趁热取样挑起，出现“挂旗”现象；②取样将膏液蘸于示指与拇指上共捻，能拉出约 2cm 左右的白丝（俗称“打白丝”）；③用细棒趁热蘸取膏液滴于桑皮纸上，不现水迹等。收膏时膏的稠度经验指标，总体冬季稍稀，夏季稍稠些。

Unless otherwise specified, the volume of refined honey or sucrose added should no more than 3 times of that of the thin extract at 100℃, and the relative density of the mixture reaches around 1.4. It can also be judged by empirical method: ① On the appearance of *tortoise shell pattern* during boiling, pick the extract with a stick or board while it is hot, if there is *flagging* phenomenon; ② placing the extract on the forefinger or thumb and rubbing between, if white silk about 2 cm in length can be drawn (known as *milling white silk*); ③ dripping a small volume of extract with a stick onto a piece of mulberry paper without appearance of water stain. When it comes to the experience index of the harvest timing, the extracts are generally thinner in winter and thicker in summer.

（五）分装

(5) Subpackage

煎膏剂半流体状，黏稠度高，为便于分装和取用，多用大口瓶盛装。容器应洁净卫生。待煎膏剂冷至室温后分装，或分装后瓶口朝下放置，冷到室温后再正向存放。避免水蒸气回流到煎膏剂表面，久贮产生霉败现象。

Since the concentrated decoctions are semi-fluid with high viscosity, to facilitate filling and administration, wide-mouth bottles are frequently applied. The containers should be clean and hygienic. Concentrated decoctions should be filled after getting cooled down to the room temperature, or filled into bottles upside down and reversed after getting cooled down to the room temperature. This can prevent the steam backflowing onto the surface of the concentrated decoctions and producing mold.

四、煎膏剂的质量要求与检查

7.5.4 Quality Requirements and Inspections of Concentrated Decoction

（一）煎膏剂的质量要求

(1) Quality Requirements for Concentrated Decoctions

煎膏剂应质地细腻，无焦臭异味，无糖的结晶析出，不得霉败。检查方法：一般取煎膏剂 5g，加热水 200ml，搅拌溶化，3 分钟后观察，不得有焦屑等异物（微量细小纤维、颗粒不在此限）。

Concentrated decoctions should be exquisite in texture, without burnt or other abnormal odors, without sucrose crystal or molds. Inspection method: to 5g of concentrated decoctions add 200ml of hot water, stir to dissolve, allow to stand for 3 minutes. No foreign matters such as scorched masses, etc. should be observed.

返砂等问题的讨论：煎膏剂贮存期间常会析出一些结晶，俗称“返砂”。返砂问题与煎膏剂中的总糖量和糖的转化率有关。一般控制总糖量在 85% 以下为宜。炼糖的转化率应控制在 40%~50%，若转化率低于 35%，易出现以蔗糖为主的结晶；转化率高于 60%，易出现以葡萄糖为主的结晶。蔗糖的转化易在加热和酸性条件下进行，收膏时尽量缩短加热时间和温度，必要时调整药液的 pH 值，防止蔗糖进一步转化。

Discussion on sugar crystallization: The appearance of crystal is called sucrose crystallization. Sucrose crystallization is relevant to the total sugar amount in concentrated decoctions or the conversion rate of the sucrose. For most of the time, the total sugar amount should be controlled below 85%, or the conversion rate of sucrose within 40%-50%. If the conversion rate is lower than 35%, it tends to produce crystal that is mainly composed of sucrose; if the conversion rate is higher than 60%, it tends to produce crystal that is mainly composed of glucose. The conversion of sucrose is inclined to take place under heated and acid conditions, therefore, a shortened heating time and lowered temperature is recommended; adjust the pH value of the medicinal liquid if necessary to prevent the further conversion of the sucrose.

（二）煎膏剂的质量检查

(2) Quality Inspection of Concentrated Decoctions

1. 相对密度 除另有规定外，取供试品适量，精密称定，加水约 2 倍，精密称定，混匀，作为供试液。照现行版《中国药典》中相对密度测定法测定。凡加入饮片药粉的煎膏剂，不检查相对密度。

① **Relative density** Unless otherwise specified, weigh accurately an appropriate quantity of concentrated decoctions being examined, dilute with double quantities of water, weigh accurately and mix well as test solution. Carry out the Determination of Relative Density required by the current version of *Chinese pharmacopoeia*. Concentrated decoctions with powders of prepared slices are not for this inspection.

2. 不溶物 取供试品 5g，加热水 200ml，搅拌使溶化，放置 3 分钟后观察。加饮片细粉的煎膏剂应在未加入药粉前检查，符合规定后，方可加入药粉，加入药粉后不再检查不溶物。

② **Insoluble matter** To 5g of concentrated decoctions add 200ml of hot water, stir to dissolve, allow to stand for 3 minutes. The concentrated decoctions with fine powder of prepared slices should be examined and should comply with the requirements before the powder is added. It is not necessary to examine the insoluble matters after the powder is added.

3. 装量 照现行版《中国药典》中最低限度检测法检查。

③ **Packing volumes** Carry out the method for the Determination of the Minimum Fill by the requirement of the appendix of the current version of *Chinese Pharmacopoeia.*

4. 微生物限度 照现行版《中国药典》中微生物限度检测法检查。

④ **Microbial limit** Carry out the method for the Determination of the Microbial Limit by the requirement of the current version of *Chinese Pharmacopoeia.*

案例导入 ¦ Case example

案例 7-4 益母草膏

7-4 Yimucao Gao

处方：益母草 2500g 红糖适量

Ingredients: Leonurus japonicus 2500g; brown sugar suitable amount

功能与主治：活血调经。用于血瘀所致的月经不调、产后恶露不绝，症见月经量少、淋漓不净、产后出血时间过长；产后子宫复旧不全症见上述证候者。

Functions and indications: To promote the blood circulation and regulate menstruation. Used for menstrual irregularity and postpartum persistent flow of lochia due to blood stasis, manifested as decreased and dribbling menstruation, prolonged bleeding postpartumly; Postpartum Uterine Rehabilitation Disorder with the symptoms described above.

制法：取益母草，切碎，加水煎煮二次，每次 2 小时，合并煎液，滤过，滤液浓缩至相对密度为 1.21~1.25（80°C）的清膏。每 100g 清膏加红糖 200g，加热溶化，混匀，浓缩至规定的相对密度，即得。

Making Procedure: Cut Leonurus japonicus into pieces and decoct with water twice, 2hours for each. Combine the decoctions, filter and evaporate the filtrate until its relative density reaches 1.21-1.25 (80°C). To every 100g of the thin extract add 200g of brown sugar. Heat to dissolve, mix well and concentrate to the required relative density.

用法与用量：口服，一次 10g，一日 1~2 次。

Usage and dosage: For oral administration, 10g every time, once or twice a day.

注解：煎膏剂黏稠度高，渗透压高，不易滋生微生物，不需添加防腐剂，但分装方法要得当。

Notes: Concentrated decoctions are high in viscosity and osmosis, that's why we don't have to add preservatives to suppress the growth of microbes. But still attention should be paid during filling.

思考题 ¦ Questions:

①煎膏剂的相对密度如何测定和计算？

① How to determine and calculate the relative density of concentrated decoctions?

②煎膏剂如何分装才能避免微生物的滋生？

② How to avoid microbial pollution during packing?

PPT

第六节　酒剂与酊剂

7.6　Medicinal Wines and Tinctures

一、酒剂与酊剂的含义

7.6.1　The Definitions of Medicinal Wines and Tinctures

（一）酒剂

(1) Medicinal Wines

酒剂系指饮片用蒸馏酒提取制成的澄清液体剂型，民间俗称“药酒”。用于制备酒剂的蒸馏酒多为谷类白酒。酒剂多供内服，常酌加矫味剂和着色剂。

Medicinal wines are clear liquid preparations which are prepared by maceration and extraction of prepared slices with distilled wine, also called *Medicinal Spirit* by folks. The distilled liquor used to prepare medicinal wines is mostly grain liquor. Medicinal wines are mostly for internal use, with flavoring agents and coloring agents added.

中医认为酒甘辛大热，具有通血脉、行药势、散寒等功效，对治疗风寒湿痹，具有祛风活血、止痛散瘀作用的方剂制成酒剂应用，药借酒势，效果更佳。以酒为溶剂，大多数中药有效成分可以溶解并可减少水溶性杂质的溶出。

Spirits are regarded by TCM as sweet and pungent in taste and hot in property, and they can dredge blood vessels, promote medicinal actions and dispel coldness, so prescriptions used against wind - cold - dampness arthralgia or prescriptions used for wind dispelling and blood circulation promotion, pain arresting and blood stasis removing can be made into medicinal wines, since the actions can be promoted by spirits, which doubles the curative effects. Using spirit as solvent can dissolve the effective ingredients in most medicinal materials and meanwhile reduce the dissolution of some water-soluble impurities.

（二）酊剂

(2) Tinctures

酊剂系指饮片用规定浓度的乙醇提取或溶解制成的澄清液体制剂，也可用稀释法制备，供口服或外用。酊剂不加矫味剂或着色剂。除另有规定外，含有毒性药的酊剂，每 100ml 应相当于原饮片 10g；其他酊剂，每 100ml 相当于原饮片 20g。有效成分明确者，应根据半成品的含量加以调整，使之符合各酊剂项下的规定。

Tinctures are clear liquid preparations which extracted or dissolved in ethanol at a specified concentration. It also can be prepared by dilution method. They are intended to oral administration or external application. Flavoring agents or colorants are not added into tinctures. Unless otherwise specified, 100ml of the tinctures are equivalent to 20g of the prepared slices. Each 100ml of tinctures containing poisonous drugs are equivalent to 10g of the prepared slices. For tinctures with exact effective ingredients the contents should be adjusted according to the contents of the semi-finished products to meet the requirement under the items of tinctures.

二、酒剂和酊剂的特点
7.6.2 The Characteristics of Medicinal Wines and Tinctures

酒剂和酊剂都为含乙醇制剂，乙醇能助药势，增加水中难溶药物的溶解度，还具有使用方便、易于保存、稳定性好等优点，但由于乙醇的刺激性（生理作用），小儿、孕妇、心脏病及高血压病人不宜服用。

Both medicinal wines and tinctures contain ethanol, which can promote the effects of medicines and increase the solubility of insoluble components. What's more, they have the advantages of convenient to administration and storage, good stability. But because of the stimulant of ethanol (physiological action), children, pregnant women and patients with heart diseases or hypertension should not use them.

三、酒剂与酊剂的制法
7.6.3 Preparation of Medicinal Wines and Tinctures

（一）酒剂的制法
(1) Preparation of Medicinal Wines

酒剂可用浸渍法、回流法、渗漉法等制备，其一般流程图如图 7-5 所示。

Medicinal wines are made by maceration, percolation or reflux method, the work flow of which is shown in Figure 7-5.

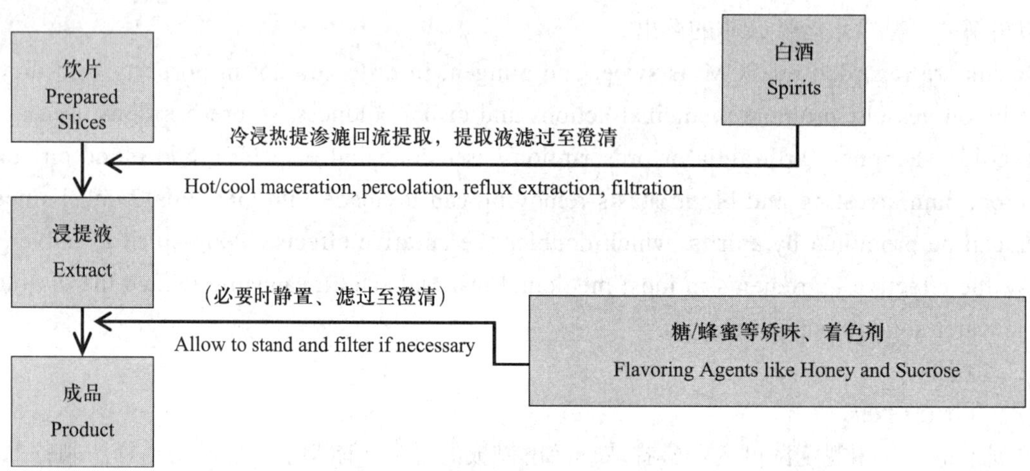

图 7-5 酒剂制备工艺流程图

Figure 7-5 Preparation Process of Medicinal Wines

1. 冷浸法 药材处理后置带盖容器中，加规定量的白酒密闭浸渍，取上清液，药渣压榨，压榨液与上清液合并，加入糖或蜂蜜，搅拌溶解，静置，滤过澄清，分装。如人参天麻药酒。

① **Cool maceration method** Medicinal materials are put into a container with a cover after predisposition, and then add certain amount of spirit, seal and macerate. Take out the supernatant, squeeze the residues, combine the supernatant with the squeezed liquid, add sucrose or honey, and stir to dissolve, leave to stand, filter, and fill, such as Renshen Tianma Medicinal Wine.

2. 热浸法 热浸法称为煮酒，是制备酒剂的传统方法。系将药材加工后置带盖容器中，加规定量的白酒，用蒸气或水浴加热，待酒欲沸时取下，连渣倾入另一带盖容器中，后续同冷浸法操作制备。

② **Hot maceration method** The hot maceration method is also called alcohol decocting, a traditional way to prepare medicinal wines. Medicinal materials are put into a container with a cover after predisposition, and then add certain amount of spirit, heat with steam or by water bath until the spirit is about to boil. Transfer all the content including residues into another container with cover. The subsequent procedures are the same as the cool maceration method.

3. 回流热浸法 即热回流法。系药材加工炮制后，以规定白酒为溶剂回流提取2~3次，滤过，合并滤液，加入糖或蜂蜜，搅拌溶解，静置，待悬浮物沉淀后，滤过即得。如参茸多鞭酒。

③ **Reflux hot maceration method** Namely reflux extraction method. Medicinal materials are processed first, and then extracted with certain amount of spirits by reflux method for 2-3 times. Filter, combine the filtrate, add sucrose or honey, and stir to dissolve, leave to stand, filter again after the suspension precipitated, such as Shenrong Duobian Medicinal wine.

4. 渗漉法 以白酒为溶媒，按渗漉方法操作，收集渗漉液，按需要加入糖和蜂蜜，搅拌，密闭静置，滤清即得。如蕲蛇酒。

④ **Percolation method** Use spirits as solvent.Operating according to the percolation method, collect the percolating liquid, add sucrose and honey if necessary, stir, seal, leave to stand and at last filter, such as Qishe Medicinal wine.

案例导入 ¦ Case example

案例 7-5 舒筋活络酒

7-5 Shujin Huoluo Medicinal Wine

处方： 木瓜 45g 桑寄生 75g 玉竹 240g 续断 30g 川牛膝 90g 当归 60g 红花 45g 独活 30g 羌活 30g 防风 60g 白术 90g 蚕沙 60g 红曲 180g 甘草 30g

Ingredients: Chaenomelis Fructus 45g; Taxilli Herba 75g; Polygonati Odorati Rhizoma 240g; Dipsaci Radix 30g; Cyathulae Radix 90g; Angelicae Sinensis Radix 60g; Carthami Flos 45g; Angelicae Pubescentis Radix 30g; Notoptterygii Rhizoma et Radix 30g; Saposhnikoviae Radix 60g; Atractylodis Macrocephalae Rhizoma 90g; excrement Silkworm 60g; Monascus 180g; Glycyrrhizae Radix et Rhizoma 30g

功能与主治： 祛风除湿，舒筋活络。用于风寒湿痹，筋骨疼痛。

Functions Indications To dispel wind and remove dampness, relax tendons and activate collaterals. Used against wind-cold-damp arthralgia, pain in tendons and bones.

制法： 以上十五味，除红曲外，其余木瓜等十四味粉碎成粗粉；另取红糖555g，溶解于白酒11100g中，按渗漉法，用红糖酒作溶剂，浸渍48小时后，以每分钟1~3ml的速度缓缓渗漉，收集漉液，静置，滤过，即得。

Making Procedure Pulverize the above ingredients, except monascus, to coarse powders. Dissolve 555g of brown sugar with 11100g of spirit, and the solution was used as extracting solution. Use percolation method, after macerating for 48hours, percolate at the speed of 1-3ml per minute. Collect the percolation, leave to stand, and filter.

用法与用量： 口服，一次 20~30ml，一日 2 次。

Usage and dosage For oral administration, 20-30ml per time, twice a day.

注解： 酒剂中可以添加矫味剂和着色剂，口感较好。

Notes: Flavoring agents and colorants can be added to improve the taste and outlooks of preparations.

思考题：酒剂和酊剂有何异同？

Questions: What are the differences between medicinal wines and tinctures?

案例导入

（二）酊剂的制法

(2) Preparation of Tinctures

不同酊剂含不同浓度的乙醇，所用醇的浓度以能将有效成分完全溶出为度，酊剂的制备方法有溶解法、稀释法、浸渍法、渗漉法，工艺流程见图 7-6。

Different tinctures contain ethanol with different concentrations which are used to dissolve the active component completely., Tinctures are made by dissolving method, diluting method, maceration or percolation method. The work flow is shown in Figure 7-6.

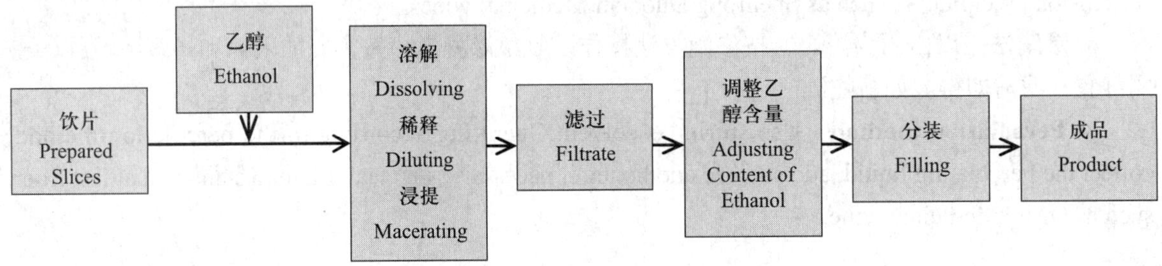

图 7-6　酊剂制备工艺流程图

Figure 7-6　Tincture Preparation Process

1. 溶解法　将药物加入规定浓度的乙醇溶解至需要量，主要适合于化学药物及中药有效部位或提纯品酊剂的制备。如复方樟脑酊等。

① **Dissolving method**　To dissolve medicines with ethanol of specified concentration, and add ethanol up to required volumes. This method is intended for the preparation of tinctures containing chemical medicines, effective fractions of Traditional Chinese Medicines or purified products, such as Fufang Zhangnao Tincture.

2. 稀释法　中药的流浸膏或浸膏加入规定浓度的乙醇，稀释至需要量，静置，滤过即得。如远志酊等。

② **Diluting method**　To dilute the fluid extracts or extracts with ethanol of specified concentration up to required volumes, leave to stand and filter, such as Yuanzhi Tincture.

3. 浸渍法　一般用冷浸法制备。

③ **Maceration method**　Cool maceration is usually used.

4. 渗漉法　此法为制备酊剂的常用方法，将饮片适当处理，用规定浓度的乙醇为溶剂，照渗漉法进行操作，调整渗漉液体积至规定量即可。如颠茄酊等。

④ **Percolation method**　This method is frequently used in tincture preparation. To percolate the prepared slices after predisposition with ethanol of specified concentration. And adjust the volume of the percolation to required volumes, such as Dianqie Tincture.

四、酒剂与酊剂的质量要求与检查
7.6.4 Quality Requirements and Inspections of Medicinal Wines and Tinctures

（一）酒剂的质量要求
(1) Quality Requirements for Medicinal Wines

酒剂中可加入适量的矫味剂和着色剂，要求澄清，贮存期间允许有少量轻摇易散的沉淀；酒剂的乙醇含量按照现行版《中国药典》进行测定，应符合该品种项下要求；对酒剂的总固体含量、甲醇量应进行限定。

Flavoring agents and colorants can be added into medicinal wines. Medicinal wines should be clear, and a small amount of dispersible precipitates during storage are allowed. The content of ethanol in medicinal wines should be inspected as is required by the current version of *Chinese Pharmacopoeia*, and should comply with the regulation under the item. Limit for total solid substance and methanol content should be established.

（二）酊剂的质量要求
(2) Quality Requirements for Tincture

酊剂中不加矫味剂和着色剂，要求澄清。成分含量或药材比量关系应符合规定。酊剂久置产生沉淀时，首先检查并调整乙醇浓度，若乙醇浓度未变，将沉淀滤除。对甲醇、乙醇含量进行严格控制。

Flavoring agents or colorants should not be added into tinctures. Tinctures should be clear. The content of components or the ratio of medicine to solvent should comply with the regulation. The ethanol concentration should be examined and adjusted first if sediments occurred in tinctures during long-time storage. If there's no change in the ethanol concentration, sediments can be filtered and removed. The content of methanol and ethanol should be strictly controlled.

（三）酒剂与酊剂的质量检查
(3) Quality Inspection of Medicinal Wines and Tinctures

1. 乙醇量 照现行版《中国药典》中乙醇量测定法测定。

① **Ethanol content** Carry out the method for Determination of Ethanol by the requirement of the current version of *Chinese Pharmacopoeia*.

2. 甲醇量 照现行版《中国药典》中甲醇量测定法检查。

② **Methanol content** Carry out the method for Determination of Methanol by the requirement of the current version of *Chinese Pharmacopoeia*.

3. 总固体量 照现行版《中国药典》中总固体量测定法检查。

③ **Total solids** Carry out the method for determination of Total solids by the requirement of the current version of *Chinese Pharmacopoeia*.

4. 装量 照现行版《中国药典》中最低限度检测法检查。

④ **Filling** Carry out the method for the Determination of the Minimum Limit Test by the requirement of the current version of *Chinese Pharmacopoeia*.

5. 微生物限度 照现行版《中国药典》中微生物限度检测法检查。

⑤ **Microbial limit** Carry out the method for the Determination of the Microbial Limit Test by the requirement of the current version of *Chinese Pharmacopoeia*.

第七节　流浸膏剂与浸膏剂

7.7 Liquid Extracts and Extracts

一、流浸膏剂及浸膏剂的含义和特点

7.7.1 The Definitions and Characteristics of Fluid Extracts and Extracts

流浸膏剂系指饮片用适宜的溶剂提取，蒸去部分或全部溶剂，调整浓度至每 1ml 相当于原饮片 1g 的制剂。浸膏剂系指药材用适宜的溶剂提取，蒸去全部溶剂，调整浓度至每 1g 相当于原饮片 2~5g 的制剂。根据干燥程度的不同，浸膏剂又分为稠膏剂与干膏剂。稠膏剂为半固体状，含水量为 15%~20%。干膏剂为粉末状，含水量约为 5%。有效成分明确的流浸膏剂或浸膏剂，经含量测定后，用溶剂或稀释剂调整至规定的规格标准。稠膏剂可用甘油、液体葡萄糖调整含量；干浸膏可用淀粉、乳糖、蔗糖、氧化锌、磷酸钙、药渣细粉等调整含量。

Liquid extracts are preparations made by soaking prepared slices in suitable solvents to extract the active ingredients and evaporating the solvents partially or completely when 1ml of a liquid extract is equivalent to 1g of the prepared slices. Extracts are preparations made by extracting prepared slices with suitable solvent and evaporating all solvent, adjusting the concentration to a degree when 1g of an extract is equivalent to 2-5g of prepared slices. Based on the degrees of drying, extracts are further divided into dense extract and dry extract. Dense extract is semi-solid, containing 15%-20% of water, while dry extract is powder-like, containing about 5% of water. Fluid extracts and extracts with definite active ingredients can be adjusted to specified standard with solvents or diluents after content determination. The content of dense extracts can be regulated with glycerin or liquid glucose; The content of dry extracts can be regulated with starch, lactose, sucrose, zinc oxide, calcium phosphate or fine powders of residues.

流浸膏剂和浸膏剂大多以不同的浓度的乙醇为溶剂，也有以水为溶剂者。以水为溶剂的流浸膏剂成品中应酌加 20%~25% 的乙醇作防腐剂。除少数品种直接用于临床外，流浸膏剂多作为配制酊剂、合剂、糖浆剂等的原料，浸膏剂一般多作为制备颗粒剂、片剂、胶囊剂、丸剂、软膏剂、栓剂等的原料。

Ethanol of distinct concentration is used as solvent of fluid extracts and extracts mostly. water can also be used as solvent and in this situation, 20%-25% of ethanol should be added as preservative. Except for a few clinical applications, most of fluid extracts are used as raw materials for tinctures, mixtures and syrups, while most of extracts are used as raw materials for granules, tablets, capsules, pills, ointments and suppositories.

二、流浸膏剂及浸膏剂的制法

7.7.2 Preparation of Fluid Extracts and Extracts

（一）流浸膏剂的制法

(1) Preparation of Fluid Extracts

除另有规定外，流浸膏剂多用渗漉法制备，工艺流程如图 7-7 所示。

Unless otherwise specified, fluid extracts are prepared with percolation method, and the process is shown in Figure 7-7.

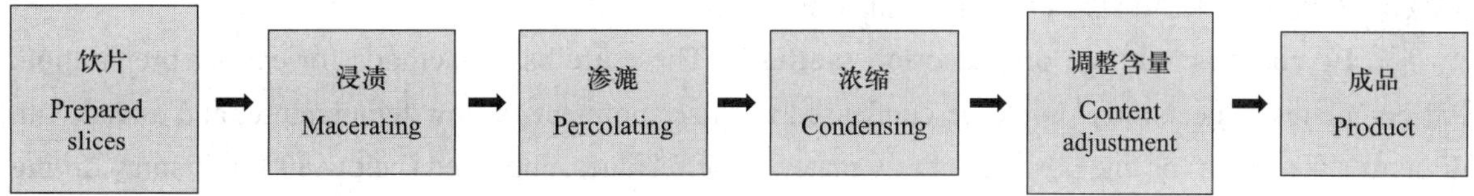

图 7-7　流浸膏剂制备工艺流程

Figure 7-7　Preparation Process of Fluid Extract

1. 渗漉法　流浸膏剂的主要制法，其操作要点：①饮片应适当粉碎，加规定的溶剂均匀润湿，密闭放置一定时间，再装入渗漉器内。饮片装入渗漉器时应均匀、松紧一致，加入溶剂时应尽量排除饮片间隙中的空气，溶剂应高出药面，密盖，浸渍适当时间后渗漉。②除另有规定外，渗漉时应先收集药材量 85% 的初渗漉液另器保存，续漉液低温浓缩至稠膏状，与初漉液合并，调整至规定量，静置，取上清液分装。③对有效成分明确者，测定含量和含醇量，调整至规定的规格标准。

① **Percolation method**　This is the predominant method to prepare fluid extract and the key points of procedures as follows: A.The prepared slices should be pulverized properly before packed into the percolator, and moistened uniformly with the specified solvent and allowed to stand in a well closed vessel for a required time. The prepared slices should be packed with uniform compactness and the solvent added to the percolator to expel most of the air in the gap of crude drug. The top of the column of prepared slices should be well covered by the solvent, allowed to stand for some time before the percolation takes place. B. Unless otherwise specified, when an amount of the initial percolate equivalent to 85% of the prepared slices in the percolator has been collected, it is set aside. The rest of the percolate should be concentrated at a low temperature and the mixed products of percolation and concentration are made up to the required volume with the solvent. Still standing, then use the supernatant for packing. C.If the active ingredients are already known, the content and ethanol content should be determined and regulated to specified standard.

2. 其他方法　流浸膏剂可用浸膏剂加规定溶剂稀释制成；也可用煎煮法或溶解法制备。

② **Other methods**　Fluid extract can also be prepared by diluting with specified solvents or decoction method, or dissolving method.

制备流浸膏剂多用不同浓度的乙醇，少数虽以水为溶媒，但最终一般都加入 20%~50% 的乙醇。若以水为溶剂，有效成分耐热，可不收集初漉液，将渗漉液全部浓缩至规定量，加适量乙醇防腐即可。也可采用煎煮法制备流浸膏剂。

Ethanol of different concentration is frequently used in fluid extract preparation. A few fluid extracts use water as solvent, and 20%-50% of ethanol is commonly added. If water is used as solvent, and the active ingredients are thermostable, it is not necessary to collect the primary percolate, but to condense all the percolate to a specified volume and add appropriate amount of ethanol as preservative. Decoction method can also be applied in the preparation of fluid extracts.

流浸膏剂应置避光容器内密封，置阴凉处贮藏。

Fluid extract should be preserved in tightly closed containers, protected from light.

（二）浸膏剂的制法

(2) Preparation of Extracts

1. 渗漉法或煎煮法　浸膏剂的基本制法。全部渗漉液或煎煮液应低温浓缩至稠膏状，再加入

适量的稀释剂（如淀粉）或原药细粉或药渣细粉直接干燥（80℃以下）至规定标准。采用喷雾干燥法可直接制得干浸膏粉。含油脂较多的饮片制备干浸膏时，须先行脱脂。采用煎煮法制备时，必要时水煎液可加乙醇处理，达到纯化的目的。

① **Percolation method or decoction method** These are basic methods for extract preparation. All percolates or decoction should be condensed to thick ointments at low temperature, and added with diluents (like starch) or fine powders of raw materials or residues, and dried (below 80℃). If spray drying is used, dry extract can be prepared directly. Prepared slices rich in grease should be degreased before preparation to dry extract. If decoction method is used to prepare extracts, ethanol can be added to purify the decoction if necessary.

2. 其他方法 根据品种和设备条件，可选用回流或浸渍法。

② **Other methods** Based on varieties and equipment conditions, reflux method or maceration method can be used.

三、流浸膏剂与浸膏剂的质量要求与检查

7.7.3 Quality Requirements and Inspections of Fluid Extracts and Extracts

（一）流浸膏剂与浸膏剂的质量要求

(1) Quality Requirements for Fluid Extracts and Extracts

流浸膏剂应符合该制剂含药量规定要求，成品中至少含20%以上的乙醇；流浸膏剂应澄清，久置若产生沉淀时，在乙醇和指标成分含量符合该药品规定的情况下，可滤过除去沉淀。含乙醇量、装量及微生物限度均应符合各品种项下的有关规定。

The content of fluid extracts should comply with the specific requirements of the very preparation. Concentration of ethanol in final product should not be less than 20%. Fluid extracts should be clear. Precipitate produced on prolonged standing of the liquid extracts may be removed by filtration, but the content of ethanol and active ingredients should comply with the requirements specified in the individual monographs. The ethanol content, filling and microbial limit should comply with regulations under each item.

浸膏剂应符合该制剂含药量规定要求；装量及微生物限度均应符合各品种项下的有关规定。应在遮光容器中密闭，置阴凉处保存。

The content of extracts should comply with the specific requirements of the very preparation. The filling and microbial limit should comply with regulations under each item. Extracts should be sealed in light resistant containers and preserved in shady and cool environment.

（二）流浸膏剂与浸膏剂的质量检查

(2) Quality Inspection of Fluid Extracts and Extracts

1. 乙醇量 照现行版《中国药典》中乙醇量测定法测定。

① **Ethanol content** Carry out the method for Determination of Ethanol Content by the requirement of the current version of *Chinese Pharmacopoeia.*

2. 装量 照现行版《中国药典》中最低限度检测法检查。

② **Packing volumes** Operate the Determination of the Minimum Limit Test by the requirement of the current version of *Chinese Pharmacopoeia.*

3. 微生物限度 照现行版《中国药典》中微生物限度检测法检查。

③ **Microbial limit** Operate the method for the Determination of the Microbial Limit Test by the requirement of the current version of *Chinese Pharmacopoeia.*

PPT

第八节　茶剂
7.8　Medicinal Tea

一、茶剂的含义
7.8.1　The Definition of Medicinal Teas

茶剂系指饮片或提取物（液）与茶叶或其他辅料混合制成的内服剂型，可分为块状茶剂、袋装茶剂（袋泡茶剂）和煎煮茶剂。

Medicinal teas are preparations for oral administration, which are made by mixing prepared slices or extracts (liquid extractives) of prepared slices with tea or other excipients. They are classified into three categories, medicinal tea lumps, medicinal bag-packed teas and medicinal teas for decoction.

二、茶剂的特点
7.8.2　The Characteristics of Medicinal Teas

茶剂可用于治疗，如利胆茶等；或保健，如三花减肥茶等。近年来新研制的茶剂以袋装茶剂为主，其体积小，利于贮存，便于携带，使用方便，适于体积较轻、质地疏松、有效成分易于浸出的中药，特别是对于含有挥发性成分的中药，能较多地保留药效成分。

Medicinal teas can be used not only for treatment, such as Lidan Medicinal Tea but also for health care, such as Sanhua Jianfei Medicinal Tea. The recently developed medicinal teas are mainly bag-packed medicinal teas, which are small in volume and easy for storage, transportation, and administration. Traditional Chinese Medicines that are large in volume, fluffy in texture and whose active ingredients are inclined to be macerated, especially those containing volatile ingredients are suitable for medicinal teas, for the effective ingredients can be better preserved.

三、茶剂的制法
7.8.3　Preparation of Medicinal Teas

茶剂外形和使用方法不同，制备方法也不同，但有相似之处：

Depending on the different outlooks and usages, medicinal teas may be prepared in different methods, but have something in common.

块状茶剂：可分不含糖块状茶剂和含糖块状茶剂。不含糖块状茶剂系指饮片粗粉、碎片与茶叶或适宜的黏合剂压制成块状的茶剂；含糖块状茶剂是指提取物、饮片细粉与蔗糖等辅料压制成块状的茶剂。

Medicinal tea lumps: medicinal tea lumps are classified into sugar free tea lumps and sugar containing tea lumps. Sugar free tea lumps are those prepared by compacting the coarse powder, broken pieces of prepared slices and tea or suitable binder. Sugar containing tea lumps are those prepared by

compacting those extracts or fine powders of prepared slices and suitable excipients such as sugar etc..

袋装茶剂：系指茶叶、饮片粗粉或部分饮片粗粉吸收提取液经干燥后，装入袋的茶剂，其中装入饮用茶袋的又称袋泡茶剂。

Medicinal bag-packed teas are those prepared by packing bags with tea, coarse powder of prepared slices or partial prepared slices absorbing liquid extractives and then dried. The medicinal bag-packed teas packed into drinking bags are called tea bags.

煎煮茶剂：系指将饮片适当碎断后，装入袋中，供煎服的茶剂。

Medicinal teas for decoction are those prepared by packing bags with slices, pieces, sections, slivers or coarse powder of the prepared slices, and decocted for drinking.

四、茶剂的质量要求与检查
7.8.4 Quality Requirements and Inspections of Medicinal Teas

（一）茶剂的质量要求
(1) Quality Requirements for Medicinal Tea

茶剂应洁净，色泽均匀，气味纯正，饮片的细度应控制在一定的范围。茶叶的饮用茶袋均应符合饮用茶标准的有关要求。

Medicinal tea should be clean, of uniform color and pure smell; the grain size of prepared slices should be controlled in a certain degree. The tea bag should comply with the relative requirements for drinking teas.

除另有规定外，不含糖块状茶剂、煎煮茶剂和袋装茶剂的水分均不得过 12.0%，含糖块状茶剂水分不得过 3.0%。含糖块状茶剂溶化性检查应全部溶化，可有轻微浑浊，不得有焦屑等。

Unless otherwise specified, the water content in sugar-free tea lumps, bag-packed teas and teas for decoction should no more than 12%; the water content in sugar containing tea lumps should no more than 3%. The Dispersibility Test for sugar containing teas should be carried out, which should be completely dissolved, without burned charings, ect. (slight turbidity is acceptable).

块状茶剂重量差异检查，供试品每块的重量与标示重量相比，10 块中超出重量差异限度的不得多于 2 块，并不得有 1 块超出限度 1 倍。装量差异除另有规定外，煎煮茶剂或袋装茶剂内容物重量，每袋（盒）装量与标示装量相比，超出装量差异限度的不得多于 2 袋（盒），并不得有 1 袋（盒）超出限度 1 倍。微生物限度等均应符合相应要求。

The variation test for tea lumps: weigh 10 lumps of medicinal tea respectively, and compare the weight of each with the labelled weight. Of all the 10 lumps, not more than 2 lumps should deviate from the limit, and none should deviate by more than twice of the limit. Unless otherwise specified, the filling of medicinal bag-packed teas and medicinal teas for decoction should be compared with the labelled filling. No more than 2 packs should deviate from the limit and none should deviate by more than twice of the limit. The microbial limit should comply with the corresponding requirements.

（二）茶剂的质量检查
(2) Quality Inspection of Medicinal Tea

1. 水分 取供试品（不含糖块状茶剂研碎，含糖块状茶剂破碎成 3mm 的颗粒），照现行版《中国药典》中水分测定法测定。

① **Water content** Carry out the Determination of Water Content by the requirements of the current version *Chinese Pharmacopoeia* (sugar-free tea lumps should be ground and sugar containing tea lumps should be ground into particles about 3mm in diameter).

2. 溶化性 取含糖块状茶剂1块，加20倍量热水，搅拌15分钟，应符合规定。

② **Dispersibility** Take one lump, add hot water at 20 times of its weight and stir for 5 minutes. The dispersibility should comply with the requirements.

3. 重量差异 取块状茶剂10块，分别称定重量，每块的重量与标示量相比（标示重量6g以下、6g以上其重量差异限度分别为 ±7%和 ±5%）。

③ **Weight variation** Weigh 10 lumps of medicinal tea respectively, and compare the weight of each with the labelled weight (For the labeled weight lower than 6g and higher than 6g, the limit of weight variations are respectively ±7% and ±5%).

4. 装量差异 取煎煮茶剂或袋装茶剂10袋（盒），分别称定每袋（盒）内容物重量，每袋（盒）装量与标示装量相比（标示重量2g及2g以下、2g以上至5g、5g以上至10g、10g以上至20g、20g以上至40g、40g以上者重量或装量差异限度分别为 ±15%、±12%、±10%、±6%、±5%、±4%）。

④ **Content uniformity** Weigh the content of 10 packs(boxes) respectively, and compare the filling of each pack(box) with the labelled filling (For the labeled filling 2g or lower than 2g, 2-5g, 5-10g, 10-20g, 20-40g, and higher than 40g, the limit of filling variations should be ±15%, ±12%, ±10%, ±6%, ±5% and ±4%respectively).

5. 微生物限度 照现行版《中国药典》中微生物限度检测法检查。

⑤ **Microbial limit** Carry out the method for the Determination of the Microbial Limit Test by the requirement of the current version of *Chinese Pharmacopoeia.*

第九节 浸出药剂容易出现的质量问题

7.9 Quality Problems of Extractions

PPT

浸出药剂成分组成复杂，属于混合分散体系，在贮存过程中易发生各种物理和化学变化，影响制剂的安全性和有效性。

The components in extractions are complicated, which belong to mixed dispersion system. Therefore, various chemical and physical changes are tented to take place during storage, which may influence the safety and effectiveness of preparations.

一、长霉发酵

7.9.1 Mildew and Fermentation

糖浆剂、合剂、口服液等含有糖、蛋白质等微生物的营养物质，且水分含量大，在适宜的温度、pH值等条件下，微生物易大量繁殖。应严格生产工艺管理，采取严格的防菌措施，避免微生物的污染；必要时可适当加入防腐剂。

Syrups, mixtures and oral liquids, etc. contain sugar and proteins that are regarded as nutrients for microbial, and contain large amount of water, therefore it is easy for microbial to proliferate under

suitable temperature and pH value. To avoid the microbial pollution, the manufacture procedures should be strictly supervised and rigid anti-bacterial measures should be taken; preservatives can be added if necessary.

含乙醇制剂，乙醇含量在 20% 以上可以达到防腐效果。

Ethanol can be anti-bacterial if the content of which reaches no less than 20% in ethanol containing preparations.

二、浑浊沉淀
7.9.2 Turbidity and Precipitation

液体浸出药剂成分复杂，既含有高分子杂质，也含有溶解度不同的各类小分子物质，因而在贮存过程中存在胶体分子的陈化和难溶性成分的析出现象；含乙醇药剂，因乙醇挥发导致醇度下降，溶解范围发生改变而产生浑浊或沉淀；因包装材料或光线、温度等因素的影响，导致成分发生水解或其他反应；药剂的 pH 值改变，也会使某些成分的溶解度下降。

Liquid extractives are complicated in component, containing both polymer impurities and various small molecular impurities of distinct solubility. Therefore, the aging of colloid molecules and crystallization of insoluble ingredients may occur during storage. Ethanol containing preparations may produce turbidity or precipitation due to the alteration of solubility range caused by the decrease of ethanol because of the volatilization. Meanwhile, the decrease of solubility can also be found when hydrolysis or other reactions take place due to the influence of package materials or light, temperature, the change of pH values of preparations.

为减少浑浊或沉淀，应加强精制，除杂彻底；制剂密闭包装，减少含乙醇药剂乙醇的挥发；溶解度小的药物成分可以加辅助溶剂或 β- 环糊精包合；包装材料使用前进行内表面的处理等。根据沉淀出现的原因，有针对性地采取措施。

To reduce the turbidity or precipitation, purification should be emphasized to completely remove the impurities; preparations should be sealed to reduce the volatilization of ethanol in ethanol containing preparations; secondary solvent or beta-cyclodextrin inclusion can be applied for ingredients with small solubility; the inner side of package materials should be processed before put into use. In one word, particular measures should be taken according to the reasons of the appearance of precipitation.

三、成分水解
7.9.3 Hydrolysis

有些中药成分在水中易水解，导致疗效降低或失效。水解往往与 pH 值、酶、温度等因素有关。调整药液的 pH 值、加热以杀灭酶的活性、低温保存、添加乙醇或其他有机溶剂等可抑制水解的进行。

Some ingredients in the Traditional Chinese Medicines tend to be hydrolyzed lead to reduce the effects or lose efficacy. Hydrolysis is generally associated with the factors such as pH value, enzyme,

and temperature. Therefore, the adjustment of pH value of the liquid extractives, inactivation of enzyme by heating, storage at low temperature, addition of ethanol or other organic solvents can inhibit the progression of hydrolysis.

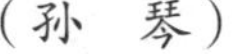

（孙 琴）

岗位对接

重点小结

题库

第八章　液体药剂
Chapter 8　Liquid Preparations

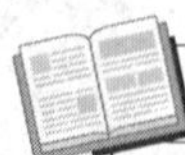

学习目标 ¦ Learning Goals

知识要求：

1. 掌握　液体药剂的含义、分类与特点；表面活性剂的含义、分类、基本性质与选用；药剂中增加药物溶解度的方法；真溶液型、胶体溶液型、乳状液型及混悬液型液体药剂的含义、特点与制法。

2. 熟悉　溶解、增溶、助溶、潜溶、乳化、混悬的概念；增溶原理；胶体溶液稳定性及其影响因素；乳剂稳定性及乳化剂的选用；混悬剂的稳定性；液体药剂的质量检查。

3. 了解　灌肠剂、洗剂、搽剂、滴鼻剂、滴耳剂等液体剂型的含义与特点；液体药剂的色、香、味及包装贮藏。

能力要求：

学会各类液体药剂的制备与质量检测方法，能制备不同类型的液体药剂，并检查和评价液体药剂的产品质量。

Knowledge requirements:

1. To master the meaning, classification and characteristics of liquid preparations; the meaning, classification, basic properties and selection of surfactants; the method of increasing drug solubility; the meaning, characteristics and preparation of true solution, colloidal solution, emulsions and suspensions.

2. To be familiar with the concepts of dissolution, solubilization, hydrotropy, cosolvency, emulsification and suspension; principle of solubilization; stability of colloidal solution and its influencing factors; stability of emulsions and selection of emulsifier; stability of suspension; quality inspection of liquid preparations.

3. To know the meaning and characteristics of liquid preparations such as enema, lotion, liniments, nasal drops and ear drops, and the color, fragrance, taste, packaging and storage of liquid preparations.

Ability requirements:

Learn the preparation and quality test methods of various liquid preparations, how to prepare different types of liquid preparations, check and evaluate the product quality of liquid preparations.

第一节 概述
8.1 Overview

一、液体药剂的含义与特点
8.1.1 The Definition and Characteristics of Liquid Preparations

液体药剂系指药物分散在液体分散介质（溶剂）中制成的液态剂型，可供内服或外用。

Liquid preparations refer to the liquid dosage forms made by medicine dispersed in liquid dispersion medium (solvent), which can be used for internal or external.

液体药剂的特点：①吸收快，作用较迅速；②给药途径广泛；③使用方便，易于分剂量，尤其适用于婴幼儿和老年患者；④能减少某些药物的刺激性；⑤某些固体药物制成液体制剂，可提高其生物利用度；⑥药物分散度较大，易引起药物的化学降解，降低药效甚至失效；⑦体积较大，携带、运输、贮存不方便；⑧水性液体药剂易霉变，非均相液体药剂易出现物理稳定性问题等。

Liquid preparations have the following characteristics: ① quick absorption and quick action; ② wide administration way; ③ convenient use and easy dosage division, especially suitable for infants and elderly patients; ④ reducing the irritation of some drugs; ⑤ making some solid drugs into liquid preparations can improve the bioavailability; ⑥ large dispersion of drugs, easily causing chemical degradation of drugs, reducing the efficacy and even invalid; ⑦ carrying, transporting and storage are inconvenient because of large volume; ⑧ liquid preparations with water as dispersion medium are prone to mildew, and non-homogeneous liquid agents are prone to physical stability problems.

二、液体药剂的分类
8.1.2 The Classifications of Liquid Preparations

（一）按分散系统分类
(1) Classifications by Decentralized System

分为溶液型、胶体溶液型、混悬液型、乳状液型四类，具体见表 8-1。

It can be divided into solutions, colloidal solutions, suspensions and emulsions, Table 8-1 for details.

表 8-1 分散体系的分类

类型		分散相大小（nm）	特征
真溶液型（低分子溶液剂）		<1	以小分子或离子状态分散的澄清溶液；稳定体系
胶体溶液型	高分子溶液剂	<100	以高分子状态分散的澄清溶液；稳定体系
	溶胶剂	1~100	以胶态分散形成的多相体系；热力学不稳定体系
混悬液型（混悬剂）		>500	以固体微粒分散形成的多相体系；热力学和动力学不稳定体系
乳状液型（乳剂）		>100	以液体微粒分散形成的多相体系；热力学和动力学不稳定体系

Table 8-1 Classifications of Dispersion System

Type		Dispersed phase size (nm)	Characteristics
True solutions (small molecule solvent)		<1	A clear solution dispersed as a small molecule or ion, with a stable system
Colloidal solutions	Polymer solutions	<100	A clear solution dispersed in a polymer state, with a stable system
	Sols	1~100	A heterogeneous system formed by colloidal dispersion, with an unstable thermodynamic system
Suspensions		>500	A heterogeneous system formed by dispersion of solid particles, with an unstable thermodynamic and dynamic system
Emulsions		>100	A heterogeneous system formed by dispersion of liquid particles, with an unstable thermodynamic and dynamic system

（二）按给药途径分类

(2) Classifications according to Administration Routes

1. 内服液体药剂

① **Oral liquid preparations**

2. 外用液体药剂 ①皮肤用液体药剂；②五官科用液体药剂；③直肠、阴道或尿道用液体药剂。

② **External liquid preparations** A.liquid preparations for skin; B. liquid preparations for ophthalmology and otorhinolaryngology; C.liquid preparations for rectum, vagina or urethra.

三、液体药剂常用的溶剂

8.1.3 Common Solvents for Liquid Preparations

液体药剂的溶剂对药物起溶解和分散作用，同时影响制剂的制备和稳定性。

The solvent of the liquid preparations can dissolve and disperse the medicine, simultaneously affect the preparation and stability of the preparations.

1. 水 水是最常用的溶剂，能与乙醇、甘油、丙二醇等以任意比例混合，能溶解中药中如生物碱盐、苷类、糖类、蛋白质及色素等。配制水性液体制剂通常使用纯化水。

(1) Water is the most common solvent, which can be mixed with ethanol, glycerin, propylene glycol, etc. in any proportion. It can dissolve alkaloid salts, glycosides, saccharides, proteins and pigments in Traditional Chinese Medicine (TCM). Purified water is usually employed to prepare liquid preparations.

2. 乙醇 乙醇是常用溶剂，能与水、甘油、丙二醇等以任意比例混合，能溶解药材中如生物碱及其盐类、苷类、挥发油、树脂、鞣质、有机酸和色素等。20% 以上的乙醇具有防腐作用。但乙醇有一定的生理作用，且易挥发、易燃烧。

(2) Ethanol is a common solvent, which can be mixed with water, glycerin and propylene glycol in any proportion. It can dissolve the alkaloids and their salts, glycosides, volatile oil, resins, tannins, organic acids and pigments in TCM. More than 20% ethanol has antiseptic effect. But ethanol has certain physiological function, and it is volatile and flammable.

3. 甘油 为黏稠性液体，能与水、乙醇、丙二醇混合。甘油黏度较大，毒性小，且有防腐性，故常将一些外用药制成甘油剂，也可用作外用制剂的保湿剂。

(3) Glycerin is a viscous liquid, which can be mixed with water, ethanol and propylene glycol. Glycerin is of high viscosity, low toxicity and antiseptic. And it is often made into glycerin by some external drugs. And it can also be used as humectant of external preparations.

4. 丙二醇 丙二醇兼有甘油的优点，刺激性与毒性均较小，能溶解很多有机药物，如磺胺类药、维生素 A、D 及性激素等。

(4) Propylene glycol has the advantages of glycerin, which is less irritating and toxic. And it can dissolve diverse organic drugs, such as sulfonamides, vitamin A, vitamin D and sex hormones, etc.

5. 聚乙二醇 常用 PEG300~600，能与水、乙醇、甘油等以任何比例混合，并能溶解许多水溶性无机盐和水不溶性有机药物。本品对易水解的药物具有一定的稳定作用，亦具有保湿作用。

(5) Polyethylene glycol (PEG) 300-600 is commonly used which can be mixed with water, ethanol, glycerin in any proportion, and can dissolve many water-soluble inorganic salts and water-insoluble organic drugs. In addition, it has a certain stable effect to the drugs which are easy to hydrolyze and moisturizing effect.

6. 脂肪油 主要指植物油类，如花生油、麻油、大豆油等。能溶解生物碱、挥发油及许多芳香族药物。多用于外用制剂，如洗剂、搽剂等。

(6) Fatty oil mainly refers to vegetable oil, such as peanut oil, sesame oil, soybean oil, etc. It can dissolve alkaloids, volatile oil and many aromatic drugs. It is mainly used in external preparations, such as lotions, liniments, etc.

其他常用溶剂还有油酸乙酯、肉豆蔻酸异丙酯等。

Other commonly used solvents include ethyl oleate, isopropyl myristate, etc.

第二节 表面活性剂

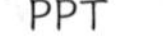
PPT

英文翻译

一、表面活性剂的含义、组成与特点

能显著降低两相间界面张力（或表面张力）的物质称为表面活性剂。

表面活性剂分子结构中同时含有亲水基团如—OH、—COOH、—NH_2 等和疏水基团如碳氢链，如图 8-1 所示。

将表面活性剂加入水中，低浓度时可被吸附在溶液的表面，亲水基团朝向水中，亲油基团（或疏水相）朝向空气中，在表面（或界面）上定向排列，从而改变了液体的表面性质，使表面张力降低，如图 8-2 所示。

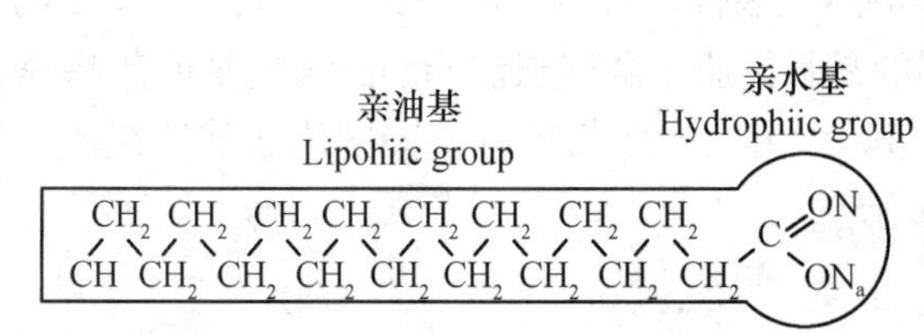

图 8-1 表面活性剂的化学结构示意图

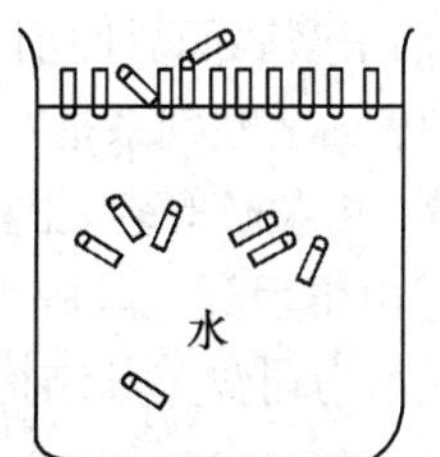

图 8-2 表面活性剂分子在水 - 空气界面的吸附作用

二、常用的表面活性剂

表面活性剂通常按其在水中的解离情况分为离子型和非离子型两大类，离子型表面活性剂按其离子所带电荷可分为阴离子型、阳离子型和两性离子型表面活性剂。

（一）阴离子型表面活性剂

阴离子型表面活性剂起表面活性作用的是其阴离子部分。

1. 肥皂类 系高级脂肪酸的盐，通式为（$RCOO^-)_n M^{n+}$。其脂肪酸烃链一般在 C_{11}~C_{18} 之间，以硬脂酸、油酸、月桂酸等较常用。根据 M 的不同，有碱金属皂、碱土金属皂和有机胺皂（如三乙醇胺皂）等。一般用于皮肤用药剂。

2. 硫酸化物 系硫酸化油和高级脂肪醇硫酸酯类，通式为 $R\cdot O\cdot SO_3^-M^+$，脂肪烃链 R 通常在 C_{12}~C_{18} 之间。硫酸化油的代表是硫酸化蓖麻油，俗称为土耳其红油，高级脂肪醇硫酸酯类中常用的是十二烷基硫酸钠（月桂醇硫酸钠）等。其乳化性较强，且较肥皂类稳定，主要用作软膏剂的乳化剂。

3. 磺酸化物 系指脂肪族磺酸化物、烷基芳基磺酸化物和烷基萘磺酸化物等，通式为 $R\cdot SO_3^-M^+$，常用作洗涤剂。

（二）阳离子型表面活性剂

阳离子型表面活性剂起表面活性作用的是阳离子部分，也称为季铵化合物，主要用于杀菌与防腐。常用的有氯苄烷铵（商品名为洁尔灭）、溴苄烷铵（商品名为新洁尔灭）等。

（三）两性离子型表面活性剂

两性离子型表面活性剂分子中同时具有正、负电荷基团，可随介质 pH 的不同而成为阳离子型或阴离子型。

1. 卵磷脂 卵磷脂是天然的两性离子型表面活性剂，目前是制备注射用乳剂的主要附加剂。其结构式如图 8-3 所示。

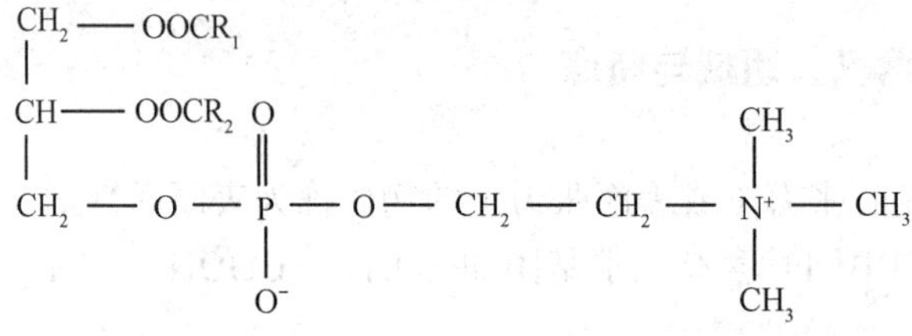

图 8-3 卵磷脂结构式

2. 合成的两性离子型表面活性剂 构成阳离子部分的是胺盐或季铵盐，阴离子部分主要是羧酸盐，也有硫酸酯、磷酸酯、磺酸盐等。羧酸盐型又分为氨基酸型和甜菜碱型两类。

（四）非离子型表面活性剂

非离子型表面活性剂系指在水溶液中不解离的一类表面活性剂，其分子中构成亲水基团的是甘油、聚乙二醇、山梨醇等多元醇，构成亲油基团的是长链脂肪酸或长链脂肪醇及烷基或芳基等。

1. 脂肪酸山梨坦类 系脱水山梨醇脂肪酸酯类，由山梨醇与各种不同的脂肪酸所组成的酯类化合物，商品名为司盘。其结构通式如图 8-4 所示。

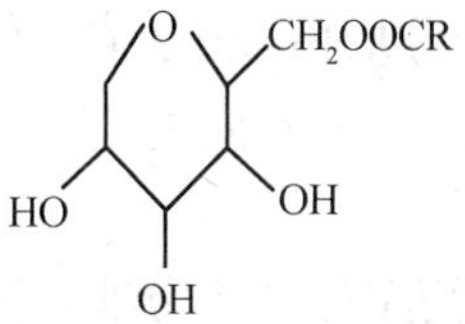

CH_2OOCR　HO　OH　OH

RCOO-为脂肪酸根，山梨醇为六元醇，因脱水而环合

图 8-4　脂肪酸山梨坦结构通式

其 *HLB* 值在 4.3~8.6 之间，亲油性较强，故一般用作 W/O 型乳剂的乳化剂，或 O/W 型乳剂的辅助乳化剂。

2. 聚山梨酯类　系聚氧乙烯脱水山梨醇脂肪酸酯类，系在司盘类的剩余—OH 上，再结合聚氧乙烯基而制得的醚类化合物，商品名为吐温。其结构通式如图 8-5 所示。

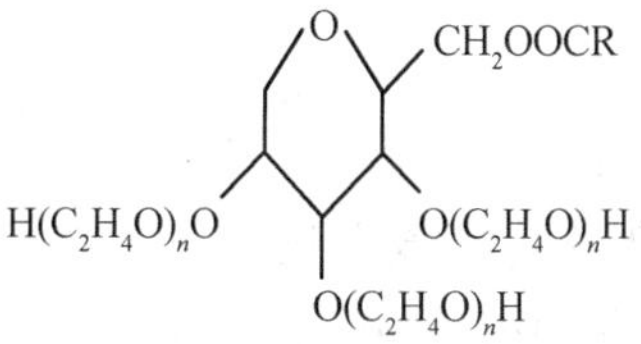

CH_2OOCR　$H(C_2H_4O)_nO$　$O(C_2H_4O)_nH$　$O(C_2H_4O)_nH$

式中—$(C_2H_4O)_nO^-$为聚氧乙烯基

图 8-5　聚山梨酯结构通式

亲水性增加，广泛用作增溶剂或 O/W 型乳化剂。

3. 聚氧乙烯脂肪酸酯类　系由聚乙二醇与长链脂肪酸缩合而成，商品名为卖泽。该类表面活性剂的乳化能力很强，常用作 O/W 型乳化剂。

4. 聚氧乙烯脂肪醇醚类　系由聚乙二醇与脂肪醇缩合而成的醚类，商品名为苄泽。该类表面活性剂常用作乳化剂或增溶剂。

5. 聚氧乙烯 - 聚氧丙烯共聚物　系由聚氧乙烯和聚氧丙烯聚合而成。最常用的有普流罗尼克，又称为泊洛沙姆。

三、表面活性剂的基本性质

（一）胶束与临界胶束浓度

表面活性剂水溶液达到一定浓度后，表面层表面活性剂已基本饱和，浓度再增大，表面活性剂分子进入溶液内部，形成亲水基向水、疏水基在内的缔合体，这种缔合体称为胶团或胶束。表面活性剂开始形成胶束时的浓度称为临界胶束浓度。

当缔合数增加，胶束的形态结构也随之变化。如图 8-6 所示。

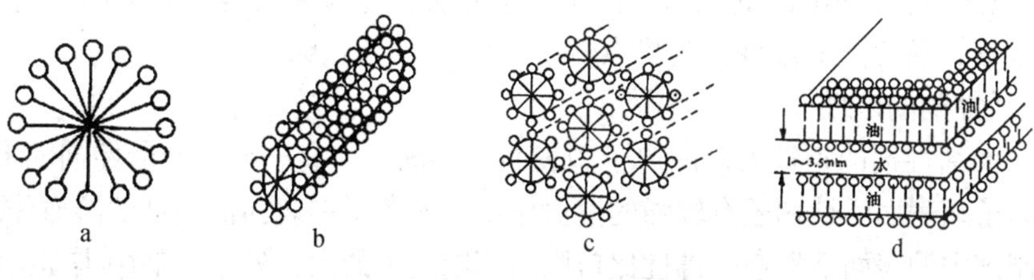

图 8-6　胶束的形态

a. 球状胶束　b. 棒状胶束　c. 束状胶束　d. 层状胶束

（二）亲水亲油平衡值

表面活性剂分子中同时含有亲水基团和亲油基团，其亲水亲油性的强弱可以用亲水亲油平衡值（*HLB* 值）表示。根据经验，将表面活性剂的 *HLB* 值范围限定在 0~40，其中非离子型表面活

性剂的 *HLB* 值范围为 0~20。*HLB* 值越高，其亲水性越强；*HLB* 值越低，其亲油性越强。不同 *HLB* 值的表面活性剂适合于不同的用途，如图 8-7 所示。

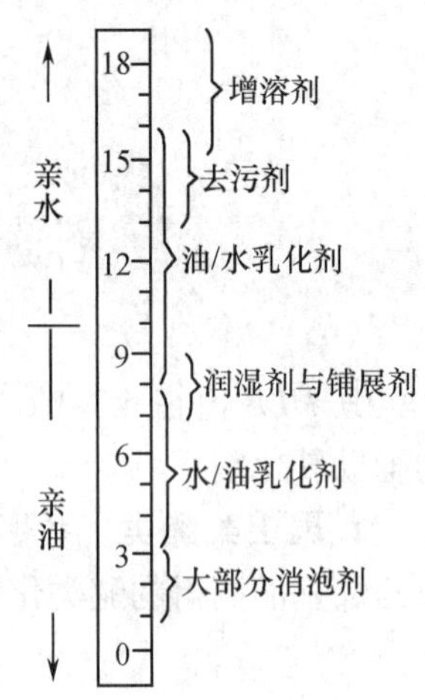

图 8-7 不同 *HLB* 值表面活性剂的适用范围

非离子型表面活性剂的 *HLB* 值具有加和性。如简单的二组分非离子型表面活性剂混合体系的 *HLB* 值可按式（8-1）计算，但此公式不能用于混合离子型表面活性剂 *HLB* 值的计算。

$$HLB_{混合乳化剂}=\frac{W_A \cdot HLB_A + W_B \cdot HLB_B}{W_A + W_B} \tag{8-1}$$

式中，W_A、W_B 为表面活性剂 A、B 的重量；HLB_A、HLB_B 为乳化剂 A、B 的 *HLB* 值。

（三）Krafft 点

图 8-8 为十二烷基硫酸钠在水中的溶解度随温度变化曲线。从图可知，随温度升高至某一温度，其溶解度急剧升高，该温度称为 Krafft 点，相对应的溶解度即为该离子表面活性剂的 *CMC*（图中虚线）。

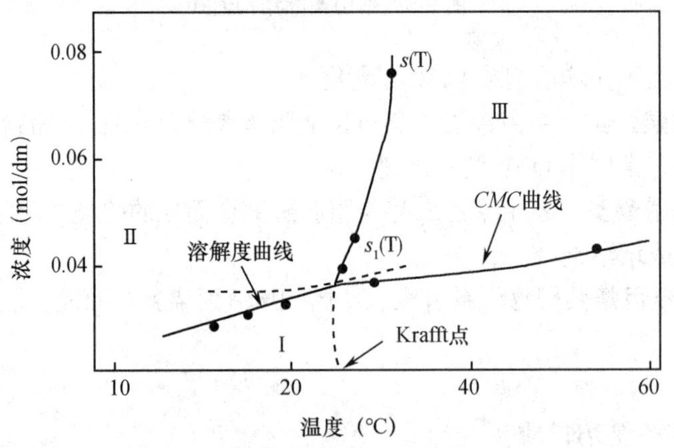

图 8-8 十二烷基硫酸钠的溶解度曲线

Krafft 点是离子型表面活性剂的特征值，Krafft 点越高，*CMC* 越小。Krafft 点是表面活性剂使用温度的下限。

（四）起昙与昙点

一些含聚氧乙烯基的非离子型表面活性剂的溶解度开始随温度上升而增大，达到某一温度后，其溶解度急剧下降，使溶液变混浊，甚至产生分层，冷却后又能恢复澄明。这种由澄明变混浊的现象称为起昙，转变点的温度称为昙点。

（五）表面活性剂的毒性

阳离子型表面活性剂的毒性大于阴离子型表面活性剂，非离子型表面活性剂的毒性相对较小。阳离子型和阴离子型表面活性剂还有较强的溶血作用，非离子型表面活性剂的溶血作用一般比较轻微。静脉给药制剂中的表面活性剂的毒性比口服给药制剂中的大，外用制剂中表面活性剂的毒性相对较小。

四、表面活性剂在药剂中的应用

（一）增溶剂

药物在水中因加入表面活性剂而溶解度增加的现象称为增溶。具有增溶作用的表面活性剂称为增溶剂。

案例导入

如前所述，当表面活性剂水溶液达到临界胶束浓度后，表面活性剂分子缔合形成胶束，被增溶物以不同方式与胶束结合而使其溶解度增大。非极性物质如苯、甲苯等可完全进入胶束内核的非极性区而被增溶；水杨酸等带极性基团的分子，其非极性基团如苯环插入胶束内核中，极性基团如羧基则伸入胶束外层的极性区；极性物如对羟基苯甲酸由于分子两端都有极性基团，可完全被胶束外聚氧乙烯链所吸引而被增溶，如图 8-9 所示。

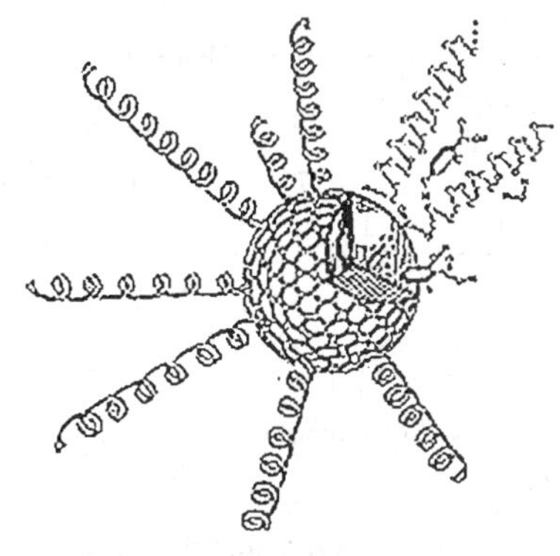

图 8-9 表面活性剂的球形胶束及其增溶模型

（二）乳化剂

表面活性剂可以用作乳化剂，其乳化作用机制主要是形成界面膜、降低界面张力或形成扩散双电层等。

（三）润湿剂

促进液体在固体表面铺展或渗透的作用称为润湿，能起润湿作用的表面活性剂称为润湿剂。润湿剂的作用原理是降低固 - 液两相界面张力和接触角。

（四）起泡剂与消泡剂

具有表面活性的高分子物质通常有较强的亲水性和较高的 *HLB* 值，在溶液中可降低液体的界面张力而使泡沫稳定，这些物质即称为起泡剂。

一些 *HLB* 值为 1~3 的亲油性较强的表面活性剂加入泡沫体系中时，其可与泡沫液层的起泡物质争夺液膜上空间，降低表面黏度，促使液膜液体流失而消泡，这些表面活性剂即称为消泡剂。

（五）杀菌剂

大多数阳离子型表面活性剂和两性离子型表面活性剂及少数阴离子型表面活性剂可用作杀菌剂。其杀菌机制是由于表面活性剂与细菌生物膜的蛋白质发生相互作用，使蛋白质变性或破坏。

（六）去污剂

去污剂，也称洗涤剂，是用于去除污垢的表面活性剂。去污作用是表面活性剂润湿、渗透分散、乳化或增溶等各种作用的综合结果。

PPT

第三节 溶解度与增加药物溶解度的方法

一、溶解度及其影响因素

1. 溶解度的概念

溶解度系指在一定温度（气体在一定压力）下，在一定量溶剂中溶解药物达到饱和时的最大量，现行版《中国药典》关于溶解度有 7 种描述：极易溶解、易溶、溶解、略溶、微溶、极微

溶解、几乎不溶或不溶。这些概念仅表示药物大致溶解性能，准确的溶解度以一份溶质（1g 或 1ml）溶于若干毫升溶剂中表示。

2. 影响溶解度的因素

（1）温度　取决于溶解过程是吸热过程还是放热过程。当溶解过程为吸热过程，溶解度随温度升高而增加；反之，溶解度随温度升高而降低。

（2）溶剂　药物在溶剂中的溶解度是药物分子与溶剂分子间相互作用的结果。即药物的极性与溶剂的极性相似，则药物溶解度大；反之，则溶解度小，即所谓的“相似相溶”规律。

（3）药物性质　不同的药物在同一溶剂中具有不同的溶解度。主要因极性有差异，也与晶型和晶格引力的大小有关。结晶型药物由于晶格能的存在，与无定型药物溶解度差别很大。

（4）粒子大小　一般情况下溶解度与药物粒子大小无关，但当药物粒子的粒径处于微粉状态时，根据 Ostwald – Freundlich 公式，药物溶解度随粒径减小而增加。

二、增加药物溶解度的方法

1. 增溶　详见本章第二节。

2. 助溶　系指一些难溶于水的药物由于第二种物质的加入而使其在水中溶解度增加的现象。加入的第二种物质称为助溶剂。

难溶性药物与助溶剂形成可溶性的络合物、有机分子复合物或通过复分解反应生成可溶性盐类而产生助溶作用。助溶机制有：①助溶剂与难溶性药物形成可溶性络合物；②形成有机分子复合物；③通过复分解而形成可溶性盐类。

常用的助溶剂可分为两类：一类是某些有机酸及其钠盐，如苯甲酸钠、水杨酸钠、对氨基苯甲酸钠等；另一类是酰胺化合物，如乌拉坦、尿素、烟酰胺、乙酰胺等。

3. 使用潜溶剂　有时溶质在混合溶剂中的溶解度要比其在各单一溶剂中的溶解度大，这种现象称为潜溶，具有这种性质的混合溶剂称为潜溶剂。常与水组成潜溶剂的有：乙醇、丙二醇、甘油、聚乙二醇 300 或 400 等。

4. 制成盐类　一些难溶性弱酸、弱碱，可制成盐而增加其溶解度。选用盐类时除考虑溶解度因素、满足临床要求外，还需考虑溶液的 pH 值、稳定性、吸湿性、毒性及刺激性等因素。

此外，提高温度可促进药物的溶解；应用微粉化技术可降低粒径以提高药物的溶解度；包合技术、固体分散技术等新技术的应用也可促进药物的溶解。

第四节　真溶液型液体药剂
8.4　True Solution Liquid Preparations

PPT

一、概述
8.4.1　Overview

真溶液型液体制剂系指药物以小分子或离子状态分散在溶剂中形成的供内服或外用的液体制

剂。主要包括溶液剂、芳香水剂、甘油剂、醑剂等剂型。真溶液型液体制剂为澄明液体，药物的分散度高，因而药物吸收快。

True solution liquid preparations refer to the liquid preparations that the drug in the solvent with the form of small molecules or ions and it can be used internal or external. It mainly includes solutions, aromatic water agents, glycerins, spirits, etc. True solution liquid preparations are the clear liquid with high drug dispersion and fast absorption.

二、溶液剂
8.4.2 Solution

溶液剂系指药物溶解于溶剂中所形成的澄明液体制剂，供内服或外用。

The solution refers to the clear liquid preparation that the drug is dissolved in solvent for oral or external use.

溶液剂的制备方法有：溶解法、稀释法与化学反应法。

The solution is prepared by dissolution method, dilution method, chemical reaction method.

案例导入 ¦ Case example

案例 8-1 复方碘溶液

8-1 Compound iodine solution

处方：碘 50g 碘化钾 100g 蒸馏水适量 共制成 1000ml

Ingredients: Iodine 50g, potassium iodide 100g, distilled water appropriate amount. It is prepared totally 1000ml.

作用与用途：调节甲状腺功能，用于甲状腺功能亢进的辅助治疗。外用作黏膜消毒剂。

Functions and indications: Regulates thyroid function, for the auxiliary treatment of hyperthyroidism. External as a mucosal disinfectant.

制法：取碘与碘化钾，加蒸馏水 100ml 溶解后，再加蒸馏水至 1000ml，搅匀即得。

Making Procedure: Take iodine and potassium iodide, add 100ml of distilled water to dissolve, add distilled water to 1000ml, and stir, obtain.

用法与用量：口服，一次 0.1~0.5ml，一日 0.3~0.8ml。极量，一次 1ml，一日 3ml。

Usage and dosage: For oral administration, 0.1-0.5ml per time, 0.3-0.8ml a day. Extreme amount, 1ml per time, 3ml a day.

注解：（1）碘在水中极微溶解（1∶2950），而且具有挥发性。本品中，碘化钾为助溶剂，可与碘生成易溶性络合物而溶解，且生成络合物后可降低碘的刺激性。

Notes: ① Iodine is very slightly soluble in water (1∶2950) and volatile. In this product, potassium iodide is a hydrotropic agent, which can be dissolved by forming a soluble complex with iodine. The stimulation of iodine can be reduced after forming a complex.

（2）制备时，应先用少量水溶解碘化钾成浓溶液，易与碘形成络合物而溶解。

② In preparation, potassium iodide should be dissolved in a small amount of water to form a concentrated solution which is conducive to the complex formation of iodine and dissolution.

思考题：使用助溶剂与增溶剂增加药物的溶解度后形成的体系有什么不同？

Question: What is the difference between using hydrotropic agent and cosolvent to increase the solubility of drugs?

案例导入

三、芳香水剂与露剂

8.4.3 Aromatic Water and Distillate

芳香水剂系指挥发油或其他挥发性芳香药物的过饱和或近饱和的澄明水溶液。个别芳香水剂可用水和乙醇的混合液作溶剂。含挥发性成分的药材用水蒸气蒸馏法制成的芳香水剂称露剂或药露。

The aromatic water refers to the clear aqueous solution that contains supersaturated or near-saturated essential oil or other volatile aromatic drugs. Ethanol solution can be used as solvent in special aromatic water. The aromatic water contains medicinal materials with volatile ingredients which made by steam distillation is called distillate.

芳香水剂常用溶解法、稀释法、蒸馏法制备。通常制成浓芳香水剂，临用时再稀释。

The aromatic water is usually prepared by dissolution, dilution and distillation. It is generally prepared to the concentrated aromatic water, then diluted before use.

案例导入

四、甘油剂

8.4.4 Glycerins

甘油剂系指药物溶于甘油中制成专供外用的溶液剂。

Glycerins refer to the solution which is dissolved in glycerine for external use.

甘油具有黏稠性、防腐性和吸湿性，对皮肤黏膜有柔润和保护作用，附着于皮肤黏膜能使药物滞留患处而起延效作用，且具有一定的防腐作用。甘油剂的引湿性较大，故应密闭保存。

Glycerine has viscous, antiseptic and hygroscopic properties, which can soften and protect the skin mucosa. Glycerine can make the drug lodge in the affected area and prolong the effect because of adhesion to the skin mucosa.It also has an effect of antisepsis. Glycerins has a high hygroscopicity, so it should be kept in a closed place.

甘油剂常用溶解法与化学反应法制备。

The glycerins are usually prepared by dissolving method and chemical reaction method.

案例导入

五、醑剂

8.4.5 Spirits

醑剂系指挥发性药物的浓乙醇溶液。凡用于制备芳香水剂的药物一般都可以制成醑剂，供外用或内服。醑剂含乙醇量一般为60%~90%。醑剂应贮藏于密闭容器中，置冷暗处保存。由于醑剂中的挥发油易氧化、酯化或聚合，久贮易变色，甚至出现黏性树脂物沉淀，故不宜长期贮藏。

Spirits refer to the concentrated ethanol solution of volatile drug. The drug used to prepare aromatic water can usually be made into spirit for internal or external use. Generally, the ethanol content is 60%-90%. The spirit should be stored in a closed container, and in a cold dark place. The volatile oil in spirit is easily oxidized, esterified or polymerized. It is easily to change color with long storage, even with the appearence of the viscos rosin precipitation, so it is not suitable for long-term storage.

醑剂常用溶解法及蒸馏法制备。

The spirt is usually prepared by dissolution and distillation.

PPT

英文翻译

第五节 胶体溶液型液体药剂

一、概述

胶体溶液型液体药剂系指大小在 1~100nm 范围的分散相质点分散于分散介质中形成的溶液。分散介质大多为水，少数为非水溶剂

二、胶体溶液的性质

1. 高分子溶液 高分子化合物以单分子形式分散于溶剂中形成的均相药剂称为高分子溶液，又称为亲水溶液。高分子溶液具有以下性质：①荷电性：溶液中的高分子化合物因解离而带电，有的带正电，有的带负电；②渗透压：亲水性高分子溶液与溶胶不同，有较高的渗透压，渗透压的大小与高分子溶液的浓度有关；③黏度：高分子溶液是黏稠性流体，黏稠性大小用黏度表示，可根据黏度测定高分子化合物的分子量；④胶凝性：有些高分子溶液，在温热条件下为黏稠性流动液体，当温度降低时形成网状结构，形成了不流动的半固体状物，称为凝胶。

2. 溶胶 溶胶是由多分子聚集体作为分散相的质点，分散在液体分散介质中组成的胶体分散体系。溶胶胶粒上既有使其带电的离子，也含有一部分反离子，形成的带电层称为吸附层；另一部分反离子散布在吸附层的外围，形成与吸附层电荷相反的扩散层。这种由吸附层和扩散层构成的电性相反的电层称双电层，又称扩散双电层。由于双电层的存在，溶胶具有以下性质：

（1）光学性质 当强光线通过溶胶时从侧面可见到圆锥形光束，即丁达尔效应。这是由于胶粒粒度小于自然光波长引起光散射所致。溶胶的浑浊程度用浊度表示，浊度愈大表明散射光愈强。

（2）电学性质 溶胶由于双电层结构而荷电，或正或负。在电场的作用下，胶粒或分散介质产生移动，产生电位差，称界面动电现象。

（3）动力学性质 溶胶中的胶粒在分散介质中有不规则的运动，即布朗运动。是由于胶粒受溶剂水分子不规则的撞击产生的，胶粒愈小，运动速度愈快。

三、胶体溶液的稳定性

1. 高分子溶液的稳定性 高分子化合物含有大量亲水基团，能与水形成牢固的水化膜，可阻止高分子化合物分子之间的相互凝聚，这种性质对高分子化合物的稳定性起重要作用。亲水胶体溶液的稳定性主要与水化作用有关。如向高分子溶液中加入少量电解质，不会由于反离子的作用（ξ 电位降低）而聚集。但若破坏其水化膜，则会发生聚集而引起沉淀。

2. 溶胶的稳定性 溶胶属热力学不稳定和动力学不稳定体系。热力学不稳定性主要表现为聚结，但由于胶粒表面电荷产生静电斥力，以及胶粒荷电所形成的水化膜，都增加了溶胶的聚结稳定性。动力学不稳定性主要表现为重力沉降，但由于胶粒的布朗运动又使其沉降速度变得缓

慢，增加了动力稳定性。

案例导入

四、胶体溶液的制法

1. 高分子溶液的制法 多采用溶解法制备。取天然或合成的高分子物质，加水浸泡、溶胀，必要时采用研磨、搅拌或加热等方法使之溶解，即得。高分子溶解时首先要经过有限溶胀过程，使高分子空隙间充满水分子，再经过无限溶胀过程，使高分子化合物完全分散在水中形成高分子溶液。整个制备过程称为胶溶，其快慢取决于所用高分子的性质以及工艺条件。

2. 溶胶的制法 ①分散法：常采用机械分散法、胶溶分散法、超声波分散法制备。②凝聚法：通过适当改变药物在溶液中的物理条件或通过化学反应（氧化、还原、复分解等）使形成的质点符合溶胶分散相质点大小的要求。

第六节 乳状液型液体药剂

8.6 Emulsion Liquid Preparations

PPT

一、概述

8.6.1 Overview

乳浊液系指两种互不相溶的液体，经乳化制成的一种液体以液滴状态分散于另一相液体中形成的非均相分散体系的液体制剂，又称乳剂。其中形成液滴的液体称为分散相、内相或非连续相，另一相液体则称为分散介质、外相或连续相。乳剂由水相（W）、油相（O）和乳化剂组成。

An emulsion is a heterogenous system comprising two immiscible liquid phases, one of which is dispersed to the other in the form of fine droplets. The phase that is present as fine droplets is called the dispersed (internal, discontinuous) phase, and the phase in which the droplets are suspended is the continuous (external) phase or dispersion medium. Emulsions usually consist of water phase(W), oil phase(O) and emulsifiers.

根据乳化剂的种类、性质及相比形成水包油（O/W）型或油包水（W/O）型，也可制备复乳，如 W/O/W 型或 O/W/O 型；根据乳滴粒径大小不同，乳剂可分为普通乳（1~100μm）、亚微乳（0.1~1.0μm）和纳米乳（1~100mm）。

There are two main types of emulsions, oil-in-water (O/W) and water-in-oil (W/O), according to the classification, property and phase proportion. An oil droplet enclosing a water droplet may be suspended in water to form a water-in-oil-in-water emulsion (W/O/W). Such systems, and their o/w/o counterparts, are termed multiple emulsions. Emulsions can be classified into three types according to their droplet size, ordinary emulsion (1-100μm), sub-microemulsion (0.1-1.0μm) and nano-emulsion (1-100mm).

乳剂可以口服、外用、肌内注射和静脉注射。乳剂中的液滴的分散度大，有利于提高生物利用度；油性药物制成乳剂能保证剂量准确，而且使用方便；水包油型乳剂可掩盖药物的不良臭味；外用乳剂能改善对皮肤、黏膜的渗透性，减少刺激性。

Emulsions can be administered orally, externally, intramuscularly and intravenously. The small particle size of the drugs present in emulsions results in a higher bioavailability. Oil and drugs can have an objectionable taste, accurate dose and be convenient to use by formulating into O/W emulsions. External emulsions can improve permeability of the skin or the mucous membranes and can reduce the irritation of some drugs.

二、常用的乳化剂种类与选用

8.6.2 Commonly Used Emulsifiers and the Selection of Emulsifiers

乳化剂是乳剂的重要组成部分，主要通过降低界面张力，在分散相液滴周围形成坚固的界面膜或形成双电层，增加乳剂的黏度等作用的发挥，促使乳剂形成并保持稳定。

Emulsifiers can significantly increase the stability of emulsions through decreasing the interfacial tension, forming interfacial film and double electric layer around the dispersed phase droplet, increasing the viscosity of emulsion.

（一）乳化剂的种类

(1) Types of Emulsifiers

根据性质不同，乳化剂可分为表面活性剂、高分子溶液和固体粉末三类。

Based on different properties, emulsifier can be divided into three categories.

1. 表面活性剂 显著降低界面表面张力，吸附在油 - 水界面形成单分子乳化膜。详细内容见本章第二节。

① Surfactants Surfactants can significantly reduce the interfacial tension, at the meanwhile adsorb at the oil-water interface and form monomolecular film. See chapter 8.2 for details.

2. 天然高分子材料 包括阿拉伯胶、西黄蓍胶、明胶、酪蛋白、果胶、琼脂、海藻酸盐及甲基纤维素等。这类材料降低油 – 水界面张力的能力较弱，但能增加分散介质黏度。

② Natural macromolecular materials These include acacia, tragacanth, gelatin, gelatin, casein, pectin, agar, sodium alginate, methylcellulose. The materials which generally exhibit little surface activity, absorb at the oil-water interface and form multimolecular films. They have the desirable effect of increasing the viscosity of the dispersion medium.

3. 固体粉末 能被油水两相润湿到一定程度，而聚集在两相间形成固体微粒膜。O/W 型乳化剂有氢氧化镁、氢氧化铝、二氧化硅、硅藻土等；W/O 型乳化剂有氢氧化钙、氢氧化锌、硬脂酸镁、碳黑等。

③ Solid powder Emulsions may be stabilized by finely divided solid particles if they are preferentially wetted by one phase and possess sufficient adhesion for one another such that they form a film around the dispersed droplets. Aluminum hydroxide, silicon dioxide and diatomite are preferentially wetted by water and thus stabilize O/W emulsions. calcium hydroxide, zinc hydroxide, magnesium stearate, carbon black are more readily wetted by oils and stabilize W/O emulsions.

（二）乳化剂的选用

(2) Selection of Emulsifiers

在选择乳化剂时，应根据药物的性质、油的类型、电解质是否存在、欲制备的乳剂类型、乳剂的黏度等综合考虑。

When selecting emulsifier, it should be considered according to the nature of the drug, the type of oil, the presence or absence of electrolyte, the desired type and viscosity of the emulsion.

1. 根据乳剂类型选择 一般 O/W 型乳剂应选择 O/W 型乳化剂，W/O 型乳剂应选择 W/O 型

乳化剂。

① **According to emulsion types** In general, O/W type emulsion should choose O/W type emulsifier, W/O type emulsion should choose W/O type emulsifier.

2. 根据乳剂给药途径选择 一般口服乳剂应选择无毒的天然乳化剂或某些亲水性高分子化合物类乳化剂；外用乳剂应选择无刺激性、无过敏性的乳化剂；注射用乳剂应选择磷脂、泊洛沙姆等无毒、无溶血性的乳化剂。

② **According to administration route of emulsion** Generally, non-toxic natural emulsifier or some hydrophilic polymer compound emulsifier should be selected for oral emulsion. Emulsifier without irritation and allergy should be selected for external emulsion. Emulsions for injection should select non-toxic and non-hemolytic emulsifiers such as lecithin and poloxamer.

3. 根据乳剂的性能选择 应选择乳化能力强，性质稳定，受外界因素如酸、碱、盐等影响小、无毒、无刺激性的乳化剂。

③ **According to properties of emulsifier** Emulsifiers with strong emulsifying efficacy, stable properties, little influence by external factors such as acid, alkali and salt, non-toxic and non-irritating should be selected.

4. 混合乳化剂的使用 为使乳化剂发挥较好的效果，可将几种乳化剂混合使用，但要注意相互间的配伍禁忌。乳化剂混合使用必须符合油相对 *HLB* 值的要求，见表 8-2。若油的 *HLB* 值为未知，可通过实验加以确定。

④ **According to combined use of emulsifiers** In order to make the emulsifiers exert better effect, several emulsifiers can be mixed, but the incompatibility between them should be paid attention to. Care must be taken to ensure the compatibility between the different emulsifiers. *HLB* values required for emulsification of commonly used oils are given in Table 8-2. If the *HLB* value of the oil is unknown, it can be determined through experiments.

表 8-2 乳化油相所需 *HLB* 值

名称	所需 *HLB* 值		名称	所需 *HLB* 值	
	W/O 型	O/W 型		W/O 型	O/W 型
液体石蜡（轻）	4	10.5	鲸蜡醇	—	15
液体石蜡（重）	4	10~12	硬脂醇	—	14
棉籽油	5	10	硬脂酸	—	15
植物油	—	7~12	精制羊毛脂	8	15
挥发油	—	9~16	蜂蜡	5	10~16

Table 8-2 *HLB* Values Required for Emulsification of Commonly Used Oils

Name	The required *HLB* value		Name	The required *HLB* value	
	W/O type	O/W type		W/O type	O/W type
Liquid paraffin (light)	4	10.5	Cetyl alcohol	—	15
Liquid paraffin (heavy)	4	10~12	Stearyl alcohol	—	14
Cottonseed oil	5	10	Stearic acid	—	15
Vegetable oil	—	7~12	Refined lanolin	8	15
The essential oil	—	9~16	beeswax	5	10~16

三、乳剂的稳定性
8.6.3 Stability of Emulsions

（一）影响乳剂稳定性的因素
(1) Factors Affecting Emulsion Stability

1. 乳化剂的性质 适宜 *HLB* 值的乳化剂是乳剂形成的关键，任何改变原乳剂中乳化剂 *HLB* 值的因素均影响乳剂的稳定性。

① **Properties of emulsifier** Emulsifiers with suitable *HLB* value are the key to the formation of emulsion, and any factors that can change the *HLB* value of emulsifier in the original emulsion will affect the stability of emulsion.

2. 乳化剂的用量 一般应控制在 0.5%~10%，用量不足则乳化不完全，用量过大则乳剂过于黏稠。

② **Dosage of emulsifier** Generally, it should be controlled at 0.5%-10%. If the dosage is insufficient, the emulsion is incomplete; if the dosage is too large, the emulsion is too thick.

3. 分散相的浓度 一般最稳定的分散相浓度为 50% 左右，25% 以下和 74% 以上均不利于乳剂的稳定。

③ **Concentration of dispersed phase** Generally, the most stable dispersed phase concentration is about 50%, below 25% and above 74% are not conducive to the stability of emulsion.

4. 分散介质的黏度 适当增加分散介质的黏度可提高乳剂的稳定性。

④ **Viscosity of dispersion medium** Increasing the viscosity of dispersion medium properly can improve the stability of emulsion.

5. 乳化及贮藏时的温度 一般认为适宜的乳化温度为 50~70℃，贮藏期间过冷或过热均不利于乳剂的稳定。

⑤ **Temperature during emulsification and storage** It is generally believed that the appropriate emulsifying temperature is 50-70℃, and supercooling or overheating during storage is not conducive to the stability of the emulsion.

6. 制备方法及乳化器械 油相、水相、乳化剂的混合次序及药物的加入方法影响乳剂的形成及稳定性，乳化器械所产生的机械能在制备过程中转化成乳剂形成所必需的乳化功，且决定了乳滴的大小。

⑥ **Preparation method and emulsifying apparatus** The mixing sequence of oil phase, water phase and emulsifier and the method of adding drugs affect the formation and stability of the emulsion. The mechanical energy generated by the emulsifying apparatus is converted into the emulsifying work necessary for emulsion formation during the preparation process, which determines the size of the emulsion droplet.

7. 其他 应避免制备过程的微生物污染，加适量的防腐剂。

⑦ **Others** Microbial contamination in the preparation process should be avoided by adding appropriate amount of preservatives.

（二）乳剂的不稳定现象
(2) Types of Instability

乳剂属于热力学不稳定的非均相体系，常出现的不稳定现象包括分层、絮凝、转相、破裂以及酸败等。

Emulsions belong to thermodynamically unstable heterogeneous systems, and the unstable phenomena often occur include creaming, flocculation, phase inversion, breaking, rancidification.

1. 乳析 在放置过程中，乳滴出现的上浮或下沉的现象称为分层。经过振摇后，分层的乳剂应能很快再均匀分散。乳剂的分层速度符合 Stokes 定律，降低乳滴的粒径、增加连续相的黏度、降低分散相与连续相之间的密度差等均可降低分层速度。其中最常用的方法是适当增加连续相的黏度。

① **Creaming(Delamination)** The disperse phase, according to its density relative to that of the continuous phase, rises to the top or sinks to the bottom of the emulsion, forming a layer of more concentrated emulsion. After shaking, the creaming emulsion should be able to disperse quickly and evenly. The rate of creaming conforms to Stokes law. According to this law, reducing the droplet sizes, thickening the continuous phase and decreasing in the density difference between the two phases can minimize the rate of creaming. The most common method is to increase the viscosity of continuous phase appropriately.

2. 絮凝 由于乳剂中电解质和离子型乳化剂的存在，使乳滴带电荷减少，ξ 电位降低，而出现的乳滴聚集成团的现象称为絮凝。由于乳滴仍保留液滴及其乳化膜的完整性，此时的聚集和分散是可逆的，但通常是乳剂破裂的前奏。

② **Flocculation** Flocculation is best defined as the association of particles within an emulsion to form large aggregates, which can easily be redispersed upon shaking. Flocculation is generally regarded as a precursor to the irreversible process of coalescence. It differs from coalescence primarily in that the interfacial film and individual droplets remain intact.

3. 转相 由于某些条件的变化而改变乳剂类型的现象称为转相。转相往往是由于外加物质使乳化剂的性质改变或油、水相容积发生变化所致。例如钠肥皂可以形成 O/W 型的乳剂，但加入足量的氯化钙溶液后，生成的钙肥皂可使其转变成 W/O 型。

③ **Phase inversion** Phase inversion refers to conversion of an O/W emulsion to W/O emulsion or vice versa. The phase inversion is usually caused by altering the phase volume ratio or the emulsifier type. For example, addition of calcium chloride(W/O emulsifier) to an emulsion stabilized with sodium soap(O/W emulsifier) will cause the emulsion to crack or invert.

4. 合并和破裂 乳剂中乳滴周围有乳化膜存在，但乳化膜破裂导致乳滴变大，称为合并，分散相乳滴合并且与连续相分离成不相混溶的两层液体的现象称为破裂。破裂后的乳剂再振摇，也不能恢复原来状态，因此破裂是不可逆的。

④ **Coalescence and breaking(cracking)** Coalescence is a much more serious type of instability. It occurs when the the interfacial film is insufficient to prevent the formation of progressively larger droplets, which can finally lead to breaking. Separation of an emulsion into its constituent phases is termed cracking or breaking. The breaking is irreversible.

5. 酸败 受外界因素（光、热、空气等）及微生物影响，使体系中油或乳化剂发生变化而引起的变质的现象称为酸败，通常可以加抗氧剂、防腐剂等方法加以抑制。

⑤ **Rancidification** The deterioration caused by changes in oil or emulsifier due to external factors (light, heat, air, etc.) and microorganisms is called rancidification, which can usually be suppressed by adding antioxidant, preservative and other methods.

四、乳剂的制备
8.6.4 Preparation of Emulsions

（一）干胶法
(1) Emulsifier in Oil Method

干胶法系将乳化剂（胶）分散于油相中，研匀，按比例加水，用力研磨制成初乳，再加水稀释至全量的方法。在初乳中油、水、胶有一定的比例，若用植物油，其比例为 4∶2∶1；若用挥发油比例为 2∶2∶1；而用液体石蜡比例为 3∶2∶1。本法适用于阿拉伯胶或阿拉伯胶与西黄蓍胶的混合胶。

It is a method of dispersing emulsifier (glue) in oil phase, grinding evenly, adding water in proportion, grinding hard to form primary emulsion, and then adding water to dilute to full volume. There is a certain proportion of oil, water and glue in primary emulsion. The proportion of oil, water and colloid is 4∶2∶1 for vegetable oil, 2∶2∶1 for volatile oil, 3∶2∶1 for liquid paraffin. This method is applicable to acacia or acacia mixed with tragacanth.

案例导入 ¦ Case example

案例 8-2 鱼肝油乳

8-2 Cod Liver Oil Emulsion

处方：鱼肝油 50.0ml，阿拉伯胶 12.50g，西黄蓍胶 0.70g，糖精钠 0.01g，挥发杏仁油 0.1ml，羟苯乙酯 0.05g，纯化水加至 100ml

Ingredients:Cod liver oil 50.0ml, acacia 12.50g, Tragacanth 0.70g, Saccharin sodium 0.01g, Volatile almond oil from prunus dulcis 0.1ml, Ethylparaben 0.05g, Purified water is added to 100ml

功能与主治：用于预防和治疗成人维生素 A 和 D 缺乏症。

Functions and indications: To prevent and treat vitamin A and D deficiency in adults.

制法：将阿拉伯胶、西黄蓍胶与鱼肝油研匀；一次性加入 25.0ml 纯化水，用力沿一个方向研磨制成初乳；加糖精钠水溶液、挥发杏仁油、尼泊金乙酯溶液，再加纯化水至全量，搅匀，即得。

Making Procedure: Grinding acacia, tragacanth and cod liver oil 25.0ml of purified water is added at one time, and the primary emulsion is prepared by hard grinding along one direction. Add sodium saccharin aqueous solution, volatile almond oil from prunus dulcis, ethylparaben solution, adding purified water to the full amount, stir well.

用法与用量：口服。预防：成人一日 15ml，分 1~2 次以温开水调服；治疗，成人一日 35~65ml，分 1~3 次以温开水调服，服用 1~2 周后剂量可减至一日 15ml，分 1~2 次服用。

Usage and dosage: Oral administration. Prevention: Adults take with 15ml of warm boiled water 1-2 times a day. For treatment, adults take with 35-65ml of warm boiled water 1-3 times a day, and the dosage can be reduced to 15ml of warm boiled water 1-2 times a day after taking for 1-2 weeks.

注解：处方中鱼肝油为药物、油相；阿拉伯胶为乳化剂；西黄蓍胶为辅助乳化剂（增加连续相黏度）；糖精钠、杏仁油为矫味剂；羟苯乙酯为防腐剂。

Notes: In the prescription, cod liver oil is the medicine and oil phase, acacia is emulsifier, tragacanth is auxiliary emulsifier (increasing viscosity of continuous phase), sodium saccharin and almond oil from

prunus dulcis is flavoring agents, ethylparaben is preservative.

思考题：干胶法制备乳剂时，初乳的形成是关键，初乳形成的判断标准是什么？制备初乳时有哪些注意事项？

Questions: When preparing emulsion by emulsifier in oil method, the key is the formation of primary emulsions. What is the judgment standard of primary emulsions formation? What should we pay attention to when preparing primary emulsions?

（二）湿胶法

(2) Emulsifier in Water Method

湿胶法也需制备初乳，初乳中油：水：胶的比例与干胶法相同。先将乳化剂分散于水相中，然后加入油相，用力研磨使成初乳，再加水稀释至全量，混匀，即得。

This method also requires the preparation of primary emulsion. The ratio of oil: water: colloid in primary emulsion is the same as that in the above method. Disperse emulsifier in water phase, add oil phase, grind hard to obtain primary emulsion, dilute with water to full volume, and mix.

（三）新生皂法

(3) Nascent Soap Method

油水两相混合时，两相界面生成新生态皂类乳化剂，经搅拌制成乳剂。植物油中含有硬脂酸、油酸等有机酸，加入氢氧化钠、氢氧化钙、三乙醇胺等，在高温下（70℃以上）或振摇，可生成新生皂为乳化剂，形成乳剂。钠盐可形成 O/W 型乳剂，钙盐可形成 W/O 型乳剂。

When oil and water are mixed, a nascent soap emulsifier is generated at the interface of the two phases, and the emulsion is prepared by stirring. Vegetable oil contains organic acids such as stearic acid and oleic acid, adding sodium hydroxide, calcium hydroxide, triethanolamine, etc., under high temperature (70℃ or above) or shaking, can generate nascent soap as emulsifier, forming emulsion. Sodium salt can form O/W emulsion, calcium salt can form W/O emulsion.

案例导入 ¦ Case example

案例 8-3　石灰搽剂

8-3　Lime Liniment

处方：花生油 500ml，氢氧化钙饱和水溶液 500ml

Ingredients: Peanut oil 500ml, Calcium hydroxide saturated solution 500ml

功能与主治：收敛、消炎。用于治疗烫伤。

Functions and indications: Convergence, anti-inflammatory. Used for treating scald.

制法：将花生油与氢氧化钙溶液混合，用力振摇，制成 W/O 型乳剂。

Making Procedure: Peanut oil and calcium hydroxide solution are mixed and shaken vigorously to prepare W/O emulsion.

用法与用量：外用。以消毒棉蘸取，涂布于患处。

Usage and dosage: External use. Apply to the affected part with the sterilized cotton.

注解：花生油中含有游离脂肪酸，与氢氧化钙生成脂肪酸钙，为 W/O 型乳剂。本法也称"新生皂法"，也可加无水羊毛脂作乳化剂，以克服分层现象。

Notes: Peanut oil contains free fatty acid, which forms fatty acid calcium with calcium hydroxide. It is a W/O emulsion. This method is also called "nascent soap method" and anhydrous lanolin can also be added as emulsifier to overcome the creaming.

思考题：新生皂法制备乳剂时，影响制成乳剂类型的主要因素是什么？

Question: What are the main factors that affect the type of emulsion prepared by the nascent soap method?

（四）两相交替加入法

(4) Alternate Addition Method

向乳化剂中每次少量交替地加入水或油，边加边搅拌，也可形成乳剂。天然胶类、固体微粒乳化剂等可用本法制备乳剂。适用于乳化剂用量较大的乳剂制备。

Alternate addition of the two phases to the emulsifier. In this method, the water and oil are added alternatively, in small portions, to the emulsifier. This method is especially suitable for natural macromolecular materials or solid particle emulsifiers and the preparation of emulsions with large amount of emulsifier.

（五）机械法

(5) Mechanical Method

将油相、水相、乳化剂混合后，利用乳化机械（乳匀机、胶体磨、超声波乳化装置等）所提供的强大的乳化能制成乳剂。此法制备乳剂时可不考虑混合顺序。

After the oil phase, water phase and emulsifier are mixed, the emulsion can be prepared by using the powerful emulsifying energy provided by emulsifying machinery, such as emulsion homogenizer, colloid mill, ultrasonic emulsifying device, etc. The mixing sequence may not be considered when preparing emulsion by this method.

（六）乳剂中添加其他药物的方法

(6) Method of Incorporation of Drugs

处方中的药物可根据其溶解性能先加于可溶解的相中，然后制成乳剂；若药物不溶于两相时，可用亲和性大的液相研磨，再制成乳剂；也可以在制成的乳剂中研磨药物，使药物混悬均匀。有的成分（如浓醇或大量电解质）可使胶类脱水，影响乳剂的形成，应先将这些成分稀释，然后逐渐加入。

The drugs in the prescription can be added into the soluble phase according to their solubility, and then made into an emulsion. If the drug is insoluble in the two phases, it can be ground by liquid phase with high affinity, and then made into emulsions. The medicine can also be ground in the prepared emulsion to make the medicine suspension uniform. Some components (such as concentrated alcohol or a large amount of electrolyte) can dehydrate colloid and affect the formation of emulsion. These components should be diluted first and then added gradually.

第七节 混悬液型液体药剂
8.7 Suspension Liquid Preparations

一、概述
8.7.1 Overview

混悬型液体制剂系指难溶性固体药物以微粒状态分散于分散介质中形成的非均相的液体制剂，也包括干混悬剂。干混悬剂系指难溶性固体药物与适宜辅料制成粉末状或粒状物，临用时加水振摇即可分散成混悬液的制剂。混悬剂属于粗分散体系，药物微粒一般在 0.5~10μm。

Suspensions are heterogeneous liquid preparations made of insoluble solid drugs substances dispersed in a liquid medium. Suspensions also include dried suspensions made of insoluble solid drugs and appropriate excipients, which are dry powder or granular mixture that require the addition of water. Suspensions belong to the coarse dispersion system. The particle diameter of suspensions lies between 0.5 and 10μm.

适宜制成混悬型液体制剂的药物有：难溶性药物、为了发挥长效作用或提高在水溶液中稳定性的药物。但剧毒药或剂量小的药物不应制成混悬液。

Suitable drugs for preparing suspension liquid preparations include: poorly soluble drugs, drugs for long-acting effect or for improving stability in aqueous solution. However, highly toxic drugs or drugs with small doses should not be made into suspension.

二、影响混悬剂稳定性的因素
8.7.2 Factors Affecting the Stability of Suspension

混悬型液体制剂的分散相微粒的布朗运动不显著，为动力学不稳定体系。因微粒有较大的界面能，容易聚集，又属于热力学不稳定体系。

The Brownian motion of dispersed phase particles of suspension liquid preparation is not significant, and it is a kinetically unstable system. Because particles have large interfacial energy and are easy to aggregate, they also belong to thermodynamically unstable systems.

1. 混悬微粒的荷电与水化 混悬液中的微粒因解离或吸附等而带电，微粒与周围分散媒之间存在电位差，即 ξ 电势。由于微粒表面荷电而与水分子发生水化作用，形成水化膜，且水化作用的强弱随双电层厚度变化，微粒荷电使微粒间产生排斥作用，加之有水化膜的存在，阻止了微粒间的相互聚集而使得混悬剂稳定。加入少量电解质可以改变混悬微粒的双电层结构和厚度，影响混悬剂的聚结特性而产生絮凝。

(1) Charge and hydration of suspended particles The particles in the suspension are charged due to dissociation or adsorption, and there is a potential difference between the particles and the surrounding dispersion medium, namely ξ potential. Due to the surface charge of the particles, hydration occurs with water molecules to form a hydration film. The strength of hydration varies with the thickness of the electric double layer. The particle charge causes repulsion between the particles. In addition, the existence

of the hydration film prevents the particles from aggregating and stabilizes the suspension. The addition of a small amount of electrolyte can change the structure and thickness of the electric double layer of the suspended particles and affect the coalescence characteristics of the suspension agent to generate flocculation.

2. 混悬微粒的沉降 在一定条件下，微粒的沉降速度遵循 Stokes 定律：

(2) Sedimentation Sedimentation is the downward movement of particles under gravity. Sedimentation is described by Stokes equation:

$$v=\frac{2r^2(\rho_1-\rho_2)g}{9\eta} \tag{8-2}$$

式中，v 为微粒沉降速度（cm/s）；r 为微粒半径（cm）；ρ_1、ρ_2 分别为微粒和分散介质的密度（g/ml）；g 为重力加速度常数（cm/s）；η 为分散介质的黏度 [g/（cm・s）]。

where v is the sedimentation velocity (cm/s); r is the particle radius (cm); ρ_1 and ρ_2 are the densities of the particles and the medium respectively (g/ml); g is the acceleration due to gravity (cm/s); and η is the viscosity of the medium [g/(cm・s)].

由式 (8-2) 可见，微粒沉降速度 v 与微粒半径的平方 r^2、微粒与分散介质的密度差（$\rho_1-\rho_2$）成正比，与分散介质的黏度 η 成反比。可采取下列措施提高混悬液的稳定性：减小微粒粒径；增加分散介质的黏度；减小固体微粒与分散介质间的密度差。

From the above formula, it can be seen that the particle settling velocity v is directly proportional to the square r^2 of the particle radius, the density difference (ρ_1-ρ_2) between the particle and the dispersion medium, and inversely proportional to the viscosity η of the dispersion medium. The following measures can be taken to improve the stability of suspension: decreasing particle size; increasing the viscosity of the disperse phase and decreasing the difference between the density of the particle and the disperse phase.

3. 微粒增大与晶型转变 难溶性药物制成混悬剂时，药物粒子大小不可能完全一致。当药物粒子处于微粉状态时，药物溶解度随粒径减小而增加，在混悬剂中将出现小微粒逐渐溶解变得越来越小，大微粒变得越来越大，沉降速度加快，造成混悬剂的稳定性降低。因此，在制备时，减少微粒粒径的同时，还要考虑其大小的一致性。

(3) Crystal growth and Polymorphism When insoluble drugs are made into suspensions, the drug particle sizes cannot be completely consistent. When drug particles are in micropowder state, drug solubility increases with the decrease of particle size, small particles appearing in the suspension gradually dissolve and become smaller and smaller, large particles become larger and larger, and the settling speed is accelerated, resulting in the decrease of stability of the suspension. Therefore, in preparation, the consistency of particle size should be considered while reducing particle size.

同质多晶型药物，其亚稳定型的溶出速度与溶解度比稳定型大，且体内吸收好。亚稳定型在贮藏过程中逐步转化为稳定型而产生结块、沉降，从而不仅可能影响混悬型液体制剂的稳定性，还可能降低药效。可以通过增加分散介质黏度或加入抑制剂等方法克服。

Polymorphism refers to the different internal crystal structures of a chemically identical compound. The dissolution rate and solubility of metastable drugs are higher than that of stable drugs and they are well absorbed in vivo. In the process of storage, the metastable type is gradually transformed into the stable type, resulting in caking and settling, which may not only affect the stability of the suspension liquid preparation, but also reduce the efficacy. It can be overcome by increasing the viscosity of

dispersion medium or adding inhibitors.

4. 分散相的浓度和温度的影响 在同一分散介质中，分散相的浓度增加，混悬剂的稳定性降低。温度的变化对混悬剂的影响更大，不仅改变药物溶解度和分解速度，还能改变微粒的沉降速度、絮凝速度、沉降容积，从而改变混悬剂的稳定性。

(4) The concentration and temperature of the dispersed phase In the same dispersion medium, the concentration of dispersed phase increases and the stability of suspension decreases. The change of temperature has greater influence on the suspension, not only changing the drug solubility and decomposition speed, but also changing the settling speed, flocculation speed and settling volume of particles, thus changing the stability of the suspension.

三、混悬剂的稳定剂
8.7.3 Stabilizer of Suspensions

为了增加混悬剂的物理稳定性，在制备时需加入助悬剂、润湿剂、絮凝剂和反絮凝剂等。

In order to increase the physical stability of suspensions, a number of formulation components can be incorporated to maintain the solid particles in dispersed state. These substances can be classified as suspending agent, wetting agent, flocculating agent and deflocculating agent.

（一）润湿剂
(1) Wetting Agents

疏水性药物（如硫黄、阿司匹林等）制备混悬剂时，常加入润湿剂以利于分散。常用的润湿剂有 *HLB* 值在 7~11 的表面活性剂，如聚山梨酯、聚氧乙烯脂肪醇醚等。

When preparing suspensions of hydrophobic drugs (such as sulfur, aspirin, etc.), wetting agents are often added to facilitate particle dispersion. Common wetting agents include surfactants with an *HLB* value of 7 to 11, such as polysorbate, Polyoxyethylene fatty alcohol ether, etc.

（二）助悬剂
(2) Suspending Agents

助悬剂能增加分散介质的黏度、降低微粒的沉降速度，同时能被药物微粒表面吸附形成机械性或电性保护膜，防止微粒间互相聚聚或产生晶型转变，或使混悬液具有触变性，从而增加其稳定性。

Suspension agents can increase the viscosity of dispersion medium and reduce the settling velocity of particle，at the same time，the agents can be adsorpted on the surface of mechanical，then form a mechanical or electrical protective film to prevent particles get together with each other or crystal transformation，or make suspension has thixotropy，thus increase the stability.

常用的助悬剂有：①低分子助悬剂，如甘油、糖浆剂等。②高分子助悬剂，主要分为天然和合成两类。常用的天然高分子助悬剂有阿拉伯胶、西黄蓍胶、琼脂、海藻酸钠、果胶等。常用的合成高分子助悬剂有甲基纤维素、羧甲基纤维素钠、羟乙基纤维素、聚维酮、聚乙烯醇等。③硅酸类，如胶体二氧化硅、硅酸铝、硅皂土等。④触变胶，利用触变胶的触变性提高混悬剂的稳定性，如单硬脂酸铝溶解于植物油中可形成典型的触变胶，在静置时形成凝胶，可防止微粒沉降，振摇时变成溶胶，有利于混悬剂的倾倒。

Commonly used suspending agents are: ① Low molecular suspending agents, such as glycerol, syrup, etc. ② Polymer suspending agents, mainly divided into natural and synthetic two categories. Commonly used natural polymer assistant suspending agents are acacia, tragacanth, agar, sodium alginate, pectin, etc. Commonly used synthetic polymer suspending agents are methyl cellulose, sodium carboxymethyl cellulose, hydroxyethyl cellulose, polyvinyl pyrrolidone, polyvinyl alcohol, etc. ③ Silicate, such as colloidal silica, aluminum silicate, bentonite, ect. ④ Thixotrope, which can improve the stability of suspensions by using thixotropic adhesive. For example, aluminum monostearate dissolved in vegetable oil can form a typical thixotrope, which can prevent the particles from settling and turn into sol when shaking, which is conducive to the toppling of suspension.

（三）絮凝剂与反絮凝剂

(3) Flocculatings Agents and Deflocculatings Agents

加入适量的电解质可使混悬型液体药剂中微粒周围双电层形成的ζ电位降低到一定程度，使得微粒间吸引力稍大于排斥力，形成疏松的絮状聚集体，经振摇又可恢复成分散均匀混悬液的现象叫絮凝，所加入的电解质称为絮凝剂。加入电解质后使ζ电位升高，阻碍微粒之间碰撞聚集的现象称为反絮凝，能起反絮凝作用的电解质称为反絮凝剂，加入适宜的反絮凝剂也能提高混悬剂的稳定性。

Adding an appropriate amount of electrolyte can reduce the ζ potential formed by the electric double layer around the particles in the suspension liquid medicament to a certain extent, so that the attraction force between the particles is slightly greater than the repulsive force, forming loose flocculent aggregates, which can be restored to a uniformly dispersed suspension after shaking. The phenomenon of forming a uniformly dispersed suspension is called flocculation, and the electrolyte added is called a flocculating agent. The added electrolyte is called flocculation. The ζ potential increases after adding electrolyte, and the phenomenon of blocking collision and aggregation between particles is called deflocculation. The electrolyte capable of deflocculation is called deflocculating agents. Adding appropriate deflocculating agent can also improve the stability of suspension.

同一电解质可因用量不同起絮凝作用或发絮凝作用，如枸橼酸盐、枸橼酸氢盐、酒石酸盐、酒石酸氢盐、磷酸盐及一些氯化物等。

The same electrolyte can be flocculated or deflocculated according to different dosage, such as citrate, hydrogen citrate, tartrate, hydrogen tartrate, phosphate and some chlorides.

四、混悬剂的制法

8.7.4 Preparation of Suspensions

（一）分散法

(1) Dispersing Method

将固体药物粉碎后，混悬于分散介质中。其中，亲水性药物（氧化锌、炉甘石、碱式碳酸铋、碳酸钙、碳酸镁、磺胺类等）一般与分散介质加液体研磨至适宜的分散度，然后加入剩余液体至全量。疏水性药物应先加润湿剂研匀，再加其他液体研磨，最后加入亲水性液体稀释至全量。

The solid drug is pulverized and suspended in a dispersion medium. Among them, hydrophilic drugs (zinc oxide, calamine, basic bismuth carbonate, calcium carbonate, magnesium carbonate, sulfonamides, etc.) are generally added with dispersion medium to grind to a proper dispersion degree, and then the remaining liquid is added to the full amount. Hydrophobic drugs should be first ground with wetting agent, then ground with other liquids, and finally diluted to full volume with hydrophilic liquid.

案例导入 ¦ Case example

案例 8-4 炉甘石洗剂

8-4 Calamine Lotion

处方：炉甘石 150g，氧化锌 50g，甘油 50ml，羧甲基纤维素钠 2.5g，蒸馏水加至 1000ml。

Ingredients: Calamine 150g, zinc oxide 50g, glycerol 50ml, sodium carboxymethyl cellulose (CMC-Na) 2.5g, distilled water was added to 1000ml.

功能与主治：用于急性瘙痒性皮肤病，如湿疹和痱子。

Functions and indications: Used for treating acute pruritus dermatoses such as eczema and miliaria.

制法：取炉甘石、氧化锌，加甘油和适量蒸馏水共研成糊状；另取羧甲基纤维素钠加蒸馏水溶胀后，分次加入上述糊状液中，随加随搅拌，再加蒸馏水使成 1000ml，搅匀，即得。

Making Procedure: Take calamine, zinc oxide, add glycerin and appropriate amount of distilled water, grind into paste. In addition, CMC-Na is added into the paste solution after being dissolved in distilled water for swelling, and is added into the paste solution in batches, stirred with the addition, distilled water is added into the paste solution to make the paste solution 1000ml, and stirred evenly to obtain the final product.

用法与用量：局部外用，用时摇匀，取适量涂于患处，每日 2~3 次。

Usage and dosage: For topical application, shake well and apply appropriate amount to the affected part 2-3 times daily.

注解：炉甘石和氧化锌均为水中不溶的亲水性药物，能被水润湿。故先加甘油研成细糊状，再与羧甲基纤维素钠水溶液混合，使粉末周围形成保护膜，以阻碍颗粒的聚合，振摇时易悬浮。

Notes: Calamine and zinc oxide are hydrophilic drugs insoluble in water and can be wetted by water. Therefore, glycerin is first added and ground into a fine paste, and then mixed with CMC-Na aqueous solution to form a protective film around the powder to hinder the polymerization of particles, which is easy to suspend during shaking.

思考题：本品除采用羧甲基纤维素钠为助悬剂外，还可以采用哪些助悬剂？

Question: Besides CMC-Na as suspending agents, which suspending agents can be used for this product?

（二）凝聚法

(2) Agglomeration

1. 物理凝聚法 药物溶解在适当的溶剂中制成饱和溶液，然后加入另一不相混溶的溶剂，使之迅速析出结晶微粒，再分散于分散介质中制得的混悬液。

① **Physical agglomeration** The drug is dissolved in a suitable solvent to form a saturated solution, then a miscible nonsolvent is added and a precipitation is formed. Disperse the precipitation in the dispersion medium to form suspensions.

2. 化学凝聚法 采用化学反应法使两种或两种以上的药物生成难溶性的药物微粒，再混悬于分散介质中制成混悬剂。为使微粒细小均匀，化学反应宜在稀溶液中进行，并应急速搅拌。

② **Chemical agglomeration** A chemical reaction method is used to make two or more drugs into insoluble drug particles, and then suspend them in a dispersion medium to make suspensions. In order to make the particles fine and uniform, the chemical reaction is carried out in a dilute solution, and stirred quickly.

第八节 其他液体药剂

8.8 Other Liquid Medicinal Preparations

PPT

除用于口服外，液体药剂还有应用于皮肤、五官科及人体腔道部位的，包括灌肠剂、洗剂、搽剂、滴耳剂、滴鼻剂和含漱剂等。

In addition to oral administration, liquid preparations are also applied to skin, ear-nose-throat and body cavity, including enemas, lotions, liniments, ear drops, nasal drops and gargarismas.

一、灌肠剂

8.8.1 Enemas

灌肠剂系指灌注于直肠的水性、油性溶液、乳状液和混悬液，以治疗、诊断或营养为目的的液体制剂。灌肠剂具有直肠给药特点，尤适用于昏迷患者、婴幼儿及不能服药或服药困难者。

Enemas are liquid preparations of aqueous or oily solutions, emulsions or suspensions, intended to be perfused into the rectum for treatment, diagnosis or nutrition. Enema has the characteristics of rectal administration. It is especially suitable for comatose patients, infants and person who cannot take medicine orally or take medicine with difficulty.

二、洗剂

8.8.2 Lotions

洗剂系指含原料药物的溶液、乳状液或混悬液，供清洗无破损皮肤或腔道用的液体制剂，常具有消毒、消炎、止痒、收敛、保护等局部作用。

Lotions are liquid preparations in the form of solutions, suspensions or emulsions containing drug substances, intended for bathing the unbroken skin or cavities. It generally has the functions of disinfection, anti-inflammatory, antipruritic, astringency, and protective action.

三、搽剂

8.8.3 Liniments

搽剂系指原料药物用乙醇、油或适宜的溶剂制成的液体制剂，供无破损皮肤揉擦用，常具有镇痛、保护和抗刺激的作用。用时可加在绒布或其他柔软物料上，轻轻涂裹患处。

Liniments are liquid preparations made of drug substances and suitable solvents such as ethanol oil etc., intend for external use to rub on unbroken skin. It has the functions of analgesia, protection and

decreasing of the irritation. When used, it can be added to flannelette or other soft materials, and gently applied to the affected area.

四、滴耳剂
8.8.4 Ear Drops

滴耳剂系指由原料药物与适宜辅料制成的水溶液，或由甘油或其他适宜溶剂制成的澄明溶液、混悬液或乳状液，供滴入外耳道用的液体制剂，一般具有消毒、止痒、收敛、消炎或润滑局部作用。

Ear drops are clear solutions, suspensions or emulsions made of drug substances, suitable excipients and suitable solvents such as water or glycerol, etc., intended for instillation in external auditory meatus. It has the functions of disinfection, antipruritic, astringency, anti-inflammatory or lubricating local areas.

五、滴鼻剂
8.8.5 Nasal Drops

滴鼻剂系指由原料药物与适宜辅料制成的澄明溶液、混悬液或乳状液，供滴入鼻腔用的鼻用液体制剂，主要供局部消毒、消炎、收缩血管和麻醉之用，也能起全身治疗作用。

Nasal drops are liquid nasal preparations in the form of clear solutions, suspensions or emulsions made of drug substances and suitable excipients, intended for administrations to the nasal cavities. It is mainly used for local disinfection, anti-inflammatory, vasoconstriction and anesthesia, and also for general treatment.

六、含漱剂
8.8.6 Gargarismas

含漱剂系指用于清洁咽喉、口腔用的液体制剂，具有清洗、防腐、杀菌、消毒及收敛等作用。常含有适量染料着色，以示外用。

Gargarismas are liquid preparations used to clean the throat and mouth, which has the functions of cleaning, antisepsis, sterilization, disinfection and convergence. Often contains the right amount of dye coloring, for external use.

第九节 液体药剂的质量要求与检查
8.9 Quality Requirements and Inspection of Liquid Medicinal Preparations

PPT

一、口服溶液剂、口服乳剂、口服混悬剂的质量要求
8.9.1 Quality Requirements of Oral Solutions, Emulsions and Oral Suspensions

1. 装量 单剂量包装的口服溶液剂、口服混悬剂和口服乳剂的装量，每支装量与标示装量相

比较，均不得少于其标示量。凡规定检查含量均匀度者，一般不再进行装量检查。多剂量包装的口服溶液剂、口服混悬剂、口服乳剂和干混悬剂照最低装量检查法，应符合规定。

(1) Filling Volume of single-dose oral solutions, oral suspensions and oral emulsions, the content in each container should not be less than the labeled quantity of the solutions, suspensions and emulsions. Where the test for content uniformity is specified, the test for weight variation may not be required. Multi-dose oral solutions, oral suspensions, oral emulsions and oral droppings should comply with the test of Minimum Fill.

2. 装量差异 单剂量包装的干混悬剂，每袋（支）装量与平均装量相比较，装量差异限度应在平均装量的 ±10% 以内，超出装量差异限度的不得多于 2 袋（支），并不得有 1 袋（支）超出限度 1 倍。凡规定检查含量均匀度者，一般不再进行装量差异检查。

(2) Weight variation For Single-dose dry suspensions, not more than 2 of the individual weights should deviate from the average weight by more than ± 10% and none more than ± 20%. Where the test for content uniformity is specified, the test for weight variation may not be required.

3. 干燥失重 干混悬剂减失重量不得过 2.0%。

(3) Loss on drying The weight loss of dry suspensions should be not more than 2.0%.

4. 沉降体积比 口服混悬剂沉降体积比应不低于 0.90。干混悬剂沉降体积比，应符合规定。

(4) Ratio of sedimental volume The ratio of sedimental volume of oral suspension should be not less than 0.90. The ratio of sedimental volume of oral suspension should comply with the requirements.

5. 微生物限度 非无菌产品微生物限度检查应符合规定。

(5) Microbial limit Microbiological examination of nonsterile products should comply with the requirements.

二、口服溶液剂、口服乳剂、口服混悬剂的质量检查
8.9.2 Quality Inspections of Oral Solutions, Emulsions and Suspensions

装量（单剂量包装的口服溶液剂、口服混悬剂和口服乳剂）、装量差异（单剂量包装的干混悬剂）、干燥失重、沉降体积比、微生物限度检查等应符合现行版《中国药典》质量要求。

The filling (single-dose oral solution, oral suspension and oral emulsion), weight variation (single-dose dry suspension), loss on drying, ratio of sedimental volume, microbial limit inspection, etc. should comply with the requirements of the current edition of *Chinese Pharmacopoeia*.

第十节 液体药剂的矫味、矫臭与着色
8.10 Taste Modifying, Odor Modifying and Coloration of Liquid Medicinal Preparations

PPT

许多有不良臭味的药物制成液体药剂时常需要加入矫味剂和着色剂改善口感和色泽，提高患者用药顺应性。

Many drugs with bad odor need to be added with flavoring agents and coloring agents to improve the taste and color and improve the compliance of patients.

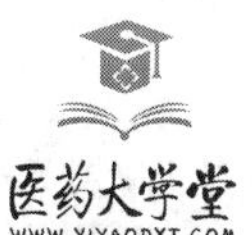

一、矫味剂
8.10.1 Flavoring Agents

矫味剂系指能改善制剂的味道和气味的物质。

Flavoring agents are substances that improve the taste and odor of preparations.

1. 甜味剂 分为天然和合成两大类。天然甜味剂有糖类、糖醇类、苷类，以糖类最常用。合成甜味剂有糖精钠、阿斯帕坦等。

(1) Sweeteners Sweeteners are divided into two categories, natural and synthetic. Natural sweetening agents are sucrose, sugar alcohols, glycosides, with sucrose being the most commonly used. Synthetic sweeteners include sodium saccharin and aspartame, etc.

2. 芳香剂 分为天然和合成两大类。天然芳香剂有挥发性芳香油（如薄荷油、橙皮油等）及其制剂。人工合成香精有香蕉香精、菠萝香精等。

(2) Fragrances Fragrances are divided into natural and synthetic categories. Natural aromatic agents include volatile aromatic oils (such as peppermint oil, orange peel oil, etc.) and their preparations. Synthetic essences include banana essence, pineapple essence, etc.

3. 胶浆剂 高分子胶浆黏稠，可以干扰味蕾的味觉而矫味。常用的胶浆剂有淀粉、羧甲基纤维素钠、甲基纤维素、海藻酸钠、阿拉伯胶胶浆等。

(3) Thickening agents Polymer mucilage is thick and can disturb taste buds and correct taste. Commonly used mucilage include starch, CMC-Na, methyl cellulose, sodium alginate, acacia, etc.

4. 泡腾剂 酸式碳酸盐与有机酸（枸橼酸、赖氨酸等）混合后，产生二氧化碳，溶于水呈酸性，能麻痹味蕾而矫味。

(4) Effervescent agents Carbon dioxide can be produced by mixing acid carbonate and organic acids (citric acid, lysine, etc.). The solution is acidic when carbon dioxide is dissolved in water, which can paralyze the taste buds and correct the taste.

5. 化学调味剂 麸氨酸钠能矫正鱼肝油的腥味，消除铁盐制剂的铁金属味。

(5) The chemical flavoring agent Sodium glutamate can correct fishy smell of cod liver oil and eliminate iron metal taste of iron salt preparation.

二、着色剂
8.10.2 Coloring Agents

着色剂能改善制剂的外观颜色，可用来识别制剂的品种，区分应用方法以及减少患者对服药的厌恶感。一般着色剂与矫味剂配合协调。分为天然色素和人工合成色素两大类。天然色素又分为植物色素（如甜菜红、姜黄、胡萝卜素、焦糖等）和矿物色素（如氧化钛等）。我国目前批准的合成食用色素有胭脂红、苋菜红、柠檬黄、靛蓝、日落黄等。外用液体药剂中常用的着色剂有伊红、品红以及美蓝等合成色素。

Coloring agents can improve the appearance and color of the preparations, which can be used to identify the varieties of preparations, distinguish application methods and reduce patients' aversion to medication. General coloring agents are coordinated with flavoring agents. It is divided into natural pigments and synthetic pigments. Natural pigments are divided into plant pigments（such as red beet,

turmeric, carotene, caramel, etc.) and mineral pigments (such as titanium oxide, etc.). At present, the synthetic edible pigments approved in China include carmine, amaranth, lemon yellow, indigo, sunset yellow, etc. There are synthetic pigments such as eosin, magenta and methylene blue in the liquid pharmaceutical preparations. Coloring agents commonly used in liquid medicines for external use include synthetic pigments such as eosin, magenta and methylene blue.

第十一节　液体药剂的包装与贮藏

8.11　Packing and Storage of Liquid Preparations

PPT

一、液体药剂的包装

8.11.1　Packing of Liquid Preparations

液体药剂的包装材料包括容器（玻璃瓶、塑料瓶等）、瓶塞（软木塞、橡胶塞、塑料塞等）、瓶盖（金属盖、电木盖等）、标签、硬纸盒、塑料盒、说明书、纸箱、木箱等。

Packaging materials for liquid preparations include containers (glass bottles, plastic bottles, etc.), bottle stoppers (cork stoppers, rubber stoppers, plastic stoppers, etc.), bottle caps (metal caps, bakelite caps, etc.), labels, cardboard boxes, plastic boxes, instructions, carton, wooden box, etc.

岗位对接

二、液体药剂的贮藏

8.11.2　Storage of Liquid Preparations

重点小结

液体药剂特别是以水为分散媒者，在贮存中容易水解、氧化或污染微生物，而产生沉淀、变色或腐败，一般都是临时调配。大量生产须采取防止微生物的措施，而且需添加防腐剂；一般应密闭，贮藏于阴凉、干燥处。

题库

Liquid preparations, especially for the dispersion medium is water, are easily to hydrolyze, oxidize or pollute microorganisms during storage, due to precipitation, discoloration or corruption, which are usually prepared temporarily. Measures to prevent microorganisms should be taken in mass production, and preservatives should be added. Generally, it should be sealed and stored in a cool and dry place.

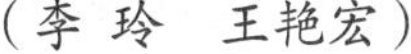

第九章　注射剂
Chapter 9　Injections

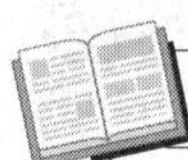

学习目标 | Learning Goals

知识要求：

1. 掌握　中药注射剂、输液剂的含义、特点、分类和质量检查；中药注射用原液的制备；中药注射剂制备的工艺过程与技术关键；热原的性质、污染途径及除去方法，热原的检查方法。

2. 熟悉　注射剂常用溶剂的种类；注射用水的质量要求及蒸馏法制备注射用水；注射用油的质量要求及精制法；注射剂常用附加剂的种类、性质、选用和质量要求及处理；热原的组成；中药注射剂存在的问题及解决途径。

3. 了解　中药注射剂的发展概况；注射剂容器的种类；血浆代用液、粉针剂、混悬液型及乳状液型注射剂的制备要点和质量检查；细菌内毒素的检查方法。

能力要求：

学会中药注射剂的制备与质量检测方法，注射剂溶剂和附加剂的选择，以及中药注射剂制备的关键技术。

Knowledge requirements:

1. To master the definition, characteristic, classification, quality inspection of Chinese medicine injections and infusions. The manufacture processes and key points of Chinese medicine injections. The characteristic, contamination route, removal method and inspection method of the pyrogen.

2. To be familiar with the common solvents. The quality requirements of water for injection and the preparation of water for injection by distillation. Or the quality requirements and the refining methods of oil for injection. Types, properties, selection, quality requirements and treatment of common additives for injection. The composition of the pyrogen. Problems and solutions of Chinese medicine injections.

3. To know the development of Chinese medicine injections. The types of containers. The key points of preparation and quality inspections of plasma substitute, powders for injection, suspension for injection and emulsion for injection. The testing methods of bacterial endotoxin.

Ability requirements:

Learn the manufacture processes and quality control methods of Chinese medicine injections, and be able to choose the solvents and additives of injections. Learn the key technology of the preparation of Chinese medicine injections.

第一节 概述

9.1 Overview

一、注射剂的含义

9.1.1 The Definition of the Injections

中药注射剂系指饮片经提取、纯化后制成的供注入人体内的溶液、乳状液，以及供临用前配制成溶液的粉末或浓溶液的无菌制剂，是临床应用最为广泛的剂型之一。

Traditional Chinese medicine injections is a kind of sterile preparations made of decoction pieces after being extracted and purified, which are classified as solutions, emulsions, or powders, concentrated solutions dissolved or diluted before injecting into the body. It is one of the most widely used dosage forms in clinic.

二、注射剂的特点

9.1.2 The Characteristic of the Injections

1. 药效迅速，作用可靠。

(1) It works quickly and has reliable effect.

2. 适用于不宜口服给药的药物。

(2) Suitable for drugs that are not available for oral administration.

3. 适用于不能口服给药的病人。

(3) Suitable for patients of whom oral administration is not convenient.

4. 可以发挥定位定向的局部作用。

(4) It can play local roles of positioning orientation.

注射剂也存在不足之处。如注射时会产生疼痛；作用不可逆转；使用不便；制造过程复杂，生产成本及价格较高。

There are also deficiencies in injections. Such as the pain caused by injecting, irreversible effect, inconvenience when injecting. And the manufacturing process is complicated, which cause the high cost of the injections.

三、注射剂的分类

9.1.3 The Classification of the Injections

注射剂可分为注射液、注射用无菌粉末与注射用浓溶液。

Injections are classified as liquids for injection, sterile powders for injection and concentrated solutions for injection.

1. 注射液 包括溶液型、乳状液型注射液。

(1) Liquids for injection Liquids for injection includes solutions and emulsions injections.

2. 注射用无菌粉末 亦称为粉针剂。系指供临床前用适宜的无菌溶液配制成澄清溶液或均匀

混悬液的无菌粉末或无菌块状物。

(2) Sterile powder for injection Sterile powder for injection are also known as powder injection, which refers to sterile powder or sterile block prepared into a clarified solution or a uniform suspension with an appropriate sterile solution before using.

3. 注射用浓溶液 系指供临床前稀释后静脉滴注用的无菌浓溶液。

(3) Concentrated solutions for injection Concentrated solutions for injection are sterile concentrated solutions for intravenous drip after preclinical dilution.

四、注射剂的给药途径

9.1.4 Administration Routes of Injections

根据医疗的需要，注射剂有不同的给药途径。

There are different administration routes of injections according to the clinical demand.

1. 皮内注射 注射于表皮与真皮之间。一般注射剂量在 0.2ml 以下。

(1) Intradermal route (i.d.) It is injected between the epidermis and the dermis. The dosage for injection is generally below 0.2ml for one time.

2. 皮下注射 注射于真皮与肌肉之间。一般注射量为 1~2ml。

(2) Subcutaneous route (s.c.) It is injected between the dermis and the muscle. The dosage for injection is generally 1 to 2ml for one time.

3. 肌内注射 注射于肌肉组织中，一次注射量在 5ml 以下。

(3) Intramuscular route (i.m.) It is injected into muscle tissue. The dosage for injection is below 5ml for one time.

4. 静脉注射 注射于静脉内，有静脉注射和静脉滴注两种方式。

(4) Intravenous route (i.v.) It is injected into vein, including intravenous bolus and drip.

5. 脊椎腔注射 注射于脊椎四周蛛网膜下腔内，一次注射量在 10ml 以下。

(5) Vertebra caval route It is injected into subarachnoid space around the spine. The dosage for injection is below 10ml for one time.

6. 其他 包括动脉注射、脑池内注射、心内注射、关节腔注射、滑膜腔注射、鞘内注射及穴位注射等给药途径。

(6) Others Other administration routes of injections include intra-arterial injection, brain pool injection, intracardiac injection, articular injection, synovial cavity injection, intrathecal injection and acupoint injection etc.

PPT

英文翻译

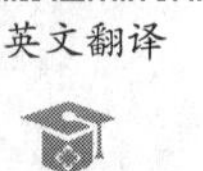

第二节 热原

一、热原的含义与组成

热原系指注射后能引起恒温动物体温异常升高的致热物质。药剂学里所指的“热原”，是指细菌性热原，是某些细菌的代谢产物、细菌尸体及内毒素。致热能力最强的是革兰阴性杆菌，霉菌、酵母菌，甚至病毒也能产生热原。

微生物代谢产物中内毒素是产生热原反应的最主要致热物质。内毒素是由磷脂、脂多糖和蛋白质所组成的复合物，其中脂多糖具有极强的致热活性。

二、热原的基本性质

1. 水溶性 热原能溶于水，是水会被热原污染的原因。

2. 不挥发性 热原本身不挥发，但因溶于水，在蒸馏时，可随水蒸气雾滴进入蒸馏水中，故蒸馏水器均应有完好的隔沫装置，以防止热原污染。

3. 耐热性 热原的耐热性较强，一般经 60℃ 加热 1 小时不受影响，100℃ 也不会发生热解，180℃、3~4 小时，250℃、30~45 分钟或 650℃、1 分钟可使热原彻底破坏。因此，常用灭菌条件不能破坏热原。

4. 滤过性 热原体积较小，在 1~5nm 之间，可通过常规滤器，但超滤膜可截留。

5. 被吸附性 热原可被活性炭吸附，也可被某些离子交换树脂所吸附。

6. 其他性质 热原能被强酸、强碱、强氧化剂（如高锰酸钾、过氧化氢）以及超声波破坏。

三、注射剂热原的污染途径

1. 溶剂带入 是注射剂出现热原的主要原因。注射用水或注射用油应新鲜使用，蒸馏器质量要好，环境应洁净。

2. 原辅料带入 有些中药原料中带有大量微生物，如果提取、浓缩的处理条件不当，易因微生物污染而导致热原的产生。用微生物方法制造的辅料如乳糖等，容易产生热原，应用时应当注意。

3. 容器或用具等带入 注射剂制备时所用的用具、管道、装置、灌装注射剂的容器，如果未按 GMP 要求认真清洗处理，均易使药液污染而导致热原产生。

4. 制备过程带入 注射剂的制备过程复杂，操作时间较长，每个环节都可能被污染而带入热原，因此，在注射剂制备的各个环节，都必须严格按 GMP 规定的操作规程操作。

5. 灭菌后带入 输液瓶经灭菌后，其铝盖轧口不严或松盖，使其在储藏过程中受微生物污染而带入热原。

6. 输液器带入 有些输液器被微生物污染而带有热原，使原本不含热原的药液被污染。

7. 使用过程带入 在加药过程中被污染的情况有两种：①在输液中加入其他药物时，所加药物本身已污染热原；②加药时操作室的洁净度达不到标准，消毒及操作不严格。

四、除去注射剂中热原的方法

（一）除去药液或溶剂中热原的方法

1. 吸附法 活性炭是常用的吸附剂，具有吸附热原、脱色、助滤等作用。除去热原需用针用规格活性炭，可与白陶土合用除去热原。

2. 离子交换法 热原分子上含有磷酸根与羧酸根，带有负电荷，因而可以被碱性阴离子交换树脂吸附。用离子交换树脂吸附除去注射剂中热原，并在大生产中应用。

3. 凝胶滤过法 也称分子筛滤过法，是利用凝胶物质作为滤过介质，当溶液通过凝胶柱时，分子量较小的成分渗入到凝胶颗粒内部而被阻滞，分子量较大的成分则沿凝胶颗粒间隙随溶剂流

出。制备的注射剂，其药物分子量明显大于热原分子时，可用此法除去热原。

4. 超滤法 本法利用高分子薄膜的选择性与渗透性，在常温条件下，依靠一定的压力和流速，达到除去溶液中热原的目的。

5. 反渗透法 本法通过三醋酸纤维素膜或聚酰胺膜除去热原，效果好，具有较高的实用价值。

6. 其他方法 采用二次以上湿热灭菌法，或适当提高灭菌温度和时间，处理含有热原的葡萄糖或甘露醇注射液亦能得到热原合格的产品。微波也可破坏热原。

以上方法联合使用，可提高热原去除率。

（二）除去容器或用具上热原的方法

1. 高温法 对于耐高温的容器或用具，如注射用针筒及其他玻璃器皿，在洗涤干燥后，经180℃加热2小时或250℃加热30分钟，可以破坏热原。

2. 酸碱法 对于耐酸碱的玻璃容器、瓷器或塑料制品，用强酸强碱溶液处理，可有效地破坏热原，常用的酸碱液为重铬酸钾硫酸洗液、硝酸硫酸洗液或稀氢氧化钠溶液。

上述方法可除去注射剂溶液、溶剂中或容器、用具上的热原，应根据实际情况合理选用。

五、热原与细菌内毒素的检查方法

1. 热原检查法 亦称家兔法，属于体内检查法。具体方法和结果判断标准见现行版《中国药典》。

2. 细菌内毒素检查法 亦称鲎试剂法，系利用鲎试剂来检测或量化由革兰阴性菌产生的细菌内毒素，以判断供试品中热原的限度是否符合规定的一种方法。具体实验方法和结果判断见现行版《中国药典》。

第三节 注射剂的溶剂

9.3 The Solvent of the Injection

PPT

注射剂所用溶剂一般分为水溶性溶剂和非水性溶剂。

Aqueous solvents and non-aqueous solvents are generally solvents used for injections.

（一）注射用水

(1) Water for Injection

1. 制药用水 制药用水分为饮用水、纯化水、注射用水及灭菌注射用水。一般应根据各生产工序或使用目的与要求选用适宜的制药用水。

① Pharmaceutical water Pharmaceutical water is divided into tap water, purified water, water for injection and sterilized water for injection. Appropriate pharmaceutical water should be selected according to the production process or the purpose and requirements.

（1）饮用水 为天然水经净化所得的水，饮用水可用于饮片净制时的漂洗、制药用具的粗洗。除另有规定外，也可作为非灭菌制剂饮片的提取溶剂。

a. Tap water It is purified from natural water. Tap water can be used to rinse decoction pieces and

wash pharmaceutical equipment roughly. Unless otherwise specified, it can also be used as an extraction solvent for the preparations of non-sterilizing decoction pieces.

（2）纯化水　为饮用水经蒸馏法、离子交换法、反渗透法或其他适宜的方法制备的制药用水。纯化水可作为配制普通药物制剂用的溶剂或试验用水；可作为中药注射剂、滴眼剂等灭菌制剂所用饮片的提取溶剂；口服、外用制剂配制用溶剂或稀释剂；非灭菌制剂用器具的精洗用水；也用作非灭菌制剂所用饮片的提取溶剂。

b. Purified water　It is the pharmaceutical water prepared from tap water by distillation, ion exchange method, reverse osmosis or other suitable methods. Purified water can be used as solvents to prepare normal drug preparation or trial water, and an extraction solvent for sterilizing preparations such as Chinese medicine injections and the eye drops. It can also be used for the solvents to prepare oral or external preparations. It is used for refined washing for containers of non-sterilizing preparations and also used as extraction solvent for non-sterilizing preparations.

（3）注射用水　为纯化水经蒸馏所得的水，应符合细菌内毒素试验要求。注射用水必须在防止细菌内毒素产生的条件下生产、贮藏和分装。可作为配制注射剂、滴眼剂等溶剂或稀释剂及容器的精洗用水。

c. Water for injection　It is distilled from purified water, which should meet the requirements of bacterial endotoxin test. Water for injection must be prepared, conserved and separated under conditions of preventing the production of bacterial endotoxin. Water for injection can be used as solvents or diluents to prepare injections and the eye drops, etc., as well as the water for fine washing of containers.

（4）灭菌注射用水　为注射用水按照注射剂生产工艺制备所得。不含任何添加剂。主要用作注射用灭菌粉末的溶剂或注射剂的稀释剂。

d. Sterilized water for injection　It is prepared according to the production process of the injection from water for injection and free of any additives. It is mainly used for solvents of the sterilized powders or diluents of the injections.

2. 注射用水的质量要求　注射用水的质量在现行版《中国药典》中有严格的规定，其性状应为无色透明液体；无臭，无味。pH 应为 5.0~7.0。氨含量不超过 0.00002%。每 1ml 含细菌内毒素的量应小于 0.25 内毒素单位（EU）。微生物限度，细菌、霉菌和酵母菌总数每 100ml 不得过 10 个。除此之外，硝酸盐与亚硝酸盐、电导率、总有机碳、不挥发物与重金属照现行版《中国药典》纯化水项下的方法检查，应符合规定。

② Quality requirements of the water for injections　Quality of water for injection is strictly stipulated in the current edition of *Chinese Pharmacopoeia*, and it should be colorless, transparent, odorless and tasteless liquid. The pH value should be 5.0 to 7.0. The ammonia content does not exceed 0.00002%. The amount of bacterial endotoxin per 1ml should be less than 0.25 endotoxin units (EU). Microbial limits (the total number of bacteria, mold and yeast) cannot exceed 10 per 100ml. In addition, nitrate and nitrite, conductivity, total organic carbon, non-volatiles and heavy metals shall be inspected in accordance with the methods under the purified water in the current edition of *Chinese Pharmacopoeia*, and should comply with the provisions.

3. 注射用水的制备　注射用水的制备常在饮用水基础上，综合应用电渗析、反渗透、离子交换树脂等方法先制备纯化水，纯化水再经蒸馏法制备成注射用水。注射用水的制备工艺流程如图 9-1 所示。

③ Preparation of water for injection　Preparation of water for injection is often based on tap water. At first, the purified water is prepared by electrodialysis, reverse osmosis, ion exchange resin and so on. Then the water for injection is prepared by distillation from the purified water. The preparation process is shown in Figure 9-1.

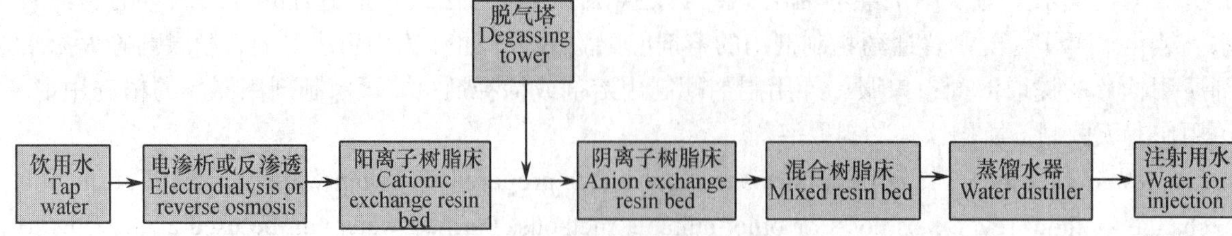

图 9-1 制备注射用水工艺流程

Figure 9-1 Process Flow Figure of Preparation of Water for Injection

（1）纯化水的制备　常用制备方法有离子交换法、电渗析法和反渗透法等。

a. Preparation of purified water　Common preparation methods include ion exchange method, electrodialysis method and reverse osmosis method.

离子交换法系指利用阴、阳离子交换树脂除去水中存在的离子，达到纯化水的目的。本法的主要特点是制得的水化学纯度高、设备简单、节约燃料和冷却水、成本低。

Ion exchange method refers to the use of anion and cation exchange resins to remove ions present in the water to achieve the purpose of purifying water. The main features of this method are the high chemistry purity of water, simple equipment, energy and cooling water saving and low cost.

反渗透法具有能耗低、水质好、设备使用与保养方便等优点。常用的反渗透膜有醋酸纤维膜（如三醋酸纤维素膜）和聚酰胺膜。

Reverse osmosis method has the advantages of low energy consumption, sound water quality, convenient use and maintenance of equipment. Commonly used reverse osmosis membranes are cellulose acetate membranes (such as cellulose triacetate) and polyamide membranes.

电渗析法对原水的净化处理较离子交换法经济，节约酸碱。常与离子交换法联用，以提高净化处理原水的效率。

Electrodialysis treatment of raw water purification is more economic and acid/alkali saving than that of the ion exchange. It is often used in combination with ion exchange to increase the efficiency of raw water purification.

（2）注射用水的制备　蒸馏法是现行版《中国药典》规定的制备注射用水的方法。制得的注射用水质量可靠，但制备过程耗能较多。蒸馏法制备注射用水的蒸馏设备，主要有下列几种：

b. Preparation of water for injection　Distillation is the method for preparing water for injection prescribed in the current edition of *Chinese Pharmacopoeia*. The quality of water for injection produced is reliable, but more energy consumption during the preparation process. The distillation equipment applied for water preparation, can be cataloged into the following types:

①塔式蒸馏水器　基本结构如图 9-2 所示。

Tower Water Distiller　The basic structure is shown in Figure 9-2.

②多效蒸馏水器　多效蒸馏水器的最大特点是节能效果显著，热效率高，能耗仅为单蒸馏水器的 1/3，并且出水快、纯度高、水质稳定，配有自动控制系统，为目前药品生产企业制备注射用水的重要设备。多效蒸馏水器通常有三效、四效、五效。五效蒸馏水器的基本结构如图 9-3 所示。

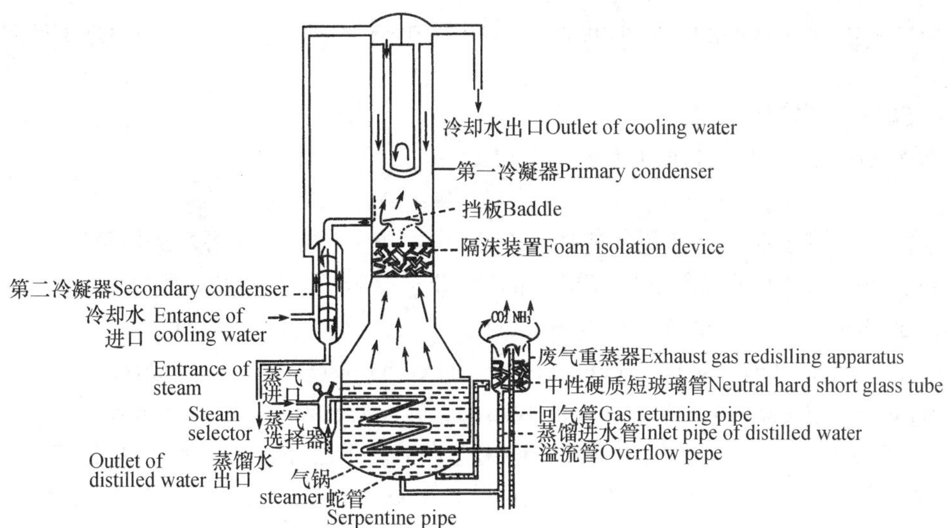

图 9-2 塔式蒸馏水器结构示意图

Figure 9-2 Tower Water Distiller Structure Diagram

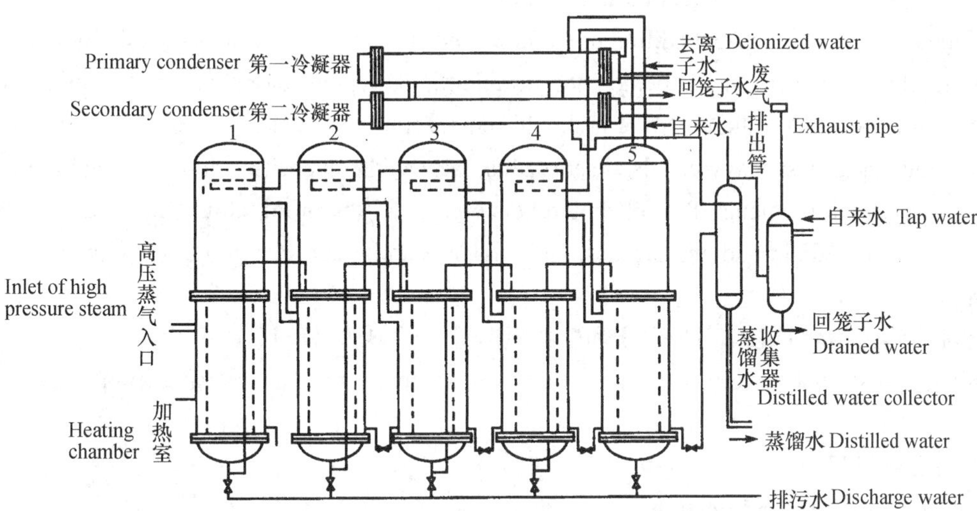

图 9-3 五效蒸馏水器结构示意图

Figure 9-3 Five-effect Water Distiller Structure Diagram

Multi-effect Water Distiller The most important features of the multi-effect water distiller are the significant energy-saving and high thermal efficiency. The energy consumption is only one-third of that of a single water distiller. Besides those mentioned above, it also has the advantages of high water production efficiency and purity, stable water quality and having automatic control system. It is considered as one of the key equipment used for water for injection preparation in the current pharmaceutical production companies. Usually, there are three, four or five effects of multi-effect water distiller. The basic structure of a five-effect water distiller is shown in Figure 9-3.

③气压式蒸馏水器 该设备具有多效蒸馏器的优点，利用离心泵将蒸汽加压，提高了蒸汽利用率，而且不需要冷却水，但使用过程中电能消耗较大。

Vapor compression still The device has the advantages as those of a multi-effect distiller. The centrifugal pump is used to pressurize the steam to increase the steam utilization rate, while no cooling

water is required in the whole process. However, the electricity consumption worth consideration.

（二）注射用非水溶剂

(2) Non-Aqueous Solvent for Injections

对于不溶或难溶于水，或在水溶液中不稳定或有特殊用途（如水溶性药物制备混悬型注射液等）的药物，可选用非水溶剂制备注射剂。常用的非水溶剂有以下几种。

For drugs that are insoluble or poorly soluble in water, or unstable in aqueous solution as well as having special uses (such as suspension injections prepared by water-soluble drugs), can be prepared into injections with non-aqueous solvents. Commonly used non-aqueous solvents as follows.

1. 油 常用的为注射用大豆油，另外，还用芝麻油、茶油等。现行版《中国药典》对注射用油的质量要求有明确规定：应无异臭、无酸败味；色泽不得深于黄色 6 号标准比色液；在 10℃时应保持澄明，过氧化物、不皂化物、碱性杂质、重金属、砷盐、脂肪酸组成和微生物限度等应符合要求，应贮于避光密闭洁净容器中，避免日光、空气接触，还可考虑加入抗氧剂等。油性注射剂只能供肌内注射。

① **Oil** Soya-bean oil for injection is the commonly used oil solvent. Besides, sesame oil and tea oil are applied as well. The current edition of *Chinese Pharmacopoeia* stipulates the quality requirements for injection oil clearly: there should be no odor, no acid rancidity; the color should not be deeper than the yellow standard colorimetric liquid No.6; it should remain transparent at 10°C. Peroxide, unsaponifiable matter, alkaline impurities, heavy metals, arsenic salts, fatty acid composition and microbial limits should meet the presented requirements. The oil should be stored in a light-proof, closed, and clean container to avoid contact with sunlight and air. Besides, antioxidants can be considered. Oil injections can be only given intramuscularly.

植物油因含游离脂肪酸、各种色素和植物蛋白等，必须加以精制。

Vegetable oils must be refined because they contain free fatty acids, various pigments, and plant proteins.

2. 其他注射用溶剂

② **Others Solvents for Injection**

（1）乙醇 采用乙醇溶液作注射剂溶剂时，乙醇浓度不宜过大。

a. Ethanol The ethanol concentration should not be too high when it is used as the injection solvent.

（2）甘油 由于甘油的黏度、刺激性等原因，不能单独作为注射剂的溶剂，常与乙醇、水等组成复合溶剂应用

b. Glycerol Due to the viscosity and irritation, the glycerin cannot be used as a solvent for injections alone. It is often used in combination with ethanol, water, etc. as the composite solvent.

（3）丙二醇 丙二醇性质稳定，能溶解多种挥发油及多种类型药物，广泛用作注射剂的溶剂，可供肌内注射或静脉注射。

c. Propanediol The property of propanediol is stable. It could dissolve a variety of volatile oils and types of drugs. It is a widely used injectable solvent for intramuscular injection or intravenous injection.

（4）聚乙二醇（PEG） 本品可用作注射剂的溶剂，其中 PEG400 最常用，在注射剂中最大浓度为 30%，超过 40% 则产生溶血作用。

d. Polyethylene glycol (PEG) This product can be used as a solvent for injections, of which PEG400 is the most commonly used. The maximum concentration of PEG in the injection is 30%. It

would cause hemolysis if the concentration is more than 40%.

此外，还有油酸乙酯、苯甲酸苄酯、二甲基乙酰胺、肉豆蔻异丙基酯、乳酸乙酯等可选作注射剂的混合溶剂。

In addition, ethyl oleate, benzyl benzoate, dimethylacetamide, isopropyl myristate, ethyl lactate and so on can be used as a mixed solvent for injections.

第四节　注射剂的附加剂

9.4　The Additives of Injections

PPT

注射剂除主药和溶剂外还可适当加入其他物质以增加注射剂的稳定性和有效性，这些物质统称为注射剂的附加剂。

Besides the drugs and solvents, other substances can be added to increase the stability and effectiveness of injections, which named additives of injections.

一、增加主药溶解度的附加剂

9.4.1　Enhancing the Solubility of the Drug Substance

1. 聚山梨酯 -80（吐温 -80） 为中药注射剂常用的增溶剂，肌内注射液中应用较多，由于吐温 -80 有降压作用与轻微的溶血作用，在静脉注射液中应慎用。常用量为 0.5%~1%。

(1) Polysorbate 80 (Tween 80) It is a commonly used solubilizer in Chinese medicine injections, mostly in intramuscular injection. Due to the hypotensive effect and slight hemolysis of tween -80, it should be used with caution in intravenous injection. The normal dosage is 0.5%-1%.

案例导入 ¦ Case example

案例 9-1　柴胡注射液

9-1　Chaihu Injection

处方： 北柴胡 1000g　氯化钠 8.5g　吐温 –80 10ml　注射用水 适量

Formula: *Bupleurum chinese* DC	1000g
NaCl	8.5g
Tween 80	10ml
Water for injection	appropriate amount

功能与主治： 退热解表。用于外感发热。

Functions and Indications: allay fever and relieve exterior syndrome. Use for exogenous fever.

制法： 取北柴胡（粗粉或饮片）1000g 加 10 倍量水，蒸馏法加热回流 6 小时；收集初蒸馏液 6000ml，将初蒸馏液重蒸馏，收集 1000ml，作含量测定，再加氯化钠及吐温 –80，使全部溶解，滤过，灌封，100℃ 灭菌 30 分钟即得。

Making Procedure: Take *Bupleurum chinese* DC (coarse powder or herbal pieces) 1000g with water

for ten times heated to reflux for six hours and then distilled. Gather the initial distillation liquid 6000ml and be distilled again. Gather the last distillation liquid 1000ml and do the content determination. Then add NaCl and Tween 80 in to make them all dissolved before the liquid was filtrated, filled and sealed and sterilized under 100℃ for 30 minutes.

用法与用量：肌内注射，一次 2ml，每日 1~2 次。

Usage and Dosages: intramuscular injection, 2ml each time, 1-2 times per day.

注解：本品采用的柴胡为伞形科植物柴胡 *Bupleurum chinense* DC. 的干燥根，习称“北柴胡”。

Notes: The dried root of *Bupleurum chinese* DC of umbelliferae herb is used in this injection and commonly known as “Bei Chai Hu”.

思考题：（1）吐温 -80 在处方中有何作用？

Questions: ① What is the role of Tween 80 in the formula?

（2）柴胡注射液的质量应达到什么标准？

② What quality standard should Chaihu injection measure up?

---

2. 甘油　甘油是鞣质和酚性物质良好的溶剂，一些以鞣质为主要成分的中药注射剂，用适当浓度的甘油作溶剂，可有效提高溶解度，保持药液的澄明度，用量一般为 15%~20%。

(2) Glycerin　Glycerin is a good solvent for tannin and phenolic substances. For some Chinese medicine injections with tannin as the main component, adding appropriate concentration of glycerol as solvent can effectively improve the solubility and maintain the clarity of the liquid. And the dosage is usually 15%-20%.

3. 其他　一些“助溶剂”可用于中药注射剂的配制，以提高药物的溶解度，如有机酸及其钠盐、酰胺与胺类。也可应用复合溶剂系统，以提高药物的浓度、确保注射剂的澄明度。

(3) Others　Some “cosolvent” could be used in Chinese medicine injection to improve the solubility of the medicaments, such as organic acids and their sodium salts, amides and amines. It is available to use the compound solvent system to enhance drug concentration and ensure the clarify of the injections.

二、帮助主药混悬或乳化的附加剂

9.4.2 Emulsifying Agents and Suspending Agents

这类附加剂主要是指助悬剂或乳化剂，添加的目的是为了使注射用混悬剂和注射用乳状液具有足够的稳定性。

This kind of additive mainly refers to suspending agents or emulsifiers, the purpose of which is to provide sufficient stability for the emulsion and suspension for injection.

常用于注射剂的助悬剂有明胶、聚维酮、羧甲基纤维素钠及甲基纤维素等。常用的乳化剂有聚山梨酯 -80、油酸山梨坦 -80（司盘 -80）、普流罗尼克（Pluronic, F-68）、卵磷脂、豆磷脂等。

Commonly used suspending agents for injection are gelatin, PVP, CMC-Na and MC. Commonly used emulsifying agents are Tween 80, Span 80, Pluronic F-68, Lecithin, Soybean Phospholipids, and so on.

三、防止主药氧化的附加剂
9.4.3 The Additives for Avoiding the Main Drug Oxidation

这类附加剂包括抗氧剂、惰性气体和金属络合剂，添加的目的是为了防止注射剂中由于主药的氧化产生的不稳定现象。

These additives contain antioxidants, inert gas and metal complexing agents. The purpose of the additions is to prevent instability due to oxidation of the main drug in the injection.

1. 抗氧剂 抗氧剂为一类易氧化的还原剂。抗氧剂保护药物免遭氧化，保证药品的稳定。

(1) Antioxidants Antioxidant is a kind of reductant which is easily to oxidize. Antioxidants protect drugs from oxidation and ensure the stability.

注射剂中抗氧剂的选用，应综合考虑主药的理化性质和药液的 pH 等因素，注射剂中常用抗氧剂的性质、用量及其适用范围如表 9-1 所示。

The physicochemical properties and pH of the liquid should be taken into consideration when choose the antioxidants in injections. The properties, dosage, and application scope of commonly used antioxidants in injections shown in Table 9-1 as follows.

表 9-1 注射剂中常用的抗氧剂

名称	溶解性	常用量	适用范围
亚硫酸钠	水溶性	0.1%~0.2%	水溶液偏碱性，常用于偏碱性药液
亚硫酸氢钠	水溶性	0.1%~0.2%	水溶液偏酸性，常用于偏酸性药液
焦亚硫酸钠	水溶性	0.1%~0.2%	水溶液偏酸性，常用于偏酸性药液
硫代硫酸钠	水溶性	0.1%	水溶液呈中性或微碱性，常用于偏碱性药液
硫脲	水溶性	0.05%~0.2%	水溶液呈中性，常用于中性或偏酸性药液
维生素 C	水溶性	0.1%~0.2%	水溶液呈中性，常用于偏酸性或微碱性药液
二丁基苯酚（BHT）	油溶性	0.005%~0.02%	油性药液
叔丁基对羟基茴香醚（BHA）	油溶性	0.005%~0.02%	油性药液
维生素 E（α-生育酚）	油溶性	0.05%~0.075%	油性药液，对热和碱稳定

Table 9-1 Common Antioxidants Used in Injections

Name	Solubility	Usual dose	Scope of application
Sodium sulfite	water-solubility	0.1%-0.2%	The aqueous solution is slightly alkaline, and is often used in alkaline liquor
Sodium bisulfite	water-solubility	0.1%-0.2%	The aqueous solution is slightly acidic, and is often used in acidic liquor
Sodium pyrosulfite	water-solubility	0.1%-0.2%	The aqueous solution is slightly acidic, and is often used in acidic liquor
Sodium thiosulfate	water-solubility	0.1%	The aqueous solution is neutral or slightly alkaline, and is often used in alkaline liquor

(continued)

Name	Solubility	Usual dose	Scope of application
Hiourea	water-solubility	0.05%-0.2%	The aqueous solution is neutral, and is often used in neutral and alkaline liquor
Vitamin C	water-solubility	0.1%-0.2%	The aqueous solution is neutral, and is often used in acidic or alkalescent liquor
Diisobutyl phenol (BHT)	oil solubility	0.005%-0.02%	Oily liquid
Butylated hydroxyanisole(BHA)	oil solubility	0.005%-0.02%	Oily liquid
Vitamin E (α-tocopherol)	oil solubility	0.05%-0.075%	Oily liquid, stability to heat and alkali

2. 惰性气体 注射剂制备过程中常用高纯度的N_2或CO_2置换药液和容器中的空气，可避免主药的氧化，一般统称为惰性气体。惰性气体可在配液时直接通入药液，或在灌注时通入容器中。

(2) Inert gas In the preparation of injections, high purity N_2 or CO_2 which called inert gas is often used to replace the air in the liquid and container, in order to avoid oxidation of the main medicaments. Inert gas can be directly injected into the liquid when mixing, or into the container when perfusing.

3. 金属络合物 药液中由于微量金属离子的存在，往往会加速其中某些化学成分的氧化分解，因此需要加入金属络合剂，使之与金属离子生成稳定的络合物，避免金属离子对药物成分氧化的催化作用，产生抗氧化的效果。注射剂中常用的金属络合剂有乙二胺四乙酸（EDTA）、乙二胺四乙酸二钠（$EDTA\text{-}Na_2$）等，常用量为0.03%~0.05%。

(3) Metal complexing agents It tends to accelerate the oxidation of some of chemicals, because there are metal ions in the liquid. Therefore, metal complexing agent is required, which can react with metal ions to produce stable complexes, can avoid catalytic oxidation effect between metal ions and the medicaments. The commonly used metal complexing agents in injections are EDTA and $EDTA\text{-}Na_2$.The usual dosage is 0.03%-0.05%.

四、调整渗透压的附加剂
9.4.4 Additives Regulating the Osmotic Pressure

常用的渗透压调节剂有氯化钠、葡萄糖等。渗透压的调整方法有冰点降低数据法和氯化钠等渗当量法。

The commonly used osmotic pressure regulator are sodium chloride and glucose, etc. The adjustment method of osmotic pressure include freezing point data reduction method and sodium chloride iso-osmotic equivalent method.

1. 冰点降低数据法 一般情况下，血浆冰点值为−0.52℃。根据物理化学原理，任何溶液其冰点降低到−0.52℃，即与血浆等渗。等渗调节剂的用量可用式（9-1）计算。

(1) Freezing point reduction method In general, plasma freezing point value is −0.52℃. According to the principle of physical chemistry, any solution whose freezing point is depressed to

−0.52℃ is isotonic with plasma. The dosage of iso-osmotic adjustment agents can be calculated by formula (9-1).

$$W = \frac{0.52 - a}{b} \tag{9-1}$$

式中，W 为配制等渗溶液需加入的等渗调节剂的量（%，g/ml）；a 为 1% 药物溶液的冰点下降度；b 为用以调节的等渗剂 1% 溶液的冰点下降度。

Within formula, W is the amount of iso-osmotic adjustment agents to be added when preparing the iso-osmotic solution (%, g/ml); a is the freezing point reducing degree of 1% drug solution; b is the freezing point reducing degree of 1% solution of isoosmotic adjustment agents which is used for regulating.

案例导入 ¦ Case example

案例 9-2 配制成分不明或无冰点降低数据的等渗溶液

9-2 Prepare the Iso-Osmotic Solution with Indefinite Composition or Unknown Freezing Point Reducing Data

配制 100ml 的 50% 金银花注射液，需加多少氯化钠才能使之成为等渗溶液？

How much sodium chloride should be added in 100ml 50% Flos Lonicerae Japonicae injection to be the iso-osmotic solution?

经试验测定，50% 金银花注射液的冰点下降度为 0.05℃，代入式（9-1）得：

Through testing, the Freezing point reducing data of 50% Honeysuckle injection is 0.05℃, substituting in formula (9-1):

$$W = (0.52 - 0.05)/0.58 = 0.81\ (\text{g}/100\text{ml})$$

即需加入 0.81g 氯化钠，才能使 100ml 的 50% 的金银花注射液成为等渗溶液。

In order to make 100ml 50% of Honeysuckle injection be the iso-osmotic solution, add sodium chloride 0.81g.

案例导入

2. 氯化钠等渗当量法 氯化钠等渗当量是指与 1g 药物呈等渗效应的氯化钠克数，用 E 表示。一些药物的 E 值见表 9-2。如硫酸阿托品的 E 值为 0.13，即 1g 硫酸阿托品与 0.13g 氯化钠具有相同的渗透压效应。按式 (9-2) 可计算等渗调节剂的用量。

(2) Sodium chloride isoosmotic equivalent method Sodium chloride isoosmotic equivalent is the number of grams of sodium chloride that are equal to the osmotic effect of 1g drugs, E is used to stand for the dosage of sodium chloride. E value of some drugs are shown in table 9-2. For instance, E value of atropine sulfate is 0.13, that is 1g atropine sulfate has the same osmotic pressure effect as 0.13g sodium chloride. Use the following formula to calculate the amount of the isoosmotic adjustment agents.

$$X = 0.009V - (G_1 \cdot E_1 + G_2 \cdot E_2 + \cdots + G_n \cdot E_n) \tag{9-2}$$

式中，X 为 Vml 药液中应加氯化钠克数；G_1、G_2、G_n 为药液中溶质的克数；E_1、E_2、E_n 分别是第 1 种、第 2 种、第 n 种药物的 E 值。

Within formula, X is the grams of sodium chloride to be added in V ml liquid, G_1、G_2、G_n is the grams of solute in the liquid, E_1、E_2、E_n is the first, second, n th E value of the drug.

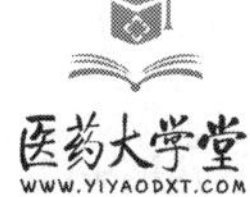

表 9-2 某些药物水溶液的冰点降低数据与氯化钠等渗当量

名称	1% 水溶液（kg/L）冰点降低值（℃）	1g 药物氯化钠等渗当量（E）	等渗浓度溶液的溶血情况		
			浓度（%）	溶血（%）	pH
硼酸	0.28	0.47	1.9	100	4.6
盐酸乙基吗啡	0.19	0.15	6.18	38	4.7
硫酸阿托品	0.08	0.1	8.85	0	5.0
盐酸可卡因	0.09	0.14	6.33	47	4.4
氯霉素	0.06	—	—	—	—
依地酸钙钠	0.12	0.21	4.50	0	6.1
盐酸麻黄碱	0.16	0.28	3.2	96	5.9
无水葡萄糖	0.10	0.18	5.05	0	6.0
葡萄糖（含 H_2O）	0.091	0.16	5.51	0	5.9
氢溴酸后马托品	0.097	0.17	5.67	92	5.0
盐酸吗啡	0.086	0.15	—	—	—
碳酸氢钠	0.381	0.65	1.39	0	8.3
氯化钠	0.58	—	0.9	0	6.7
青霉素 G 钾	—	0.16	5.48	0	6.2
硝酸毛果芸香碱	0.133	0.22	—	—	—
吐温 -80	0.01	0.02	—	—	—
盐酸普鲁卡因	0.12	0.18	5.05	91	5.6
盐酸丁卡因	0.109	0.18	—	—	—

Table 9-2 Freezing Point Reducing Data and Sodium Chloride Iso-osmotic Equivalent of Some Drug Solutions

Name	Freezing point reducing data (℃) of 1% aqueous solution (kg/L)	sodium chloride iso-osmotic equivalent of 1g drug (E)	Hemolysis of the iso-osmotic solution		
			Concentration (%)	hemolysis (%)	pH value
Boric acid	0.28	0.47	1.9	100	4.6
Ethylmorphine Hydrochloride	0.19	0.15	6.18	38	4.7
Atropine sulfate	0.08	0.1	8.85	0	5.0
Cocaine hydrochloride	0.09	0.14	6.33	47	4.4
Chloramphenicol	0.06	—	—	—	—
Calcium Disodium Edetate	0.12	0.21	4.50	0	6.1
Ephedrine Hydrochloride	0.16	0.28	3.2	96	5.9
Glucosum Anhydricum	0.10	0.18	5.05	0	6.0
Glucose (containing H_2O)	0.091	0.16	5.51	0	5.9
Homatropine Hydrobromide	0.097	0.17	5.67	92	5.0

(continued)

Name	Freezing point reducing data (℃) of 1% aqueous solution (kg/L)	sodium chloride iso-osmotic equivalent of 1g drug (*E*)	Hemolysis of the iso-osmotic solution		
			Concentration (%)	hemolysis (%)	pH value
Morphine Hydrochloride	0.086	0.15	—	—	—
Sodium bicarbonate	0.381	0.65	1.39	0	8.3
Sodium chloride	0.58	—	0.9	0	6.7
Potassium penicillin G	—	0.16	5.48	0	6.2
Pilocarpine nitrate	0.133	0.22	—	—	—
Tween-80	0.01	0.02	—	—	—
Procaine Hydrochloride	0.12	0.18	5.05	91	5.6
Dicaine hydrochloride	0.109	0.18	—	—	—

3. 等渗溶液与等张溶液　等渗溶液系指与血浆渗透压相等的溶液。等张溶液系指与红细胞膜张力相等的溶液，在等张溶液中既不发生红细胞体积改变，也不发生溶血。

(3) Isoosmotic solution and isotonic solution　The isotonic solution is the solution of which osmotic pressure is equal to plasma osmotic pressure. The isotonic solution is a solution that has the same tension as the erythrocyte membrane. In the isotonic solution, neither erythrocyte volume changes nor hemolysis occurs.

高于或低于血浆渗透压的溶液相应地称为高渗溶液或低渗溶液。在静脉注射时当大量低渗溶液注入血液后，水分子穿过细胞膜进入红细胞内，使红细胞胀破，造成溶血现象。而当静脉注入高渗溶液时，红细胞内水分因渗出而发生细胞萎缩，尽管只要注射速度缓慢，机体血液可自行调节使渗透压恢复正常，但在一定时间内也会影响正常的红细胞功能。因此，静脉注射必须注意渗透压的调整。对于脊椎腔内注射，由于脊椎液量少，循环缓慢，渗透压的紊乱很快就会引起头痛、呕吐等不良反应，所以也必须使用等渗溶液。

Osmotic pressure of solution above or below the plasma osmotic pressure is correspondingly called hypertonic or hypotonic solution. After a lot of hypotonic solution is intravenous injected into the blood, the water molecules pass through the cell membrane into the red cells to burst the red cell and cause hemolysis. When hypertonic solution is intravenous injected into the blood, the red cells will atrophy because of the exudation. If the injection rate is slow, the osmotic pressure of blood can adjust themselves to normal, but it also affects the function of red cells in a period of time. Therefore, intravenous injection must be aware of osmotic pressure adjustment. For vertebra caval injection, due to the low volume of spinal fluid and slow circulation, the disturbance of osmotic pressure will soon cause adverse reactions, such as headache and vomiting, etc., so iso-osmotic solution must be used as well.

五、抑制微生物增殖的附加剂
9.4.5　An Additive that Inhibits Microbial Proliferation

这类附加剂也称为抑菌剂，添加的目的是防止注射剂制备或多次使用过程中微生物的污染和生长繁殖。一般多剂量注射剂、滤过除菌或无菌操作法制备的单剂量注射剂，均可加入一定量的

抑菌剂，以确保用药安全。而用于静脉注射或脊椎腔注射的注射剂一律不得添加抑菌剂，剂量超过 5ml 的注射液在添加抑菌剂时，应当特别谨慎。

These additives are also known as antimicrobial preservatives. The purpose is to prevent the contamination and prohibit the growth of micro-organisms during the preparation or multiple use process of the injections. Generally, multiple dose injections and single dose of sterilization by filtration or aseptic manipulation injections may add an appropriate concentration of suitable antimicrobial preservatives to ensure the safety of medication. No anti-microbial preservatives should be added to intravenous or spinal injections. Pay more attention to using antimicrobial preservatives if the dosage is more than 5ml.

注射剂常用的抑菌剂见表 9-3。

The commonly used antimicrobial preservatives in the injections are shown in table 9-3.

表 9-3　注射剂常用的抑菌剂

名称	溶解性	常用量	适用范围
苯酚	室温时稍溶于水，65℃以上能与水混溶	0.5%	偏酸性药液
甲酚	难溶于水，易溶于脂肪油	0.25%~0.3%	与一般生物碱有配伍禁忌
氯甲酚	极微溶于水	0.05%~0.2%	与少数生物碱及甲基纤维素有配伍禁忌
三氯叔丁醇	微溶于水	0.25%~0.5%	微酸性药液
苯甲醇	溶于水	1%~3%	偏碱性药液，对热稳定
苯乙醇	溶于水	0.25%~0.5%	偏酸性药液

Table 9-3　Commonly Used Antimicrobial Preservatives in the Injections

Name	Solubility	Usual dose	Scope of Application
Phenol	It is slightly soluble in water at room temperature and soluble in water above 65℃	0.5%	Acidic solution
Cresol	It is poorly soluble in water and soluble in fatty oil	0.25%-0.3%	It has incompatibility with general alkaoids
Chlorocresol	It is very slightly soluble in water	0.05%-0.2%	It has incompatibility with few alkaloids and MC
Chlorobutanol	It is slightly soluble in water	0.25%-0.5%	Micro-acidic solution
Phenylcarbinol	It is soluble in water	1%-3%	Alkaline liquor, stable to heat
Phenethyl alcohol	It is soluble in water	0.25%-0.5%	Acidic solution

六、调整 pH 的附加剂

9.4.6 The Additives Which are Used for Adjusting the pH

这类附加剂包括酸、碱和缓冲剂，添加的目的是为了减少注射剂由于 pH 不当而对机体造成局部刺激，增加药液的稳定性以及加快药液的吸收。

These additives include acids, bases and buffers, in order to reduce the local irritation caused by the improper pH value of the injection, increase the stability of the liquid and accelerate the absorpt of the injections.

原则上尽可能使药液接近人体血液的 pH（7.4 左右），一般应控制 pH 在 4.0~9.0，同一品种的 pH 允许差异范围应不得超过 2.0，大容量注射液 pH 应近中性。

In principle, make the solution is as far as possible close to the pH value of human blood (about 7.4). Generally, the pH value should be controlled between 4.0 and 9.0. The allowable range of the same variety pH value should not exceed 2.0. The pH value of large volume injections are as far as possible close to neutral.

注射剂中常用的 pH 调节剂有盐酸、枸橼酸、氢氧化钾（钠）、枸橼酸钠及缓冲剂磷酸二氢钠和磷酸氢二钠等。

The commonly used pH adjusting agents in the injections is hydrochloric acid, citric acid, potassium hydroxide(sodium), sodium citrate, sodium dihydrogen phosphate and sodium phosphate dibasic, etc.

七、减轻疼痛的附加剂
9.4.7 The Additives to Alleviate Pain

经皮下或肌内注射时易产生疼痛的注射剂，为减轻药物本身或其他原因引起的刺激性，可酌加止痛剂。常用止痛剂有苯甲醇、盐酸普鲁卡因、三氯叔丁醇、盐酸利多卡因等。

Subcutaneous or intramuscular injecting is easily to cause pain. To reduce the irritation caused by the medicaments or other causes, the additives to alleviate pain may be applied. Benzyl alcohol, Procaine hydrochloride, Chlorobutanol, Lidocaine hydrochloride are usually used analgetic.

第五节 注射剂的制备
9.5 Preparation of the Injections

PPT

一、注射剂制备的工艺流程
9.5.1 Technological Process Flow of the Preparation of Injections

注射剂的生成过程包括原辅料和容器的前处理、配制、灌封、灭菌、质量检查和包装等步骤。制备不同类型的注射剂，其具体操作方法和生产条件有区别。

The manufacturing process of injections includes the steps of pretreatment for raw materials and containers, preparation, filling and sealing, sterilization, quality inspection and packaging. There are differences in the specific operating methods as well as production conditions when preparing different types of injections.

一般工艺流程见图 9-4。

The general process flow are shown in Figure 9-4.

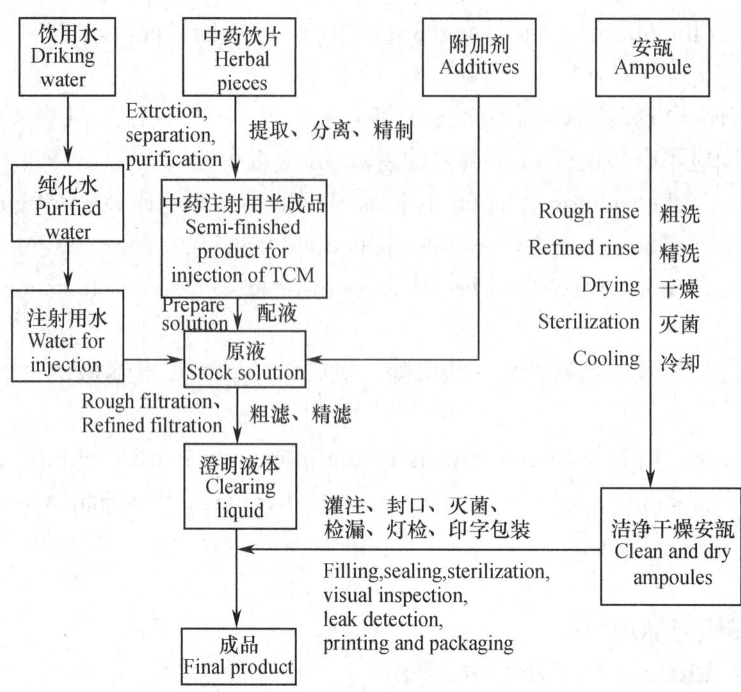

图 9-4 注射剂制备的工艺流程

Figure 9-4 Technological Process Flow Figure of Injection Preparation

二、中药注射用半成品

9.5.2 Semi-Finished Product for TCM Injections

用半成品通常包括从中药饮片中提取的有效成分、有效组分混合物。按照《中药、天然药物注射剂基本技术要求》的规定，以有效成分制成的中药注射剂，其有效成分的纯度应达到 90% 以上；以多成分制备的中药注射剂，在测定总固体量（mg/ml）基础上，其中结构明确的成分含量应不低于总固体量的 60%。

Semi-finished products usually include active ingredients and active ingredient mixtures extracted from the Chinese medicine decoction pieces. According to the provisions given in the *Basic technical requirements for traditional Chinese medicine and natural medicine injections*, the purity of active ingredients for traditional Chinese medicine injections that are made with active ingredients should be more than 90%; whilst for the traditional Chinese medicine injections prepared with multi-components, being that it is measured on the basis of total solids(mg/ml), the content of its well-defined components should not be less than 60% of the total solids.

（一）中药注射用原液的制备

(1) Preparation of Stock Solution for Chinese Medicine Injections

根据处方中药物所含成分的基本理化性质，结合中医药理论确定的功能主治，并考虑该处方的传统用法、剂量，以及制成注射剂后注射的部位和作用时间等，选择合适的溶剂，确定提取与纯化方法，以最大限度地除去杂质，保留有效成分，制成可供配制注射剂成品用的原液或相应的干燥品，通常也称为半成品或提取物。

On the grounds of the basic physical and chemical properties of the ingredients contained in the prescription, combined with the functional indications determined by the theory of traditional Chinese

medicine, and taking into consideration of traditional usage of the prescription and its dosage, as well as the injection site and action time after injection, etc., a suitable solvent is to be selected, as well as the extraction and purification methods which are supposed to maximize the removal of impurities and conserve the active ingredients, in order to make a stock solution or a corresponding dried product which is also usually called semi-finished product or extract.

目前常用的制备方法如下：

The commonly used preparation methods are as follows:

1. 蒸馏法 是提取挥发性成分常用方法，适用于处方组成中含有挥发油或其他挥发性成分的药物。

① **Distillation** It is a commonly used method for extracting volatile components, which is suitable for the prescription containing volatile oil or the drugs having other volatile components.

2. 综合法 根据有效成分的性质，采用水醇法进行提取分离，并在此基础上，结合有效成分的性质，选择适宜方法进一步精制以达到注射用半成品的质量要求。分别有溶剂萃取法、酸碱沉淀法、吸附分离法、超滤法等。

② **Comprehensive method** Based on the nature of the active ingredients, the hydroalcoholic method is used for extraction and separation. And on this basis, in combination with the nature of the active ingredients, a suitable method is selected for further refinement in order to meet the quality requirements of semi-finished products used for the injection. There are solvent extraction method, acid-base precipitation method, adsorption separation method, ultrafiltration method and so on.

（二）除去注射剂原液中鞣质的方法

(2) Methods for Removing Tannin from the Injection Stock Solution

中药注射用原液除去鞣质，是中药注射剂临床应用安全有效的保证。目前常用的除鞣质方法如下。

The removal of tannins from TCM injection liquid is a guarantee for safe and effective clinical application of Chinese medicine injections. Currently, the commonly used methods for removing tannins are:

1. 改良明胶法（胶醇法） 在水提浓缩液中加入明胶生成鞣酸蛋白沉淀后，不滤过，直接加乙醇处理，可减少明胶对某些有效成分的吸附。

① **Modified gelatin method (Gelatin alcohol method)** After adding gelatin to the water concentrated solution to induce tannic acid protein precipitation, and directly adding ethanol without filtering, it is possible to reduce the adsorption of certain active ingredients by gelatin.

2. 醇溶液调 pH 法 利用鞣质可与碱成盐，在高浓度乙醇中难溶而沉淀除去。

② **Alcohol solution adjusting pH method** The tannin can be used to form salt with alkali, making it difficult to dissolve in highly concentrated ethanol and being removed by precipitation.

3. 聚酰胺吸附法 利用聚酰胺分子内的酰胺键，可与酚类、酸类、醌类、硝基化合物等形成氢键而有吸附作用的性质，以达到去除鞣质的目的。

③ **Polyamide adsorption method** The amide bond in polyamide molecule can form hydrogen bond with phenols, acids, quinones, nitro compounds, etc. and having the property of adsorption, so as to achieve the purpose of removing tannin.

根据实际情况，除去鞣质还可采用酸性水溶液沉淀法、超滤法、铅盐沉淀法等。

According to the actual situation, tannins can be removed by acidic aqueous solution precipitation method, ultrafiltration method, lead salt precipitation method, etc.

三、注射剂的容器与处理

9.5.3 The Containers and Handling of Injections

（一）注射剂容器

(1) Injection Containers

1. 种类 注射剂常用容器有玻璃安瓿、玻璃瓶、塑料安瓿、塑料瓶（袋）等。

① Types Containers commonly used for injections include glass ampoules, glass bottles, plastic ampoules, plastic bottles (bags), etc.

2. 规格 按盛装剂量分为单剂量、多剂量和大剂量容器。单剂量玻璃小容器，俗称安瓿，其形状分为有颈安瓿和粉末安瓿，其容积通常有 1ml、2ml、5ml、10ml、20ml 等规格。此外，还有曲颈安瓿。粉末安瓿供分装注射用粉末和结晶性药物用。多剂量容器系指玻璃小瓶以橡胶塞封口，瓶口胶塞上另有铝盖密封，常用的有 5ml、10ml、20ml、30ml 及 50ml 等规格。大剂量容器常见的为输液瓶、输液袋，有 500ml、1000ml 等规格。

② Specifications According to the contained dose, they are divided into single-dose, multi-dose and high-dose containers. Single-dose small glass containers, commonly known as ampoules, are divided by its shape into ampoules with neck and powder ampoules, its volume usually goes by 1ml, 2ml, 5ml, 10ml, 20ml etc. There are also curved neck ampoules. Powder ampoules are used to contain dispense powder for injections and crystalline drugs. Multi-dose container refers to a glass vial sealed with a rubber stopper, and be hermetically sealed with an aluminum cap. Commonly used specifications are 5ml, 10ml, 20ml, 30ml and 50ml. Large-dose containers are usually infusion bottles and infusion bags. There are 500ml, 1000ml and other sizes.

3. 质量要求 除另有规定外，容器应符合有关药用玻璃容器、塑料容器、胶塞的国家标准规定。

③ Quality requirements Unless otherwise specified, the containers should comply with the related requirements of the National Standards about medical glass containers, plastic containers, and rubber stoppers.

（二）安瓿的处理

(2) Handling of Ampoules

1. 安瓿的洗涤 安瓿洗涤前，一般使用离子交换水灌瓶蒸煮，质量较差的安瓿用 0.1%~0.5% 的盐酸或 0.5% 醋酸水溶液，以 100℃ 蒸煮 30 分钟，以除去微量的碱和金属离子。洗涤方法一般有甩水洗涤法和加压喷射气水洗涤法。

① Ampoules washing Before washing the ampoules, they are usually cooked in ion-exchange water bottles. Poor quality ampoules are cooked with 0.1% to 0.5% hydrochloric acid or 0.5% acetic acid solution at 100℃ for 30 minutes to remove traces of alkali and metals ion. The washing method generally includes throwing water washing method and the pressurized jet gas water washing method.

2. 安瓿的干燥与灭菌 安瓿洗涤后，一般置于 120~140℃ 烘箱内干燥。用于无菌操作或低温灭菌的安瓿应在 200℃ 以上干热灭菌 40 分钟或 180℃ 干热灭菌 3 小时。大生产中多采用隧道式烘箱。安瓿干燥灭菌后，应密封保存并及时应用。

② Drying and sterilization of ampoules After being washed, ampoules are generally put into an oven at 120-140℃ for drying. The ampoules used for aseptic operations or low temperature sterilization should be dry heat sterilized above 200℃ for 40min or at 180℃ dry heat sterilized for 3h. When it comes to large production, tunnel ovens are mostly used. After the ampoule is dried and sterilized, it should be

sealed and applied in time.

四、注射剂的配液与滤过

9.5.4 Compounding and Filtration of Injections

（一）注射剂的配液

(1) Injection Compounding

1. 原辅料的质量要求与投料量计算 供注射用的原辅料，应符合“注射用”规格，并经检验合格方能投料；辅料应符合药用标准，若有注射用规格，应选用注射用规格。

① Quality requirements for raw materials and additives and the feeding calculating Raw materials and additives for injections which should comply with the stipulated standard requirements for “injections” are feeded after comfirming to standard by inspection it is possible to perform material feeding. The auxiliary materials should meet the pharmaceutical standards, if there are specific injection standards, then these are the ones that should be used.

在投料之前，应根据处方规定用量、原料实际含量、成品含量及损耗等计算所有成分的实际投料量。

Before feeding material, the actual feeding amount of all the ingredients should be calculated according to the prescribed dosage, the actual content of raw materials, the content of finished products and loss etc.

2. 配制用具的选择与处理 配液用具须采用化学稳定性好的材料制成，常用的有玻璃、不锈钢、耐酸碱搪瓷或无毒聚氯乙烯塑料等，不宜选用铝制容器。大量生产可选用有夹层的不锈钢锅，并装有搅拌器。

② Selection and treatment of preparation utensils Liquid preparation utensils must be made of materials with good chemical stability, the ones that are commonly used are glass, stainless steel, acid and alkali resistant enamel or non-toxic polyvinyl chloride plastics, while aluminum containers are not suitable. Mass production could select stainless steel pots with interlayers, and which are also equipped with agitators.

3. 药液配制方法 配液方式有两种。一种是稀配法，即将原料加入溶剂中一次配成规定的浓度，本法适用于原料质量好，小剂量注射剂的配制。另一种是浓配法，即将原料加入部分溶剂中，配成浓溶液，加热滤过后再加溶剂稀释至全量，本法可进一步除去中药注射用半成品中的杂质，提高注射剂的澄明度。

③ Preparation method of medicinal solution There are two methods of preparing the solution. One is the dilute solution preparing method, meaning that the raw materials are added to the solvent to prepare a prescribed concentration all at once. This method is suitable for the preparation of small-dose injections with good raw material quality. The other method is the concentrated solution preparing method, which implies adding raw materials to one part of the solvent to prepare a concentrated solution. After being heating and filtering, solvent is added to dilute the full amount, this method can furthermore remove impurities in the semi-finished product for Chinese medicine injections and improve the clarity of the injection.

为提高注射剂的澄明度和稳定性，配制时常采取以下措施：①水处理，冷藏：中药提取液中加一定量注射用水后，破坏了原提取液中成分之间所形成的增溶体系，而使部分被增溶的杂质进一步沉降；②热处理，冷藏：将配制的注射液加热至95℃以上，维持30分钟，冷却后再冷藏，

使成胶体分散状态的杂质沉淀；③活性炭处理：选用经 150℃ 干燥活化 3~4 小时的针用活性炭，用量为 0.1%~1.0%，应用时应注意考察活性炭对有效成分吸附的影响；④加入附加剂：如 pH 调节剂、抗氧剂和止痛剂。

In order to improve the clarity and stability of injections, these following measures are often taken during preparations: ① Water treatment and refrigeration: after adding a certain amount of water for injection to Chinese herbal extract, the solubilized system formed between the components in the original extract gets destroyed, allowing for the partially solubilized impurities to be further settled; ② Heat treatment and refrigeration: heat up the prepared injection solution above 95℃ for 30 minutes, and then refrigerate so that the colloidal dispersion of impurities precipitation; ③ Activated carbon treatment: using dry activated carbon for 3 to 4hours at 150℃, and the dosage is 0.1% to 1.0%. During its application, carefully observe the effect of activated carbon on the adsorption of active ingredients; ④ Adding additional agents: such as pH regulators, antioxidants and analgesics.

若为油溶液，注射用油应在用前经 150~160℃ 干热灭菌 1~2 小时后冷却待用。

If it is an oil solution, the oil for injection should be sterilized by dry heating at 150-160℃ for 1-2h, then cool down to use.

药液配好后，应进行半成品质量检查，包括 pH、含量等项目，合格后才能滤过灌封。

After the liquid medicine has been prepared, the quality of the semi-finished product should be verified, including pH value, content and other parameters. And only after proven to be up to standard, it can be filtered, filled and sealed.

（二）注射剂的滤过

(2) Filtration of Injections

注射剂的滤过一般分两步完成，即先粗滤再精滤。粗滤常用的滤材有滤纸、长纤维脱脂棉、绸布、纸浆、滤板等。常用的滤器有布氏漏斗、板框压滤机等。精滤常用滤器有垂熔玻璃滤器，其中 G_3 用于常压过滤，G_4 用于加压或减压过滤，G_6 用于滤过除菌；微孔滤膜滤器，常用 0.8μm、0.45μm 的微孔滤膜。0.22μm 以下的微孔滤膜也可用于滤过除菌。

Filtration of injection liquid is generally completed in two steps, that is to say through rough filtration and refined filtration. Filter materials commonly used for rough filtration are filter paper, long-fiber absorbent cotton, silk cloth, pulp, filter plate etc. Commonly used filters are Buchner funnels, plate and frame filter presses, etc. Sintered glass filter are commonly used refined filter, of which G_3 is used for atmospheric pressure filtration, G_4 is used for pressure or decompression filtration, and G6 is used for filtration to remove bacteria; microporous membrane filters sizes that are commonly used are 0.8μm and 0.45μm. Microporous filters size below 0.22μm can also be used for filtration to remove bacteria.

注射剂的滤过通常有高位静压滤过、减压滤过及加压滤过等方法，其具体装置有以下几种：

The filtration of injections usually includes high static pressure filtration, decompression filtration, and pressure filtration method. The specific devices are as follows:

1. 高位静压滤过装置 利用药液本身的静压差在管道中进行滤过，该法压力稳定，滤过质量好，但滤速较慢。

① High static pressure filtration device This device uses the static pressure's difference of the medicinal solution itself to perform filtration in the pipeline. This method has stable pressure and good filtration quality, but its filtration speed is slow.

2. 减压滤过装置 此种装置适用于各种滤器，设备要求简单，但压力不够稳定，操作不当，

易引起滤层松动，直接影响滤过质量。一般可采用减压连续滤过装置。

② **Decompression filtration device** This device is suitable for various filters, and the equipment requirements are simple. However the pressure is not stable enough, and with improper handling it is easy to cause filter layer to get loose, which directly affects the filtration quality. Normally can use decompression continuous filtration devices.

3. 加压滤过装置 此种装置在药厂大生产时普遍采用，其特点是压力稳定、滤速快，由于全部装置保持正压，操作过程对滤层的影响较小，外界空气不易漏入滤过系统，滤过质量好而且稳定。

③ **Pressure filtration device** This device is commonly used in large-scale production in pharmaceutical factories. It is characterized by stable pressure and fast filtration speed. Being that all devices maintain positive pressure, the operating process has small impact on the filter layer. Therefore external air can't easily leak into the filter system, and the quality of filtration is good and stable.

五、注射剂的灌封
9.5.5 Filling/Sealing of Injections

灌封包括灌注药液和封口两步，是将滤净的药液，定量地灌装到安瓿中，灌后立即封口，以免污染。是注射剂生产中保证无菌的最关键操作。

The filling/sealing includes two steps of filling the liquid medicine and sealing. The filtered liquid medicine is quantitatively filled into the ampoule and sealed immediately after filling in order to prevent contamination. It is the most critical operation to ensure sterility in the production process of injections.

（一）灌注
(1) Filling

药液的灌装要求剂量准确，药液不沾瓶口，不受污染。灌装时按《中国药典》中要求适当增加药液量，以保证注射用量不少于标示量。除另有规定外，多剂量包装的注射液，每一容器的装量不得超过 10 次注射量。

The filling of the medicinal solution requires accurate dosage, as well as that the medicinal solution does not stick to the bottle's mouth and not contaminated. According to the requirements given in the *Chinese Pharmacopoeia*, the content in each container is not less than the labelled quantity of the injection. Unless otherwise specified, for multi-dose injections, the quantity in each container shall not exceed 10 doses..

接触空气易变质的药物，在灌装过程中，应排除容器内的空气，可填充二氧化碳和氮气等气体，立即用适宜的方法熔封或严封。

The containers for filling the drug substances, which are readily deterioration when exposure to air, should be evacuated and displaced of carbon dioxide or nitrogen, etc., during filling, and melt or seal immediately with appropriate method.

（二）熔封
(2) Sealing

安瓿的熔封应严密，无缝隙，不漏气，顶端圆整光滑，无尖锐易断的尖头及易破碎的球状小泡。

The sealing of the ampoule should be tight, seamless, airtight, round and smooth at the top, without sharp and fragile pointed tips or fragile spherical bubbles.

六、注射剂的灭菌与检漏
9.5.6 Sterilization and Leak Detection of Injections

（一）灭菌
(1) Sterilization

除无菌操作生产的注射剂外，所有的注射剂灌封后都应及时灭菌。一般1~5ml安瓿多用流通蒸汽100℃/30分钟灭菌；10~20ml安瓿采用100℃/45分钟灭菌；对热不稳定的产品，可适当缩短灭菌时间；对热稳定的品种、输液，均应采用热压灭菌。以油为溶剂的注射剂，选用干热灭菌。

All injections, except those produced aseptically, should be promptly sterilized after sealing. Generally, 1-5ml ampoules are sterilized by circulation steam at 100℃/30min; 10-20ml ampoules are sterilized at 100℃/45min; for heat unstable products, the sterilization time can be appropriately shortened; heat-stable types and infusions should be autoclaved. Oil-based solvent injections are sterilized by dry heating.

（二）检漏
(2) Leak Detection

注射剂灭菌后要进行检漏，检漏一般应用灭菌检漏两用的灭菌器，灭菌后待温度稍降，抽气至真空度85.3~90.6kPa，停止抽气。将有色溶液吸入灭菌锅中至盖过安瓿，关闭色水阀，打开气阀。由于漏气安瓿中的空气被抽出，当空气放入时，有色溶液即借大气压力压入漏气安瓿内而被检出。

Leakage detection should be carried out after sterilization of injection. Generally, a sterilizer with dual purpose of sterilization and leakage detection should be used for leakage detection. After sterilization, wait for temperature to be slightly lowered, extract gas up until vacuum degree is 85.3-90.6 kPa and finish the gas extraction. Inject the colored solution into the sterilizer until it covers up the ampoule, close the colored water valve and open the air valve. Being that the air in the leaked ampoule gets drawn out, after the air is released, the colored solution gets pressed into the leaked ampoule under high atmospheric pressure and is therefore detected.

七、注射剂的印字与包装
9.5.7 Injections Printing and Packaging

注射剂经质量检测合格后方可印字、包装。每支注射剂均需印上品名、规格、批号等。

Injections can be printed on and packaged only after passing the quality inspection. Each injection should be printed with the product name, specifications, batch number etc.

在标签或说明书中，应标明注射剂所用的辅料名称，加有抑菌剂的注射剂，应标明所加抑菌剂的浓度。

The name of the excipient used in the injection shall be indicated on the label or in the instruction manual. For injections with antibacterial agent, the concentration of the antibacterial agent shall be indicated.

案例导入 ¦ Case example

案例 9-3 参麦注射液
9-3 Shenmai Injection

处方： 红参 100g 麦冬 200g 10% 氢氧化钠溶液 适量 聚山梨酯-80 适量 注射用水适量

Formula:	
Red ginseng 100g	Radix ophiopogon 200g
10% Sodium hydroxide solution	appropriate amount
Polysorbate 80	appropriate amount
Water for injection	appropriate amount

功能与主治： 益气固脱，养阴生津，生脉。用于治疗气阴两虚性休克，冠心病，病毒性心肌炎，慢性肺心病，粒细胞减少症。

Functions and indications: Tonify qi for relieve desertion, nourish yin and promote the production of body fluid, promote pulse activation. It is used to treat both qi-yin deficiency shock, coronary heart disease, viral myocarditis, chronic pulmonary heart disease, and granulocytopenia.

制法： 取红参、麦冬，用 80% 乙醇 600ml，回流提取两次，每次 2 小时，滤过，药渣用 80% 乙醇 200ml 分次洗涤，合并上述滤液和洗涤液，冷藏，静置 12 小时，滤过，于滤液中按体积加入 1% 活性炭，搅拌 1 小时，滤过，滤液减压回收乙醇至无醇味，添加注射用水至约 1000ml，于 100℃ 灭菌 30 分钟，加 10% 氢氧化钠溶液调节 pH 至 7.5，冷藏 48 小时以上，滤过，滤液加聚山梨酯-80 适量，并调 pH 至 7.5，加注射用水至 1000ml，滤过，灌封，100℃ 流通蒸汽灭菌，即得。

Making Procedures: Take Red ginseng(ginseng radix rubra) and Radix ophiopogon and 600ml of 80% ethanol, then extract twice under reflux for 2h each time, filter and wash the drug residue gradually with 200ml of 80% ethanol. Combine the above filtrate and washing liquid and refrigerate, leave still for 12h, filter it, add 1% activated carbon to the filtrate according to its volume, stir for one hour, filter, recover ethanol from the filtrate under reduced pressure until there is no alcohol odor, add water for injection to about 1000ml, sterilize at 100℃ for 30min, add 10% sodium hydroxide solution to adjust pH value to 7.5, refrigerate for more than 48h, filter it, add the appropriate amount of polysorbate 80, and adjust the pH value to 7.5, add 1000ml of water for injection, filter it, fill, seal and steam sterilize at 100℃ and it is obtained.

用法与用量： 肌内注射，每次 2~4ml，一日 1 次。静脉滴注，一次 20~40ml，用 5% 葡萄糖注射液稀释后应用，或遵医嘱。

Usage and Dosage: Intramuscular injection, 2-4ml each time, once a day. Intravenous infusion, 20-40ml at a time, dilute with 5% glucose and use afterwards, or as instructed by the doctor.

注解：（1）本品以醇提水沉法制备。在制备过程中，若采用大孔树脂吸附处理，则可有效提高提取物中人参皂苷的含量。

Notes: (1) This product is prepared by alcohol extraction water precipitation method. In the preparation process, if the macroporous resin adsorption treatment is adopted, it will effectively increase the content of ginsenosides in the extract.

（2）制备过程中，用活性炭吸附杂质和脱色，所用活性炭应选用针用规格，为保证吸附完全，也可用水浴适当加热。

(2) During the preparation process, activated carbon is used to adsorb impurities and decolorize, and

in order to ensure adsorb completely, needle specifications should be used for all the activated carbon, and it can also be appropriately heated in a water bath.

（3）药液中含有聚山梨酯-80，灭菌后应注意及时振摇，防止产生起昙现象而影响注射剂澄明度。

(3) If there is polysorbate 80 in the medicinal solution, it should be shaken on time after sterilization in order to prevent the occurrence of clouding formation and affect the clarity of the injection.

思考题：（1）参麦注射液处方中主药与附加剂各有什么作用？

Questions: (1) What are the effects of the main medicine and the additives respectively in Shenmai injection?

（2）参麦注射液的制备工艺采用了什么方法？

(2) What method does Shenmai injection preparation/production technology adopt?

第六节　中药注射剂的质量控制

9.6　Quality Control of Chinese Medicine Injections

PPT

一、中药注射剂的质量控制项目与方法

9.6.1　Quality Control Items and Methods of Chinese Medicine Injections

（一）制剂通则检查

(1) General Requirements for Preparations

照现行版《中国药典》注射剂项下有关规定进行检查。主要包括以下内容：

Inspect according to the relevant provisions of the Inspection under the current edition of *Chinese Pharmacopoeia* (Ch.P.) injections, which including the following items.

1. 装量及装量差异　除另有规定外，注射液、注射用浓溶液及注射用无菌粉末照现行版《中国药典》注射剂的装量及装量差异检查法检查，应符合规定。

① **Loading quantity and its deviation**　Unless otherwise specified, filling and weight variation of liquids for injection, concentrated solutions for injection and sterile powders for injection should inspected and in accordance with the requirements of the Injections in the current edition of Ch.P., and meet the requirements.

2. 可见异物　除另有规定外，照现行版《中国药典》可见异物检查法检查，应符合规定。

② **Visible particles**　Unless otherwise specified, visible foreign matters shall be inspected according to the inspection method of visible foreign matters in current edition of Ch.P., and meet the requirements.

3. 不溶性微粒　除另有规定外，用于静脉注射、静脉滴注、鞘内注射、椎管内注射的溶液型注射液、注射用无菌粉末及注射用浓溶液照现行版《中国药典》不溶性微粒检查法检查，应符合规定。

③ **Insoluble particle**　Unless otherwise specified, solutions for intravenous injection, intravenous infusion and intrathecal or intraspinal injection, sterile powders for injection and liquid concentrates for

injection should comply with the requirements of the Test for insoluble particle in the current edition of Ch.P., and meet the requirements.

4. 有关物质 除另有规定外，一般应检查蛋白质、鞣质、树脂等，静脉注射液还应检查草酸盐、钾离子等，照现行版《中国药典》注射剂规定的有关物质检查法检查，应符合规定。

④ **Related substance** Unless otherwise specified, generally should check protein, tannin, resin, etc.. Intravenous injection should also check oxalate, potassium, etc.. according to the current version of Ch.P. Injection provisions of the relevant substances inspection method, all the substances should comply with the provisions.

5. 重金属及有害元素残留量 除另有规定外，照现行版《中国药典》铅、镉、砷、汞、铜测定法检查，按各品种项下每日最大使用量计算，铅不得超过 12μg，镉不得超过 3μg，砷不得超过 6μg，汞不得超过 2μg，铜不得超过 150μg。

⑤ **Residues of heavy metals and harmful elements** Unless otherwise specified, according to the current edition of Ch.P., the determination method of lead, cadmium, arsenic, mercury and copper is used. According to the calculation of the maximum daily use of each variety, the residual plumbum content should not exceed 12μg; while cadmium content should not exceed 3μg, arsenic content should not exceed 6μg, mercury content should not exceed 2μg and copper content should not exceed 150μg.

6. pH 照现行版《中国药典》pH 测定法测定。其 pH 要求与血液相等或接近（血液的 pH 约 7.4），一般控制在 4~9 的范围内。

⑥ **pH value** According to the Determination of pH Value in the current edition of Ch.P., the pH value should be equal or close to that of blood (about 7.4), generally controlled in the range of 4-9.

7. 渗透压摩尔浓度 除另有规定外，照现行版《中国药典》渗透压摩尔浓度测定法检查，静脉输液及椎管注射用注射液按各品种项下的规定，其渗透压应与血浆的渗透压相等或接近；供静脉注射、脊椎腔注射的注射剂应为等渗、等张溶液。

⑦ **Osmolality** Unless otherwise specified, according to the Determination of Osmolality in the current edition of Ch.P., the osmotic pressure of the injection for intravenous infusion or vertebral canula injections should be equal or close to that of plasma, the intravenous injection and spinal cavity injection should be isotonic with blood.

（二）安全性检查

(2) Safety Inspection

1. 异常毒性 照现行版《中国药典》异常毒性检查法检查，应符合规定。

① **Abnormal toxicity** Comply with the requirements of the Test for Abnormal Toxicity in the current edition of Ch.P..

2. 过敏反应 照现行版《中国药典》过敏反应检查法检查，应符合规定。

② **Allergen** Comply with the requirements of the Test for Anaphylactic reaction in the current edition of Ch.P..

3. 溶血与凝聚 照现行版《中国药典》溶血与凝聚检查法检查，应符合规定。

③ **Hemolysis and agglomeration** Comply with the requirements of the Test for Hemolysis and Agglomeration in the current edition of Ch.P..

4. 热原或细菌内毒素 除另有规定外，静脉用注射剂按各品种项下的规定，照现行版《中国药典》热原检查法或细菌内毒素检查法检查，应符合规定。

④ **Pyrogens or bacterial endotoxins** Unless otherwise specified, according to the Test for

Pyrogen or Test for Bacterial endotoxin in the current edition of Ch.P., injections for intravenous use should comply with the requirements as specified in under each variety.

5. 无菌 照现行版《中国药典》无菌检查法检查，应符合规定。

⑤ **Sterility** Comply with the requirements stated in the Test for Sterility in the current edition of Ch.P..

（三）所含成分的检测

(3) Detection of Chemical Compositions

1. 总固体含量测定 精密量取注射液 10ml，置于恒重的蒸发皿中，于水浴上蒸干后，105℃干燥 3 小时，移至干燥器中冷却 30 分钟，迅速称定重量，计算出注射剂中含总固体的量（mg/ml），应符合限度范围的要求。

① **Detection of total solids content** Accurately measure 10ml of injection solution, and put it in a constant weight evaporating dish, then evaporate it in a water bath before dry at 105℃ for 3h. At last, put it in a desiccator for 30min, and quickly weigh, then calculate the total solid content (mg/ml), of which should comply with the requirements of the limit.

2. 有效成分或有效部位含量测定 以有效成分或有效部位为组分配制的注射剂，扣除注射剂中附加剂的加入量，所测有效成分或有效部位的量应不低于总固体量的 70%（静脉注射剂不低于 80%）。

② **Determination of active components or active parts content** For the injections prepared with active components or active parts, the amounts of the additional agents should be deducted, and the amounts of the active ingredients in the injections should not be less than 70% of the total solids (not less than 80% for intravenous injections).

3. 指标成分含量测定 以饮片或总提取物为组分配制的注射剂，根据所含成分的性质，应选择适宜的方法，测定其代表性的有效成分、指标成分或一类成分（如总多糖等）的含量。扣除注射剂中附加剂的加入量，所测成分的总含量应不低于总固体量的 20%（静脉注射剂不低于 25%）。

③ **Determination of marker components content** According to the properties of the components contained in the injection prepared by decoction pieces or total extracts, an appropriate method should be chosen to determine the contents of the representative active components, marker components or a class of components (such as total polysaccharides, etc.). The total content of the component measured should be not less than 20% of the total solid volume (not less than 25% of the total solid volume for intravenous injection), excluding the addition of the injection.

4. 含量表示方法 以有效成分或有效部位为组分的注射剂含量均以标示量的上下限范围表示；以饮片为组分的注射剂含量以限量表示；含有毒性药味时，必须确定有毒成分的限量范围；注射剂的组分中含有化学药品的，应单独测定该化学药品的含量，并从总固体内扣除，不计算在含量测定的比例数内。

④ **Methods of contents representation** For the injections prepared with active ingredients, the amounts of the active ingredients should be indicated by upper and lower limits of the indicated quantity. For the injections prepared with Chinese medicinal materials or extracts, the amounts of the marker substances should be indicated by limits.If the injections contains toxic medicinal materials, the limit range of toxic ingredients should be determined.If the injections contains Chinese medicinal materials and chemicals, the amounts of the chemical components should be determined separately.

目前中药注射剂含量测定的方法还不能全面地反映中药注射剂中所含相关成分的种类与数量，为了更好地进行质量控制，2000 年国家药品监督管理局又下发了《中药注射剂指纹图谱研究的技术要求》，率先要求中药注射剂推行指纹图谱的质检方法。

At present, the methods for the determination of the content of Chinese medicine injections cannot fully reflect the types and quantities of related ingredients in Chinese medicine injections. In 2000, the National Medical Products Administration(NMPA) issued *technical requirements for fingerprint study of TCM* to control the qualities of Chinese medicine injections firstly.

二、中药注射剂存在的质量问题

9.6.2　Quality Problems of Chinese Medicine Injections

目前，中药注射剂在生产和应用中还存在一些问题，主要表现为：

At present, there are still some problems in the production and application of Chinese medicine injections, which are mainly manifested as follows:

（一）可见异物与不溶性微粒问题

(1) Visible Particles and Insoluble Particulate Matter

可见异物与不溶性微粒是评价中药注射剂质量的重要指标。中药注射剂在灭菌后或在贮藏过程中产生浑浊或沉淀，出现可见异物与不溶性微粒不合格现象。一般解决的方法如下。

Visible particles and insoluble particles are important indexes to evaluate the quality of Chinese medicine injections. After sterilization or in the process of storage, the Chinese medicine injection produces turbidity or precipitation. The general solution is as follows.

1. 去除杂质　由于原料本身是多种成分的混合物，其中含有的一些高分子化合物，如鞣质、淀粉、树胶、果胶、黏液质、树脂、色素等杂质，在前处理过程中未能除尽，当温度、pH 等因素变化时，这些成分就会进一步聚合变性，使溶液呈现浑浊或出现沉淀；同时，注射剂中含的有些成分不稳定，在制备或贮藏过程中发生水解、氧化等反应，影响澄明度。

① **Removing impurities**　Chinese medicinal materials contains many components, such as tannin, starch, gum, pectin, mucilage, resin, pigment, etc.which may polymerize and make the solution turbid or sedimentary when the temperature or pH value changed.At the same time, some unstable components in the injection may undergo hydrolysis, oxidation and other reactions during preparation or storage, which may affect the clarity of the solution.

2. 调节药液的 pH　中药中某些成分的溶解性能与溶液的 pH 相关，若 pH 调节不当，则容易产生沉淀。一般碱性的有效成分（如生物碱类），药液宜调整至偏酸性；酸性、弱酸性的有效成分（如有机酸等），药液宜调整至偏碱性。

② **Adjusting pH value**　The solubility of some components in traditional Chinese medicine is related to the pH value of the solution. Generally, the solution should be adjusted to acidic of alkaline active ingredients (such as alkaloids). The solution should be adjusted to alkaline of acid or weak acid active components (such as organic acid, etc.).

3. 采取热处理冷藏措施　中药注射剂的高分子物质一般呈胶体分散状态，具有热力学不稳定性及动力学不稳定性，受温度影响，或在放置时胶体粒子的运动碰撞，导致胶粒聚结而使药液浑浊或沉淀。因此，在注射剂灌封前，先对药液进行热处理冷藏，如采用流通蒸气 100℃ 或热压处理 30 分钟，再冷藏放置一段时间，以加速药液中胶体杂质的凝结，然后滤过，除去沉淀后再灌封。

③ **Heating and refrigerating**　The high molecular substances of Chinese medicine injections are in colloidal dispersion state, the colloidal particles are easily to agglomerate and make the medicine liquids turbid or sedimentary.Before filling, the injection liquids should be heated first, then refrigerated

and filtered to remove the sediments.

4. 合理选用附加剂 有些中药注射剂本身含有的成分溶解度小，经灭菌和放置后可能会析出，加入合适的增溶剂、助溶剂（或混合使用）可改善澄明度。制备过程中使用助滤剂也有利于保证注射剂的澄明度。

④ **Choosing additives reasonably** Some chemical components in Chinese medicine injections have low solubility, which may be dissolved out after sterilization or storage for a period of time. Adding a suitable solubilizing agent, cosolvent (or mixed use) can improve the clarity. The use of filter aid during preparation also helps to ensure the clarity of the injection.

5. 应用新技术 如制备过程中应用超滤技术等，可提高注射剂的澄明度。

⑤ **Using new technologies** For example, the clarity of injection can be improved by using ultrafiltration technology in preparation.

（二）刺激性问题

(2) Irritancy

引起中药注射剂刺激性的原因很多，一般解决的方法如下。

There are many causes of irritation of Chinese medicine injections, and the general solutions are as follows.

1. 消除有效成分本身的刺激性 注射剂中的某些成分本身就有较强的刺激性，在不影响疗效的情况下，可通过降低药物浓度、调整 pH 或酌情添加止痛剂的方式来减少刺激性。而对于某些有刺激性的临床需要高浓度使用的或刺激反应严重的有效成分，则可通过改变剂型或改变注射方式消除刺激性。

① **Eliminating the irritation of the active ingredients** Some ingredients in the injection are irritant. The irritation can be reduced by reducing medicine concentration, adjusting pH value or adding analgesics, without affecting the efficacy. For some stimulating clinical ingredients that require high concentration or have severe stimulus reactions, the irritation can be eliminated by changing the dosage form or the way of injection.

2. 去除杂质 中药注射剂中存在杂质，特别是鞣质含量较高时，可使注射局部产生肿痛或硬结；药液中钾离子浓度较高，也会产生刺激性。应通过适当工艺措施除去杂质。

② **Removing impurities** The impurities in Chinese medicine injections, such as a large amount of tannin, can cause swelling, pain or induration in the injection area. The high concentration of potassium ion in the injections will also cause irritation. Impurities shall be removed by appropriate process measures.

3. 调整 pH 注射剂的 pH 过高过低，均可刺激局部，引起疼痛，应在配制药液时注意调节 pH。

③ **Adjusting pH value** Inappropriate pH value may cause irritation or pain. The suitable pH value should be adjusted when preparing the solution.

4. 调整渗透压 注射剂的渗透压不当，也会产生刺激性。应注意药液渗透压的调节，尽可能使之成为等渗溶液。

④ **Adjusting Osmolality** Inappropriate osmolality may cause irritation. So it is necessary to adjust osmolality of injection to be equal to that of the plasma as far as possible.

（三）疗效问题

(3) Curative Effect

影响中药注射剂疗效的因素，除原中药的质量差异外，组方的配伍、用药剂量、特别是提取与纯化方法的合理与否都与之相关。一般解决的方法如下。

The factors affecting the efficacy of Chinese medicine injections are not only the quality difference of the original TCM, but also the compatibility of the formula, the dosage, especially the rationality of the extraction and purification methods. The general solution is as follows.

1. 控制原料质量　由于中药来源、产地、采收、加工炮制等方面的差异，使中药注射剂的原料存在差异，应从原料控制入手，保证每批注射剂的质量稳定。

① Controlling the quality of raw materials　The qualities of Chinese medicinal materials are related to their sources, producing areas, harvesting stages and processing methods, which should be controlled to ensure the quality stability of each batch of injections.

2. 优化工艺　一般注射剂的用药量都较小，应当从提取纯化工艺入手，采用新技术、新方法提高中药注射剂中有效成分的含量。

② Optimizing process　In general, the dosage of injections is small, so the extraction and purification process should be improved. Some new technologies and methods should be used to improve the contents of effective ingredients in Chinese medicine injections.

3. 提高有效成分溶解度　有些中药的有效成分水溶性较小，不能保证注射剂中有足够的浓度，可通过增溶、助溶或其他方法，提高有效成分的溶解度。

③ Improving the solubility of active ingredients　The effective ingredients of some traditional Chinese medicines are less water-soluble and cannot be guaranteed to have sufficient concentration in the injection. The solubility of the effective ingredients can be improved by methods of solubilizing, complex solubilizing or others.

第七节　输液剂与血浆代用液

PPT

英文翻译

一、输液剂的含义

输液剂是指供静脉滴注用的大体积（除另有规定外，一般不小于 100ml）注射液，也称静脉输液。

二、输液剂的特点与分类

输液剂的使用剂量大，直接进入血循环，故能快速产生药效，是临床救治危重和急症病人的主要用药方式。其作用多样，适用范围广，临床主要用于纠正体内水和电解质的紊乱，调节体液的酸碱平衡，补充必要的营养、热能和水分，维持血容量。也常把输液剂作为一种载体，将注射液如抗生素等加入其中供静脉滴注，以使药物迅速起效，并维持稳定的血药浓度，确保临床疗效的发挥。

目前临床上常用的输液剂可分为：

1. 电解质输液　用于补充体内水分、电解质，纠正体内酸碱平衡等。如氯化钠注射液（俗称生理盐水）、乳酸钠注射液等。

2. 营养输液　用于不能口服吸收营养的患者，补充供给体内热量、蛋白质和人体必需的脂肪酸和水分等。如葡萄糖注射液、氨基酸输液、脂肪乳输液等。

3. 胶体输液 用于调节体内渗透压。是一类与血液等渗的胶体溶液，由于胶体溶液中的高分子不易通过血管壁，可使水分较长时间在血液循环系统内保持，产生增加血容量和维持血压的效果。胶体输液有多糖类、明胶类、高分子聚合物等。如右旋糖酐、淀粉衍生物、明胶、聚维酮等。

4. 含药输液 含有药液的输液，可用于临床治疗。如氧氟沙星、苦参碱等输液。

三、输液剂的制法

（一）容器的处理

常用中性硬质玻璃制成的输液瓶、聚丙烯塑料瓶或由无毒聚氯乙烯制成的输液袋。输液容器要求其物理化学性质稳定，质量符合国家规定。输液瓶的洗涤应视其洁净程度选择相应的处理方法，一般新瓶及洁净度较好的输液瓶可先用水洗去表面灰尘，然后用冲瓶机以70℃左右的3%碳酸钠或2%氢氧化钠溶液冲洗10秒以上，再以纯水冲洗去碱液，注射用水冲洗，最后再以微孔滤膜滤过的注射用水洗净。

橡胶塞能耐高温高压灭菌，并具有高度的化学稳定性、吸附性小等性能。橡胶塞的处理流程为：制药纯水洗净→0.5%的氢氧化钠煮沸30分钟→制药纯水洗去碱液→注射用水洗净→1%的盐酸煮沸30分钟→制药纯水洗去酸液→注射用水洗净，加塞前用滤过的注射用水随冲随塞。

涤纶薄膜和聚丙烯薄膜做衬垫薄膜，可使药液与橡胶塞隔阂，以防药液被胶塞污染。其处理方法如下：用注射用水煮沸或115℃加热处理30分钟，再用滤清的注射用水动态漂洗至澄清；临用时用滤过的注射用水逐张冲洗后覆盖在瓶口上，立即加上胶塞。

（二）制备要点

1. 配制 常采用浓配法，即先将原料加新鲜注射用水配制成较高浓度的溶液，经过滤过等处理后再稀释至规定体积。原料质量好的药物可采用稀配法，即将原料药物直接加新鲜注射用水配制成所需浓度。

2. 滤过 应在封闭系统内进行，以减少污染，先用一般滤器粗滤，再用垂熔玻璃滤器（G_4）或微孔滤膜（0.45μm、0.65μm）等精滤。

3. 灌封 输液瓶用滤过的注射用水冲洗后再灌入药液，盖上用注射用水冲洗过的衬垫薄膜，再用注射用水冲洗的橡胶塞塞紧，最后加上铝盖轧紧密封。

4. 灭菌 灌封后的输液应及时灭菌，一般采用热压灭菌，即68.7kPa，115℃保持30分钟。

5. 质量检查与包装 按照现行版《中国药典》有关规定进行检查，应符合规定。质量检查合格的输液，应逐瓶贴上标签，再装箱。

四、输液剂质量问题讨论

（一）输液剂存在的问题

1. 染菌问题 由于生产过程中污染、灭菌不彻底、瓶塞松动、漏气等原因，致使输液剂出现浑浊、霉团、云雾状、产气等染菌现象，使用这种输液可能会引发败血症、热原反应等，甚至导致死亡。

2. 热原问题 关于热原的污染途径和防止办法在本章第二节已有详述。但输液使用过程中的污染引起的热原反应不容忽视，如输液器等的污染。因此尽量使用已经灭菌处理的一次性全套输液器，包括插管、导管、调速与加药装置、末端滤器、针头等。特定患者群（例如新生儿）对热

原反应可能比根据正常健康成年人体重确定的限度预期反应更危险，这使GMP控制内毒素变得更为重要。

3. 可见异物与不溶性微粒的问题 输液中的微粒包括碳黑、碳酸钙、氧化锌、纤维素、纸屑、黏土、玻璃屑、细菌、真菌、真菌芽胞和结晶体等。若输液中如含有大量肉眼看不见的微粒、异物，其对人体的危害是潜在的、长期的，可引起过敏反应、热原样反应等。较大的微粒，可造成局部循环障碍，引起血管栓塞；微粒过多，会造成局部堵塞和供血不足，组织缺氧，产生水肿和静脉炎；异物侵入组织，由于巨噬细胞的包围和增殖而引起肉芽肿。

微粒产生的原因有：

（1）原料与附加剂质量问题 原料与附加剂质量对澄明度影响较显著，如注射用葡萄糖有时含有水解不完全的产物糊精、蛋白质、钙盐等杂质；氯化钠、碳酸氢钠中含有较高的钙盐、镁盐和硫酸盐；氯化钙中含有较多的碱性物质。这些杂质的存在，可使输液产生乳光、小白点、浑浊等。活性炭杂质含量多，不仅影响输液的可见异物检查指标，而且还影响药液的稳定性。

（2）容器质量问题 胶塞与输液容器质量不好，在储存中有杂质脱落而污染药液。如输液中的“小白点”经分析表明为钙、锌、硅酸盐与铁等物质；储存多年的氯化钠输液检测出钙、镁。对聚氯乙烯袋装输液与玻璃瓶装输液进行对比试验，将检品持续振摇2小时，发现前者产生的微粒比后者多5倍，分析表明，微粒为对人体有害的增塑剂二乙基邻苯二甲酸酯（DEHP)。另丁基胶塞的硅油污染亦可产生微粒。

（3）工艺操作中的问题 如生产车间空气洁净度差，输液瓶、丁基胶塞等容器和附件洗涤不净，滤器选择不当，滤过方法不好，灌封操作不合要求，工序安排不合理等。

（4）医院输液操作以及静脉滴注装置的问题 无菌操作不严、静脉滴注装置不净或不恰当的输液配伍等。

（二）解决办法

1. 输液用的原辅料及输液容器与附件应符合质量要求。

2. 减少制备生产过程中的污染，严格控制灭菌条件，严密包装。

3. 合理安排工序，加强工艺过程管理，采取单向层流净化空气，及时除去制备过程中新产生的污染微粒，采用微孔滤膜滤过等。

4. 在输液器中安置终端滤过器（0.8μm孔径的薄膜），可防止使用过程中微粒的污染。

五、血浆代用液

（一）血浆代用液的含义

血浆代用液也称血浆扩张剂，是指与血浆等渗而无毒的胶体溶液。血浆代用液由高分子聚合物制成，静脉注射后能暂时维持血压或增加血容量，可用于因出血、烫伤、外伤等所引起的休克或失血之症，但不能代替全血。

（二）血浆代用液的质量要求

1. 渗透压应与血浆相近。

2. 无毒性，无蓄积作用，不发生发热、抗原性、过敏性或其他反应。

3. 在血液循环系统中，能保留较长的时间，半衰期为5~7小时，无利尿作用。

4. 在血液中停留期间，不影响人体组织与血液正常的生理功能。

5. 溶液pH应为6~8，其中所含的电解质不得超过下列浓度：钾6mmol/L，钠156mmol/L，钙3mmol/L，镁1.5mmol/L，无机磷1.4mmol/L，氯离子110mmol/L。

6. 无菌，无热原反应。

7. 性质稳定，能经受较高温度的灭菌。

（三）血浆代用液的种类

1. 多糖类 包括右旋糖酐、淀粉衍生物、缩合葡萄糖等。

2. 蛋白质类 包括变性明胶、氧化明胶、聚明胶等。

3. 合成高分子聚合物类 包括聚维酮、氧乙烯 - 聚丙烯二醇缩合物等。

PPT

第八节 粉针剂与其他注射剂

一、粉针剂

粉针剂为注射用无菌粉末的简称，是指药物制成的供临用前用适宜的无菌溶液配制成澄清溶液或均匀混悬液的无菌粉末或块状物。凡对热不稳定或在水溶液中易分解失效的药物，如一些抗生素、医用酶制剂及生化制品，均需用无菌操作法制成粉针剂。粉针剂可用适宜的注射用溶剂配制后注射，也可用静脉输液配制后静脉滴注。

粉针剂的生产必须在无菌室内进行。其质量要求与溶液型注射剂基本一致。

粉针剂的制法如下：

1. 无菌粉末直接分装法

（1）原材料准备 对直接无菌分装的原料，应了解药物粉末的理化性质，测定物料的热稳定性、临界相对湿度、粉末的晶形和松密度，以便确定适宜的分装工艺。

无菌原料可用灭菌溶剂结晶法、喷雾干燥法或冷冻干燥法制得，必要时进行粉碎和过筛。

（2）容器的处理 安瓿或小瓶、丁基胶塞处理及相应的质量要求同注射剂和输液剂。各种分装容器洗净后，需经干热灭菌或红外线灭菌后备用。已灭菌好的空瓶应存放在有净化空气保护的贮存柜中，存放时间不超过 24 小时。

（3）分装 必须在高度洁净的灭菌室中按照灭菌操作法进行。根据药物的性质控制分装条件。分装后，小瓶立即加塞并用铝盖密封。安瓿也应立即熔封。

（4）灭菌 能耐热品种，可选用适宜灭菌方法进行补充灭菌，以保证用药安全。对不耐热品种，应严格无菌操作，控制分装过程不被污染，成品不再灭菌处理。

2. 无菌水溶液冷冻干燥法 冷冻干燥法是先将药物配制成注射溶液，再按规定方法进行除菌滤过，滤液在无菌条件下立即灌入相应的容器中，经冷冻干燥，得干燥粉末，最后在无菌条件下封口即得。

本法制得的粉针剂，常会出现含水量过高、喷瓶、产品外观萎缩或成团等问题。这些问题可通过改进冷冻干燥的工艺条件或添加适量的填充剂得到解决。目前，粉针剂中常用的填充剂（又称支架剂）主要有葡萄糖、甘露醇、氯化钠等。

二、混悬液型注射剂

将不溶性固体药物分散于液体分散介质中，可供肌内注射或静脉注射的药剂称为混悬液型注射剂。对于无适当溶剂可溶解的不溶性固体药物，或在水溶液中不稳定而制成的水不溶性衍

生物，或希望固体微粒在机体内定向分布及需要长效的药物均可采用适当的方法制成混悬液型注射剂。

（一）混悬液型注射剂的质量要求

混悬液属固液分散的不稳定体系，混悬液型注射剂的质量要求除了应符合一般注射剂的规定以外，必须注意分散微粒的大小及微粒在分散介质中的分散程度，以确保体系的稳定。一般注射剂，混悬颗粒应小于 15μm，15~20μm 的颗粒应不超过 10%。供静脉注射用的注射剂，其混悬颗粒应更小，2μm 以下的颗粒应占 99%，否则易引起静脉栓塞。混悬颗粒应具有良好的分散性和通针性，在分散介质中不能沉降太快。贮存期间一旦下沉，经振摇即可重新分散而无结块现象。

（二）混悬液型注射剂的制法

混悬液型注射剂的制法与一般混悬剂的制法相似。首先应根据药物的性质及注射剂给药的要求，选择合适的溶剂、润湿剂与助悬剂。溶剂一般选用注射用水或注射用油；制备水性混悬剂所需的润湿剂，一般选用聚山梨酯 -80，常用量为 0.1%~0.2% (g/ml)；助悬剂一般选用羧甲基纤维素钠、甲基纤维素、低聚海藻酸钠等，用量为 0.5%~1% (g/ml)。

混悬液型注射剂中固体药物的分散方法有微粒结晶法、机械粉碎法、溶剂化合物法。制备时将药物微晶混悬于含有稳定剂（润滑剂及助悬剂）的溶液中，用超声波处理使其分散均匀，滤过，调 pH，灌封，灭菌即得。

三、乳状液型注射剂

乳状液型注射剂是以挥发油、植物油或脂溶性药物为原料，加入乳化剂和注射用水经乳化制成的供注射给药的乳状液。包括油 / 水（O/W）型与水 / 油（W/O）型或水 / 油 / 水（W/O/W）型复乳。

乳状液型注射剂应无菌，无毒，无热原，具有适宜的 pH，分散相微粒大小在 1~10μm 范围内，W/O 型及 O/W 型乳状液注射剂可供肌内或组织注射用。外相为水的乳状液可作静脉注射，但微粒大小必须严格控制，一般应≤ 1μm，而且应大小均匀，能耐高压灭菌，化学和生物学稳定性好。此类供静脉注射用乳状液，除补充能量外，还具有对某些脏器的定向分布作用和淋巴系统的指向性，因此，将抗癌药物制成乳状液型注射剂供静脉注射应用，可提高疗效。

（一）静脉乳剂原辅料的质量要求

乳状液型注射剂的原辅料包括溶剂、脂肪油、乳化剂、等渗调节剂等。静脉乳剂所选用的原辅料均应符合注射要求，尤其是乳化剂的选择，以天然品纯化的豆磷脂、卵磷脂及合成品普流罗尼克 F-68 为好。

（二）静脉乳剂的制法

乳状液为热不稳定体系，在高温下易聚合成大油滴。为保证体系的稳定性，乳状液型注射剂的制备方法应使分散相微粒大小适当，粒度均匀。制备过程中常采用乳化器械帮助乳化。

PPT

第九节 眼用液体制剂

一、概述

眼用液体制剂系指治疗或诊断眼部疾病的液体药剂，分为滴眼剂、洗眼剂和眼内注射溶液三类。眼用液体制剂也有以固态药物形式包装，另备溶剂，临用前配成溶液或混悬液的剂型。

滴眼剂系指由药物与适宜辅料制成的供滴入眼内的无菌液体制剂。可分为水性或油性溶液、混悬液或乳状液。

洗眼剂系指由药物制成的无菌澄明水溶液，供冲洗眼部异物或分泌液、中和外来化学物质的眼用液体剂型。

眼内注射溶液系指由药物与适宜辅料制成的无菌澄明溶液，供眼周围组织（包括球结膜下、筋膜下及球后等）或眼内注射（包括前房注射、前房冲洗、玻璃体内注射、玻璃体内灌注等）的无菌眼用液体剂型。

眼用液体制剂在生产与储存中应符合下列规定：

1. 滴眼剂中可加入调节渗透压、pH、黏度及增加药物溶解度和制剂稳定性的辅料，并可加适宜浓度的抑菌剂和抗氧剂。所用辅料不应降低药效或产生局部刺激。

2. 除另有规定外，滴眼剂应与泪液等渗。混悬型滴眼剂的沉降物经振摇应易再分散。

3. 洗眼剂属用量较大的眼用制剂，应尽可能与泪液等渗并具相近的 pH。多剂量的洗眼剂一般应加适当的抑菌剂。

4. 眼内注射溶液、眼内插入剂、供外科手术用和急救用的眼用制剂，均不得加抑菌剂、抗氧剂或不适当的缓冲剂，且应包装于无菌容器内供一次性使用。

5. 除另有规定外，滴眼剂每个容器的装量应不超过 10ml；洗眼剂每个容器的装量应不超过 200ml。包装容器应无菌、不易破裂，其透明度应不影响可见异物的检查。

6. 眼用制剂应遮光密封贮存，启用后最多可使用 4 周。

二、眼用液体制剂的附加剂

1. pH 调节剂　常用的有磷酸缓冲液、硼酸缓冲液等。

2. 渗透压调节剂　常用的有氯化钠、硼酸、葡萄糖等。

3. 抑菌剂　滴眼剂是多剂量外用制剂，制剂中应加入作用迅速而有效的抑菌剂。常用抑菌剂有硝酸苯汞（0.002%~0.005%）、硫柳汞（0.005%~0.01%）、苯扎氯铵（0.001%~0.002%）、苯乙醇（0.5%）、三氯叔丁醇（0.35%~0.5%）等。

4. 黏度调节剂　适当增加滴眼剂的黏度，可以减小刺激性，延长药液的眼内滞留时间，增强药效。合适的黏度是 4.0~5.0cPa · s。常用的黏度调节剂有甲基纤维素、羧甲基纤维素钠，其他如聚乙烯醇、聚乙二醇、聚乙烯吡咯烷酮等亦可选用。

5. 其他附加剂　根据主药性质和制备需要，还可加入抗氧剂、增溶剂、助溶剂等。

三、眼用液体制剂的制法

眼用液体制剂的制备工艺流程一般如图 9-5 所示。

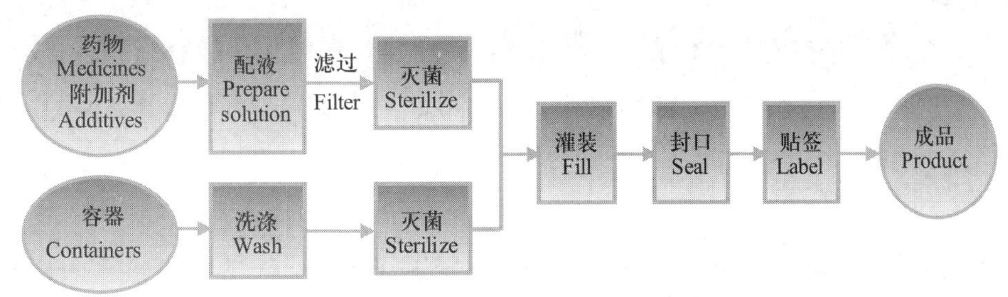

图 9-5 眼用液体制剂制备工艺流程图

用于手术、伤口、角膜穿通伤的滴眼剂及眼用注射溶液按注射剂生产工艺制备，分装于单剂量容器中密封或熔封，最后灭菌，不加抑菌剂，一次用后弃去。洗眼剂用输液瓶包装，其清洁方法同输液包装容器。药物不稳定者，全部以严格的无菌生产工艺操作。若药物稳定，可在大瓶装后灭菌，然后再在无菌操作条件下分装。

四、眼用液体制剂的质量要求与检查

眼用液体制剂的质量要求类似于注射剂，在 pH、渗透压、无菌、可见异物等方面都有相应的要求与检查。

（一）质量要求

1. pH 人体正常泪液的 pH 为 7.4，正常眼可耐受的 pH 为 5.0~9.0，pH 为 6.0~8.0 时无不适感觉，小于 5.0 或大于 11.4 时有明显的刺激性。

2. 渗透压 应与泪液等渗。眼球能适应的渗透压范围相当于浓度为 0.6%~1.5% 的氯化钠溶液，超过 2% 就有明显的不适。

3. 无菌 对于眼部有外伤或手术的患者，所用的眼用制剂必须无菌，并不得加入抑菌剂，成品必须严格灭菌，多采用单剂量包装，一经打开使用后，不得放置再用。用于眼部无外伤的眼用制剂，一般要求无致病菌，不得检出铜绿假单胞菌和金黄色葡萄球菌。滴眼剂是一种多剂量剂型，为避免多次使用后染菌，应添加适当的抑菌剂。

4. 可见异物 溶液型的眼用液体制剂应澄明无异物，特别不得有碎玻璃屑。混悬液型的眼用液体制剂其混悬颗粒要求小于 50μm，其中含 15μm 以下的颗粒不得少于 90%，且颗粒不得结块，易摇匀。

5. 黏度 滴眼剂的黏度适当增大可使药物在眼内停留时间延长，从而增强药物的作用。合适的黏度为 4.0~5.0cPa · s。

6. 其他 眼用溶液类似注射剂，也要注意稳定性问题。很多眼用药物是不稳定的，例如毒豆碱、后马托品、乙基吗啡等。

（二）检查

为确保眼用液体制剂的成品质量，根据上述质量要求，必须逐项进行质量检查。其他照现行版《中国药典》进行检查，应符合相关规定。

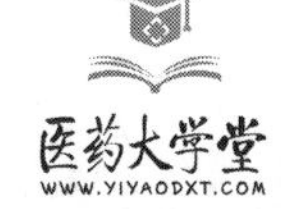

（李 文 杨军宣）

第十章　外用膏剂

Chapter 10　External Ointments

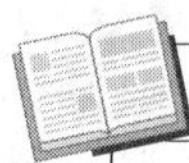

学习目标 | Learning Goals

知识要求：

1. **掌握**　软膏剂、膏药、橡胶膏剂的含义、特点与制法。

2. **熟悉**　外用膏剂的透皮吸收机制及影响因素；凝胶剂、凝胶膏剂、糊剂、涂膜剂及贴剂的含义、特点及制法；软膏与黑膏药基质的种类和性质。

3. **了解**　外用膏剂的质量检查。

能力要求：

学会各类外用膏剂的制备与质量检测方法，能制备不同类型的外用膏剂，并检查和评价外用膏剂的产品质量。

Knowledge requirements:

1. **To master** the meaning, characteristics and preparation method of ointments, plasters and rubber plasters.

2. **To be familiar with** transdermal absorption mechanism and influencing factors of external ointments, the meaning, characteristics and preparation method of gels, gel pastes, pastes, coatings and patches, types and properties of ointments and black plaster bases.

3. **To know** the quality inspection of external ointments.

Ability requirements:

To be able to to use various preparation methods to manufacture different external ointments, and quality testing methods to evaluate and control the quality of external ointments.

第一节　概述

10.1　Overview

PPT

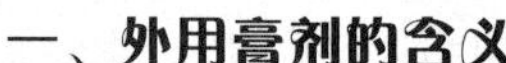

10.1.1　The Definition of External Ointments

外用膏剂系指药物与适宜的基质制成专供外用的半固体或近似固体的一类剂型，包括软膏

剂、硬膏剂（膏药）以及贴膏剂（橡胶膏剂、凝胶膏剂、贴剂），此外还有糊剂、涂膜剂、凝胶剂、透皮贴片剂等。

External ointments refer to drugs and suitable matrices which are formulated as semi-solid or near-solid dosage forms for external use, including ointments, hard plasters(plasters) and cataplasms (adhesive plasters, hydrogel plasters, patches), as well as pastes, pigments, gels, transdermal patch tablets, etc.

软膏剂和膏药（铅硬膏）在我国应用较早，橡胶膏剂起源于国外，贴剂近年来发展迅猛，凝胶膏剂和凝胶剂因能容纳多量中药提取物而受到重视，传统的铅硬膏通过穴位经络发挥药物通经活络、行滞祛瘀、开窍透骨、祛风散寒的作用。2020 年版《中国药典》一部收载的中药成方制剂中收录外用膏剂 35 种，其中软膏剂 14 种，橡胶膏剂 14 种，膏药 7 种。

Ointments and plasters (lead plasters) were used early in China. Adhesive plasters originated abroad, and patches have developed rapidly in recent years. Hydrogel plasters and gels are valued for their ability to hold large amounts of Chinese herbal extracts. The traditional lead plaster has the functions of meridian activation, stasis removal, opening orifices, wind and cold dispersal through acupoints and meridians. The 2020 edition of the *Chinese Pharmacopoeia* contained 35 types of external ointments, including 14 ointments, 14 adhesive plasters, and 7 poultices.

二、外用膏剂的特点
10.1.2 The Characteristics of External Ointments

外用膏剂广泛应用于皮肤科与外科，易涂布或黏附于皮肤、黏膜或创面上，具有保护创面、润滑皮肤和局部治疗作用，也可以透过皮肤和黏膜起全身治疗作用。药物透过皮肤起全身治疗作用具有以下优点：①能避免肝脏的首过效应；②避免药物对胃肠道产生刺激；③维持恒定持久的释药速率；④减少给药次数等。

External ointments are widely used in dermatology and surgery. They can be easily applied or adhered to the skin, mucous membranes, or wounds. They can protect the wounds, lubricate the skin, and treat the skin, as well as treat the whole body through the skin and mucous membranes. Medication administered through the skin for systemic treatment has the following advantages: ① Can avoid the first pass effect of the liver; ② Avoid irritating the gastrointestinal tract; ③ Maintain a constant and sustained release rate; ④ Reduce the number of administration, etc.

三、外用膏剂的分类
10.1.3 The Classification of External Ointments

外用膏剂按基质及形态可分为两类：

External ointments can be divided into two types according to their matrix and morphology:

软膏剂 系指将原料药物与适宜基质混匀制成的易涂抹于皮肤或黏膜上的半固体外用剂型。类似软膏的有糊剂、凝胶剂，与软膏剂应用类似的还有涂膜剂。

Ointments refer to a semi-solid external dosage form prepared by mixing the raw material drug with a suitable base, which is easy to apply to the skin or mucous membranes. Pastes and gels are similar to ointments, and applications of coating agents are also similar to ointments.

硬膏剂 系指将原料药物溶解或混合于黏性基质中，摊涂于背衬材料上制成的供贴敷使用的近似固体的外用剂型，药物可以透过皮肤起全身治疗作用。

Hard plasters refer to an approximately solid external dosage form prepared by dissolving or mixing raw drug in a viscous matrix and spreading it on a backing material for application. The drug can pass through the skin for systemic treatment.

按基质组成可分为两类：

According to the matrix composition, it can be divided into two categories:

膏药 系指以高级脂肪酸铅盐（红丹或宫粉）为基质的硬膏剂，如黑膏药、白膏药等。

Plasters refer to plasters based on higher fatty acid lead salts (red lead oxide or ceruse), such as black plaster, white plaster, etc.

贴膏剂 系指以适宜的基质和基材制成的供皮肤贴敷的一类片状外用制剂。包括：①橡胶膏剂：以橡胶为主要基质，涂布于背衬材料上制成。②凝胶膏剂：以亲水材料为基质，涂布于背衬材料上制成。③贴剂：以适宜高分子材料为基质制成。

Cataplasms refer to a sheet-type external preparation for skin application made from a suitable matrix and substrate. Including: ① Adhesive plasters: rubber is used as the main substrate and coated on the backing material. ② Hydrogel plasters: based on a hydrophilic material and coated on a backing material. ③ Patches: made with suitable polymer materials as the matrix.

四、药物经皮吸收机制与影响因素
10.1.4 Drug Transdermal Absorption Mechanism and Influencing Factors

（一）药物经皮吸收机制
(1) Drug Transdermal Absorption Mechanism

外用膏剂的透皮吸收系指其中的药物通过皮肤进入血液的过程，包括释放、渗透及吸收进入血液循环三个阶段。释放系指药物从基质中脱离出来并扩散到皮肤或黏膜表面；渗透系指药物通过表皮进入真皮、皮下组织，对局部组织起治疗作用；吸收是指药物通过皮肤微循环或与黏膜接触后通过血管或淋巴管进入体循环而产生全身作用的过程。

The transdermal absorption of an external ointment refers to the process by which the drug enters the blood through the skin, including the three stages of release, penetration and absorption into the blood circulation. Release refers to the release of the drug from the base and it being spread to the skin or mucosal surface; penetration refers to the drug entering the dermis and subcutaneous tissue through the epidermis, which has a therapeutic effect on local tissue; absorption refers to the process in which the drug passes through the skin microcirculation or enters the systemic circulation through blood vessels or lymphatic vessels after coming into contact with the mucosa, resulting in a systemic effect.

1. 皮肤的构造 正常人皮肤由表皮、真皮及皮下脂肪组织三部分组成，如图 10-1 所示。

① The structure of the skin Normal human skin is composed of epidermis, dermis and subcutaneous adipose tissue, as shown in Figure 10-1.

2. 经皮吸收途径 药物的经皮吸收主要有以下两个途径。

② Percutaneous absorption pathway There are two main ways for the transdermal absorption of drugs:

（1）完整的表皮途径 是药物经皮吸收的主要途径。完整表皮的角质层细胞及其细胞间隙具有类脂膜性质，有利于脂溶性药物以非解离型透过皮肤，而解离型药物较难透过。

a. *Intact epidermal pathway* This pathway is the main route of drug transdermal absorption. Keratinocytes of the intact epidermis and their intercellular spaces have lipid-like membrane properties, which is beneficial for fat-soluble drugs to penetrate the skin in a non-dissociated type, while dissociated

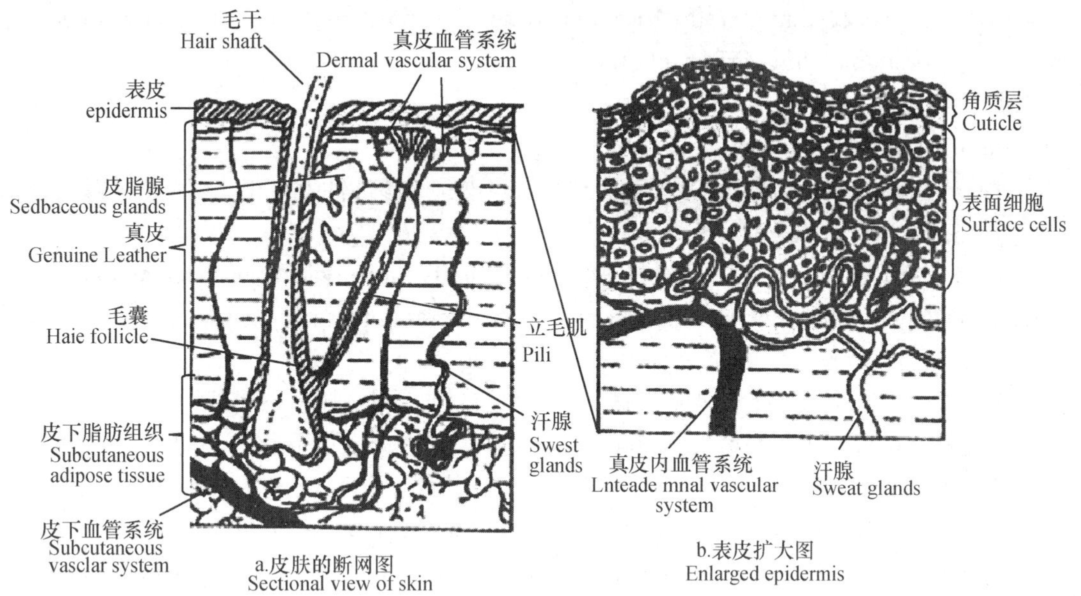

图 10-1　皮肤的构造

Figure 10-1　The Structure of the Skin

drugs are more difficult to penetrate.

（2）皮肤附属器途径　即通过皮脂腺、皮囊及汗腺吸收。在吸收初期药物穿透皮肤附属器比完整表皮快，当吸收达到稳态后，则附属器途径可忽略，且其所占面积只有皮肤总面积的 1% 左右，故不是主要吸收途径。大分子和离子型药物可能主要通过这些途径转运。

b. *Skin appendage approach*　This approach is absorbed through the sebaceous glands, skin capsules and sweat glands. In the early stage of absorption, the drug penetrates the skin appendage faster than the intact epidermis. When the absorption reaches a steady state, the appendage pathway is negligible, and its area is only about 1% of the total skin area, so it is not the main absorption pathway. Macromolecular and ionic drugs may be mainly transported through these pathways.

（二）影响因素

(2) Influencing Factors

影响经皮吸收的因素可以用式（10-1）说明：

The factors that affect transdermal absorption can be illustrated by equation (10-1):

$$dQ/dt = K \cdot C \cdot D \cdot A/T \qquad (10\text{-}1)$$

式中，dQ/dt 为达到稳定时的药物透皮速率；K 为药物皮肤 / 基质分配系数；C 为溶于基质中的药物浓度；D 为药物在皮肤屏障中的扩散系数；A 为给药面积；T 为有效屏障厚度。分配系数 K 是药物在皮肤与基质中相对溶解度的指数。当 A、D、T 不变时，C 是透皮吸收最重要的理化参数。K、C 的乘积可代表药物的热力学活性，即药物与基质亲和力越弱，在基质中浓度越高，透皮速率越大。影响药物经皮吸收的因素如下：

Where: dQ / dt is the transdermal rate of the drug when it is stable; K is the skin / base partition coefficient of the drug; C is the concentration of the drug dissolved in the base; D is the diffusion coefficient of the drug in the skin barrier; Area; T is the effective barrier thickness. Partition coefficient K is an index of the relative solubility of a drug in the skin and base. When A, D, T are unchanged, C is the most important physical and chemical parameter for transdermal absorption. The product of K and C can represent the thermodynamic activity of the drug, that is, the weaker the affinity of the drug and the

base, the higher the concentration in the base, the greater the transdermal rate. The factors affecting the percutaneous absorption of drugs are as follows:

1. 皮肤生理因素

① Skin physiological factors

（1）种属与个体差异　不同动物、动物与人之间皮肤的渗透性差异很大。同种动物性别、年龄不同，其渗透性也有较大差别。

a. Species and Individual Differences　Skin permeability varies widely between animals, animals and humans. Different animals of the same species have different sexes and ages, and their permeability varies greatly.

（2）皮肤的部位　药物的穿透吸收速度与皮肤角质层的厚度、附属器密度等有较大关系。一般角质层薄、毛孔多的部位则较易透入。不同部位的皮肤通透性大小顺序为：耳廓后部 > 腹股沟 > 颅顶盖 > 脚背 > 前下臂 > 足底。对全身作用的经皮吸收制剂宜选择角质层薄、施药方便的部位。

b. Parts of the skin　The penetration rate of the drug has a greater relationship with the thickness of the stratum corneum and the density of the appendages. Generally, the stratum corneum is thin and the pores are more easily penetrated. The order of skin permeability in different parts is as follows: posterior auricle> groin> cranial cap> instep> forearm> foot. For percutaneous absorption preparations with systemic effects, it is advisable to select a part with a thin stratum corneum and convenient administration.

（3）皮肤的状况　如皮肤患湿疹、溃疡或切伤、烧烫伤时，皮肤角质层屏障作用下降或丧失，药物易于穿透，吸收速度和吸收程度大大增加（溃疡皮肤渗透性为正常皮肤的 3~5 倍），但疼痛、过敏等副作用也会增加。而硬皮病、牛皮癣及老年角化病等皮肤病使角质层致密硬化，药物渗透性降低。

c. Skin condition　For example, when the skin suffers from eczema, ulcers, cuts, or burns, the cuticle barrier of the skin is reduced or lost, the drug can easily penetrate, and the absorption rate and degree of absorption are greatly increased (ulcer skin permeability is 3 to 5 times that of normal skin). However, side effects such as pain and allergies also increase. Skin diseases such as scleroderma, psoriasis, and senile keratosis make the stratum corneum dense and hard, reducing drug permeability.

（4）皮肤的温度与湿度　皮肤温度增加，血液循环加快，吸收增加。皮肤湿度大，有利于角质层的水合作用，引起角质层肿胀，细胞间隙疏松，药物渗透性增加。

d. Skin temperature and humidity　Increased skin temperature increases blood flow circulation and increases absorption. The high humidity of the skin is conducive to the hydration of the stratum corneum, causing swelling of the stratum corneum, loosening of intercellular spaces, and increasing drug permeability.

（5）皮肤的结合与代谢作用　药物与皮肤蛋白质或脂质等的结合是可逆性结合，可延长药物渗透时滞，也可能在皮肤内形成药物的贮库。酶代谢对多数药物在皮肤吸收不产生明显的首过效应。

e. Skin binding and metabolism　The combination of the drug with skin proteins or lipids is a reversible combination, which can prolong the time lag of drug penetration, and may also form a drug depot in the skin. Enzyme metabolism does not have a significant first-pass effect on skin absorption of most drugs.

2. 药物性质

② Drug properties

（1）油水分配系数　角质层具有类脂质特性，非极性强，一般脂溶性药物比水溶性药物易穿透皮肤，但组织液是极性的，因此既有一定脂溶性又有一定水溶性的药物（分子具有极性基团和非极性基团）更易穿透。有机弱酸或有机弱碱性药物的分子型比离子型脂溶性大，故较易透过皮肤吸收。

a. Oil-water partition coefficient The stratum corneum has lipid-like properties and is highly non-polar. Generally, fat-soluble drugs penetrate the skin more easily than water-soluble drugs, but the interstitial fluid is polar, therefore drugs with certain fat-solubility/lipophilicity and water-solubility (the molecules have extremely Sex groups and non-polar groups bonds) can penetrate more easily penetrated. Organic weak acids or organic weak alkaline drugs are more molecularly soluble than ionic fats, so it is easier for these to be absorbed through the skin.

（2）分子量 药物的扩散系数与分子量的平方根或立方根成反比，相对分子量超过 600 的药物较难透过角质层。

b. Molecular weight The diffusion coefficient of a drug is inversely proportional to the square or cubic root of its molecular weight. It is more difficult for the drugs with molecular weights above 600 are more difficult to penetrate the stratum corneum.

（3）熔点 熔点愈高的药物和水溶性药物，在角质层的渗透速率较低。

c. Melting point Drugs with higher melting points and water-soluble drugs have lower penetration rates in the stratum corneum.

3. 基质性质

③ Base properties

（1）基质的种类与组成 直接影响药物在基质中的理化性质及贴敷处皮肤的生理功能。油脂性强的基质封闭性强，如中药膏药能阻止皮肤内水分与汗液蒸发，有利于角质层的水合作用，从而加快药物吸收，透皮吸收效果较好。而水溶性的基质对药物释放虽快，但几乎不能阻止水分的蒸发（如聚乙二醇），故不利于药物穿透与透皮吸收。

a. Type and composition of base It directly affects the physicochemical properties of the drug in the base and the physiological function of the skin at the application site. The oily base has strong sealing properties. For example, Chinese medicinal plasters can prevent the moisture and sweat in the skin from evaporating, which is beneficial to for the hydration of the stratum corneum, thereby accelerating the absorption of the drug, and the effect of transdermal absorption is better. While the water-soluble base releases the drug fast, it can hardly prevent the evaporation of water (such as polyethylene glycol), which is not conducive to drug penetration and transdermal absorption.

（2）基质对药物的亲和力 若两者亲和力大，药物的皮肤 / 基质分配系数小，药物难以从基质向皮肤转移，不利于吸收。

b. Base affinity for drugs If the two have high affinity, the skin / base partition coefficient of the drug is small, and it is difficult for the drug to transfer from the base to the skin, which is not conducive to absorption.

（3）基质的 pH 值 pH 值影响弱酸性和弱碱性药物的分子形式，当基质的 pH 值小于弱酸性药物的 pK_a 或大于弱碱性药物的 pK_a 时，这些药物的分子型（非离子型）增加，脂溶性加大有利于穿透皮肤或黏膜。故可根据药物的 pK_a 值来调节基质的 pH 值，增加非离子型的比例，提高渗透性。

c. Base pH The pH value affects the molecular form of weakly acidic and weakly basic drugs. When the pH of the base is less than the pK_a of weakly acidic drugs or greater than the pK_a of weakly basic drugs, the molecular type (non-ionic) of these drugs increases which is beneficial for penetrating

the skin or mucous membranes. Therefore, the pH value of the base can be adjusted according to the pK_a value of the drugs, the proportion of non-ionic type can be increased, and the permeability can be improved.

4. 附加剂

④ Additives

（1）表面活性剂　自身可以渗入皮肤与皮肤成分相互作用，促进药物渗透。通常非离子型表面活性剂的作用大于阴离子型表面活性剂，且刺激性小。但表面活性剂的用量与药物的渗透作用不一定成正比，用量高，药物被增溶在胶团中，反而不易释放，一般以 1%~2% 为宜。

a. Surfactant　It can penetrate into the skin and interact with skin components to promote drug penetration. Generally, the effect of non-ionic surfactants is greater than that of anionic surfactants, and it is less irritating. However, the amount of surfactant is not necessarily proportional to the penetrating effect of the drug, the amount is high, the drug is solubilized in the micelle, but it is not easily released, generally 1% to 2% is appropriate.

（2）透皮促进剂　系指能加速药物穿透皮肤的一类物质。它们能可逆地降低皮肤的屏障性能，增加药物的渗透性，从而增强药物的经皮吸收。促渗机制包括溶解角质层类脂、干扰脂质分子的有序排列、增加其流动性，或提高皮肤的水合作用等。常用的透皮吸收促进剂有表面活性剂、有机溶剂类、月桂氮酮及其同系物、有机酸、角质保湿剂及萜烯类。

b. Skin penetration enhancer　It is a substance that accelerates the penetration of drugs into the skin. They can reversibly reduce the barrier properties of the skin, increase the permeability of the drug, and enhance the transdermal absorption of the drug. Permeation-promoting mechanisms include dissolving the stratum corneum lipids, interfering with the ordered arrangement of lipid molecules, increasing their fluidity, or improving the hydration of the skin. Commonly used transdermal absorption enhancers are surfactants, organic solvents, laurone and its homologs, organic acids, humectants, and terpenes.

月桂氮酮又称氮酮，是一种新型透皮促进剂。对皮肤、黏膜的刺激性小，毒性小。本品对亲水性药物的渗透作用强于亲脂性药物。其他促进剂如乙醇、丙二醇、油酸等能加强其促渗透作用。氮酮的透皮作用具有浓度依赖性，有效浓度常在 1%~6%，其促渗透作用常不随浓度升高而增加，最佳浓度应根据实验确定。

Lauzone, also known as Azone, is a new transdermal enhancer with the chemical name 1-dodecylazacycloheptan-2-one. It causes little irritation to the skin and mucous membranes and it has low toxicity. This product has stronger penetrating effect on hydrophilic drugs than lipophilic drugs. Other accelerators such as ethanol, propylene glycol, and oleic acid can enhance its penetration promoting effect. The transdermal effect of Azone is concentration-dependent. The effective concentration is usually 1% -6%. Its penetration-promoting effect does not increase with increasing concentration. The optimal concentration should be determined experimentally.

其他透皮促进剂尚有丙二醇、甘油、聚乙二醇等多元醇，角质保湿剂尿素、吡咯酮类等，一般单独应用效果较差，常配伍使用。中药挥发油经实验证明具有较强的透皮促进能力，如薄荷油、桉叶油、松节油等。

Other transdermal enhancers include propylene glycol, glycerin, polyethylene glycol and other polyhydric alcohols, keratin humectants urea, pyrrolidone, etc. Generally, the effect is poor when used alone, and it is often used in combination. It has been proved that traditional Chinese medicine volatile oils, such as peppermint oil, eucalyptus leaf oil, turpentine and so on have strong transdermal promotion ability.

5. 其他因素 制剂中药物浓度、用药面积、应用次数及应用时间等一般与药物的吸收量成正比。其他如气温、相对湿度、局部摩擦、脱脂及离子导入应用等均有助于药物的透皮吸收。

⑤ Other factors The concentration of the drug, the skin area of the drug covers, and the times and time of application are generally proportional to the absorption of the drug. Other factors such as air temperature, relative humidity, local friction, degreasing, and iontophoresis all contribute to the transdermal absorption of the drug.

第二节 软膏剂

10.2 Ointments

PPT

一、概述

10.2.1 Overview

软膏剂系指提取物、饮片细粉与适宜基质均匀混合制成的半固体外用剂型。主要起润滑、保护和局部治疗作用，少数能经皮吸收产生全身治疗作用，多用于慢性皮肤病，禁用于急性皮肤损害部位。常用基质类型分为油脂性、乳剂型和水溶性基质。其中油脂性基质软膏常称为油膏；乳剂型基质软膏也称为乳膏剂，可分为水包油型（O/W）和油包水型（W/O）两类。

Ointments refers to a semi-solid external dosage form made by uniformly mixing extracts, decoction pieces and suitable bases. It is mainly used for lubrication, protection and local treatment. A few can be absorbed through the skin to produce systemic treatment. Most of them are used for chronic skin diseases and are prohibited in the area of acute skin damage. Common base types are divided into greasy, emulsion and water-soluble bases. Among them, the greasy base ointment is often referred to as an ointment; the emulsion-based base ointment is also referred to as a cream, it can be divided into two types: oil-in-water (O/W) and water-in-oil (W/O).

二、基质

10.2.2 Bases

基质是软膏剂形成和发挥药效的重要组成部分。软膏基质的性质对软膏剂的质量影响很大，理想的软膏基质具有以下特点：①应有适当稠度，润滑，无刺激性；②性质稳定，能与多种药物配伍，不发生配伍禁忌；③不妨碍皮肤的正常功能，有利于药物的释放吸收；④有吸水性，能吸收伤口分泌物；⑤易清洗，不污染衣物。但实际应用中，很少有基质能完全符合上述要求，应根据医疗用途及皮肤的生理病理状况，使用混合基质或添加附加剂，以保证制剂的质量。

Bases are an important part of ointment formation and achieving therapeutic effects. The nature of the ointment base greatly affects the quality of the ointment. An ideal ointment base has the following characteristics: ① Should have appropriate consistency, be smooth and non-irritating; ② Stable in nature, compatible with many drugs, no contraindications; ③ Does not hinder the normal function of the skin, which is conducive to the release and absorption of the drug; ④ Absorbs water and absorbs wound

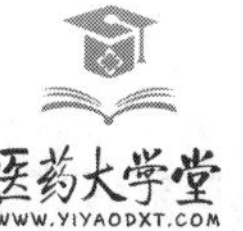

secretions; ⑤ Easy to clean and does not contaminate clothing. However, in practice, very few matrices can fully meet the above requirements. According to medical uses and physiological and pathological conditions of the skin, a mixed base or an additional agent should be used to ensure the quality of the preparation.

软膏基质的吸收能力常用水值表示，水值系指在规定温度下（20℃）100g 基质能容纳的最大水量（以 g 表示）。如白凡士林的水值为 9.5，羊毛脂为 150。

The absorption capacity of the ointment base is usually expressed by the water value. The water value refers to the maximum amount of water (in g) that 100g of the base can hold at a specified temperature (20℃). For example, the water value of white petrolatum is 9.5 and the lanolin is 150.

（一）油脂性基质

(1) Oleaginous Bases

油脂性基质包括动植物油脂类、类脂类及烃类等疏水性物质。共同的特点是润滑、无刺激性，对皮肤的保护及软化作用强；能防止水分蒸发，促进水合作用，对表皮增厚、角化、皲裂有软化保护作用；能与大多数药物配伍。但油腻性与疏水性大，不易用水洗除，不宜用于急性且有多量渗出液的皮肤疾病，对药物的释放穿透作用较差。

The greasy base includes hydrophobic substances such as animal and vegetable fats, lipids, and hydrocarbons. Common features are lubrication, non-irritanting, strong protection and softening effect on the skin; can prevent water evaporation, promote hydration, soften and protect the epidermis thickening, keratosis, and cleft palate; compatible with most drugs However, it is greasy and hydrophobic, and it is not easy to wash off with water. It is not suitable for acute skin diseases with a large amount of exudate, and has a poor penetration effect on drug release.

1. 油脂类 系从动物或植物中得到的高级脂肪酸甘油酯及其混合物。易受温度、光线、氧气等影响而引起分解、氧化和酸败，可加抗氧剂和防腐剂改善。常用的有动物油、植物油、氢化植物油等。中药油膏常以麻油与蜂蜡融合为基质。

① **Oil or fat** It is a higher fatty acid glyceride obtained from animals or plants and mixtures thereof. It is susceptible to temperature, light, oxygen, which can cause decomposition, oxidation and rancidity. It can be improved by adding antioxidants and preservatives. Commonly used are animal oils, vegetable oils, and hydrogenated vegetable oils. Traditional Chinese medicine ointment is usually based on the fusion of sesame oil and beeswax.

2. 类脂类 系高级脂肪酸与高级醇化合而成的酯类，其物理性质与油脂类似，化学性质较油脂稳定，常与油脂类基质合用。

② **Lipoid** It is an ester of higher fatty acids and higher alcohols. Its physical properties are similar to oils and fats, and its chemical properties are more stable than those of oils and fats.

（1）羊毛脂 又称无水羊毛脂，有良好的吸水性，可吸水 150%、甘油 140%。羊毛脂与皮脂组成接近，故有利于药物渗透；但过于黏稠而不宜单用，常与凡士林合用，以提高凡士林的吸水性和渗透性。

a. Lanum Also known as anhydrous lanolin, it has good water absorption, and can absorb 150% of water, 140% of glycerol. The composition of lanolin and sebum is close, which is conducive to drug penetration; however, it is too thick and should not be used alone. It is often used in combination with vaseline to improve the water absorption and permeability of vaseline.

（2）蜂蜡 主要成分为棕榈酸蜂蜡醇酯，含少量游离的高级脂肪醇，可作为 W/O 型辅助乳化剂，调节软膏的稠度。熔点为 62~67℃。

b. Bee wax The main component is beeswax palmitate, which contains a small amount of free higher fatty alcohols, and can be used as a W/O-type auxiliary emulsifier to adjust the consistency of the ointment. The melting point is 62 to 67℃.

（3）鲸蜡 主要为棕榈酸鲸蜡醇酯，并含少量高级脂肪酸酯，有辅助乳化作用，熔点42~50℃，不易酸败，有较好的润滑性，主要用于调节基质的稠度。

c. Spermaceti wax It is mainly cetyl palmitate, and contains a small amount of higher fatty acid esters. It has an auxiliary emulsification effect. Its melting point is 42-50℃. It is not easy for it to rancidify and has good lubricity. It is mainly used to adjust the consistency of the substrate.

3. 烃类 系石油分馏得到的各种烃的混合物，大部分为饱和烃类，不易被皮肤吸收，适用于保护性软膏；不溶于水，能与多数植物油、挥发油混合。

③ Hydrocarbon It is a mixture of various hydrocarbons obtained from the distillation of petroleum. Most of them are saturated hydrocarbons, which are not easily absorbed by the skin, and are suitable for protective ointments. They are insoluble in water and can be mixed with most vegetable oils and volatile oils.

（1）凡士林 又称软石蜡，为多种分子量烃类组成的半固体混合物，熔点为38~60℃，能与大多数药物配伍，具有适宜的稠度和涂展性，无刺激性，能与蜂蜡、脂肪、植物油（除蓖麻油外）熔合。本品油腻性大，吸水能力差，能吸收其重量5%的水，故不适用于有多量渗出液的患处。凡士林中加入适量羊毛脂、某些高级醇类或表面活性剂可增加其吸水性和释药性。

a. Vaseline Also known as soft paraffin, it is a semi-solid mixture composed of a variety of molecular weight hydrocarbons, with a melting point of 38-60℃. It is compatible with most drugs, has a suitable consistency and spreadability, has no irritation, and it can be fused with beeswax, fat, Vegetable oils (except castor oil) has. This product is very greasy and has poor water absorption capacity. It can absorb 5% of its weight of water, so it is not suitable for affected areas with a large amount of exudate. Adding proper amount of lanolin, certain higher alcohols or surfactants to petrolatum can increase its water absorption and drug release.

（2）固体石蜡与液体石蜡 前者为各种固体烃的混合物，后者为液体烃的混合物。用于调节软膏剂的稠度。其优点是结构均匀，与其他基质熔合后不会析出，故优于蜂蜡。

b. Solid paraffin and Liquid paraffin The former is a mixture of various solid hydrocarbons, and the latter is a mixture of liquid hydrocarbons. It is used to adjust the consistency of ointments. Its advantage is that the structure is uniform, and it will not precipitate after fusion with other substrates, so it is better than beeswax.

4. 硅酮类 为不同分子量的聚二甲基硅氧烷的总称，简称硅油。黏度随分子量增大而增加。其最大优点是在应用温度范围内（−40~150℃）黏度变化极小。本品润滑作用好，易于涂布，无刺激性，疏水性强，与羊毛脂、硬脂酸、聚山梨酯、脂肪酸山梨坦等均能混合，用于乳膏剂作润滑剂；也常与油脂性基质合用制成防护性软膏。本品对眼有刺激性，不宜用作眼膏基质。

④ Silicone It is a general term for polydimethylsiloxanes of different molecular weight, referred to as silicone oil for short. The viscosity increases with increasing molecular weight. Its biggest advantage is that the viscosity change is very small in the application temperature range (−40 ~ 150℃). This product has good lubricating effect, easy to apply, non-irritating, and strong hydrophobicity. It can be mixed with lanolin, stearic acid, polysorbate, fatty acid sorbitan, etc., and it is used as a lubricant for creams; it is also often used together with grease base to make a protective ointment. This product can cause eyes irritation and should not be used as an ointment base.

（二）乳剂型基质（乳膏剂）

(2) Emulsion Base (Creams)

乳剂型基质（乳膏剂）是由水相、油相和乳化剂的在一定温度下乳化而成的半固体基质，形成基质的类型及原理与乳剂相似。可分为O/W和W/O两类。油相多为固体或半固体，如硬脂酸、蜂蜡、石蜡、高级醇等，为调节稠度而加入液状石蜡、凡士林、植物油等。水相为蒸馏水或药物水溶液及水溶性的附加剂。

Emulsion type base (cream) is a semi-solid base emulsified by water phase, oil phase and emulsifier at a certain temperature, the type and principle of forming a base are similar to emulsions. It can be divided into two types of oil-in-water (O/W) and water-in-oil (W/O). The oil phase is mostly solid or semi-solid, such as stearic acid, beeswax, paraffin, higher alcohol, etc. In order to adjust the consistency, liquid paraffin, petrolatum, vegetable oil, etc. are added. The water phase is distilled water or aqueous drug solution and water-soluble additives.

乳剂型基质对油、水均具有一定亲和力，能与创面渗出液混合，对皮肤正常功能影响小；W/O型乳剂油腻性比油脂性基质小，能吸收部分水分，水分从皮肤表面蒸发时有缓和的冷却作用，习称“冷霜”。O/W型乳剂，能与水混合，无油腻性，易洗除，习称“雪花膏”。O/W型乳剂可促使药物与皮肤接触，药物释放、透皮吸收较快，但也可促使病变处分泌物反向吸收而致炎症恶化，故湿疹等分泌物较多的病变部位不宜使用；易干燥、发霉，需加入保湿剂和防腐剂。遇水不稳定的药物不宜制成乳剂型软膏。乳剂型基质常用的乳化剂及稳定剂如下：

The emulsion base has a certain affinity for oil and water, can be mixed with wound exudate, and has little effect on the normal function of the skin; W/O emulsions are less greasy than oily bases, and can absorb part of the water, and when the water evaporates from the skin surface. It has a mild cooling effect which is called “cold cream”. O/W emulsions, can be mixed with water, they are not greasy, easy to wash off, commonly known as “vanishing cream”. O/W emulsion can help the drug to contact the skin, hence causing faster drug release and transdermal absorption are faster, but it can also promote the reverse absorption of the secretions at the wound lesion and worsen the inflammation, therefore it should not be used for the lesions with more secretions such as eczema; It is prone to dryness and mold, necessary to add humectants and preservatives. Drugs that are unstable in contact with water should not be made into creams. The emulsifiers and stabilizers commonly used in emulsion bases are as follows:

1. 阴离子表面活性剂

① Anionic surfactant

（1）一价皂　常用钠、钾、铵的氢氧化物或三乙醇胺等有机碱与脂肪酸（如硬脂酸）作用生成的新生皂配制软膏，为O/W型乳化剂。硬脂酸用量中仅一部分与碱反应生成肥皂，未皂化的硬脂酸与油相物质一起被乳化形成分散相，可增加基质的稠度。用硬脂酸制成的O/W型乳化剂基质光滑美观，水分蒸发后留有一层硬脂酸薄膜而具有保护作用，常加入适量的凡士林、液体石蜡等油脂性基质，以调节其稠度和涂展性。

a. Monovalent soap　Commonly used sodium, potassium, ammonium hydroxide or triethanolamine and other organic bases and fatty acids (such as stearic acid) to produce ointment, is an O/W emulsifier. Only a part of the amount of stearic acid reacts with alkali to form soap. Unsaponified stearic acid is emulsified with the oil phase substance to form a dispersed phase, which can increase the consistency of the base. The O/W emulsifier base made of stearic acid is smooth and beautiful. After the water evaporates, a layer of stearic acid is left for protection. A suitable amount of oily bases such as vaseline and liquid paraffin are often added to adjust its consistency and Spreadability.

此类基质的缺点是易被酸、碱、钙离子、镁离子或电解质破坏。制备用水宜用蒸馏水或离子交换水，制成的软膏在 pH 值 5~6 以下时不稳定。

The disadvantage of such matrices is that they are easily destroyed by acids, bases, calcium ions, magnesium ions or electrolytes. Distilled water or ion-exchanged water is suitable for the preparation water. The ointment produced is unstable when the pH value is 5-6.

（2）高级脂肪醇硫酸酯类　常用十二烷基硫酸钠（月桂醇硫酸钠），其水溶液呈中性，对皮肤刺激小，pH 值 4~8 之内稳定，不受硬水影响，能与肥皂、碱类、钙镁离子配伍，但与阳离子表面活性剂可形成沉淀而失效。常用量为 0.5%~2.0%。

案例导入

b. Higher fatty alcohol sulfates　Commonly used sodium dodecyl sulfate (sodium lauryl sulfate), its aqueous solution is neutral, has little irritation to the skin, it has stable 4-8 pH range, is not affected by hard water, and is compatible with soap, alkalis, calcium and magnesium. However, it can form a precipitate with cationic surfactant and fail. The commonly used amount is 0.5% to 2.0%.

（3）多价皂　由二价、三价金属如钙、镁、铝与脂肪酸作用形成的多价皂，在水中溶解度小，形成的 W/O 型基质较一价皂形成的 O/W 型基质更稳定。如硬脂酸铝或氢氧化钙与处方中脂肪酸（如硬脂酸）作用生成的脂肪酸铝钙皂。

c. Multivalent soap　Polyvalent soaps formed by the interaction of divalent and trivalent metals such as calcium, magnesium, aluminum and fatty acids have low solubility in water, and the formed W/O base is more stable than the O/W base formed by monovalent soap. Such as aluminum, calcium soaps of fatty acids produced by the action of either aluminum stearate or calcium hydroxide and fatty acids from the prescription (such as stearic acid).

2. 非离子表面活性剂

② Non-ionic surfactant

（1）聚山梨酯类　O/W 型乳化剂。对黏膜和皮肤刺激性小，并能与电解质配伍。为调节制品的 *HLB* 值与稳定性，此类表面活性剂常与其他乳化剂（如脂肪酸山梨坦、十二烷基硫酸钠）合用。

a. Polysorbates　O/W type emulsifier. It causes less irritation to mucous membranes and skin and is compatible with electrolytes. In order to adjust the HLB value and stability of the products, such surfactants are often combined with other emulsifiers (such as fatty acid sorbitan, sodium dodecyl sulfate).

案例导入 ¦ Case example

案例 10-1　含聚山梨酯 -80 的乳剂型基质

10-1　Emulsion base containing polysorbate-80

处方：硬脂酸 150g　白凡士林 100g　单硬脂酸甘油酯 100g　聚山梨酯–80 50g　硬脂山梨坦–60 20g　尼泊金乙酯 1g　蒸馏水 479ml

Ingredients: Stearic acid 150g; white petrolatum 100g; glyceryl monostearate 100g; polysorbate-80 50g; Stearyl sorbitan-60 20g; ethyl paraben 1g; distilled water 479ml.

制法：取硬脂酸、白凡士林、单硬脂酸甘油酯水浴上加热熔融，保温于 70°C 左右，加入硬脂酸山梨坦–60 与尼泊金乙酯使溶解；另取蒸馏水加热至 80°C，加入聚山梨酯–80 溶解混匀，将上述油相缓缓加入水相，边加边搅拌至冷凝，即得。

Making Procedure: Take stearic acid, white petrolatum and glyceryl monostearate on a water bath to heat and melt, keep the temperature at about 70°C, add sorbitan-60 stearate and ethyl paraben to dissolve; then take the distilled water and heat up to 80℃ Add Polysorbate-80 to dissolve and mix evenly. Add the above oil phase to the water phase slowly. Stir until condensed while adding.

注解：处方中聚山梨酯-80为主要乳化剂，硬脂酸山梨坦-60为W/O型乳化剂，用以调节适宜的*HLB*值而形成稳定的O/W型乳化膜。硬脂酸、单硬脂酸甘油酯为增稠剂与稳定剂，并使制得的基质细腻光亮。

Notes: Polysorbate-80 is the main emulsifier and sorbitan-60 stearate is the W/O type emulsifier in the prescription, which is used to adjust the appropriate HLB value to form a stable O/W type emulsified film. Stearic acid and glyceryl monostearate are thickeners and stabilizers, and make the base delicate and bright.

（2）聚氧乙烯醚的衍生物类　①平平加O为O/W型乳化剂，*HLB*值为15.9，在冷水中溶解度比热水中大，溶液pH值为6~7，对皮肤无刺激性，有良好的乳化、分散性能。本品性质稳定。但能与羟基和羧基形成络合物，故不宜与苯酚、水杨酸等配伍。②硬脂酸聚氧乙烯酯，为O/W型乳化剂，可溶于水，pH值近中性，渗透性较大，常与平平加O等混合应用。③烷基酚聚氧乙烯醚类，为O/W型乳化剂，可溶于水，用量一般为油相总量的2%~10%。

b. Polyoxyethylene ether derivatives　I. Leveling agent O is an O/W emulsifier with an HLB value of 15.9. Its solubility in cold water is greater than that in hot water. The pH of the solution is 6-7. It does not cause irritation to skin and has good emulsification and dispersion properties. This product is stable in nature. However, it can form complexes with hydroxyl and carboxyl groups, so it is not compatible with phenol, salicylic acid, etc. II. Polyoxyethylene stearate, O/W emulsifier, soluble in water, almost neutral pH, high permeability, often mixed with ordinary addition of O and other applications. III. Alkylphenol polyoxyethylene, O/W type emulsifier, soluble in water, the amount is generally 2% to 10% of the total oil phase.

案例导入

（3）脂肪酸山梨坦类系　W/O型乳化剂。常与O/W型乳化剂如聚山梨酯类合用于O/W型基质中，用于调节*HLB*值并使之稳定；或与高级脂肪醇等合用于W/O型基质中，能吸收少量水分，对皮肤黏膜刺激性小。

c. Fatty acid sorbitans　W/O type emulsifier. Often used with O/W type emulsifiers such as Tween in O/W type substrates to adjust and stabilize the HLB value; or used with higher fatty alcohols in W/O type substrates to absorb small amounts of moisture, little irritation to the skin and mucous membranes.

3. 高级脂肪醇类及其他弱W/O乳化剂　主要作为W/O乳化剂，有一定吸水作用，也常作为O/W型乳化剂基质的辅助乳化剂，以调整适当的*HLB*值达到油相所需范围，并有稳定与增稠作用。常用的品种有十六醇（鲸蜡醇）、十八醇（硬脂醇）、单硬脂酸甘油酯、蜂蜡、羊毛脂、胆甾醇等。

③ Higher fatty alcohols and other weak W/O emulsifiers　It is mainly used as a W/O emulsifier and they have a certain water absorption effect. These are also often used as an auxiliary emulsifier for the O/W type emulsifier base in order to adjust the appropriate HLB value to reach the range required for the oil phase, and they have the function of stabilization and thickening. Commonly used varieties are cetyl alcohol (cetyl alcohol), stearyl alcohol (stearyl alcohol), glyceryl monostearate, beeswax, lanolin, cholesterol and so on.

（三）水溶性基质

(3) Water-Soluble Base

水溶性基质由天然或合成的水溶性高分子物质组成。高分子物质溶解后形成凝胶，则属凝胶剂，如羧甲基纤维素钠、明胶等。目前常用的水溶性基质主要是聚乙二醇类。水溶性基质易涂展，能吸收组织渗出液，一般释放药物较快，无油腻性，易洗除。对皮肤、黏膜无刺激性，可用于糜烂创面及腔道黏膜。其缺点是润滑作用较差。

The water-soluble base consists of natural or synthetic high-molecular water-soluble substances. Gels are formed by dissolving high-molecular substances, which are gelling agents, such as sodium carboxymethyl cellulose and gelatin. Water-soluble base commonly used so far has mainly been polyethylene glycol. The water-soluble base is easy to spread, it can absorb tissue exudate, generally releases the drug quickly, is non-greasy, and easy to wash away. It does not irritate the skin and mucous membranes, and it can be used for erosion wounds and mucosa of the cavity. The disadvantage is poor lubrication.

聚乙二醇为乙二醇的高分子聚合物，常用的平均相对分子量为 300~6000。PEG-700 以下均是液体，PEG-1000 至 1500 是半固体，PEG 2000 至 6000 是固体。若取不同平均分子量的聚乙二醇以适当比例相混合，可制成稠度适宜的基质，PEG 化学性质稳定，可与多数药物配伍，耐高温，不易霉败。易溶于水，能与乙醇、丙酮、三氯甲烷混溶。吸湿性强，可吸收分泌液，对皮肤有一定刺激性，长期使用可致皮肤脱水干燥。

PEG is a high molecular polymer of ethylene glycol, and the average molecular weight of the commonly used one is 300-6000. PEG-700 and below are all liquids, PEG-1000 to 1500 are semi-solids, and PEG 2000 to 6000 are solids. If polyethylene glycols with different average molecular weights are mixed in an appropriate ratio, a base with an appropriate consistency can be prepared. PEG is chemically stable, compatible with most drugs, resistant to high temperatures and not prone to mildew. Soluble in water, miscible with ethanol, acetone, and chloroform it has strong hygroscopicity, can absorb secretions, have a certain irritation effect onto the skin, long-term use can cause skin dehydration and dryness.

三、软膏剂的制法
10.2.3 Preparation Method of Ointments

（一）工艺流程（图 10-2）
(1) Flow Chart (Figure 10-2)

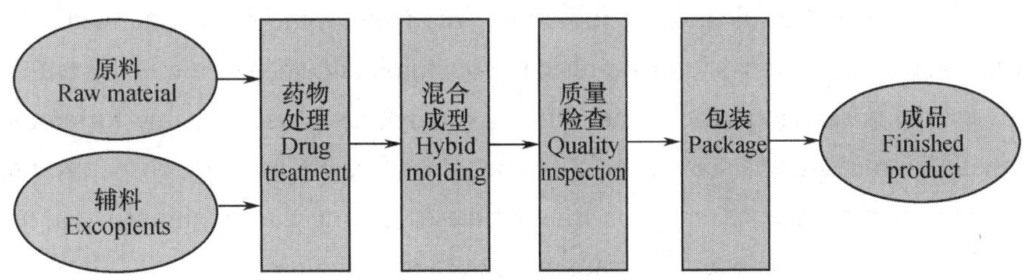

图 10-2 软膏的制备工艺流程图

Figure 10-2 Ointment Preparation Process Flow Chart

（二）制法
(2) Manufacturing Method

1. 基质的处理 油脂性基质应先加热熔融，再于 150°C 灭菌 1 小时并除去水分。

① **Treatment for bases** The greasy substrate should be heated and melted first, and then sterilized at 150°C for 1hour and removed from moisture from water.

2. 制备

② **preparation**

（1）研和法　将药物细粉用少量基质研匀或用适宜液体研磨成细糊状，再递加其余基质研匀的制备方法。适用于软膏基质较软、在常温下通过研磨即可与药物均匀混合，或不宜加热、不溶性及少量的药物的制备。

a. Grinding method　A preparation method of grinding the medicine which is in the form of fine powder with a small amount of bases or grinding into a fine paste with suitable liquid, and then adding the remaining base and grinding uniformly. It is suitable for the ointment base which is soft and can be mixed with the drug uniformly by grinding at normal temperature; or preparation of drugs which are not suitable for heating, insolubility and small amount.

（2）熔合法　指将基质加热熔化，再将药物分次加入，边加边搅拌直至冷凝的方法。适用于软膏处方中基质熔点不同，常温下不能混合均匀者，先加温熔化高熔点基质，再加入其他低熔点成分，然后加入药物，搅拌均匀冷却即可。

b. Fusion method　Refers to the method of heating and melting the base, and then adding the drug in portions, and stirring while adding until it condenses. It is suitable for those with different melting points of the base in the ointment prescription, which cannot be mixed uniformly at normal temperature, first heat and melt the high melting point bases, then add other low melting point ingredients, then add the drug, stir and cool uniformly.

（3）乳化法　基质为乳剂型时用乳化法。将处方中的油溶性组分一起加热至80℃左右，另将水溶性组分溶于水中，加热至80℃左右，两相混合，搅拌至乳化完全并冷凝。乳化法中油、水两相有三种混合方法：①两相同时混合，适用于连续的或大批量的操作，需要一定的设备，如输送泵、连续混合装置等；②分散相加到连续相中，适用于含小体积分散相的乳剂系统；③连续相加到分散相中，适用于多数乳剂系统，在混合过程中引起乳剂转型，能产生更为细小的分散相粒子，使乳膏更为均匀细腻。

c. Emulsification method　Emulsification method is used when the base is an emulsion type, an emulsification method is used. The oil-soluble components in the prescription are heated together to about 80℃, and the water-soluble components are dissolved in water, heated to about 80℃, the two phases are mixed, stirred until the emulsification is complete and condensed. There are three mixing methods for oil and water phases in the emulsification method: two are mixed at the same time, which is suitable for continuous or large-scale operations, and requires certain equipment, such as a transfer pump, continuous mixing device, etc; the dispersed phase is added to the continuous phase, suitable for emulsion systems containing a small volume of dispersed phase; continuous phase is added to the dispersed phase, suitable for most emulsion systems, causing emulsion transformation during the mixing process, it can produce finer dispersed phase particles, making the cream more even and smooth.

3. 包装与贮藏　生产中多采用密封性好的铝制或塑料软膏管包装，软膏剂的容器应不与药物或基质发生理化作用。软膏应密封包装，贮藏于阴凉干燥处。

③ **Packaging and storage**　Aluminum or plastic ointment tubes with good sealing properties are often used for packaging. Ointment containers should not have physical or chemical reactions with drugs or bases. The ointment should be sealed and stored in a cool and dry place.

（三）药物加入方法

(3) Method for Adding Drugs

1. 不溶性药物或直接加入的饮片　制成细粉、最细粉、极细粉或超微粉。制备时取药粉先与少量基质或液体成分如液状石蜡等研成糊状，再不断递加其余基质；或将药物细粉在不断搅拌下加到熔融的基质中，继续搅拌至冷凝。

① **Insoluble drugs or directly added pieces** Regrind into fine powder, finest powder, superfine powder or ultrafine powder. When preparing the medicine powder, first grind it into a paste with a small amount of base or liquid ingredients such as liquid paraffin, etc., and then continuously add the remaining base; or add the drug fine powder to the molten base under constant stirring and continue stirring until it condenses.

2. 可溶于基质的药物 应溶解于基质或基质组分中。饮片可以先用适宜方法提取，滤过后将油提取液与油相基质混合；水溶性药物一般先用少量水溶解，以羊毛脂吸收，再与油脂性基质混匀；或直接溶解于水相，再与水溶性基质混合。遇水不稳定的药物不宜选用水溶性基质或O/W型乳剂。

② **Base-soluble drugs** Should be dissolved in the base or base components. The decoction pieces can be extracted by a suitable method, and the oil extract is mixed with the oil phase base after filtering. The water-soluble drugs are generally dissolved with a small amount of water, absorbed with lanolin, and mixed with the oily base; or dissolved directly in the water phase, and then mixed with water-soluble base. It is not suitable to use water-soluble base or O/W emulsion for drugs that are unstable in water.

3. 中药煎剂、浸膏等 可先浓缩至稠膏状，再与基质混合。固体浸膏可加少量溶剂如水、稀醇等使之软化或研成糊状，再与基质混匀。

③ **Chinese medicine decoction, extract, etc.** It can firstly be concentrated to a thick paste and mixed with the base. The solid extract can be softened or made into a paste by adding a small amount of solvent such as water and dilute alcohol, and then mixed with the base.

4. 共熔组分 应先共熔再与基质混合，如樟脑、薄荷脑等并存时，可先研磨至共熔后，再与冷却至40℃左右的基质混匀。

④ **Eutectic component** Should be co-melted and then mixed with the base, such as camphor, menthol, etc., can be ground to co-melted first, and then mixed with the base cooled to about 40℃.

5. 挥发性、易升华的药物，或树脂类药物 应使基质降温至40℃左右，再与药物混合均匀。

⑤ **Volatile, sublimable drugs, or resin drugs** The base should be cooled to about 40℃ and mixed with the drug evenly.

案例导入 ¦ Case example

案例 10-2 老鹳草软膏

10-2 Geranium ointment

处方：老鹳草 1000g 对羟基苯甲酸乙酯 0.3g 羊毛脂 50g 凡士林 适量

Formula: Geranium 1000g; ethyl paraben 0.3g; lanolin 50g; vaseline appropriate amount.

功能与主治：除湿解毒，收敛生肌。用于湿毒蕴结所致的湿疹、痈、疔、疮及小面积水、火烫伤。

Functions and indications: Remove dampness and detoxify, promote tissue regeneration. It is used for eczema, scabies, sores as well as burns and scalding on small skin areas.

制法：取老鹳草加水煎煮两次，每次1小时，合并煎液，滤过，滤液浓缩后加一倍量乙醇使之沉淀，静置12~24小时，滤取上清液，浓缩至相对密度为1.20，加对羟基苯甲酸乙酯、羊毛脂与凡士林，混匀，即得。

Making Procedure: Take geranium and cook twice with water for 1 hour each time. Combine the decoction and filter. After the filtrate is concentrated, add twice the amount of ethanol to precipitate it. Let it sit for 12 to 24 hours. take the supernatant, concentrate to a relative density of 1.20, add ethyl paraben, lanolin and petrolatum, mix well and it is done.

用法与用量：外用，涂敷患处，一日 1 次。

Usage and dosage: For external use, apply to the affected area once a day.

注解：①本品为油脂性软膏，原料药物水提醇沉后可除去杂质，提高有效成分的含量。

Notes: ① This product is a greasy ointment, the impurities can be removed by water extraction and alcohol precipitation of the raw drug, increasing the content of active ingredients can be increased.

②处方中对羟基苯甲酸乙酯作为防腐剂，羊毛脂与凡士林合用，可以提高凡士林的吸水性和渗透性。

② Ethyl p-hydroxybenzoate is used as a preservative in prescriptions. Lanolin combined with vaseline can improve the water absorption and permeability of vaseline.

四、软膏剂的质量检查

10.2.4 Ointment Quality Inspection

1. 外观 软膏剂应均匀、细腻，具有适当的黏稠性，易涂布于皮肤或黏膜上，无刺激性。应无酸败、变色、变硬、融化、油水分离等变质现象。

(1) Exterior The ointment should be uniform and delicate, has appropriate viscosity, and be easy to apply on the skin or mucous membrane without irritation. There should be no deterioration such as rancidity, discoloration, hardening, melting, oil-water separation, etc.

2. 稠度 一般软膏要求常温下插入度在 100~300 之间，乳膏为 200~300。

(2) Consistency The general ointment requires an insertion degree between 100 and 300 at room temperature, and a cream of 200 to 300.

3. 粒度 取含药材细粉的软膏剂供试品适量，置于载玻片上，涂成薄层，覆以盖玻片，共涂 3 片，按现行版《中国药典》中粒度测定法（第一法，即显微镜法）测定，均不得检出大于 180μm 的粒子。

(3) Particle size Take an appropriate amount of the ointment containing the fine powder of the medicinal material, place it on a glass slide, apply a thin layer, cover it with a cover slip, and apply a total of 3 layers. According to the particle size determination method in the current edition of *Chinese Pharmacopoeia* (the first method, that is, the microscope method), no particles larger than 180μm can be detected.

4. 装量差异 按现行版《中国药典》中最低装量检查法（重量法）检查，求出每个容器内容物的装量与平均装量，均应符合药典规定。如有 1 个容器装量不符合规定，则另取 5 个（50g 以上者 3 个）复试，均应符合规定。

(4) Weight variation Check the minimum filling method (weight method) regulated by the current edition of the *Chinese Pharmacopoeia*, and determine the amount and average filling content of each container, which should meet the requirements of the *Chinese Pharmacopoeia*. If the amount of one container does not meet the requirements, take another five (three above 50g) and repeat the test, making sure they meet the requirements.

5. 无菌　用于烧伤或严重创伤的软膏剂，按现行版《中国药典》中无菌检查法检查，应符合规定。

(5) Sterility　Ointments used for burns or severe trauma should be inspected in accordance with the sterility inspection method in the current edition of the *Chinese Pharmacopoeia*, and they should meet the requirements.

6. 微生物限度　按现行版《中国药典》中微生物限度检查法检查，应符合规定。

(6) Microbial Limit　Inspection in accordance with the microbial limit inspection method in the current edition of the *Chinese Pharmacopoeia* shall comply with the regulations.

7. 稳定性　将软膏分别置恒温箱（39℃ ± 1℃）、室温（25℃ ± 1℃）及冰箱（0 ± 1℃）中1~3个月，进行加速试验，应符合相关规定。将乳膏剂分别放置于55℃恒温6小时与–15℃恒温24小时进行耐热、耐寒检查，一般O/W型基质能耐热，但不耐寒；而W/O型基质不耐热，常于38~40℃即有油分离出。或将软膏10g置于离心管中，以2500r/min离心30分钟，不应有分层现象。

(7) stability　Place the ointment in a thermostat (39℃±1℃), room temperature (25℃±1℃), and refrigerator (0℃±1℃) for 1 to 3 months for accelerated testing, which should comply with relevant regulations. Place the cream at a constant temperature of 55℃ for 6h and a constant temperature of –15℃ for 24h to check the heat and cold resistance. Generally, O/W type substrates can be heat resistant, but not cold resistant; while W/O type substrates are not heat resistant, oil often gets separated at 38-40℃. Or put 10g ointment in a centrifuge tube and centrifugalize at 2500r / min for 30min, there should be no delamination.

8. 刺激性　包括皮肤测定法（家兔）、贴敷实验法与黏膜测定法（家兔眼黏膜）。

(8) Irritating　Including skin test (rabbit), application test and mucous membrane test (rabbit eye mucosa).

9. 药物含量测定　主药有效成分明确的软膏应当用适宜方法测定有效成分。

(9) Drug content determination　Ointments with well-defined active ingredients of the main drug should be determined by an appropriate method.

五、眼膏剂
10.2.5　Eye Ointments

（一）概述
(1) Overviews

眼膏剂系指原料药物与适宜基质制成供眼用的灭菌软膏剂，眼膏剂较一般滴眼剂的疗效持久且能减轻对眼球的摩擦。常用基质为凡士林、液状石蜡、羊毛脂（8：1：1）混合而成。羊毛脂具有较强的吸水性和黏附性，较单用凡士林更易与药液及泪液混合和附着在眼黏膜上，促进药物渗透。基质应均匀、细腻、无刺激性，并易涂布于眼部，便于药物分散和吸收。基质在配制前应滤过并灭菌。

Eye ointments refer to a sterilized ointment for ophthalmic use made of raw materials and a suitable base. Eye ointments have a longer lasting effect than ordinary eye drops and can reduce eye friction. The commonly used base is made of petroleum jelly, liquid paraffin, and lanolin (8：1：1). Lanolin has strong water absorption and adhesion, and is easier to mix with medicinal solution and tears and adhere to the ocular mucosa than Vaseline alone, and promote drug penetration. The base should be uniform,

案例导入

delicate, non-irritating, and easy to apply to the eyes, to facilitate drug dispersion and absorption. The base should be filtered and sterilized before preparation.

（二）制法

(2) Manufacturing Method

眼膏剂的制备应在灭菌条件下进行。基质用前必须加热滤过，并于 150℃ 干热灭菌 1 小时，必要时可酌加适宜抑菌剂和抗氧剂等。基质与药物的混合方法基本同软膏剂。除另有规定外，每个容器的装量应不超过 5g。

Eye ointments should be prepared under sterilized conditions. The substrate must be filtered through heating before use, and sterilized by dry heat at 150℃ for 1hour. If necessary, suitable bacteriostatic agents and antioxidants can be added. The method of mixing the base and the drug is basically the same as that of the ointment. Unless otherwise specified, the volume of each container should not exceed 5g.

（三）质量检查

(3) Quality Inspection

眼膏剂的质量检查与普通软膏剂基本一致，还应检查粒度、无菌、金属性异物等。

The quality inspection of eye ointments is basically the same as that of ordinary ointments. The particle size, sterility, and metallic foreign bodies should also be checked.

1. 粒度 按现行版《中国药典》中粒度检查法，应符合规定。

① **Particle size** should meet the requirements in accordance with the current edition of *Chinese Pharmacopoeia*, should meet the requirements

2. 金属性异物 按现行版《中国药典》中金属性异物检查法检查，应符合规定。

② **Metallic foreign body** The inspection should be in accordance with the metal foreign body inspection method of the current edition of the *Chinese Pharmacopoeia*.

3. 无菌 用于伤口的眼用制剂按现行版《中国药典》中无菌检查法检查应该符合规定。

③ **Sterility** The ophthalmic preparations used for wound should be tested according to the sterility test of the current edition of *Chinese Pharmacopoeia*.

第三节 膏药

10.3 Plasters

PPT

一、概述

10.3.1 Overview

膏药系指饮片、食用植物油与红丹（铅丹）或宫粉（铅粉）炼制成膏料，摊涂于裱背材料上制成的供皮肤贴敷的外用剂型，前者称为黑膏药，后者称为白膏药。膏药属于硬膏药，为传统剂型。近年来以黑膏药居多。膏药可发挥局部或全身治疗作用，外治可消肿、拔毒、生肌，主治皮肤红肿、痈疽，疮疡等症状；内治可以活血通络、驱风止痛、消痞，主治跌打损伤、风湿痹痛等。其作用比软膏剂持久，并可随时终止给药，安全可靠。清代吴师机的《理瀹骈文》为膏药专著，全面论述了膏药的应用和制备。

Plasters refer to external preparations made of decoction pieces, edible vegetable oils and red lead oxide or ceruse. The former is called black plasters, the latter white plasters. Plasters are hard plasters and are traditional dosage forms. In recent years, the majority used are black plasters. The plasters can exert local or systemic treatment effects. External treatment can reduce swelling, detoxification, and muscle regeneration. It can treat skin redness, swelling, ulcers, and sores. Internal treatment can invigorate blood circulation and open meridians, dispel wind and relieve pain, as well as treat bruises and injuries by falling, or arthralgia due to wind and dampness. Its effect is longer than that of ointment, and it can be terminated at any time, which is safe and reliable. *Li-yue-pian-wen* written by Wu Shiji (Qing Dynasty) is a plaster monograph, which comprehensively discusses the application and preparation of plaster.

二、黑膏药
10.3.2 Black Plasters

（一）概述
(1) Overview

黑膏药的基质是食用植物油与红丹经高温炼制的铅硬膏，黑膏药一般为黑色坚韧固体，用前须烘热软化后贴于皮肤上。

The base of the black plaster is a high-temperature lead plaster made from edible vegetable oil and red dan. The black plaster is generally a black, tough solid, which must be dried and softened before being use and applied to the skin.

（二）基质
(2) Matrix

1. 植物油 应选用质地纯净、沸点低、熬炼时泡沫少、制成品软化点及黏着力适当的植物油。以麻油最好，棉籽油、豆油等亦可应用，但炼制时易产生泡沫。

① Edible vegetable oil Vegetable oil should be used with pure texture, low boiling point, low foam during refining, softening point of finished products and proper adhesion should be used. Sesame oil is the best. Cottonseed oil, soybean oil, etc. can also be used, but it is easy to produce foam during refining.

2. 红丹 又称樟丹、黄丹、铅丹等，为橘红色粉末，质重，主要成分为四氧化铅（Pb_3O_4），含量应在 95% 以上。红丹使用前应炒除水分，过五号筛，以防聚成颗粒沉底，不易与油充分反应。

② Red lead oxide Also known as zhang dan, yellow dan, and lead dan, they are orange-red powder, heavy in weight, and the main component is lead tetroxide (Pb_3O_4). Whose content should be above 95%. Before being used, Hongdan should fried to remove the water and pass through a No.5 sieve to prevent it from forming into particles and sinking to the bottom, and not to react fully with oil.

（三）制法

(3) Manufacturing Method

1. 工艺流程（图 10-3）

① Flow chart (Figure 10-3)

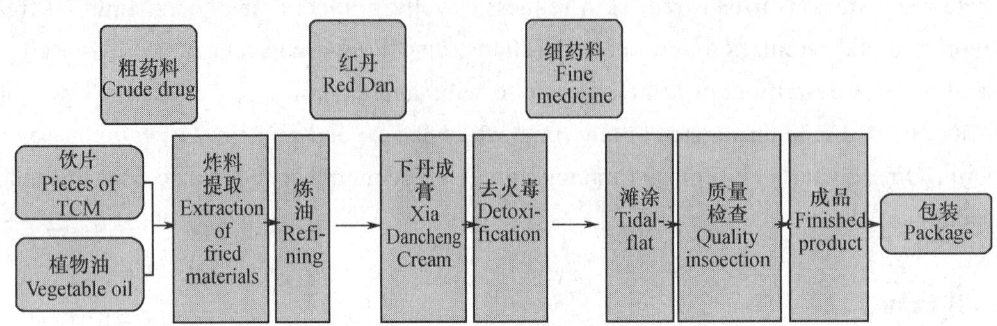

图 10-3 黑膏药的制法

Figure 10-3 Preparation Method of Black Plasters

2. 制法

② Manufacturing method

（1）药料提取　药料的提取按其质地有先炸后下之分，将药料中质地坚硬的饮片、含水量高的肉质类、鲜药类中药置铁丝笼内移置炼油器中，加盖，加热先炸，油温控制在 200~220℃；质地疏松的花、草、叶、皮等饮片宜在上述饮片炸至枯黄后入锅，炸至饮片表面呈深褐色，内部焦黄色。炸好后将药渣连笼移出，得到药油。提取中，应用水洗器喷淋逸出的油烟，残余烟气由排气管排出室外。提取时需防止泡沫溢出。

a. Extraction of herbs According to its texture, the extraction of medicinal materials is done by frying first and divided into the following steps, the hardened pieces of medicinal materials, succulent and fresh Chinese medicine with high water contents are placed in a wire cage and moved to a oil refiner utensil, covered (with lid), heated and fried first, and the oil temperature is controlled at 200-220℃. The loose pieces of flowers, grass, leaves, skin, etc. should be put into the pot after the pieces mentioned above become yellow and dry, and fried until the surface of the pieces is dark brown and its interior is light brown. After being fried, the medicine residue is removed from the cage to obtain medicated oil. During extraction, wet scrubber is used to spray the diffused oil fume, and the residual fume is exhausted from the exhaust pipe to the outside. Avoid foam overflow during extraction.

药料与油经高温处理，有效成分可能破坏较多。现也有采用适宜的溶剂和方法提取有效成分，例如将部分饮片用乙醇提取，浓缩成浸膏后再加入膏药中，可减少成分的损失。

The medicinal materials and oil are subjected to high temperature treatment, and the active ingredients may be destroyed. There are also suitable solvents and methods for extracting active ingredients, such as extracting some decoction pieces with ethanol, concentrating them into extracts, and then adding them to the plaster, which can reduce the loss of ingredients.

（2）炼油　将去渣后的药油于 270~320℃ 继续加热熬炼，使油脂在高温下氧化聚合、增稠，炼至“滴水成珠”，即取油少许滴于水中，以药油聚集成珠不散为度。炼油为制备膏药的关键，炼油过“老”则膏药质脆，黏着力小，贴于皮肤易脱落。炼油过“嫩”则膏药质软，贴于皮肤易移动。

b. Refining The slag-removed medicinal oil is continuously heated and smelted at 270-320℃ to oxidize, polymerize and thicken the fat at high temperature, and refine it to “drip water into beads”, that is, drip a bit of oil into the water, and aggregate the medicated oil into bead-like non scattered form. Refining is the key to making plasters. If the refining is “old”, the plasters are brittle, have low adhesion, and fall off easily when applied to the skin. If the refining is “tender”, the plaster is soft and moves easily on the skin.

（3）下丹成膏　系指在练成的油中加入红丹反应生成脂肪酸铅盐的过程。下丹时将炼成的油送入下丹锅中，加热至近 300℃ 时，在搅拌下缓慢加入红丹，保证油与红丹充分反应，至成为黑褐色稠厚状液体。油丹用量比一般为 500：150~（200）（冬少夏多）。为检查膏药老、嫩程度，可取少量样品滴入水中数秒钟后取出，若膏黏手，拉之有丝则太嫩，应继续熬炼。若拉之发脆则过老。膏不黏手，稠度适中，表示合格。膏药亦可用软化点测定仪测定，以判断膏药老嫩程度。

c. Xia Dan cheng gao　Refers to the process of adding red salvia lead to the refined oil to produce lead salts of fatty acids. Xiadan means putting the refined oil into the xiadan pot, when the dandan is lowered, the refined oil is sent to the lower dandan pot. When it is heated to nearly 300℃, red dandan is slowly added under stirring to ensure that the oil and red dandan fully react until it becomes a dark brown thick liquid. The ratio of oil dandan is generally 500：(150-200) (more in winter, less in summer). In order to check the degree of softness of the plaster, a small amount of sample can be dropped into the water for a few seconds and then taken out. If the plaster sticks to your hands, or if pulled it has silky feel to it meaning it is too soft, you should continue to refine it. If it is brittle when pulled, it means it is “aged”. If paste is not sticky, and its consistency is moderate, it is up to standard. Softening point tester can also be used to measure and determine the plaster’s degree of consistency.

（4）去“火毒”　油丹炼合而成的膏药若直接应用，常对皮肤局部产生刺激性，轻者出现红斑、瘙痒，重者出现发疱、溃疡，这种刺激俗称“火毒”。传统视为经高温熬炼后膏药产生的“燥性”，在水中浸泡或久置阴凉处可除去。现代认为是油在高温下氧化聚合反应生成的低分子分解产物，如醛、酮、低级脂肪酸等。通常将炼成的膏药以细流倒入冷水中，不断强烈搅拌，待冷却凝结取出，反复揉搓，制成团块并浸于冷水中去尽“火毒”。

d. Eliminate “Fire toxin”　If you apply the dan plaster directly, it will often cause local irritation to the skin, such as erythema and itching in mild cases, or blisters and ulcers in severe cases, this kind of irritation is commonly known as “fire toxin”. Traditional view is that, the “dryness” of plasters after high-temperature refining can be removed by soaking in water or leaving in a cool place for a long time. Modern thinking is that low molecular decomposition products, such as aldehydes, ketones, lower fatty acids, etc., are formed by the oxidative polymerization of oil at high temperatures. Usually, the smelted plaster is poured into cold water in a thin stream, and continuously stirred vigorously. After cooling and coagulating, it is taken out, rubbed against repeatedly, made into lumps and immersed in cold water to completely eliminate “fire toxin”.

（5）摊涂膏药　将去“火毒”的膏药团块用文火熔化，如有挥发性的贵重药材细粉应在不超过 70℃ 的温度下加入，混合均匀。按规定量涂于皮革、布或多层韧皮纸制成的裱背材料上，膏面覆盖衬纸或折合包装，于干燥阴凉处密闭贮藏。

e. Tantu plaster　Take eliminate fire toxin plaster clumps and melt with at low fire/gentle fire, if volatile precious medicinal powder is added, it should be added at a temperature not exceeding 70℃, and mixed well. Smear a specified amount to the backing material made of leather, cloth or multi-layer bast paper, making sure the surface smeared with paste is covered with the interleaving paper or packaging is folded, after which it is sealed and stored in a dry and cool place.

三、白膏药
10.3.3 White Plasters

白膏药系指原料药物、食用植物油与宫粉［碱式碳酸铅 $2PbCO_3 \cdot Pb(OH)_2$］炼制成的膏药，摊涂于裱背材料上制成的供皮肤贴敷的外用制剂。

白膏药的制法与黑膏药基本相同，唯一不同是下丹时油温要冷却到100℃左右，缓缓递加宫粉，以防止产生大量的二氧化碳气体使药油溢出。宫粉的氧化作用不如红丹剧烈。宫粉用量较红丹多，与油的比例为1∶1或1.5∶1，允许有部分多余的宫粉存在。加入宫粉后需搅拌，在将要变黑时投入冷水中，成品为黄白色。

White plasters refer to plasters made from raw materials, edible vegetable oils, and ceruse [$2PbCO_3 \cdot Pb(OH)_2$], external preparations which are spread on the backing material for skin application. The manufacturing method of white plaster is basically the same as that of black plaster. The only difference is that the temperature of the oil should be cooled to about 100℃ during the time of xiadan, and the ceruse is slowly added to prevent the large amount of carbon dioxide gas from causing the oil to overflow. The oxidative effect of ceruse is not as severe as that of red lead oxide. The amount of ceruse is more than that of red lead oxide. The ratio of ceruse to oil is 1∶1 or 1.5∶1. Some excess ceruse is allowed to exist. After adding the ceruse, it needs to be stirred and put into cold water when it is going to be black. The finished product is yellow-white.

四、膏药的质量检查
10.3.4 Quality Inspection of Plasters

1. 外观 膏药的膏体应油润细腻，光亮，老嫩适宜，摊涂均匀，无飞边缺口。黑膏药应乌黑、无红斑；白膏药应无白点。加温后能粘贴于皮肤上且不移动。

(1) Exterior The form of the plaster should be oily and delicate, bright, suitable consistency,, spread out evenly, and have no burrs. Black plaster should be dark and without red spots; white plaster should have no white spots. After heating, it should stick to the skin without moving.

2. 软化点 用于测定膏药在规定条件下受热软化时的温度情况以检测膏药的老嫩程度，并可间接反映膏药的黏性。按现行版《中国药典》中膏药的软化点测定法，采用软化点测定仪，测定膏药因受热下坠达25mm时的温度的平均值，应符合规定。

(2) Softening point It is used to determine the temperature of the plaster when it is softened by heat under specified conditions to detect the degree of consistency of the plaster, and it can indirectly reflect the viscosity of the plaster. According to the method of measuring the softening point of the plaster of the current edition of the *Chinese Pharmacopoeia*, the softening point measuring instrument is used to measure the average temperature of the plaster when it drops to 25mm due to heat, which should meet the requirements.

3. 重量差异限度 取供试品5张，分别称定总重量。剪取单位面积（cm^2）的裱背，折算出裱背的重量。膏药总重量减去裱背重量即为膏药重量，与标示量相比较不得超出表10-1中的规定。

(3) Weight difference limit Take 5 test samples and weigh the total weight. Cut the backing per unit of skin area (cm^2) and calculate the weight of the backing. The total weight of the plaster minus the weight of the backing is the weight of the plaster, and it must not exceed the requirements in Table 10-1 when compared with the labeled amount.

表 10-1 膏药重量差异限度

Table 10-1 Plaster Weight Difference Limits

标示重量（Labelled weight）	重量差异限度（Weight variation limit）
3g 或 3g 以下 (3g or less)	± 10%
3g 以上至 12g (More than 3g to 12g)	± 7%
12g 以上至 30g (More than 12g to 30g)	± 6%
30g 以上 (More than 30g)	± 5%

第四节 贴膏剂

10.4 Cataplasms

PPT

贴膏剂系指提取物、饮片细粉或化学药物与适宜的基质和基材制成的供皮肤贴敷，可产生局部或全身性作用的一类片状外用制剂，包括橡胶膏剂、凝胶膏剂（原巴布膏剂）和贴剂等。

Cataplasms are lamellar external preparations for local or systemic effects, made by extracts, prepared slices powders or chemicals and suitable matrices. They include adhesive plasters, hydrogel plasters (formerly known as Babu plasters), and patches.

一、橡胶膏剂

10.4.1 Adhesive Plasters

（一）概述

(1) Overview

橡胶膏剂系指中药提取物或化学药物与橡胶等基质混匀后，涂布于背衬材料上制成的贴膏剂，包括不含药者（如橡皮膏即胶布）和含药者（如伤湿止痛膏）两类。

Adhesive plasters are pastes made by mixing traditional Chinese medicine extracts or chemicals with rubber and other substrates and then coating them on a backing material. It includes those who do not contain medicines (such as plaster is also called adhesive tape) and those who contain medicines (such as shangshi zhitong plaster).

橡胶膏剂黏着力强，与黑药膏相比可直接贴于皮肤，不污染衣物，携带使用方便。含药者常用于治疗风湿痛、跌打损伤等；不含药者可保护伤口、防止皮肤皲裂。但贴膏剂膏层薄，容纳药物量少，维持时间较短。

The adhesive plasters have strong adhesive force, can be directly applied to the skin compared with the black ointment, do not contaminate clothing, and are convenient to carry and use. Those with medicines are often used to treat rheumatic pain and bruises; those without medicines can protect wounds and prevent skin cracking. However, because of the thin layer of the plaster, the amounts of medicine contained is small, and the maintenance time is short.

（二）组成

(2) Composition

1. 膏料层 由药物和基质组成，为橡胶膏剂的主要部分。基质主要由以下成分组成：

① **Paste layer** It is composed of medicine and matrix and is the main part of rubber pasters. The matrix is mainly composed of the following components:

（1）橡胶 为基质的主要原料，常用未经硫化的生橡胶以及热可塑性橡胶，具有较好的黏性、弹性。不透气，不透水。

a. Rubbers It is the main raw material of matrix. It is often used as raw rubber without vulcanization and thermoplastic rubber, with good viscosity and elasticity. It's impermeable.

（2）软化剂 可使生胶软化，增加可塑性，增加成品柔软性、耐寒性及黏性。常用的软化剂有凡士林、羊毛脂、液状石蜡、植物油等。

b. Softeners It can soften raw rubber, increase plasticity, and increase the softness, cold resistance and stickiness of the finished product. Commonly used softeners are vaseline, lanolin, liquid paraffin, and vegetable oil.

（3）增黏剂 可增加膏体的黏性，常用松香，因松香中含有的松香酸可加速橡胶膏剂的老化。可采用甘油松香酯、氢化松香、β-蒎烯等新型材料取代天然松香作增黏剂，具有抗氧化、耐光、耐老化和抗过敏等性能。

c. Tackifiers It can increase the viscosity of the paste. Rosin is commonly used. Because the rosin acid contained in rosin can accelerate the aging of rubber pastes.

Glycerol rosin ester, hydrogenated rosin, β-pinene and other new materials are widely used to replace natural rosin as a tackifier, which has properties of anti-oxidation, light resistance, aging resistance and anti-allergy.

（4）填充剂 常用氧化锌。其有缓和的收敛作用，并能增加膏料与裱背材料间的黏着性。氧化锌与松香酸生成的松香酸锌盐，能降低松香酸对皮肤的刺激性。锌钡白（俗称立德粉）常用作热压法制备橡胶膏剂的填充剂，其特点是遮盖力强，胶料硬度大。

d. Fillers Commonly used zinc oxide. It has a mild astringent effect and can increase the adhesion between the paste and the backing material. Zinc oxide and abietic acid zinc salts of abietic acid can reduce the skin irritation caused by abietic acid. Barium sulfate zinc sulfide (commonly known as lithopone) is often used as a filler for the preparation of rubber pastes by hot pressing, which is characterized by strong hiding power and high rubber hardness.

2. 背衬材料 一般采用漂白细布。

② **Backing material** Bleached fine cloth is usually used.

3. 膏面覆盖物 多用塑料薄膜或玻璃纸等，以避免膏片互相黏着及防止挥发性成分的挥散。

③ **Plaster cover** It uses plastic film, or cellophane to avoid paste layers from sticking to each other and prevent the volatile components from scattering.

（三）制法

(3) Making Method

橡胶膏剂常用制法有溶剂法与热压法。

Solvent method and hot-pressing method are commonly used in rubber paste.

1. 橡胶膏剂溶剂法工艺流程 见图 10-4（Figure 10-4）。

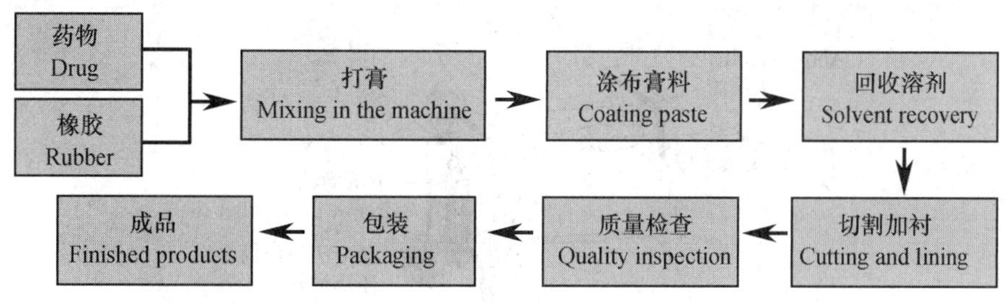

图 10-4 橡胶膏剂制备工艺流程图

Figure 10-4 Process Flow Chart of Rubber Paste Preparation

2. 制法

（1）提取药料 药料常用适当的有机溶剂提取。能溶于橡胶基质中的药物如薄荷脑、冰片、樟脑等可直接加入。

① *Extraction of medicinal materials* The medicinal materials are usually extracted with appropriate organic solvents. Drugs soluble in the rubber matrix such as menthol, borneol, camphor, etc. can be added directly.

（2）制备胶浆 胶浆由药物和基质混合制成，一般制法如下：

② *Preparation of glue* The glue is made of a mixture of a drug and a base. The general method is as follows:

①压胶：取生橡胶洗净，50~60°C 干燥后切成大小适宜的条块，在炼胶机中压成网状胶片，摊在铁丝网上去静电。

a. Pressing rubber: Wash the raw rubber, dry it at 50-60ºC, cut it into suitable size pieces, press it into a mesh film in a rubber mixer, and spread it on a wire mesh to remove static electricity.

②浸胶：将网状胶片浸入适量汽油中，浸泡 18~24 小时至完全溶胀成凝胶状。浸泡时需密闭，以防汽油挥发引起火灾。

b. Dipping rubber: Immerse the mesh film in an appropriate amount of gasoline and soak it for 18 to 24 hours until it swells into a gelatinous form. It must be sealed when soaking to prevent fire caused by volatilization of gasoline.

③打膏：将胶浆移入打膏机中搅拌 3~4 小时后，依次加入凡士林、羊毛脂、液状石蜡、松香、氧化锌等制成基质，再加入药物浸膏或细粉，继续搅拌成均匀胶浆，在滤胶机上压过筛网，即得药膏料。

c. Plastering: After moving the glue into the paste machine and stirring for 3 to 4 hours, add petroleum jelly, lanolin, liquid paraffin, rosin, zinc oxide, etc. to make a base, and then add drug extract or fine powder, and continue stirring to form a uniform glue. The slurry is pressed through a sieve on a rubber filter to obtain an ointment.

（3）涂布膏料 将膏料置于装好细白布的涂料机上，如图 10-5 所示，利用上下滚筒将膏料均匀涂布在缓慢向上移动的布面上，通过调节两滚筒间的距离来控制涂膏量。

③ *Coating paste* Put the paste on the coating machine equipped with a fine white cloth, as shown in Figure 10-5, use the upper and lower rollers to evenly spread the paste on the slowly moving cloth surface, and control the paste by adjusting the distance between the two rollers the amount.

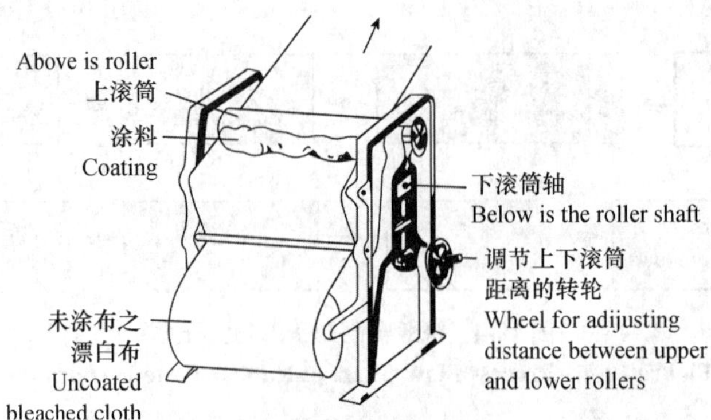

图 10-5　橡胶膏涂料机的涂布部分

Figure 10-5　Coating Part of Rubber Paste Coating Machine

（4）回收溶剂　胶布上涂以膏料后，以一定速度进入封闭的溶剂回收装置，见图 10-6，经蒸汽加热管加热，溶剂（汽油）沿罩管及溶剂蒸汽导管，经鼓风机送入冷凝系统吸收和排出。

④ *Solvent recovery*　After the plaster is coated with paste, it enters the closed solvent recovery device at a certain speed, as shown in Figure 10-6. It is heated by the steam heating tube, and the solvent (gasoline) is sent along the hood tube and the solvent vapor duct, and sent to the condensation system by a blower to absorb discharge.

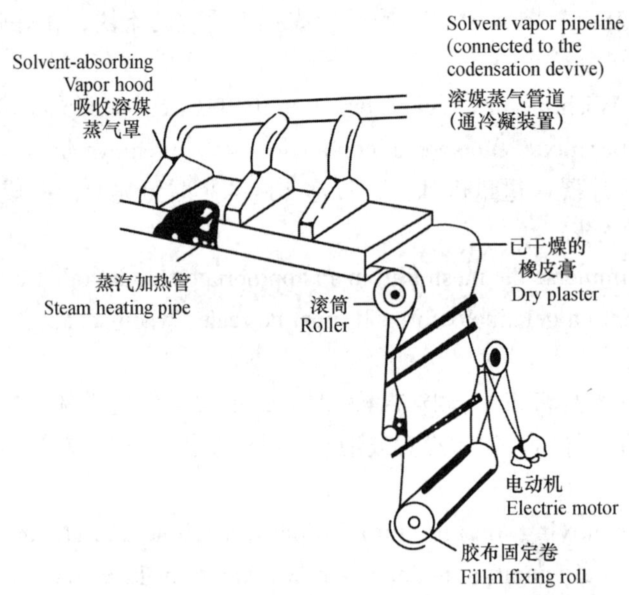

图 10-6　橡胶膏涂料机的溶剂回收装置与拉布部分

Figure 10-6　Solvent Recovery Device and Cloth Drawing Part of Rubber Paste Coating Machine

（5）切割加衬与包装　将膏布在切割机上切成规定的宽度，再移至纱布卷筒装置上，见图 10-7，使膏面覆上脱脂硬纱布或塑料薄膜等以避免黏合，最后切成小块后包装。

⑤ *Cutting, lining and packaging*　Cut the paste into a predetermined width on the cutting machine, and then move it to the gauze roll device, as shown in Figure 10-7, so that the paste surface is covered with degreased hard gauze or plastic film to avoid sticking, and finally cut into small pieces after packaging.

橡胶膏剂还可用热压法制备，将胶片用处方中的油脂性药材等浸泡，待溶胀后再加入其他药物和立德粉或氧化锌、松香等，炼压均匀，涂膏盖衬。此法不用汽油，无需回收装置，但成品欠

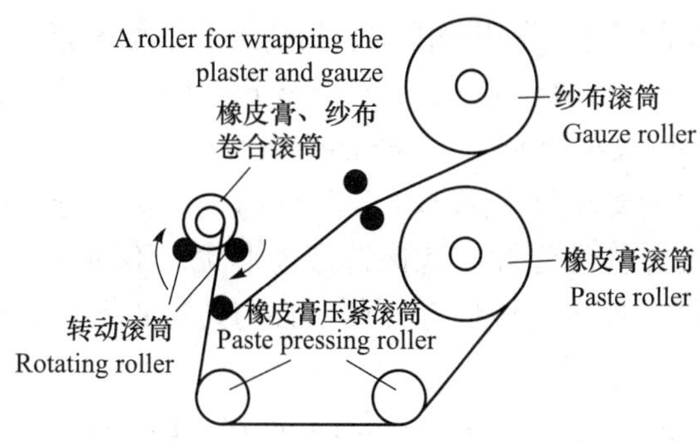

图 10-7 橡胶膏纱布卷筒装置

Figure 10-7 Rubber Paste Gauze Roll Device

光滑。

The rubber paste can also be prepared by hot pressing. The film is soaked with the oily medicinal materials in the prescription. After swelling, other drugs and lithopone or zinc oxide and rosin are added. This method does not use gasoline and does not require a recovery device, but the finished product is not smooth.

二、凝胶膏剂

10.4.2 Hydrogel Plasters

（一）概述

(1) Overview

凝胶膏剂，原称巴布膏剂，系指提取物、饮片细粉和化学药物与适宜的亲水性基质混匀后，涂布于背衬材料上制成的贴膏剂。

Hydrogel plasters, formerly known as Babu paste, refers to the extract, powder and chemical powder mixed with suitable hydrophilic base, paste coated on the backing material made of paste.

凝胶膏剂与传统中药黑膏药和橡胶膏剂相比，具有以下特点：①载药量大，尤其适用于中药浸膏。②与皮肤生物相容性好，透气、耐汗、无致敏性、无刺激性。③释药性好，有利于药物透皮吸收，能提高角质层的水化作用。④采用透皮吸收控释技术，使血药浓度平稳，药效持久。⑤使用方便，不污染衣物，易洗除，反复揭贴仍能保持黏性。

Compared with black plaster and adhesive plasters, hydrogel plasters has the following characteristics: ① it has large drug loading, especially for Chinese medicine extract. ② It has good biocompatibility with the skin, breathable, sweat-resistant, non-allergenic and non-irritating. ③ it has good drug release, is conducive to drug transdermal absorption, and can improve the hydration of the cuticle. ④ it adopts the technology of transdermal absorption and controlled release to make the blood concentration stable and the effect lasting. ⑤ it is easy to use, does not pollute clothes, is easy to wash and remove, and can remain sticky after being repeatedly lifted off.

（二）组成

(2) Composition

1. 背衬层 为基质的载体，常用无纺布、人造棉布等。

① Backing layer It is the carrier of base, commonly used ones are non-woven fabric, artificial cotton and so on.

2. 防黏层　起保护膏体的作用，常用聚丙烯、聚乙烯及聚酯薄膜等。

② **Anti-adhesive layer**　It plays the role of protecting paste, commonly used ones are polypropylene, polyethylene, polyester film, cellophane and so on.

3. 膏体　为凝胶膏剂的主要部分，由基质和药物构成。基质选用的条件是：不影响主药稳定性，无副作用；有适当的黏性和弹性；能保持膏体形状，不因汗水、温度作用而软化，也不残留在皮肤上；具有一定稳定性与保湿性，无刺激性与过敏性等。基质的原料主要有以下几个部分：

③ **Paste**　It is a major part of gel paste, consisting of base and drugs. The conditions for base selection are: it does not affect the stability of the main drug and has no side effects; it has appropriate viscosity and elasticity; it can maintain the shape of the paste, will not soften due to the effect of sweat and temperature, nor will it remain on the skin; it has certain stability and moisture retention, no irritation and allergy, etc. The raw materials of base mainly include the following parts:

（1）黏合剂　是基质骨架材料，也是影响持黏力与剥离强度的主要因素。包括天然、半合成或合成的高分子材料，如阿拉伯胶、海藻酸钠、西黄蓍胶、明胶、羟丙甲基纤维素、聚丙烯酸及其钠盐、聚乙烯醇、聚维酮等。

a. Adhesives　It is not only a base material, but also a main factor affecting the adhesion and peel strength. It includes natural, semi synthetic or synthetic polymer materials, such as Arabic gum, sodium alginate, tragacanth gum, gelatin, hydroxypropyl Methyl cellulose, polyacrylic acid and its sodium salt, polyvinyl alcohol, povidone, etc.

（2）保湿剂　决定基质的柔韧性和初黏力。凝胶膏剂基质为亲水性，含水量大，选择合适的保湿剂很重要。常用甘油、丙二醇、聚乙二醇、山梨醇以及它们的混合物。

b. Moisturizers　It determines the flexibility and initial adhesion of the base. Gel paste base is hydrophilic and has high water content. It is very important to choose suitable moisturizing agents. Commonly used ones, are propylene glycol, polyethylene glycol, sorbitol and their mixtures.

（3）填充剂　影响膏体成型性，常用微粉硅胶、二氧化钛、碳酸钙等。

c. Fillers　It affects the paste formability, commonly used ones are silica gel, titanium dioxide, calcium carbonate.

（4）渗透促进剂　提高药物经皮渗透性能。可用氮酮、尿素、中药挥发性物质如薄荷脑、冰片、桉叶油等。

d. Penetration enhancers　It improves the transdermal permeability of drugs. Azone, dimethyl sulfoxide, urea, volatile substances in traditional Chinese medicines such as menthol, borneol, eucalyptus oil, etc. can be used. The combination of azone and propylene glycol can improve the permeability of Azone. Volatile substances in traditional Chinese medicines such as menthol, borneol, eucalyptus oil, etc. can also promote penetration.

根据药物的性质，还可以加入表面活性剂、液状石蜡等其他附加剂。

According to the properties of the drugs, surfactants, liquid paraffin and other additives can also be added.

（三）制法

(3) Making Method

1. 工艺流程　如图 10-8（Figure 10-8）所示。

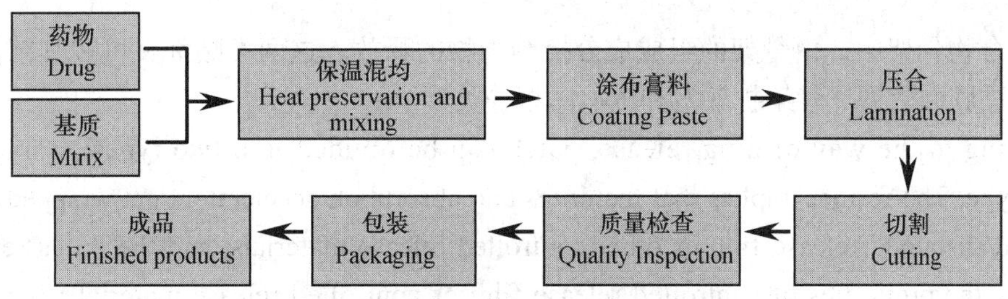

图 10-8　凝胶膏剂制备工艺流程图

Figure 10-8　Process Chart of Gel Paste Preparation

2. 制法　凝胶膏剂的制备工艺主要包括原料药物前处理、基质成型与制剂的成型三部分。基质原料类型及其比例、基质与药物的比例、配制程序等均影响凝胶膏剂的成型。

The preparation process of the gel paste mainly includes three parts: pretreatment of raw materials, base molding, and formulation molding. The type of base material, its ratio, the ratio of base to drug, and the formulation process all affect the molding of the gel paste.

三、贴剂
10.4.3　Patches

（一）概述
(1) Overview

贴剂系指提取物和化学药物与适宜的高分子材料制成的一种薄片状贴膏剂，也称经皮给药系统或经皮治疗系统。这类制剂为一些慢性病提供了简单有效的给药方法，与常规剂型相比，具有延长作用时间、维持恒定的血药浓度、减少胃肠道副作用以及避免肝脏首过效应等优点，但由于皮肤的屏障性能，贴剂仅适合于药理作用强、相对分子量低于 1000、在水和油中有适宜溶解度（>1mg/ml）的药物。贴剂主要由背衬层、药物贮库层，黏贴层以及防黏层组成。透皮贴剂中除药物、透皮促进剂外，还需要控制药物释放速率的高分子物质、固定贴剂的压敏胶、背衬材料与保护膜等。对皮肤有刺激性、过敏性的药物不宜制成贴剂。贴剂的制备比较复杂，成本较高。

Patches refer to a kind of thin patch made of extracts and chemicals and suitable polymer materials, also known as transdermal delivery system or transdermal treatment system. This kind of preparation provides a simple and effective drug delivery method for some chronic diseases. Compared with the conventional dosage form, it has the advantages of prolonging the action time, maintaining a constant blood concentration, reducing gastrointestinal side effects and avoiding the first pass effect of liver. However, due to the barrier performance of skin, the patch is only suitable for drugs with strong pharmacological effect, molecular weight less than 1000, and suitable solubility in water and oil (>1mg/ml). The sticking agent is mainly composed of backing layer, drug storage layer, sticking layer and anti sticking layer. In addition to drugs and transdermal enhancers, the transdermal patches also need polymer materials to control drug release rate, as well as pressure-sensitive adhesives for fixed patches, backing materials and protective films. The patch is not suitable for the drugs which cause skin irritation and allergies. The preparation of patch is complex and the cost is high.

（二）分类
(2) Classification

贴剂按释药方式可分为贮库型与骨架型两大类，前者是药物和吸收促进剂等被控释膜或其他控释材料包裹成为贮库，由控释膜或控释材料的性质控制药物的释放速率；后者是药物溶解或均

匀分散在聚合物骨架中，由骨架的组成成分控制药物的释放。这两类贴剂又可按其结构特点分成膜控释型、黏胶分散型、骨架扩散型和微贮库型等类型。

According to the way of drug release, patch can be divided into two types: storage type and framework type. The former implies that the drugs and absorption accelerators get wrapped into storage by controlled/sustained release film or other controlled release materials, and the drugs release rate is controlled by the properties of controlled release film or controlled release materials; the latter is the dissolution or even dispersion of drugs in the polymer framework, and the release of drugs is controlled by the components of the framework. According to their structural characteristics, these two kinds of patches can be divided into membrane controlled release type, adhesive dispersion type, framework diffusion type and micro storage type.

（三）制法

(3) Manufacturing Method

根据其类型与组成可分为骨架黏合工艺、涂膜复合工艺、充填热合工艺等三种类型。

According to its type and composition, it can be divided into three types: framework bonding process, coating composite process and filling heat sealing process.

1. 骨架黏合工艺 是在骨架材料溶液中加入药物，浇铸冷却成型，切割成小圆片，黏贴于背衬膜上，加保护膜而成。

① **Skeleton bonding process** It is made by adding medicine into the skeleton material solution, casting, cooling and forming, cutting into small circles, sticking to the backing membrane and adding a protective film.

2. 涂膜复合工艺 是将药物分散在高分子材料如压敏胶溶液中，涂布于背衬膜上，加热烘干使溶解高分子材料的有机溶剂蒸发。可进行第二层或多层膜的涂布，最后覆盖上保护膜，亦可以制成含药物的高分子材料膜，再与各层膜叠合或黏合。

② **Coating film composite process** The drug is dispersed in a polymer material such as a pressure-sensitive adhesive solution, coated on a backing film, and heated and dried to evaporate an organic solvent in which the polymer material is dissolved. It can be coated with a second or multi-layer film, and finally covered with a protective film. It can also be made into a drug-containing polymer material film, and then laminated or bonded with each layer of film.

3. 充填热合工艺 是在定型机械中，于背衬膜与控释膜之间定量充填药物储库材料，热合封闭，覆盖上涂有胶黏层的保护膜。

③ **Filling and heat sealing process** It is a protective film coated with adhesive layer, which is used to quantitatively fill the drug storage material between the backing film and the controlled-release film in the setting machine.

四、贴膏剂的质量检查

10.4.4 Quality Inspection of Cataplasms

1. 外观 膏面应光洁，厚薄均匀，色泽一致，无脱膏、失黏现象。背衬面应平整、洁净、无漏膏现象。盖衬的长度和宽度应与背衬一致。

(1) Exterior The paste surface should be smooth, uniform in thickness, uniform in color, and free from unguent and viscidity. The backing surface should be flat, clean and free of leakage. The length and width of the cover lining should be consistent with the backing.

2. 含膏量 橡胶膏剂和凝胶膏剂分别按现行版《中国药典》中贴膏剂含膏量方法一与方法二检查，应符合规定。

(2) Paste content Adhesive plasters, hydrogel plasters amount should be inspected in accordance with the methods of method 1 and method 2 of the plasters in the current edition of the *Chinese Pharmacopoeia*, which should meet the requirements.

（1）橡胶膏剂 取供试品2片（每片面积大于35cm^{2}的应切取35cm^2），除去盖衬，精密称定，置于有盖玻璃容器中，加适量有机溶剂（如三氯甲烷、乙醚等）浸渍，并时时振摇，待背衬与膏体分离后，将背衬取出，用上述溶液洗涤至背衬无残附膏料，挥去溶剂，在105℃干燥30分钟，移至干燥器中，冷却30分钟，精密称定，减失重量即为膏重，按标示面积换算成100cm^{2}的含膏量。

① Take 2 test samples of rubber paste (each piece bigger than 35cm^2 should be cut to 35cm^2), remove the cover lining, weigh accurately, place it in a glass container with a cover lid, add an appropriate amount of organic solvent (such as chloroform, ether, etc.) to macerate it, shake it from time to time, after the backing and the paste are separated, take out the backing, wash with the solution mentioned above until the backing has no residual paste, evaporate the solvent, dry at 105℃ for 30min, and move to the desiccator, cool for 30min, weigh accurately, what is left after subtracting the weight loss is considered to be the paste weight, convert it to 100cm^2 paste content according to the marked area.

（2）凝胶膏剂 取供试品1片，除去盖衬，精密称定，置烧杯中，加适量水，加热煮沸至背衬与膏体分离后，将背衬取出，用水洗涤至背衬无残留膏体，晾干，在105℃干燥30分钟，移至干燥器中，冷却30分钟，精密称定，减失重量即为膏重，按标示面积换算成100cm^{2}的含膏量。

② Take one sample of the gel paste, remove the cover lining, weigh accurately, place in a beaker, add appropriate amount of water, heat and boil until the backing line separates from the paste, remove the backing line, and wash it with water until there is no residual paste, air dry, dry at 105℃ for 30min, move to a desiccator, cool for 30min, measure weight accurately, what is left after subtracting weight loss is paste weight, and convert into 100cm^2 paste amount according to the indicated area.

3. 耐热性 橡胶膏剂按现行版《中国药典》中贴膏剂耐热性试验方法检查，应符合规定。

(3) Heat-resistance Adhesive plasters shall be checked in accordance with the test method for heat-resistance in the current edition of the *Chinese Pharmacopoeia* and shall comply with the regulations.

4. 赋形性 凝胶膏剂按现行版《中国药典》中贴膏剂做赋形性试验检查，应符合规定。

(4) Excipient Hydrogel plasters should be tested for excipients according to the current edition of *Chinese Pharmacopoeia*, which should meet the requirements.

5. 黏附性 凝胶膏剂按现行版《中国药典》中黏附力测定法第一法（初黏力的测定）、橡胶膏剂照黏附力测定法第二法（持黏力的测定），贴剂照黏附性测定法第二、第三法（剥离强度的测定）测定，应符合规定。

(5) Adhesiveness The hydrogel plasters adhesive force is determined in accordance with the first method of adhesion determination(determination of initial viscosity)given in the current edition of *Chinese Pharmacopoeia*, adhesive plasters adhesive force is determined in accordance with the second method (measurement of protracted viscosity), while the patches adhesive force is determined in accordance with the second and the third methods (peeling strength measurement) and should all comply with the regulations.

6. 重量差异 取20片贴剂，按现行版《中国药典》中贴膏剂重量差异方法检查，每片重量与平均重量相比较，重量差异限度应在平均重量的±5%内，超出重量差异限度的不得多于2片，并不得有1片超出限度的1倍。

(6) Weight difference Take 20 patches and check according to the weight difference method of the patch in the current edition of *Chinese Pharmacopoeia*. Comparing the weight of each tablet with the average weight, the weight difference limit should be within ± 5% of the average weight, and no more than 2 tablets should exceed the weight difference limit, and no one tablet should exceed the limit.

7. 微生物限定 贴剂按现行版《中国药典》中微生物限度检查法检查，应符合规定。

(7) Microbial limitation The patches should be inspected according to the microbial limit inspection method in the current edition of *Chinese Pharmacopoeia*, and it should meet the requirements.

PPT

英文翻译

第五节　凝胶剂、糊剂和涂膜剂

一、凝胶剂

（一）概述

凝胶剂系指中药提取物与适宜基质制成的具有凝胶特性的半固体或稠厚液体剂型。主要供外用。凝胶剂分为水性凝胶和油性凝胶。水性凝胶的基质一般由西黄蓍胶、明胶、淀粉、纤维素衍生物等加水、甘油或丙二醇等制成；油性凝胶的基质常由液体石蜡与聚氧乙烯或脂肪油与胶体硅或铝皂、锌皂构成。在临床上应用较多的是水性凝胶，其特点为：易涂展和洗除，无油腻感，能吸收组织渗出液而不妨碍皮肤正常功能。由于黏度较小而利于药物，特别是水溶性药物的释放。缺点是润滑作用较差，易失水和霉变，常需添加保湿剂和防腐剂，且用量较大。

（二）凝胶剂的制备

1. 凝胶剂的常用水性凝胶基质

（1）卡波姆　系丙烯酸与丙烯基蔗糖交联的高分子聚合物，商品名为卡波普，按分子量不同常分为 930、934、940 等规格，本品是一种引湿性很强的白色松散粉末，可溶于水、稀乙醇和甘油，其 1% 水溶液的 pH 值约为 3.0，为黏性较低的酸性溶液。在 pH 值 6~11 有最大的黏度和稠度。其分子结构中的羧酸基团使其水溶液呈酸性，当用碱中和时，随大分子逐渐溶解，黏度也逐渐上升，在低浓度时形成澄明溶液，在浓度较大时形成半透明状的凝胶。中和使用的碱以及卡波普的浓度不同，其溶液的黏度变化也有所区别。一般中和 1g 卡波姆约消耗 1.35g 三乙醇胺或 400mg 氢氧化钠，本品制成的基质无油腻感，涂用润滑舒适，特别适宜于治疗脂溢性皮肤病。与聚丙烯酸相似，盐类电解质可使卡波姆凝胶的黏性下降，碱土金属离子以及阳离子聚合物等均可与之结合成不溶性盐，强酸也可使卡波姆失去黏性，在配伍时必须避免。

（2）纤维素衍生物　纤维素经衍生化后成为在水中可溶胀或溶解的胶性物。根据不同规格取用一定量，调节适宜的稠度可形成水溶性软膏基质。常用的品种有甲基纤维素和羧甲基纤维素钠，两者常用的浓度为 2%~6%，1% 的水溶液 pH 值均在 6~8, pH 值 2~12 时均稳定。甲基纤维素缓缓溶于冷水，不溶于热水，但湿润、放置冷却后可溶解，羧甲基纤维素钠在任何温度下均可溶解，在 pH 值小于 5 或 pH 值等于 10 的环境下黏度显著降低，与阳离子型药物有配伍禁忌，遇强酸及重金属离子能形成不溶物。本类基质涂布于皮肤时有较强黏附性，较易失水干燥而有不适感，常需加入 10%~15% 的甘油调节。制成的基质中均需加入防腐剂，常用 0.2%~0.5% 的羟苯乙酯。

2. 制法　水凝胶剂的制备，一般先按基质配制方法制成水凝胶基质，药物溶于水者常先溶于部分水或甘油中，必要时加热，加入基质中，再加水至足量搅匀即得。药物不溶于水者，可先用少量水或甘油研细，分散，再混于基质中搅匀即得。

（三）质量检查

1. 外观　凝胶剂应均匀、细腻，在常温时保持凝胶状，不干涸或液化。

2. 装置、微生物限度　同软膏剂检查，应符合规定。

3. pH 值　按规定方法检查，应符合规定。

二、糊剂

（一）概述

糊剂系指原料药物与适宜基质制成的糊状制剂，为含多量粉末与软膏剂类似的制剂，含固体粉末一般在 25% 以上，有的高达 75%，具较高稠度、较大吸水能力和较低的油腻性，一般不影响皮肤的正常功能，具收敛、消毒、吸收分泌物作用，适用于亚急性皮炎、湿疹等渗出性慢性皮肤病。

（二）分类

根据基质的不同，糊剂可分为水溶性糊剂、脂溶性糊剂两类：前者系以甘油明胶、甘油或其他水溶性物质如药汁、酒、醋等与淀粉等固体粉末调制而成。赋形剂本身具有辅助治疗作用，适用于渗出液较多的创面。后者系以凡士林、羊毛脂或其混合物为基质制成，粉末含量较高。

（三）制法

饮片需粉碎成细粉（过六号筛），或采用适当方法提取制得干浸膏并粉碎成细粉，再与基质拌匀调成糊状。基质需加热时控制在 70℃ 以下，以免淀粉糊化。

三、涂膜剂

（一）概述

涂膜剂系指原料药物与成膜材料制成的供外用涂抹，能形成薄膜的液体制剂。常以乙醇为溶剂，常用的成膜材料有：聚乙烯醇、聚乙烯吡咯烷酮、丙烯酸树脂类、聚乙烯醇缩丁醛等。增塑剂有甘油、丙二醇、邻苯二甲酸二丁酯等。必要时可加入适宜附加剂。涂膜剂用后形成的薄膜，可以保护创面，同时逐渐释放所含药物而起治疗作用。涂膜剂制备工艺简单，不用背衬材料，无需特殊设备，使用方便。对某些皮肤病有较好的防治作用。

岗位对接

（二）制法

先溶解成膜材料，若药物与附加剂溶于溶剂，可直接加入到成膜材料中。饮片应先制成乙醇提取液或其提取物的乙醇、丙酮溶液，再加入成膜材料液中，混匀。涂膜剂因含有大量有机溶剂，应密封贮藏，并注意避热、防火。

重点小结

（三）质量检查

1. 装量、微生物限度　同软膏剂检查，应符合规定。

题库

2. 其他　以水或稀乙醇为溶剂的涂膜剂一般应检查相对密度、pH 值，以乙醇为溶剂的应检查乙醇量。

（严国俊）

第十一章　栓剂
Chapter 11　Suppository

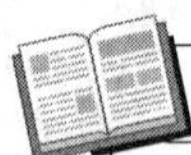

学习目标 ¦ Learning Goals

知识要求：

1. **掌握**　栓剂的含义、特点与分类；药物吸收的途径与影响吸收的因素；热熔法制备栓剂的工艺要求；置换价的含义及计算。

2. **熟悉**　栓剂常用基质的种类、特点以及栓剂的质量评价。

3. **了解**　栓剂的发展概况以及包装贮藏要求。

能力要求：

学会栓剂的制备工艺及操作要点，能制备肛门栓、阴道栓等不同类型的栓剂；能运用置换价计算栓剂生产中所需的基质用量；并检查和评价栓剂的产品质量。

Knowledge requirements:

1. To master the definition, characteristics and classification of suppositories; drug absorption pathways and factors affecting absorption; process requirements for preparing suppositories by the hot-melt method; meaning and calculation of the replacement value.

2. To be familiar with types and characteristics of common bases for suppositories, and quality evaluation of suppositories.

3. To know the development overview of suppositories and relevant requirements on packaging and storage conditions.

Ability requirements:

To be able to manufacture different types of suppositories, such as rectal suppositories, vaginal suppositories by various preparation processes and based on operation points: Use the replacement value to calculate the required amount of bases in the production of suppositories; inspect and evaluate the quality of suppositories.

第一节 概述
11.1 Overview

PPT

一、栓剂的含义
11.1.1 The Definition of Suppositories

栓剂系指原料药物与适宜基质制成供腔道给药的固体剂型。栓剂在常温下为固体，纳入人体腔道后，在体温下能迅速软化熔融或溶解于分泌液，逐渐释放药物而产生局部或全身作用。

Suppositories are solid preparations made by incorporating drug substances in suitable bases, intended for administration to cavities. The suppositories are solid at room temperature, and able to be melted, softened or dissolved quickly when inserted into the cavity, and are miscible with body fluid to release the drug substances gradually thus exert local or systemic effect.

栓剂在古代称坐药或塞药，是我国传统剂型之一，历代医籍中多有记载。张仲景的《伤寒杂病论》、葛洪的《肘后备急方》中有栓剂处方和应用的明确记载；《千金方》《证治准绳》中亦有栓剂的制备与应用的记述。明朝李时珍在《本草纲目》中记载有耳用栓、鼻用栓、肛门栓、阴道栓、尿道栓等。最初栓剂仅限于局部用药，近几十年，关于具有全身作用的栓剂的研究有了新进展，开发了双层栓、中空栓、泡腾栓、微囊栓、凝胶栓、骨架控释栓、渗透泵栓、海绵栓等多种新型栓剂，拓展了栓剂的应用范围。2020 年版《中国药典》一部收载的中药成方制剂中共有栓剂 10 种。

Suppositories were called sitting medicine or medicine for plugging in ancient times. As one of the traditional dosage forms in China, it has been recorded in most of the classical medical books through the ages, such as clear records of suppository prescription and application in *Treatise on Febrile and Miscellaneous Diseases (Shang Han Za Bing* Lun*)* written by Zhang Zhongjing and *Handbook of Prescription for Emergency (Zhou Hou Bei Ji Fang)* written by Ge Hong; description of suppository preparation and application in *Qian Jin Yao Fang* and *Standards of Diagnosis and Treatment (Zheng Zhi Zhun Sheng)*. In the Ming Dynasty, the book named *Compendium of Materia Medica (Ben Cao Gang Mu)* written by Li Shizhen also recorded ear suppositories, nasal suppositories, rectal suppositories, vaginal suppositories and urethral suppositories. Initially, suppositories were intended for local application, but have recent advances for systemic effects in recent decades, and many new suppositories have been developed, such as double-layer suppositories, hollow suppositories, effervescent suppositories, microcapsule suppositories, gel suppositories, framework controlled-release suppositories, osmotic pump suppositories, sponge suppositories, expanding the application scope of suppositories. There are a total of 10 suppositories in the traditional Chinese Medicine prescriptions included in 2020 edition of *Chinese Pharmacopoeia* (Part 1).

二、栓剂的特点
11.1.2 The Characteristics of Suppositories

栓剂最初作为肛门、阴道等部位用药，可在腔道起润滑、收敛、抗菌、杀虫、消炎、止痛、止痒等局部治疗作用，临床多用于内痔、阴道炎及直肠炎的治疗；用于全身治疗的栓剂多为直肠

栓，通过吸收入血发挥镇痛、镇静、兴奋、扩张支气管和血管等全身治疗作用。

The suppositories were originally used as medicine for anus, vagina and other parts, and exert lubrication, converging, antibacterial, insecticidal, anti-inflammatory, analgesic, antipruritic effects and other local therapeutic effects. They are commonly used for treatment of internal hemorrhoids, vaginitis and proctitis in clinical application. The suppositories used for systemic treatment are mostly rectal suppositories, which can play a systemic therapeutic role such as analgesia, sedation, excitation, dilation of bronchi and blood vessels through being absorbed into the blood.

栓剂可避免药物受胃肠 pH 值或酶的破坏而失去活性，适于不能口服的药物；可减少药物对胃肠道的刺激；可减少或避免药物受肝脏首过效应的影响，降低对肝脏毒副作用；便于不能或不愿吞服药物的患者使用。栓剂的不足之处在于使用过程中某些患者不习惯，不如口服给药方便。

Suppositories can prevent drugs from losing their activity due to the destruction of gastrointestinal pH or enzymes, and are suitable for drugs that can't be taken orally; reduce the effect of drug on gastrointestinal tract irritation; reduce or avoid the first-pass effect of the drug on the liver, and reduce toxic and side effects on the liver; are suitable for patients who can't or don't want to swallow the drugs. The disadvantages of suppositories are some patients are not used to them during application, and are not as convenient as oral administration.

三、栓剂的分类

11.1.3 The Classification of Suppositories

（一）按给药途径分类

(1) Classification by Administration Routes

栓剂按施药腔道不同，可分为肛门栓、阴道栓、尿道栓、鼻用栓、耳用栓等，其中最常用的是肛门栓和阴道栓。

Depending on the different cavities they are intended to apply to, suppositories can be divided into rectal suppositories, vaginal suppositories, urethral suppositories, nasal suppositories, ear suppositories, etc., among them rectal suppositories and vaginal suppositories are commonly used.

1. 肛门栓 肛门栓的形状有圆锥形、圆柱形、鱼雷形等，塞入肛门后，由括约肌的收缩引入直肠，每颗栓重约 2g，长 3~4cm，以鱼雷形较为常用。

① **Rectal suppositories** Rectal suppositories are in the shape of a cone, cylinder or torpedo, etc. After being inserted into the anus, they slide into the rectum with the contraction of the sphincter. Each suppository weighs about 2g and is 3-4cm long. The shape of a torpedo is commonly used.

2. 阴道栓 阴道栓的形状有球形、卵形、圆锥形、鸭嘴形等，每颗栓重 2~5g，直径约 1.5~2.5cm，以鸭嘴形较为常用。

② **Vaginal suppositories** Vaginal suppositories are in the shape of a ball, oval, cone or drawing pen, etc. Each suppository weights 2-5g and is 1.5-2.5cm in diameter. The shape of a drawing pen is commonly used.

栓剂形状如图 11-1 所示。

The shapes of suppository are shown in Figure 11-1.

（二）按制备工艺和释药特点分类

(2) Classification by Preparation Process and Characteristics of Drug Release

栓剂按制备工艺和释药特点不同，分为传统工艺制备的普通栓剂和特殊工艺制备的双层栓、中空栓、泡腾栓、缓释栓、控释栓等，特殊栓剂如图 11-2 所示。

Based on different preparation processes and characteristics of drug release, suppositories can be classified as conventional type suppositories made by traditional preparation process, and double-layer suppositories, hollow suppositories, effervescent suppositories, sustained-release suppositories and controlled-release suppositories made by special preparation process. Diagrams of same special suppositories are shown in Figure 11-2.

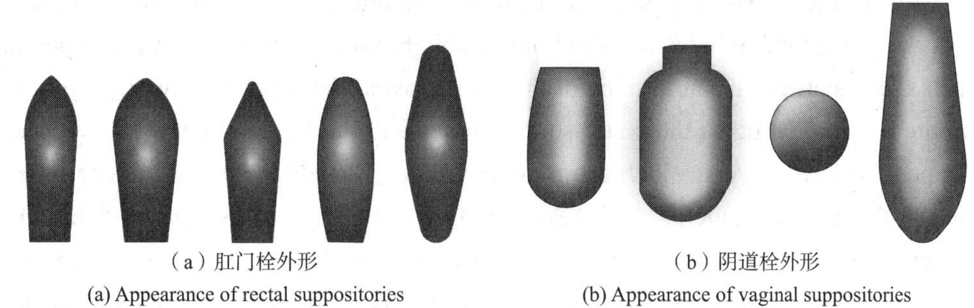

（a）肛门栓外形
(a) Appearance of rectal suppositories

（b）阴道栓外形
(b) Appearance of vaginal suppositories

图 11-1 常用栓剂的形状

Figure 11-1 Shapes of Commonly Used Suppositories

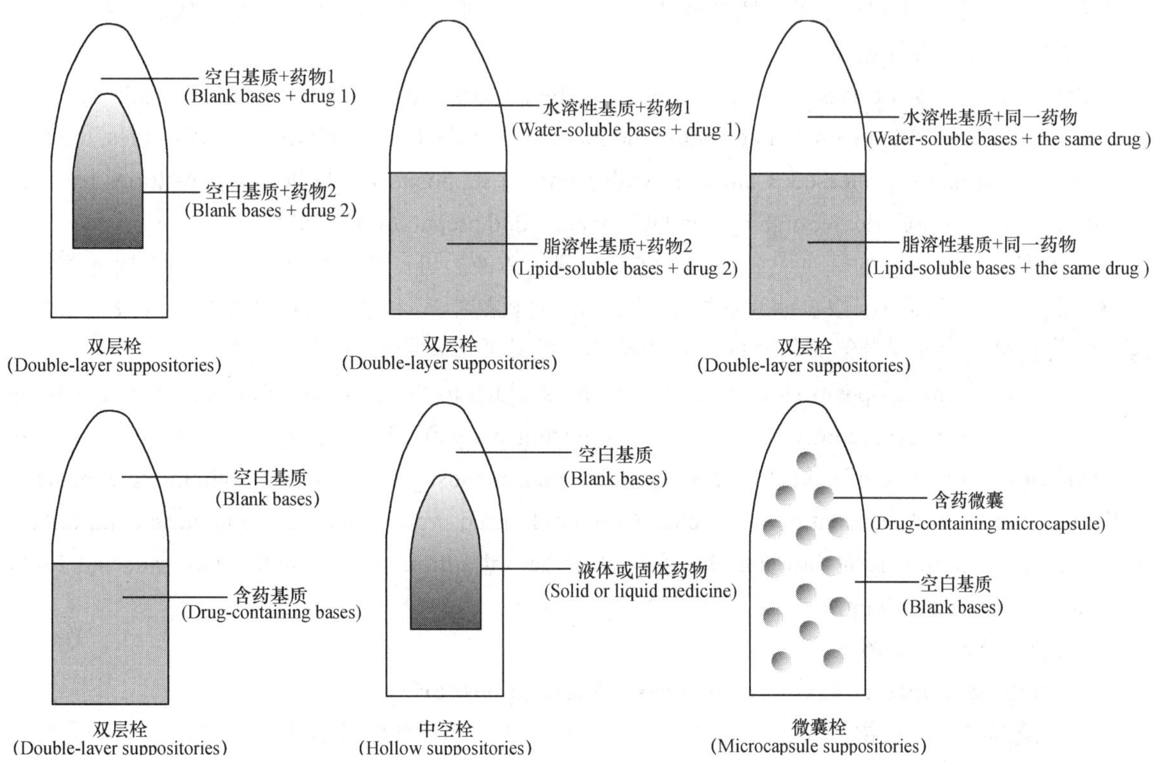

图 11-2 部分特殊栓剂示意图

Figure 11-2 Diagram of Some Special Suppositories

1. 双层栓 双层栓由两层组成，可分为内外双层栓剂和上下双层栓剂。

① Double-layer suppositories Double-layers suppositories are composed of two layers, which can be divided into internal-external double suppositories and upper-lower double suppositories.

内外双层栓剂由内、外两层组成，通常各含有不同药物，可实现药物的先后释放。上下双层栓剂通常有三种形式，第一种是将两种理化性质不同的药物分别分散于水溶性基质和脂溶性基质中，制成上、下两层，有利于药物的吸收或避免药物的配伍禁忌。第二种是将同一种药物分别分

散于水溶性基质和脂溶性基质中，制成上、下两层，同时发挥速释和缓释作用；第三种是用空白基质和含药基质制成上下两层，当空白基质熔化后，形成的液态基质屏障层可有效阻止后端所释药物向上扩散，减少药物自直肠上静脉吸收，可提高生物利用度，减少毒副作用。

Internal-external double suppositories are composed of inner and outer layers, usually containing different drugs in each layer, to achieve drug release successively. Upper-lower double suppositories are usually classified as three types. The first is to distribute two drugs with different physical and chemical properties in the water-soluble bases and the lipid-soluble bases respectively to make upper and lower layers, which is conducive to the absorption of drugs or to avoid the compatibility of drugs. The second is to distribute the same drug in the water-soluble bases and the lipid-soluble bases respectively to make the upper and lower layers, which can play the role of immediate-release and controlled-release simultaneously. The third is made of blank bases and drug-containing bases organized into two layers. When the blank bases are melted, the liquid bases barrier layer can be formed to effectively prevent upward diffusion of the drug released at the back end, reduce the absorption of the drug from the superior rectal vein, improve bioavailability and reduce toxic side effects.

2. 中空栓 中空栓外层为基质制成的壳，中间空心部位填充固体或液体药物。当外层栓壳融化或溶解后，内部的药物可快速地释放出来。相比于普通栓剂，具有释药速度快、生物利用度高、制剂稳定性好等优点。

② **Hollow suppositories** The outer layer of the hollow suppository is the shell made of bases, with the hollow area filled with solid or liquid medicine. When the outer shell melts or dissolves, the drug of inside can be quickly released. Compared with common suppositories, hollow suppositories have the advantages of fast drug release, high bioavailability and good preparation stability.

3. 泡腾栓 泡腾栓的基质中加入了发泡剂，遇到体液后可产生泡腾作用，有利于栓剂熔融和药物释放。发泡剂多由碳酸氢钠或碳酸钠与不同的有机酸组成，常用的有机酸有枸橼酸、酒石酸等。此类栓剂适合于黏膜皱襞较多的腔道内给药，尤其适用于阴道给药。

③ **Effervescent suppositories** Foaming agent is added to the bases of effervescent suppositories that can produce effervescent effect after encountering body fluids, and is beneficial to melting of suppositories and release of medicine. The foaming agent is mostly composed of sodium bicarbonate or sodium carbonate and different organic acids. Commonly used organic acids include citric acid, tartaric acid, etc. Such suppositories are suitable for intramucosal administration with more mucosal folds, especially for vaginal administration.

4. 其他缓释、控释栓

④ **Other sustained-release or controlled-release suppositories**

（1）微囊栓 将药物微囊化后与基质混合而制成的栓剂。微囊栓具有缓释作用，与普通栓剂相比，具有血药浓度稳定、维持时间长的特点。

a. Microcapsule suppositories It is a kind of suppositories that the drug is microencapsulated and mixed with bases. Microcapsule suppositories have the function of sustained release, and have the characteristics of stable blood concentration and long maintenance time compared with common suppositories.

（2）骨架控释栓 利用高分子物质为骨架材料，与药物混合制成的栓剂，具有控释作用。骨架材料在体内不溶解，体液渗入骨架内部，药物缓慢地溶解，从骨架材料中扩散、释放出来。

b. Framework controlled-release suppositories The suppositories made of macromolecular substances as framework materials and mixed with medicine have a controlled release effect. The

framework materials do not dissolve in the body, the body fluid penetrates into the framework, and the drug slowly dissolves, diffuses and is released from the framework materials.

（3）渗透泵栓 利用渗透泵原理制成的一种长效栓剂。由微孔膜、渗透压活性物质、半透膜及药物组成。纳入人体后，水分进入栓剂产生渗透压，药物透过半透膜上的微孔慢慢释放出来，可在一定时间内保持血药浓度稳定。

c. Osmotic pump suppositories It is a kind of long-acting suppositories based on the principle of osmotic pump. Osmotic pump suppositories are composed of microporous membrane, osmotic active substance, semi-permeable membrane and drugs. After entering the human body, suppositories contact with water to produce osmotic pressure, and the drug is slowly released through the micropores on the semi-permeable membrane, which can keep the blood concentration stable for a certain period of time.

（4）凝胶栓 利用凝胶为载体的栓剂，在体内逐渐吸收水分，缓慢膨胀，对生物黏膜具有黏合力，具有缓释作用，能延长药物的停留和释放时间，且柔软有弹性，无异物感。

d. Gel suppositories Refer to suppositories taking gel as carrier. They can slowly expand after absorbing water in the body, have adhesive force to biological mucosa and exert a slow-release effect that can prolong the drug retention time and release time. Such suppositories are soft and elastic, and can't cause foreign body sensation.

（5）海绵栓 系指海绵状栓剂，多为阴道用。其常用基质为明胶，所制得的栓剂在体内可以通过酶解吸收。此类栓剂可持久分散于腔道黏膜表面，药效维持时间长。

e. Sponge suppositories Refer to suppositories in the shape of a sponge and mostly used for vagina. It usually takes gelatin as bases, and the suppositories can be absorbed by enzymatic hydrolysis in human body. Such suppositories can be permanently dispersed on the mucous surface of cavity, and maintain efficacy for a long time.

四、栓剂中药物的吸收途径及其影响因素

11.1.4 Drug Absorption Pathways of Suppositories and Relevant Factors Affecting Absorption

（一）药物吸收途径

(1) Drug Absorption Pathways

以直肠给药发挥全身作用，通常通过以下两条途径：一条是经直肠上静脉经门静脉进入肝脏，肝脏代谢后进入体循环；另一条是通过直肠中、下静脉和肛门静脉，经髂内静脉绕过肝脏进入下腔静脉，直接入大循环起全身作用，如图 11-3 所示。通常而言，栓剂在应用时被塞入距肛门口约 2cm 处时，有 50%~70% 的药物可经直肠中下静脉吸收直接进入体循环，绕过肝脏，避免肝首过效应。研究表明，直肠淋巴系统也是栓剂中药物（尤其是大分子药物）吸收的一条途径。

Rectal administration can exert a systemic effect through the following two pathways: one is the drug entering liver through superior rectal vein and portal vein, and then getting into systemic circulation after liver metabolism; the other is the drug getting into inferior vena through middle rectal vein, inferior rectal vein, anal vein and internal iliac vein and bypassing the liver to enter systemic circulation for exerting systemic effect showed in Figure 11-3. The suppositories are generally inserted about 2cm from the anal opening; about 50%-70% of the drug can be absorbed through middle and inferior rectal veins, bypass the liver and directly enter the systemic circulation, and then can avoid liver first pass effect. Studies have

shown that rectal lymphatic system is also a way of absorbing drugs (especially macromolecular drugs) in suppositories.

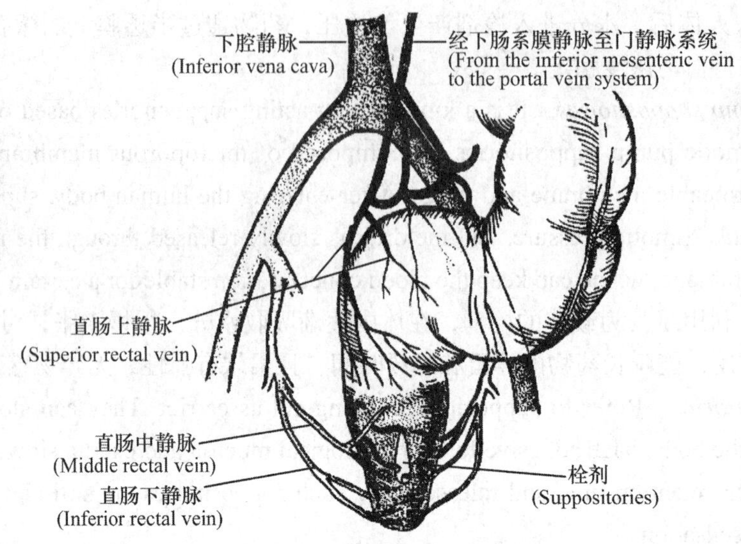

图 11-3 直肠给药的吸收途径

Figure 11-3 Absorption Pathways of Rectal Administration

（二）药物吸收的影响因素

(2) Factors Affecting Drug Absorption

1. 生理因素

① Physiological factors

直肠液中 pH 微环境对药物的吸收起着重要的作用。一般直肠液 pH 为 7.4，酶活性较低，且无缓冲能力。药物进入直肠后的 pH 取决于溶解的药物，其吸收的难易视环境 pH 对被溶解药物的影响而定。栓剂在直肠的保留时间越长，吸收越趋于完全。此外，直肠内如果存有粪便，也会影响药物的扩散从而影响药物吸收。因此给药前排便或灌肠可增加药物的吸收。

The pH microenvironment in rectal fluid plays an important role in drug absorption. The rectal solution has a pH value of 7.4, a low enzymatic activity, and no buffer capacity. The pH value after the drug entering the rectum depends on the dissolved drug, and the difficulty of absorption is subject to the effect of environmental pH value on the dissolved drug. The longer the suppository stays in the rectum, the more complete the absorption is. In addition, the presence of feces in the rectum can also affect drug diffusion and drug absorption. Therefore, defecation or enema before administration can increase drug absorption.

2. 药物因素 药物的影响因素主要有以下几个方面：①溶解度：药物水溶性较大时，易溶解于分泌液，利于吸收；溶解度小的药物则吸收少。难溶性药物应制成溶解度大的盐类或衍生物，以利于吸收；②粒度：以混悬、分散状态存在于栓剂中的药物，其粒度越小，分散度越大，越有利于吸收；③脂溶性与解离度：脂溶性药物较易吸收，非解离型药物比解离型药物容易吸收；pH 大于 4.3 的弱酸性药物或 pH 小于 8.5 的弱碱性药物，在直肠部位呈非解离型可被直肠黏膜迅速吸收。

② Drug factors The influencing factors of the drug mainly include the following aspects: ① Solubility: When the drug is more water-soluble, it can be easily dissolved in the secretion, which is

good for absorption; the drug with low solubility is less absorbed. So the insoluble drugs should be made into salts or derivatives with high solubility for absorption. ② Particle size: For the drug composition in the suppositories in suspension or dispersion state, the smaller the particle size, the greater the dispersion, and the more conducive to absorption. ③ Lipid solubility and degree of dissociation: Lipid-soluble drugs are more easily absorbed, while non-ionized drugs are more easily absorbed than ionized drugs. Weakly acidic drugs with a pH value greater than 4.3 or weakly alkaline drugs with a pH value less than 8.5 are non-dissociated in the rectal area and can be quickly absorbed by the rectal mucosa.

3. 基质因素　对于发挥全身作用的栓剂，药物要被吸收，须先从基质中释放出来。由于基质种类和性质的不同，药物释放的速度也不同。一般应根据药物性质选择与药物溶解性相反的基质，有利于药物释放，增加吸收。水溶性药物分散于油脂性基质中，药物能较快释放或分散至分泌液中，故吸收较快。如果药物是脂溶性的，则通常选择水溶性基质。

③ **Bases factors**　For suppositories exerting systemic effects, they must be released from the bases followed by being absorbed. Drugs are released at different rates depending on the type and nature of bases. Generally, the selected bases should be opposite to the solubility of the drug according to the nature of drug, which is conducive to the drug release and can increase absorption. Water-soluble drugs is dispersed in the lipid bases that the drugs can be released or dispersed into the secretion fluid relatively quickly, and therefore absorbed quickly. If the drug is lipid-soluble, the water soluble bases should be selected.

表面活性剂可增加药物的亲水性，加速药物向分泌液转移，有助于药物的释放吸收，但表面活性剂浓度不宜过高，以免形成胶束，阻碍药物释放，反而不利于吸收。

Surfactant can increase the hydrophilicity of the drug, accelerate the transfer of the drug to the secretion, and facilitate the release and absorption of the drugs. However, the concentration of surfactant should not be too high, so as to avoid the formation of micelles, which can block the release of drugs, and is not conducive to absorption.

第二节　栓剂的基质与附加剂

11.2　Bases and Additives in Suppositories

PPT

栓剂主要由药物与基质组成。药物加入后可溶于基质，也可混悬于基质。基质不仅有助于药物成型，且对药物的释放和吸收有重要影响。此外，为改变栓剂的物理性状或改善药物的吸收、提高稳定性，栓剂中往往要加入一些附加剂，如吸收促进剂、乳化剂、增塑剂、防腐剂等。

Suppositories are primarily composed of drugs and bases. The drugs are required to be soluble or uniformly suspended in bases, which has the benefit of not only yielding a positive effect on drugs shape, but also facilitates the release and absorption of the drugs. In addition, appropriate additives are contained in suppositories to change their physical properties or improve the absorption and stability of drugs; typically these are absorption promoters, emulsifiers, plasticizers, preservatives, and the like.

一、基质的要求

11.2.1 Requirements of Bases

优良的栓剂基质应符合下列要求：①在室温下具有适宜的硬度，塞入腔道时不变形、不碎裂。在体温条件下易软化、融化或溶解；②对黏膜无刺激性、毒性和过敏性；③本身性质稳定，与药物混合后不发生反应，不影响主药的作用与含量测定；④具有润湿或乳化能力，能混入较多的水；⑤油脂性基质的酸价应在 0.2 以下，皂化价应在 200~245 之间，碘价低于 7，熔点与凝固点之差要小。

A suitable suppository base should meet the following requirements: ① appropriately firm at room temperature with no deformation or chipping when inserted into the body/bodily cavity, but easily soften, melt and dissolve at body temperature; ② non-irritating, toxic or allergic to mucous membranes; ③ stable in nature, and without affecting the function and chemical content determination of the main drugs after being mixed with other supplementary drugs; ④ be able to add more water into drug content in line with with the wetting or emulsifying ability; ⑤ for oleaginous bases, the acid value should be below 0.2, the saponification value between 200 and 245, and the iodine value less than 7; the difference between melting point and freezing point needs to be small.

二、基质的种类

11.2.2 The Classification of Bases

常用的栓剂基质分为油脂性基质和水溶性基质两大类。

Bases are normally classified as oleaginous and water-soluble bases.

（一）油脂性基质

(1) Oleaginous Bases

1. 天然油脂 由某些天然植物的种仁提取精制而得。

① **Natural grease** This type is refined from the seeds of certain natural plants, such as the following:

（1）可可豆脂 系从梧桐科植物可可树种仁中得到的一种固体脂肪，主要含硬脂酸、棕榈酸、油酸、亚油酸和月桂酸的甘油酯。可可豆脂为天然产物，是最早应用的栓剂基质。常温下为白色或淡黄色脆性蜡状固体，可塑性好，无刺激性，熔点为 31~34℃，加热至 25℃开始软化，在体温下能迅速融化。

a. Cocoa butter This is a solid fat extracted from the seeds of the cocoa tree (terculiaceae family), which mainly contains stearic acid, palmitic acid, oleic acid, linoleic acid and lauric acid. Cocoa butter is a natural product and is the earliest used suppository base. At room temperature, it is a white or pale yellow brittle waxy solid with good plasticity and no irritation. The melting point is 31-34℃ and it can be softened by heating to 25℃ and melt quickly at body temperature.

可可豆脂因所含酸的比例不同，组成甘油酯混合物的熔点不同。可可豆脂具有同质多晶性，有 α、β、β′、γ 四种晶型，其中 α、γ 晶型不稳定，熔点分别为 22℃和 18℃，β 晶型较稳定，其熔点为 34℃，晶型之间可随温度不同而发生相互转化。为避免影响栓剂的成型，制备时通常缓慢升温，待基质融化至 2/3 时停止加热，利用余热使其全部融化，以避免晶型的转化。

Glyceride mixtures containing cocoa butter have different melting points due to the different proportion of acids. Cocoa butter has homogeneous polymorphism and has four crystalline forms of α, β, β′ and γ, of which α and γ are unstable with melting points of 22℃ and 18℃ respectively. While β is relatively stable with a melting point of 34℃, the crystalline forms can transform with different temperatures. The heating process is usually slow in preparation to prevent problems in suppositories moulding. The base should be removed from the heat when it melts to 2/3, and residual heat is used to make it melt completely to avoid the transformation of crystal form.

可可豆脂产量少，价格较贵，其代用品有香果脂、乌桕脂等。

With a low yield and high cost, cocoa butter is commonly substituted by oleum linderae and oleum sapii.

（2）香果脂　由樟科植物香果树的成熟种仁脂肪油精制而成。为白色结晶性粉末或淡黄色固体块状物，气微，味淡。熔点为 30~34℃，温度高于 25℃开始软化，与乌桕脂配合使用可克服易于软化的缺点。

b. Oleum Linderae　This type is refined from mature seed kernel oil of Emmenopterys Henryi (Lauraceae family). It is a white crystalline powder or a light yellow lump with faint smell and flat/plain taste. The melting point is between 30 and 34℃, and the softening starts when the temperature is higher than 25℃. The disadvantage of easy softening can be overcome when used in combination with oleum sapii.

（3）乌桕脂　由乌桕科植物乌桕树的种子外层固体脂肪精制而成。为白色或黄白色固体，味特臭而无刺激性。熔点 38~42℃，软化点 31.5~34℃。释药速度较可可豆脂缓慢。

c. Oleum Sapii　It is prepared from solid fat on the outer layer of seeds of sapium sebiferum (triadica sebifera) of family sapium sebiferum. It is a white or yellowish-white solid, with an unpleasant odour but not irritating. It's melting point is in the range 38-42℃ with a softening point between 31.5-34℃. The drug release rate of oleum sapii is slower than that of cocoa butter.

2. 半合成与全合成脂肪酸甘油酯　半合成脂肪酸甘油酯系由天然植物油（如椰子油或棕榈油等）水解、分馏所得 C_{12}~C_{18} 游离脂肪酸，经部分氢化再与甘油酯化而得的甘油三酯、二酯、一酯的混合酯。由于所含的不饱和碳链较少，不易酸败，化学性质稳定，成型性能良好，具有适宜熔点，为目前取代天然油脂较理想的栓剂基质。国内已投产的有半合成椰油酯、半合成山苍子油酯、半合成棕榈油酯等。现已广泛应用。全合成脂肪酸甘油酯有硬脂酸丙二醇酯等。

② **Semi-synthetic and full synthetic fatty glycerides**　Semi-synthetic fatty acid glycerides is a mixed ester of triglycerides, diglycerides and monoglycerides obtained by partially hydrogenating C_{12}-C_{18} free fatty acids, which are extracted from natural vegetable oils (such as coconut oil or palm oil) through the process of hydrolyzing and fractionating, and then esterifying with glycerin. Due to less unsaturated carbon chains, less rancidity, stable chemical properties, good molding performance and suitable melting point, it is an ideal suppository base to replace natural oils, at present. Domestic production as semi-synthetic coconut ester, semi-synthetic cubeba oil ester, semi-synthetic palmitate and so on, now has been widely used. Full synthetic fatty acid glycerides include glycol stearate, and the like.

（1）半合成椰油酯　由椰油、硬脂酸与甘油酯化而成。为乳白色或黄白色蜡状固体，熔点为 33~41℃，凝固点为 31~36℃，有油脂臭，刺激性小。

a. Semi-synthetic coconut ester　Coconut ester is derived from coconut oil, stearic acid and glycerin. It is a milky white or yellowish white waxy solid with melting point at 33-41℃, freezing point at 31-36℃, oily odour and little irritation.

（2）半合成山苍子油酯　由山苍子油水解、分离得月桂酸，再加硬脂酸与甘油经酯化而成。为黄色或乳白色块状物，具油脂光泽。三种单酯混合比例不同，成品的熔点也不同，有 34 型（33~35℃）、36 型（35~37℃）、38 型（37~39℃）、40 型（39~41℃）等不同规格，其中 38 型最

为常用。

b. Semi-synthetic litsea cubeba oil ester Litsea cubeba oil ester is an esterified mixture of lauric acid, stearic acid and glycerin, in which lauric acid is obtained by hydrolyzing and extracting litsea cubeba oil. It is a yellow or milky white lump with a greasy luster. Since the mixing ratios of the three monoesters vary, the melting points of the finished product are also different. They are as follows: 34 type (33-35℃), 36 type (35-37℃), 38 type (37-39℃), 40 type (39-41℃), and other different specifications, of which 38 type are most commonly used.

（3）半合成棕榈油酯 由棕榈油经碱化、酸化加入硬脂酸与甘油经酯化而得。本品为乳白色固体，熔点为 33~39℃，抗热能力强，对直肠和阴道无影响。

c. Semi-synthetic palmitate Semi-synthetic Palmitate is esterified from alkalized and acidified palm oil, stearic acid and glycerin. This product is a milky white solid with melting point in the range of 33-39℃ with strong heat resistance, and which has no undue influence on the rectum or vagina.

（4）硬脂酸丙二醇酯 由硬脂酸与 1，2- 丙二醇经酯化而得，是硬脂酸丙二醇单酯与双酯的混合物，为乳白色固体或黄色蜡状固体，略有脂肪臭。水中不溶，遇热水可膨胀，熔点 36~38℃，对腔道黏膜无明显的刺激性。

d. Glycol stearate Glycol stearate is obtained by esterification of stearic acid and 1,2-propanediol, and it is a mixture of Propylene glycol stearate and diester. It is a milky white or yellow waxy solid with slight fatty odour. It is insoluble in water, but with a melting point of 36-38℃it is easy to swell in hot water; it has no obvious irritation to lumen mucosa.

3. 氢化植物油 由植物油部分或全部氢化而得的白色固体脂肪。如氢化棉子油（熔点 40.5~41℃）、部分氢化棉子油（熔点 35~39℃）、氢化椰子油（熔点 34~37℃）、氢化花生油等。性质稳定，无毒，无刺激性，不易酸败，价廉，但释药能力较差，加入适量表面活性剂可以改善。

③ Hydrogenated vegetable oil Hydrogenated vegetable oil is a white solid fat obtained by partial or complete hydrogenation of vegetable oil. Typical examples are hydrogenated cottonseed oil (melting point 40.5-41℃), some hydrogenated cottonseed oil (melting point 35-39℃), hydrogenated coconut oil (melting point 34-37℃), hydrogenated peanut oil, etc. It is stable in nature, non-toxic, non-irritant, not easy to rancidity, low in price, but poor in drug release ability; however, if a proper amount of surfactant is added, it will be improved.

（二）水溶性基质

(2) Soluble Bases

1. 甘油明胶 系用明胶、甘油与水以一定比例加热融合，滤过，放冷，凝固而成。本品具有很好的弹性，不易折断，体温下不融化，但可软化并缓慢溶于腔道分泌液中，释放药物缓慢。其溶解速度与明胶、甘油及水三者用量有关，甘油与水含量越高越容易溶解，通常水分含量控制在 10% 以下。

① Gelatin glecerin Gelatin, glycerin and water are heated and fused in a certain proportion, and then through filtration, cooling and solidification process gelatin glecerin is made. With good elasticity, this product is hard to break; it does not melt at body temperature, but can soften and slowly dissolve in cavity fluids to release the drug slowly. The dissolution rate is related to the dosage of gelatin, glycerol and water. The higher the content of glycerol and water, the easier it is to dissolve, usually the water content is controlled below 10%.

本品多用作阴道栓剂基质，因明胶是胶原的水解产物，凡与蛋白质能产生配伍变化的药物如鞣酸、重金属盐等均不能用甘油明胶作基质。此外以本品为基质制备的栓剂在贮存时应注意其失

水性和霉菌污染，需添加适量抑菌剂。

This product is widely used as the base of vaginal suppositories. Since gelatin is the hydrolysate of collagen, glycerol gelatin cannot be used as the base for drugs that produce compatibility changes with protein, such as tannic acid and heavy metal salts. In addition, water loss and mold contamination during storage may occur to suppositories prepared with this product as the base, so appropriate amount of bacteriostatic agents should be added.

2. 聚乙二醇类 为乙二醇高分子聚合物的总称，具有不同的聚合度、分子量和物理性状。相对分子量在 200~600 者为无色透明液体，随着分子量增加逐渐呈半固体或固体，熔点也随之升高。常用的如 PEG1000、PEG1540、PEG4000、PE6000，其熔点分别为 38~40℃、42~46℃、53~56℃、55~63℃。通常用不同分子量的 PEG 以一定比例加热熔融，制得适当硬度的栓剂基质。

本品无生理作用，体温下不熔化，但能缓缓溶于体液而释放药物，对黏膜有一定刺激性，加入约 20%的水，可减轻其刺激性；吸湿性较强，应采用防潮包装并贮存于干燥处。

② **Polyethylene glycols, PEG** Polyethylene glycols, PEG is a general term for ethylene glycol polymer with different polymerization degrees, molecular weights and physical properties. If the molecular weight is 200 ~ 600, it is a colorless and transparent liquid. As the molecular weight increases, it gradually becomes semi-solid or solid, and the melting point also increases. Common varieties such as PEG1000, PEG1540, PEG4000 and PE6000 have melting points of 38-40℃, 42-46℃, 53-56℃ and 55-63℃, respectively. PEG with different molecular weights are usually heated and melted in a certain proportion to prepare suppositories bases of appropriate hardness.

3. 聚氧乙烯（40）硬脂酸酯类 商品名为 Myrj52，商品代号 S-40，系聚乙二醇的单硬脂酸酯和二硬脂酸酯的混合物，呈白色或淡黄色蜡状固体。熔点 39~45℃，可溶于水、乙醇、丙酮等，与 PEG 混合使用可制备释放性能较好、性质稳定的栓剂。

③ **Polyoxyl 40 stearate** The trade mark is Myrj52, trade number S-40, it is a mixture of monostearate and distearate of polyethylene glycol, as a white or yellowish waxy solid, with melting point of 39-45℃. It is soluble in water, ethanol, acetone, etc. Suppositories with good release and stable properties can be prepared by mixing it with PEG.

4. 泊洛沙姆 系聚氧乙烯和聚氧丙烯的嵌段聚合物，本品有多种型号，随聚合度增大，物态呈液体、半固体至蜡状固体，易溶于水。较常用型号为 188 型，商品名为 Pluronic F68，熔点为 52℃，能促进药物吸收并起到缓释与延效的作用。

④ **Poloxamer** This is a block polymer of polyoxyethylene and polypropylene oxide with many types. With the increase of the polymerization degree, it is liquid, semi-solid to waxy solid and soluble in water. The most commonly used types are model 188 (trade mark Pluronic F68); its melting point of 52℃ can promote the drug absorption as well as slow release to prolong the effect.

三、栓剂的附加剂

11.2.3 Additives in Suppositories

除基质外，栓剂的处方中，常根据不同目的需要加入一些附加剂。

Some additives are often added to the prescription of suppositories for different purposes, in addition to bases.

1. 吸收促进剂 起全身作用的栓剂，为增加药物的全身吸收，可加入吸收促进剂。常用的有：①非离子型表面活性剂：在基质中加入适量的非离子型表面活性剂，可增加药物的亲水

性，促进药物与基质的混合，改善药物的吸收，提高生物利用度，如聚山梨酯-80；②氮酮类（Azone）：氮酮作为一种常用的透皮吸收促进剂，已用于栓剂。可改变生物膜的通透性，增加药物的亲水性，有利于药物的释放、吸收；③其他：脂肪酸、脂肪醇、脂肪酸酯类、羧甲基纤维素钠、环糊精衍生物等也可作为吸收促进剂。

(1) Absorption promoters Suppositories of systemic effect can be added with absorption promoters to increase systemic absorption of drugs. Commonly used types are: ① Nonionic surfactants: a proper amount of nonionic surfactant added into the base can increase the hydrophilicity of the drug, it will promote the mixing of the drug and the base, improve the absorption of the drug, and increase the bioavailability, such as Polysorbate 80; ② Azone: Azone, as a widespread transdermal absorption promoter used in suppositories, can change the permeability of biofilms, increase the hydrophilicity of drugs, as well as facilitate the release and absorption of drugs; ③ others include: fatty acids, fatty alcohols, fatty acid esters, carboxymethylcellulose sodium(CMC-Na), cyclodextrin derivatives, etc. can also be used as absorption promoters.

2. 吸收阻滞剂 缓释栓剂的制备中可加入吸收阻滞剂，如海藻酸、羟丙基甲基纤维素、硬脂酸、蜂蜡、磷脂等。

(2) Absorption blockers Absorption blockers such as alginate acid, hydroxypropyl methyl cellulose (HPMC), stearic acid, beeswax, phospholipid, etc. can be added in the preparation of sustained release suppositories.

3. 乳化剂 当栓剂处方中含有与基质不相混溶的液相时，可考虑加入适量的乳化剂，如聚山梨酯-80、十二烷基硫酸钠等。

(3) Emulsifiers When the suppository prescription contains a liquid phase that is immiscible with the base, appropriate amounts of emulsifiers such as polysorbate 80 and sodium dodecyl sulfate can be added.

4. 增塑剂 加入适量的增塑剂可使脂肪性基质具有弹性，降低脆性，防止栓剂破裂，如聚山梨酯-80、脂肪酸甘油酯、蓖麻油、甘油、丙二醇等。

(4) Plasticizers Adding a proper volume of plasticizer will increase the elasticity of fatty bases, and reduce the brittleness to prevent the rupture of suppositories, such as polysorbate 80, fatty glycerides, castor oil, glycerin, propanediol, etc.

5. 硬度调节剂 ①硬化剂：白蜡、鲸蜡醇、硬脂酸、巴西棕榈蜡等，可防止栓剂在运输、贮存和使用过程中软化；②增稠剂：氢化蓖麻油、单硬脂酸甘油酯等可调节药物释放。

(5) Hardness modifiers ① Hardening agents: white wax, cetyl alcohol, stearic acid, carnauba wax, etc. can prevent suppositories from softening during transportation, storage and application; ② Thickening agents: hydrogenated castor oil, glyceryl monostearate, etc. can regulate the drug release.

6. 抗氧剂 易氧化的药物可加入抗氧剂，提高栓剂的稳定性，如没食子酸、间苯二酚、维生素C等。

(6) Antioxidants Antioxidants can be added to easily oxidative drugs to improve the stability of suppositories, such as gallic acid, resorcinol, vitamin C, etc.

7. 防腐剂 加入适量的防腐剂可防止水溶性基质或含有中药浸膏的栓剂霉变，如对羟基苯甲酸酯类、苯甲酸钠、三氯叔丁醇等。

(7) Preservatives Adding appropriate amounts of preservatives, such as parabens, sodium benzoate, chlorobutanol, etc., can prevent water-soluble bases from mildewing.

四、栓剂基质与附加剂的选用

11.2.4 Selection of Bases and Additives in Suppositories

栓剂基质与附加剂的选用要考虑以下几点：①用药目的，如是起局部治疗还是全身治疗作用；②用药部位，如是阴道给药还是直肠给药；③药物的理化性质，如药物的形态、在基质中的溶解或分散情况；④适宜的基质与附加剂，可控制药物的释放与吸收。

The selection of bases and additives in suppositories should consider the following points: ① the purpose of medication, whether it is local treatment or systemic treatment; ② the part of body for administration, whether the drug is administered vaginally or rectally; ③ the physiochemical nature of drugs, such as drug morphology, dissolution or dispersion in bases; ④ appropriate bases and additives can control the release and absorption of drugs.

（一）基质的选用

(1) Selection of Bases

1. 根据临床治疗目的选用基质 栓剂在临床上使用通常可起到局部治疗和全身治疗作用，用于局部作用的栓剂要求释药缓慢持久，可选用融化或溶解速度慢的基质，但基质液化时间不宜过长，否则不利于药物释放完全，同时使患者感到不适；用于全身作用的栓剂要求释药迅速，可选用融化或溶解速度快的基质。

① On the Purpose of Clinical Treatment Suppositories can exert local and systemic effects for clinical treatment. For local effect, slow and sustained drugs release is required, so bases with measured melting or dissolution speed can be selected. However, the liquefaction time of bases can't be too long, otherwise it will not be conducive to the complete release and it also makes patients feel uncomfortable. Those suppositories required for systemic effect need rapid drugs release, therefore bases with fast melting or dissolution speed can be selected.

常用基质纳入人体腔道后的液化时间，见表 11-1。

Table 11-1 below shows liquefaction times of common bases after being incorporated into human cavities.

表 11-1 常用基质纳入人体腔道后的液化时间

基质	可可豆脂	半合成椰油酯	一般脂肪性基质	甘油明胶	聚乙二醇
液化时间（min）	4~5	4~5	10	30~50	30~50

Table 11-1 Liquefaction Times of Common Bases into Human Cavities

Bases	Cocoa butter	Coconut ester	General fatty bases	Gelatin glecerin	Polyethylene glycols
Liquefaction Times (min)	4-5	4-5	10	30-50	30-50

2. 根据药物的理化性质选用基质 ①药物在基质中的溶解情况直接影响药物的释放与吸收。一般而言，药物在基质中的溶解度越大，越不利于药物释放。因此，要保证栓剂中药物的快速释放与吸收，通常应选择与药物溶解性相反的基质，即一般水溶性药物选择脂溶性基质，脂溶性药物选择水溶性基质。②含有稠浸膏的栓剂，可考虑选择水溶性基质或采用适量羊毛脂吸收后与油脂性基质混合，以利于药物的分散。

② On the Physiochemical Nature of Drugs The dissolution of drugs in bases directly affects its release and absorption. In general, the higher the solubility of the drug in the base, the more unfavorable

the drug release. Therefore, bases with the opposing drugs solubility should be selected to ensure the rapid release and absorption of drugs in suppositories, i.e. water-soluble bases should be selected for general oleaginous-soluble drugs and conversely oleaginous-soluble bases for water-soluble drugs. Suppositories containing thick extract may select water-soluble bases or choose to mix with oleaginous bases after its absorption with appropriate amounts of lanolin to facilitate drug dispersion.

（二）附加剂的选用

(2) Selection of Additives

在确定基质种类和用量的同时，以外观、色泽、光洁度、硬度、稳定性或体外释放度等为指标，选择适宜的附加剂，以筛选出适宜的基质配方。

While determining the type and dosage of bases, the appropriate additives are selected by taking the appearance, color, smoothness, hardness, stability, or release in vitro as indicators, to screen out the suitable base formula.

（三）置换价

(3) Displacement Value

置换价系指药物的重量与同体积基质的重量之比。在栓剂的生产中，通常栓剂模型的容量是固定的，但栓剂的重量随基质与药物密度的不同而有区别。为使栓剂含药量准确，必须测定置换价，从而准确计算基质用量。

Displacement value (DV) refers to the ratio of the weight of the main drugs to the weight of the same volume of bases. In suppository production, the volume of the same model is equal, but the quality of the prepared suppository varies with the density of bases and drugs. It is necessary to determine the displacement value, in order to determine the base dosage of different suppositories and ensure the accuracy of the drugs dosage.

测定方法如下：制纯基质栓，称其平均重量为 G，另制药物含量为 $X\%$ 的含药栓，得平均重量为 M，每粒平均含药量为 $W=M\times X\%$，则可计算某药物对某基质的置换价 f。置换价在栓剂生产中对保证投料的准确性有重要意义。

The determination method is as follows: After making several pure base suppositories, weigh them to get the average weight of each pure base suppository G; then prepare some suppositories with drug content of $X\%$ and the average weight of each is M, so the average drug content per pill is $W=M\times X\%$, therefore the displacement value f of drugs to bases can be calculated. Displacement value is of great significance to ensure the accuracy of dosage in suppository production.

公式（11-1）为置换价 f 的计算公式。

Formula (11-1) below can be used to calculate the displacement value f:

$$f=\frac{W}{G-(M-W)} \tag{11-1}$$

式中，G 为纯基质栓每粒平均重量，M 为含药栓每粒平均重量，$M-W$ 为含药栓中基质的重量，$G-(M-W)$ 为两种栓中基质的重量之差，W 为含药栓中每粒平均含药量，即药物同体积的基质的重量。

Wherein G is the weight of each pure base suppository, M is the weight of each drug-containing suppository, $M-W$ is the weight of the base in each drug-containing suppository, $G-(M-W)$ is the weight difference of the base in two kinds suppositories, W is the weight of the drug in each suppository, that is, the weight of the base with the same volume of the drug.

案例导入 | Case example

案例 11-1 置换价计算

11-1 The Calculation of Displacement Value

已知某厂生产的鞣酸栓，每粒含鞣酸 0.2g，以可可豆油为基质，模孔重量为 2.0g，由文献查得，鞣酸对可可豆油的置换价为 1.6。求每枚栓的实际重量是多少克？制备鞣酸栓 1000 枚，需基质多少克？

The given tannic acid suppository produced by a factory contains 0.2g of tannic acid each grain, using cocoa butter as the base, and the volume of the mould is 2.0g. From the literature, the displacement value of tannic acid to cocoa butter is 1.6. How to find the actual weight of each suppository? How many grams of the base is required to prepare 1000 tannic acid suppositories?

解：已知，$G = 2.0\text{g}$　$W = 0.2\text{g}$　$f = 1.6$

Answer: Given $G = 2.0\text{g}$　$W = 0.2\text{g}$　$f = 1.6$

①求得含药栓每粒的实际重量

① Calculate the actual weight of each drug-containing suppository

因为（Because），$f = \dfrac{W}{G-(M-W)}$

所以（So），$M = (G + W) - W/f = (2 + 0.2) - 0.2/1.6 = 2.075\text{g}$

即，每粒栓的实际重量为 2.075g。

That is, the actual weight of each suppository is 2.075g.

②生产 1000 枚鞣酸栓所需基质重量

② The weight of the base required to prepare 1000 tannic acid suppositories is:

$(2.075 - 0.2) \times 1000 = 1875\text{g}$

实际生产中还应考虑到操作过程中的损耗。

In the practical production, the loss during operation should also be taken into consideration.

第三节 栓剂的制法

11.3 Preparation of Suppositories

PPT

一、一般栓剂的制法

11.3.1 Preparation of General Suppositories

栓剂的常用制备方法有两种，即冷压法与热熔法。其中热熔法最为常用，水溶性基质与油脂性基质均可采用该法制备。

The suppositories are commonly prepared by cold molding method and fusion method, of which the latter one is the most commonly used, especially for water-soluble bases and greasy bases.

冷压法仅适用于油脂质性基质，是将药物与基质的粉末置于冷容器内，混合均匀，然后装入制栓机内压制成一定形状的栓剂。冷压法可避免加热对主药或基质所产生的稳定性影响，但目前生产上已较少采用。

Cold molding method is only applicable to the greasy bases that put the powder of drug and bases into a cold container, mix them evenly, and then put them into a suppository machine to press the suppositories in a certain shape. The cold molding method can avoid the influence of heating on the stability of the main drug or bases, but it is seldom used in production.

（一）热熔法工艺流程（图 11-4）

(1) Process Flow Chart by Fusion Method (Figure 11-4)

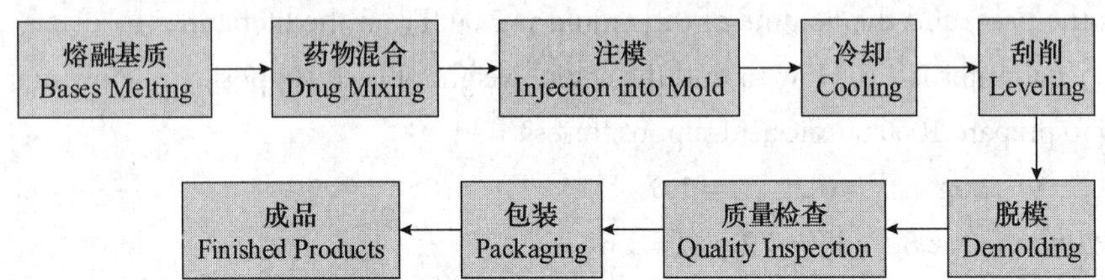

图 11-4　热熔法制备栓剂的一般工艺流程

Figure 11-4　General Preparation Process Flow of Suppositories by Fusion Method

（二）热熔法的制备过程

(2) Preparation Process by Fusion Method

1. 栓模准备

① Preparation of suppository mold

（1）栓模的选用　通常需根据不同栓剂的用药途径及制备工艺选择合适的栓模，并进行清洗干燥，备用。栓剂制备的常用模具如图 11-5 所示。

a. Selection of suppository mold　Usually, based on administration routes and preparation processes of different suppositories, the appropriate molds should be selected, washed and dried for further use. The commonly used molds are shown is Figure 11-5.

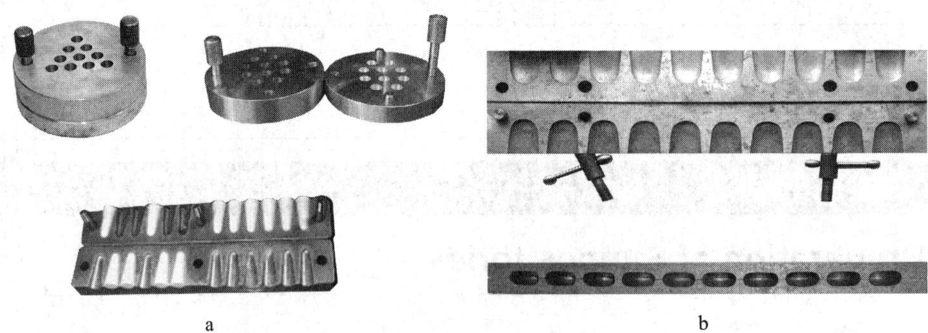

图 11-5　栓剂制备的常用模具

Figure 11-5　Common Molds for Preparation of Suppositories

a. 肛门栓模具（Molds for rectal suppositories）　b. 阴道栓模具（Molds for vaginal suppositories）

（2）润滑剂的选用　为了使栓剂冷却成型后便于脱模，制备时常在模孔内侧涂布少量润滑剂，可可豆脂、聚乙二醇类本身不黏模，可不用润滑剂。常用的润滑剂通常有两种：①用于油脂性基质的润滑剂：软肥皂、甘油各 1 份与 90% 乙醇 5 份混合制成的醇溶液；②用于水溶性基质的润滑剂：液状石蜡或植物油等油类物质。

b. Selection of lubricant In order to make the suppositories easy to take off the molds after cooling and molding, a small amount of lubricants is often applied on the inside of the mold hole during preparation. Cocoa butter and polyethylene glycol are not sticky, and lubricants are not required. There are generally two kinds of commonly used lubricants: Lubricants for greasy bases: Alcohol solution made by mixing one part of soft soap and one part of glycerin with five parts of 90% ethanol; Lubricants for water-soluble bases: Oil substances such as paraffin or vegetable oil.

2. 药物的处理与混合 在栓剂制备过程中，药物与基质混合方法及混合前药物的处理十分重要，以免混合不均匀影响栓剂的内在品质和制剂的外观。

② **Drug processing and mixing** During preparation of suppositories, the method of mixing the drug with bases and the drug processing before mixing are very important, so as to avoid uneven mixing affecting the intrinsic quality of the suppositories and the appearance of the preparations.

（1）油溶性药物 如樟脑、中药醇提物等可直接混入已熔化的油脂性基质中，使之溶解。若添加的药量过大使基质的熔点降低或使栓剂变得过软，可加入适量石蜡或蜂蜡调节硬度。

a. Oil-soluble drugs Such as camphor and Chinese medicine alcohol extracts, etc. They can be directly mixed into the melted oily bases for dissolution. If the added drug dosage is too large to reduce the melting point of the bases or make the suppositories too soft, an appropriate amount of paraffin wax or beeswax can be added to adjust the hardness.

（2）水溶性药物 水溶性稠浸膏、生物碱盐等可直接溶解于已熔化的水溶性基质中或用少量水制成浓溶液，用适量羊毛脂吸收后与油脂性基质混合。

b. Water-soluble drugs Water-soluble thickened extract and alkaloid salt can be directly dissolved in the melted water-soluble bases or prepare concentrated solution with a small amount of water, and then mix it with oily bases after being absorbed with an appropriate amount of lanolin.

（3）难溶性药物 如中药细粉、某些浸膏粉、矿物药等，应研制成最细粉，过七号筛后，再采用等量递增法与基质混合。

c. Poorly water-soluble drugs Such as traditional Chinese medicine fine powder, some extract powders, mineral drug, etc. They should be grinded into the very fine powders, sieved by No. 7 sieve, and then mixed with bases by the equal increment method.

（4）含挥发油的中药 所含的挥发油量大时可考虑加入适宜的乳化剂与水溶性基质混合，制成乳剂型栓。

d. Traditional Chinese medicine containing volatile oil When the amount of volatile oil is large, suitable emulsifier can be added to mix with water-soluble bases and prepare the suppositories in emulsion type.

3. 栓剂的成型 制备小量栓剂一般采用手工灌模的方法。将熔融的含药基质，倾入预热好并预先涂有润滑剂的栓模中（稍微溢出模口为度），静置冷却，待完全凝固后，削去溢出部分，脱模，即得栓剂。大量生产采用自动化制栓机，填充、冷却、排出、清洁模具等操作均可自动化完成。典型的自动旋转式制栓机如图 11-6 所示，产量为每小时 3500~6000 粒。

③ **Molding of suppositories** Small quantities of suppositories are usually prepared by manual mold filling. The fused drug-containing bases are poured into the pre-heated and pre-lubricated suppository mold (slightly overflow the die orifice); let it cool, wait for complete solidification, cut off the overflow part, release from the mold and get the suppositories. Automatic suppository-preparation machine is used for mass production. The operations such as filling, cooling, discharging, mold cleaning can be done automatically. The production capacity of typical automatic rotary suppository-preparation machine is 3,500-6,000 suppositories per hour, the machine is shown in Figure 11-6.

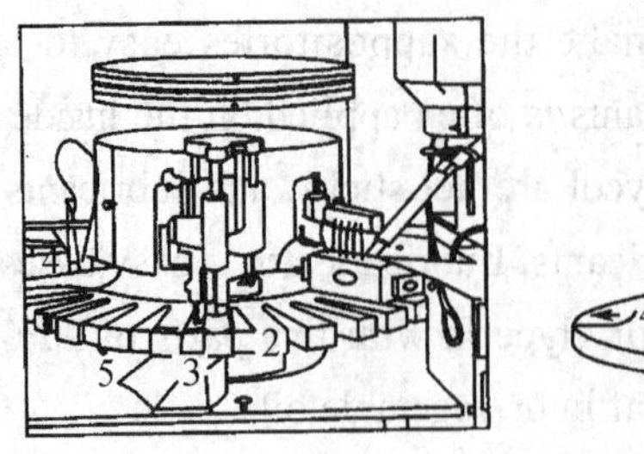

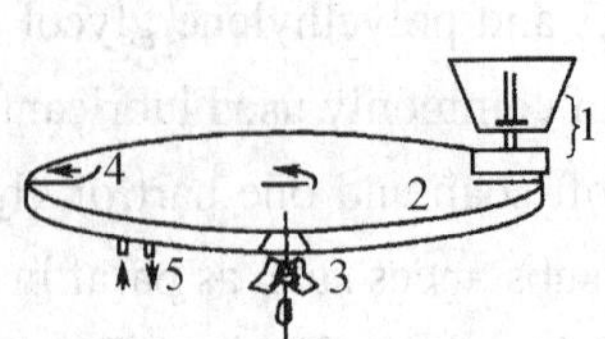

图 11-6　自动旋转式制栓机

Figure 11-6　Automatic Rotary Suppository-Preparation Machine

1. 饲料装置及加料斗　2. 旋转式冷却台　3. 栓剂抛出台　4. 刮削设备　5. 冷冻剂入口及出口

1. Feeder and hopper　2. Rotary cooling table　3. Suppository casting table　4. Scraping equipment　5. Freezer inlet and outlet

（三）注意事项

(3) Notes

1. 熔融基质温度不宜过高，熔融时最好采用水浴或蒸汽浴以免基质局部过热。加热时间不宜太长（有 2/3 量基质熔融时即可停止加热）以减少基质的物理性状改变。

① The temperature of fused bases should not be too high. It is best to use water bath or steam bath when fusing to avoid local overheating of the bases. The heating time should not be too long (stop heating when 2/3 bases is melted), so as to reduce the physical properties change of the bases.

2. 注模时温度不宜过高，防止不溶性药物及其他与基质相对密度不同的组分沉降在模孔中。注模时为避免发生液流或液层凝固，应操作迅速并一次完成。

② The temperature should not be too high during molding to prevent insoluble drugs and other components with different relative density from the bases from settling in the mold holes. The operation should be done quickly in one time, in order to avoid liquid flow or liquid layer solidification during molding.

3. 冷却温度不宜过低、冷却时间不宜过长，以防栓剂严重收缩、碎裂。

③ The cooling temperature should not be too low, and the cooling time should not be too long, so as to prevent suppositories from severe contraction or splintering.

案例导入 | Case example

案例 11-2　化痔栓

11-2　Hemorrhoid suppository

处方：次没食子酸铋 200g　苦参 370g　黄柏 92.5g　洋金花 55.5g　冰片 30g

Formula: Bismuth subgallate 200g; Sophora flavescens 370g; Phellodendron 92.5g; Datura metel 55.5g; Borneol 30g

功能与主治：清热燥湿，收涩止血。用于大肠湿热所致的内外痔、混合痔疮。

Functions and indications: Clears heat and dry dampness, has a significant effect to stop bleeding. For treatment of internal and external hemorrhoids and mixed hemorrhoids caused by damp and heat of large intestine.

制法：以上五味，苦参、黄柏、洋金花加水煎煮二次，第一次 4 小时，第二次 2 小时，合并煎液，滤过，静置 12 小时，取上清液浓缩至相对密度为 1.12(60~65℃）的清膏，干燥，粉碎成最细粉；将 2.6g 的羟苯乙酯用适量乙醇溶解；另取混合脂肪酸甘油酯、蜂蜡适量，加热熔化，加入次没食子酸铋、上述最细粉、冰片以及 16.8g 聚山梨酯 -80、羟苯乙酯乙醇液，混匀、灌注，制成 1000 粒，即得。

Making Procedure: Above five flavors: Sophora flavescens, Phellodendron and Datura metel are decocted twice with water, the first time for 4 hours, and the second time for 2 hours. Mix the decoction, filter the solution, and let it stand for 12 hours. Take the supernatant and concentrate it to a clear paste with a relative density of 1.12 (60-65℃), dry and grind it to the very fine powder; dissolve 2.6g of ethylparaben with an appropriate amount of ethanol; take an appropriate amount of mixed fatty acid glyceride and beeswax, and heated them to melt, then add bismuth hypogallate, the very fine powder mentioned above, borneol, and 16.8g polysorbate 80, and ethyl hydroxybenzoate ethanol solution; mix and fill them well to prepare 1000 suppositories.

用法与用量：患者取侧卧位，置入肛门 2~2.5cm 深处。1 次 1 粒，一日 1~2 次。

Usage and dosage: The patient gets into side-lying position and the drug is inserted into the anus to a depth of 2-2.5cm. One suppository once, 1-2 times each day.

注解：（1）本品为暗黄褐色的栓剂。

Notes: ① The product is a dark yellow brown suppository.

（2）本品中次没食子酸铋具有收敛作用。

② Bismuth hypogallate has an astringent effect in this product.

（3）为保证与基质混合均匀，浸膏粉应粉碎成最细粉；非离子型表面活性剂聚山梨酯-80 的加入，可增加药物的亲水性，有助于药物与基质的混合。

③ To ensure uniform mixing with the bases, the extract powder should be crushed into the very fine powder. The addition of polysorbate-80, a nonionic surfactant, increases the hydrophilicity of the drug and facilitates the mixing of the drug with the bases.

（4）栓剂宜存放在阴凉干燥处，防止受热变形。若因温度过高等原因致使药栓变软、熔化，但稍有变形、变软不影响疗效，仍可将药栓冷冻后再撕开使用。

④ Suppositories should be stored in a cool and dry place to prevent deformation by heat. If the suppository becomes soft and melts due to high temperature, but a little deformation and softening will not affect the curative effect, the suppository can still be frozen and then torn open for use.

二、特殊栓剂的制法

11.3.2 Preparation of Special Suppositories

（一）双层栓剂

(1) Double-Layer Suppositories

案例导入

双层栓由两层组成，可分为内外双层栓剂和上下双层栓剂。

Double-layer suppositories are composed of two layers, which can be divided into internal-external double suppositories and upper-lower double suppositories.

上下双层栓剂的制备可将同一药物或不同药物，分别分散于水溶性基质和脂溶性基质中，制成上、下两层；也可用空白基质和含药基质制成上下两层。

Upper-lower double-layer suppositories can distribute the same or different drugs in the water-soluble bases and the lipid-soluble bases respectively to make upper and lower layers; they can also be made of blank bases and drug-containing bases into two layers.

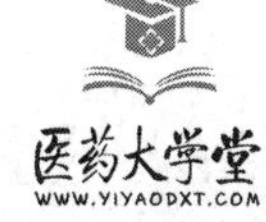

实验室小量制备的内外双层栓剂，栓模由圆锥形内模和外套组成，如图 11-7 所示。先将内模插入模型外套中固定好，将外层的基质和药物熔融混合，注入内模与外套之间，待凝固后，取出

内模，再将已熔融的基质和药物注入内层，熔封而成。

For internal-external double-layer suppositories prepared in small scale in laboratory, the suppository mold is composed of conical internal model and external coat, showed in Figure 11-7 . First, insert the internal model into the external coat and fix well, fuse and mix the external bases and drug, fill them into the area between internal model and external coat, take out the internal model after solidification, and then fill the fused bases and drug into the inner layer for heat sealing.

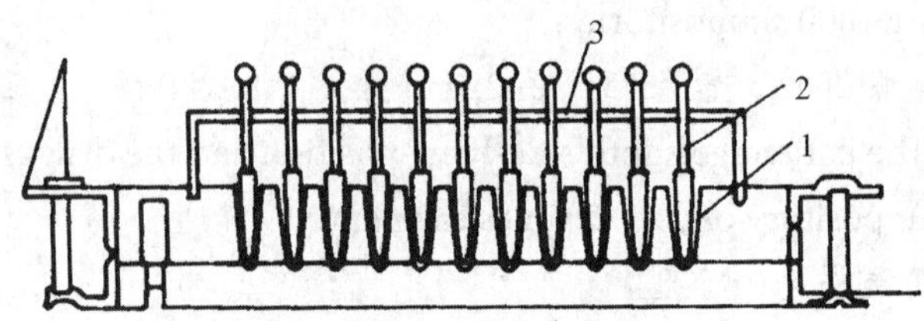

图 11-7　双层栓模型

Figure 11-7　Model of Double-Layer Suppositories

1. 外套　2. 内模　3. 升降杆

1. External coat　2. Internal model　3. Lifting poker

（二）中空栓剂

(2) Hollow Suppositories

中空栓剂的空心部分可填充药物，外层为基质制成的壳，制备过程中先将基质制成栓壳，再将药物封固在栓壳内。

The hollow area of hollow suppositories can be filled with drugs, and the outer layer is a shell made of bases. During preparation, the bases are made into the suppository shell, and then the drug is sealed in the shell.

实验室小量制备时，可在普通栓模上方插入一个不锈钢管，固定，沿边缘注入熔融的基质，待基质凝固后，拔出钢管，在栓壳的中空部分注入药物，最后用相应的基质封好尾部即得。

For small-scale preparation in laboratory, a stainless steel tube can be inserted above the ordinary suppository model, fixed well, and the fused base is injected along the margin. Pull out the steel tube after the base solidification, fill drug into the hollow part of the suppository shell, and seal the tail with the corresponding bases.

（三）泡腾栓剂

(3) Effervescent Suppositories

案例导入

泡腾栓的制备过程中，加入了发泡剂，遇到体液后可产生泡腾作用，产生大量泡沫，从而增加药物与阴道和宫颈黏膜的接触，并使药物能渗入到黏膜皱褶深部，充分发挥治疗作用。

Foaming agent is added during the preparation process of effervescent suppositories that can produce an effervescent effect after encountering body fluids and generate a large number of bubbles, so as to increase the contact of the drug with the vaginal and cervical mucosa, and allow the drug to penetrate into the deep part of the mucosal folds, give full play to the therapeutic effect.

第四节 栓剂的质量检查、包装与贮藏
11.4 The Quality Inspection, Packaging and Storage of Suppositories

PPT

一、栓剂的质量检查
11.4.1 Quality Inspection of Suppositories

（一）外观
(1) Appearance

栓剂的外形应完整光滑，色泽均匀，无裂缝，无变形、霉变等现象。有适宜的硬度，塞入腔道后能熔化、软化或溶化。

Suppositories should look intact and smooth with uniform color, and avoid cracks, deformation, mildew or other similar phenomena. Suppositories are appropriately firm and able to be melted, softened or dissolved when inserted into the cavity.

（二）重量差异
(2) Weight Variation

取供试品栓剂 10 粒，精密称定总重量，求得平均粒重后，再分别精密称定各粒的重量。每粒重量与平均粒重相比较（有标示粒重的栓剂，每粒重量应与标示粒重比较），按表 11-2 所示规定，超出重量差异限度的栓剂不得多于 1 粒，并不得超出限度 1 倍 。凡规定检查均匀度的栓剂，一般不再进行重量差异检查。

Weigh accurately together 10 suppositories and calculate the average weight; then individually weigh each of the 10 suppositories. As table 11-2 shows, not more than one of the individual weights should deviate from the average weight (or the labelled weight) by more than the weight variation limit shown in the table and not a single one should exceed double the limit. Where the test for content uniformity is specified, the test for weight variation may not be required.

表 11-2 栓剂重量差异限度

Table 11-2 Limit of Suppositories Weight Variation

标示粒重或平均粒重（Average or labelled weight）	重量差异限度（Weight variation limit）
1g 及 1g 以下（1.0g or less）	± 10%
1g 至 3g（More than 1.0g to 3.0g）	± 7.5%
3g 以上（More than 3.0g）	± 5.0%

（三）融变时限
(3) Disintegration Test

除另有规定外，按照现行版《中国药典》四部通则融变时限检查法检查，应符合规定。取栓剂 3 粒，在室温放置 1 小时后，油脂性基质的栓剂应在 30 分钟内全部融化或软化变形，水溶性基质的栓剂应在 60 分钟内全部溶解。如有 1 粒不符合规定，另取 3 粒复试，均应符合规定。缓释栓剂应进行释放度的检查，不再进行融变时限检查。

Unless otherwise specified, suppositories should comply with the requirements of Disintegration Test for Suppositories in the current edition of *Chinese Pharmacopoeia*, which is conducted as follows: take 3 suppositories and allow them to remain at room temperature for 1 hour before checking. Suppositories of oleaginous bases should be completely melted, or softened to deformation, while water-soluble suppositories should dissolve completely within 60 minutes. If there is one grain of suppository that does not conform to the requirements, take another 3grains for a second test, which should all comply to the requirements. The sustained-release suppositories should be checked for the release rate and not for disintegration test.

（四）微生物限度

(4) Microbial Limit

除另有规定外，按照现行版《中国药典》四部非无菌产品微生物限度检查法检查，应符合规定。

Unless other specified, suppositories should comply with the Microbiological Examination of Nonsterile Products in the current edition of *Chinese Pharmacopoeia* (ChP).

二、栓剂的包装与贮藏

11.4.2 The Packaging and Storage of Suppositories

岗位对接

重点小结

题库

栓剂所用包装材料或容器应无毒性，并不得与药物或基质发生理化作用。大剂量包装使用自动化机械包装设备，将栓剂置于塑料硬片（如聚乙烯）的凹槽中，再将另一张匹配的塑料硬片与其热合密封，再用外盒包装即得。

除另有规定外，栓剂应置于干燥阴凉处30℃以下密闭贮存，防止因受热、受潮而变形、发霉、变质。

Packaging materials or containers used for suppositories shall be non-toxic and have not cause any unwarranted physical or chemical reaction with the drugs or bases. Automatic mechanical packaging equipment are used for the package of mega-dose suppositories, that works like placing the suppository in the groove of a plastic hard sheet (such as polyethylene), then another matching plastic hard sheet is covered on it by heat sealing, and finally placing the finished product within an outer box to complete the packing process. Unless otherwise specified, suppositories should be stored sealed in a dry and cool place under 30℃ to prevent deformation, mildew and deterioration due to heat and moisture.

（颜　红）

第十二章　胶剂
Chapter 12　Glues

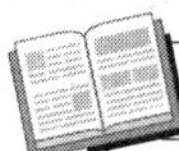

学习目标 ¦ Learning Goals

知识要求：

1. **掌握**　胶剂的含义与分类；胶剂原辅料的选择与处理。
2. **熟悉**　胶剂的制法。
3. **了解**　胶剂的一般质量检查。

能力要求：

学会各类胶剂的制备与质量检测方法，能制备不同类型的胶剂，并检查和评价胶剂的产品质量。

Knowledge requirements:

1. **To master** the definition and classification of glues; Selection and treatment of raw materials.
2. **To be familiar with** the preparation of glues.
3. **To know** the general quality inspections of glues.

Ability requirements:

Learn the preparation and quality testing methods of various glues, be able to manufacture different types of glues, check, and evaluate the product quality of glues.

第一节　概述
12.1　Overview

PPT

一、胶剂的含义
12.1.1　The Definition of Glues

胶剂系指用动物皮、骨、甲或角等为原料，水煎取胶质，浓缩成稠胶，干燥后制成的固体内服剂型。其主要成分为动物胶原蛋白及其水解产物和多种微量元素。制备时可加入一定量的糖、油及黄酒等辅料，用于去腥、矫味等。胶剂多采用“烊化”方法服用，可单独加水煎煮胶剂使之

溶化后，再与其他药煎煮液混合同服，也可将其他药煎好后去渣，取滤液与胶剂煎煮，搅拌使之溶解后服用。其主要具有滋补作用，其中皮胶类补血，角胶类温阳，甲胶类侧重滋阴，还有活血祛风等作用。

Glues are solid lump preparations intended for oral administration, prepared by decocting animal skim, bone, shell or horn with water, concentrating into thick gelatinous mass and then drying. Main components of glues are animal collagen, hydrolysis products of the collagen and various trace elements. During preparation, a certain amount of sugar, oil, yellow rice wine and other excipients can be added to eliminate fishy smell and adjust the taste. The glue is mostly taken by the melting method. It can be added with water to decoct the glue alone to dissolve it. and then decocted with other medicines and taken. It can also been taken by mixing filter fluid after have been boiled with other medicine. It main properties are include nourishing effect, such as skin glues can nourish blood, horn glues can warm yang and nail glues nourish yin, promote blood circulation, dispelling wind, etc..

胶剂作为我国的传统剂型之一，具有悠久的历史。胶的药用，始见于湖南长沙马王堆汉墓出土的古医帛书《五十二病方》，其中记载以葵种汁煮胶治疗癃病。在汉代《神农本草经》中即有“白胶”和“阿胶”的记载。

As one of China’s traditional dosage form, glues has a long history. The medicinal use was firstly recorded in an ancient medical book excavated from Hunan changsha mawangdui named “*wu shi er bing fang*”, which records to decoct glue with sunflower seed solution to treat gonorrhoea. “Bai Jiao” and “E Jiao” had been recorded in *shen nong beng cao jing* of Han dynasty.

二、胶剂的分类
12.1.2 The Classification of Glues

常用的胶剂，按原料来源不同大致可分为以下几类：

Ordinary, glues can be divided into the following categories, according to the source of raw materials:

1. 皮胶类 系以动物的皮为原料制成。常用的有驴皮及牛皮，猪皮是在驴皮资源紧缺的情况下，研制投产的代用品。现在以驴皮为原料者称阿胶，以猪皮为原料者称新阿胶，以牛皮为原料的则称黄明胶。

(1) Skin glues Skin glues are made from animal skins. Donkey skin and cattlehide are commonly used. Pigskin is a substitute for the shortage of donkey skin resources. Now, skin glues which processed from donkey skin as the raw material is called colla corii asini(E Jiao), from pigskin is called new colla corii asini(new E Jiao), and from cowhide is called yellow-bright glue.

2. 角胶类 主要指鹿角胶，其原料为雄鹿骨化的角。鹿角胶应呈白色半透明状，但目前制备鹿角胶时也会掺入一定量的阿胶，因而颜色加深呈黑褐色。熬胶所剩的角渣称为鹿角霜，也可供药用。

(2) Horn glues Horn glues mainly refers to male deer-horn glue, which raw material is the horn of the bucks ossification. Deer-horn glue should appear white and translucent. At present, a certain amount of donkey-hide glue is also added during its preparation. The glues’ color deepens to dark brown. The remaining residue of boiled glue is called deer-horn cream, which is also used as medicinal.

3. 骨胶类 系用动物的骨骼为原料制成。如鹿骨胶、狗骨胶、鱼骨胶等。

(3) Bone glues Bone glues are made from animal bones, such as deer-bone glue, dog-bone glue, dog-bone glue, fish-bone glue and so on.

4. 甲胶类 以龟科、鳖科等动物的甲壳为原料制成，如龟板胶、鳖甲胶等。

(4) Nail glues Nail glues are made from the carapace of tortoise family and turtle family animals, such as tortoise-shell glue and turtle-shell glue.

5. 其他胶类 含有蛋白质的动物药材，经水煎熬炼，一般均可制成胶剂。如以牛肉为原料可制成霞天胶。以龟甲和鹿角为原料或以龟板胶和鹿角胶为原料可制成龟鹿二仙混合胶剂。

(5) Other glues Other glues are made from animal medicine containing protein can be generally made into glue after water decoction. For example, beef can be made into Xia-tian glue. The mixture glue of tortoise-deer can be made from tortoise-shell and deer-horn or tortoise-shell glue and deer-horn glue.

第二节 胶剂的原辅料选择

12.2 Raw Materials Selection of Glues

PPT

一、原料的选择

12.2.1 Selection of Raw Material

胶剂各种来源的原料均应取自健康的动物，因原料的优劣直接影响产品的质量和产量，故原料的选择极为重要，可按下述经验选用。

The raw material of glues of all sorts of sources should be taken from the healthy animal. Raw material choice is very important because the quality of raw material affects the quality and yield of product directly. It can be chosen according to the following experience.

1. 皮类 如驴皮，以张大、毛色黑、质地肥厚、无伤无病，尤以冬季宰杀者为佳，名为“冬板”；其他以春秋季宰杀，张小、皮薄、色杂的“春秋板”次之；夏季剥取的驴皮为“伏板”，质最差。黄明胶所用的黄牛皮以毛色黄、皮张厚大、无病的北方黄牛为最佳。制新阿胶的猪皮，以质地肥厚、新鲜者为佳。

(1) Skins For example, bulky donkey skin which are black hair, thick skin texture, and healthy, especially slaughtered in winter is better, named “winter board”; Other spring or autumn slaughtered, the donkey with smaller and thinner skin texture, mixed color named “spring or autumn board”, which are worse than “winter board”. Donkey skins peeled in summer are of the worst quality. Yellow-bright glue is made of the yellow hair, thick skin, and healthy northern cattle, which is the best quality. Pigskin should be thick and fresh, which made the new donkey-hide glue is better.

2. 角类 鹿角分砍角与脱角两种。“砍角”表面呈灰黄色或灰褐色，质重，有光泽，质地坚硬，含有血质，对光照视，角尖呈粉红色者为佳。春季，鹿自脱之角称“脱角”，表面灰色，质轻、无光泽。以砍角为佳，脱角次之。若野外自然脱落之角，经受风霜侵蚀，使角质变白，有裂纹者称“霜脱角”，不宜采用。

(2) Horns There are two kinds of horns, named “cut horns” and “dehorn horns”. Cut horn, which surface is grey-yellow or grey-brown, is heavy, appears lustrous, with hard texture and contains blood. In the light, the horn which tip presents pink is better. In spring, deer takes off their horns, which are gray,

light and dull. Cut horns'quality is better than dehorn horns. Withstand the wind and frost erosion, the horn fall off in outdoors. These horn turn to white and appear crackle called "cream dehorn horn" and should not be used.

3. 龟板、鳖甲 龟板为龟科动物的腹甲及背甲，其腹甲习称"龟板"，板大质厚，颜色鲜明者称"血板"，其质佳；而产于洞庭湖一带者最为著名，俗称"汉板"，光照下微呈透明，色粉红，又称为"血片"。鳖甲为鳖之背甲，以个大、质厚、未经水煮者所取甲为佳。

(3) Tortoise shell and turtle shell Tortoise shell is the abdominal shell and back shell of the tortoise family. The abdominal shell is called "tortoise shell", with large shell, thick texture and bright color called "blood shell". Tortoise shells from Dongting lake area, are most famous known as "han shell". In the light it appears slight transparent, pink color, also known as "blood piece". These turtle shells are best, which are the back shell of the turtle, with large bulk, hard texture and unboiled.

4. 狗骨、鹿骨 以骨骼粗大、质地坚实、质润色黄的胫骨新品为最佳，陈久者产胶量低。

(4) Dog bone and deer bone The Dog bone and deer bone which are new tibia with thick bones, solid texture and yellow texture is the best. The old bone coule not yields many glues.

二、辅料的选择
12.2.2 Selection of Excipients

胶剂根据治疗需要，常加入糖、油、酒等辅料，起到矫味矫臭、辅助成型的作用，也有一定的医疗辅助作用。辅料的质量的优劣与胶剂的质量直接相关。

According to need of treatment, glues are usually added with sugar, oil, wine etc., This process plays a role in correcting the taste and odor, assisting in forming, and also has medical aid effect. The quality of excipients is directly related to the quality of glues.

1. 冰糖 以色白洁净、无杂质者为佳。加入冰糖能起到矫味作用，并能增加胶剂的硬度和透明度，也可用白糖代替。

(1) Rock sugar The good rock sugar is white, clean and pure. Adding rock sugar can adjust the smell and taste of the final product, and increase the glues' hardness and transparent. It can also be replaced with white sugar.

2. 酒类 多用黄酒，以气味芳香的绍兴酒为佳，也可用白酒代替。胶剂加酒主要为矫臭矫味。收胶时也利于包裹在胶中的气泡逸散，使成品无气泡，提高产品外观质量。

(2) The wine Yellow rice wine is mostly used, and Shaoxing wine with aromatic smell is the best. It can also be replaced by white wine. Glues add wine are mainly for adjusting odor and taste. It also conducive to loss the bubble escaping in the glue when collecting the glue, which making the finished product without bubbles and improving the appearance quality of the product.

3. 油类 制胶剂用油，常用花生油、豆油、麻油。以纯净新制油为佳，酸败者禁用。胶剂加油目的是降低胶的黏度，便于下一步切胶，而且在收胶时也有消泡作用。

(3) Oil Oil generally includes peanut oil, soybean oil, sesame oil. It is better to use pure new oil and rancid oil is forbidden. The purpose of adding oil to glue is to reduce the viscosity, which facilitates the next step of cutting the glue and also has the effect of defoaming while collecting the glue.

4. 阿胶 某些胶剂在熬炼时，常掺入少量阿胶，目的是增加胶的黏度，使之易于凝固成型，也可起到协同发挥疗效的作用。

(4) Donkey-hide glue Some glues in the refining, often mixed with a small amount of donkey-hide glue. The purpose is to increase the viscosity of the glue, which makes it easy to solidify and form, and also can play synergistic effect.

5. 明矾　以色白纯净者为佳。用明矾主要是沉淀胶液中的泥土等杂质，以保证胶块成型后，具有一定的透明度。

(5) Alum　White color and pure Alum is better. Alum is mainly precipitating the soil and other impurities in the glue solution, to ensure transparency degree after forming of the glue block.

6. 水　熬胶用水有一定选择。阿胶原出于山东"阿平郡"用阿井之水制胶而得名。现在生产胶剂，应选用纯化水。

(6) Water　Water for boiling should be optimized. Donkey-hide glue originated from "apingjun" in Shandong province and was named from Awell's water. Now the water production of glues, include for boiling, all should use purified water.

第三节　胶剂的制法

12.3　Preparation of Glues

PPT

胶剂的制备工艺流程如图 12-1 所示。

The preparation process of glues is shown in the Figure 12-1.

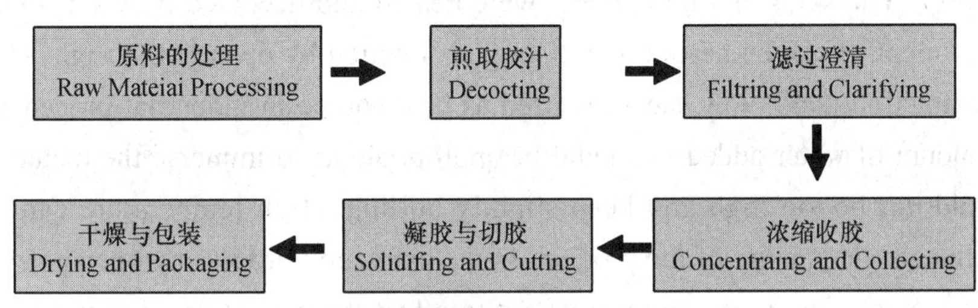

图 12-1　胶剂的制备工艺流程

Figure 12-1　Preparation Process of Glues

1. 原料的处理　胶剂的原料，如动物的皮、骨、角、甲、肉等，有一些毛、脂肪、筋、膜等附属物和其他不洁之物，必须分离除去，才能煎胶。下面以皮类、骨角类原料为例，介绍其处理方法。

(1) Raw material processing　The raw materials of glues, such as animal skin, bone, horn, nail, meatand etc., have some hair, fat, fascia, other appendages and other unclean substances, which must be separated and removed before decocting glue. raw materials of skins, bone-horns are taken as examples to introduce their preparations following.

（1）动物皮类　先浸泡 5~7 日，每日换水，待皮质变柔软后，用刀刮去皮上残存的腐肉、脂肪、筋膜及毛，工厂生产也可用蛋白分解酶。然后将动物皮切成小块，置洗皮机中反复清洗除去泥沙，再加入碳酸钠使浓度达到 1.5% 左右，清洗除去油脂，并洗至中性，加热使皮块膨胀卷缩成卷，最后再进行熬胶。

① Animal skins　Animal skins should be soaked in water for 5-7 days, and changed water daily. After the skins become soft, the remaining carrion, fat, fascia and hair are scraped off by knife.

Proteolysis enzymes can also be used in the industrial production. Then the animal skin is cut into small pieces, washed in the rinsing machine to remove the sediment repeatedly. After that, sodium carbonate is added to make the concentration at about 1.5%, and then the skin is washed with water to remove oils and to neutral. The skin block is heated to expand and shrink into a roll, and finally boiled.

（2）骨角类　先用清水浸泡 20~40 日，每日换水 1 次，用刀刮净残存的腐肉筋膜，取出后亦可用碱水洗除油脂，再以水洗至中性，以便熬胶。对于所附筋肉较多的骨类药材，可将原料放入沸水中稍煮后，用刀刮净筋肉。角中常有血质，可用清水反复冲洗干净，备用。

② Bone-horns　Bone-horns should be soaked in water for 20-40 days, and changed the water every day. The remaining carrion and fascia should be scraped off with a knife. It can also be washed with alkali water to remove the grease after removal, and then washed with water to neutral for easily boiling glue. For the bone medicines with more muscle, the raw material can be put into boiling water and cooked for a little time, then scraped off muscle and fascia by knife. There often contains blood in the horn, which can be washed by clean water repeatedly, for future use.

2. 煎取胶汁（熬胶）　处理后的皮类或骨角，用水加热煎煮提取胶液。可用敞口锅，或密闭的蒸球或多功能提取罐加热提取。现在工厂生产以蒸汽为热源进行加热，加水量要适宜，一般以浸没原料为度，煎煮的温度不宜太高，一般以保持锅内煎液微沸即可，温度太高可使原料焦化而影响产品的品质。使用敞口锅提取的，在提取过程中要随时补充因蒸发所失去的水分，以免因水分不足而影响胶汁的煎出。为了尽可能地把原料中的胶汁提取出来，煎煮时间也是一个重要的因素。根据原料的不同，一般以煎煮 10~48 小时，皮类反复煎煮 3~5 次，骨类反复煎煮 10~15 次，直至原料中的胶汁全部提取出来为止。

(2) Decocting　The skins and bone-horns were heated and decocted by water to extract the glue solution after treatment. It can be heated to extract glue solution by open pot, airtight steaming ball and multi-function extraction tank. Now, steam is used as heat source in industrial procedure. It should be noted that the amount of water added in should be appropriate as to immerse the material. The cooking temperature could not be too high and keep slightly boiling. High temperature can coking the raw materials and influence the quality of the product. In the extraction process by open pot, it should supply the water lost by evaporation at any time so as not to affect the extraction of glue solution for lack of water. In order to extract the glue solution from the raw material as much as possible, the decocting time is also an important factor. According to different kind of raw materials, generally materials are decocted 10-48h, Skins 3-5 times, bones 10-15 times repeatedly, until the glue was extracted from the raw materials completely.

3. 滤过澄清　每次煎煮提取后的胶液，应趁热滤过，否则胶液冷却后因黏度增大而滤过困难。胶液过滤并澄清后，才能浓缩。常用沉降法或沉降法、过滤法合用。为了使胶液沉淀完全，一般在胶液中加入适量的明矾溶液（每 100kg 原料加入明矾 60~90g），搅拌静置数小时，待细小杂质沉降后，取上层澄清胶液，或用细筛或棉纱过滤后，再进行浓缩。

(3) Filtering and Clarifying　The glue solution should be filtered while hot after each decoction and extraction. Otherwise it is difficult to filter for increased viscosity after cooling. The glue solution can only be concentrated after it has been filtered and clarified. Sedimentation method or combination of sedimentation method and filtration method are commonly used. Adding an appropriate amount of alum solution (about 60-90g alum per 100kg raw material) to the glue solution generally to make the glue solution precipitate completely. Stiring it and stand for fine impurities to settle for several hours. Taking the upper clarifying glue solution or filter it with thin sieve or cotton yarn, and then concentrate it.

4. 浓缩收胶 浓缩可以使胶原蛋白继续水解，并进一步除去杂质和水分。取澄清胶液，先用薄膜蒸发去除大部分水分，再移至蒸汽夹层锅中继续浓缩。浓缩时应不断搅拌，随时除去上层浮沫。随着水分不断蒸发，胶液黏度越来越大，应防止胶液粘锅，直至胶液不透纸（将胶液滴于滤纸上，四周不见水迹），含水量为26%~30%，相对密度为1.25左右时，加入豆油，搅拌，再加入糖，搅拌使全部溶解，继续浓缩至“挂旗”时，在强力搅拌下，加入黄酒，此时锅底产生大量气泡，俗称“发锅”，待胶液无水蒸气溢出时即可出锅。

(4) Concentrating and Collecting Concentration allows collagen to continuously hydrolyze and further removes impurities and moisture. Taking the clarifying glue solution to remove most of the water by thin film evaporation firstly, and then move to the steam jacket to continue the concentration. When concentrated should stir constantly to remove the upper froth at any time. As the water evaporating constantly, the glue solution viscosity is becoming bigger and bigger. To prevent glue solution sticking to the pan, when the glue solution can’t get through the filter paper (drop the glue solution on the filter paper, no water stains marks are found around), the water content is about 26%-30% and relative density is about 1.25, adding soybean oil and stiring, adding sugar, then stiring to dissolve all and continue to concentrate to “hang flag”. Adding yellow rice wine under strong mixing, while a large amount of air bubbles is generated at the bottom of the pot, commonly known as “leaven pan”. When the glue solution overflows without water vapor, it can come out of the pan.

各种胶剂浓缩的程度不同，如鹿角胶应防止“过老”，否则成品色泽不够光亮，易碎裂；而龟板胶浓缩稠度应大于驴皮胶、鹿角胶等，否则不易凝成胶块。因此，浓缩程度要适量，若含水分过多，成品在干燥过程后常出现四周高、中间低的“塌顶”现象。

The concentration degree of various glues varies, such as deer-horn glue should prevent “too old”, otherwise the color of final product is not bright enough and is easily broken. The concentration consistency of tortoise-shell glue should be greater than donkey-hide glue, deer-horn glue, etc, otherwise, it is not easy to solidify into glue. Therefore, the concentration degree should properly. If contain too much water, the finished products often appear all round tall, middle low named “collapse top” phenomenon after drying.

浓缩是使胶原蛋白继续水解、进一步除去杂质及水分的过程。随着胶原蛋白的逐渐水解，颗粒质点变小，疏水性成分与亲水性成分也逐步分离，且混悬于胶液中。由于浓缩时水分不断蒸发，胶液中金属离子浓度增大，离子的电性可中和疏水胶体粒子的电性，使其聚合成疏松的粒子团，相对密度较小而上浮。浓缩过程中不断打沫，目的是除去此类水不溶性杂质，以提高胶剂的质量。

Concentration is the process of continuing to hydrolyze the collagen and further removing impurities and moisture. With the gradual hydrolysis of collagen and granular particles become smaller, hydrophobic components and hydrophilic components are gradually separated and suspended in the glue solution. Due to the constantly evaporation of water during concentration, the concentration of metal ions in the glue solution increased and the electrical properties of ions can neutralize the electrical properties of hydrophobic colloidal particles, which made them polymerize into loose particles and floated up for smaller relatively density. Such water-insoluble impurities are removed by continuous foaming during the concentration process, thereby improving the quality of the glue.

5. 凝胶与切胶 胶液熬成后，趁热倾入凝胶盒中使其胶凝，即将胶液凝固成块状。为了防止胶液与凝胶盒粘连，在胶凝前需在凝胶盒内涂抹少量的植物油，倾入热胶液后，凝胶盒放置25~35℃的凝胶室18~24小时，然后再把凝胶盒放置在0~5℃的冷藏室中，冷藏约24小时，即可凝成胶块。凝固后的胶块切成小片状，称为“开片”。手工切片操作时，要求刀口平齐，一刀切成，以防出现重复刀口痕迹，影响胶片的外观性状。大生产时可用切胶机切割。

(5) Solidifing and Cutting The glue solution should be poured into the gel box and make into gelation while hot after boiling, which solidified the glue solution into blocks. In order to prevent glue solution and gel box adhesion, a small amount of vegetable oil should be smeared in the gel box before gelation. Pouring into the hot glue solution, the gel box is placed in the gel room of 25-35℃ for about 18-24h. Then put the gel box in the cold room of 0-5℃ and refrigerated for about 24h. Then it can be condensed into a gel block and is cut into small pieces, which called "slicing". When manual cutting operation, it requires smooth and tiny edge cut by once to prevent the repeated blade marks, which affect the appearance of the glue. Mass production can be cut by glue cutting machine.

6. 干燥与包装 胶片切成后，放置在干燥的晾胶室内晾置、干燥，把胶片整齐地摆放在晾胶床上，晾置24~48小时后，将胶片逐个翻动一次，使胶片两面的水分均匀蒸发，以免因水分蒸发不均匀而造成胶片弯曲变形。3~5日后，将晾胶床上的胶片整齐地装入整胶盒中，密闭放置2~3日，使胶片内部的水分缓缓地散发至胶片表面，称之为"闷胶"或"瓦胶"，然后打开整胶盒，把胶片取出，用棉布把胶片表面的水分擦去，再整齐地摆放在晾胶床上，晾置2~3日，后又依前法再装入整胶盒中，密闭放置2~3日后再取出，擦去表面水分，放置在晾胶床上晾置，如此反复操作3~5次，即可达到胶片干燥的目的。现在也有用微波进行胶片干燥的，可以缩短干燥时间。

(6) Drying and Packaging After cutting into pieces, it should be placed in the dry drying room for drying. The pieces are placed neatly on the drying bed for 24-48h. Then the piece is turned over one by one to make the water in both sides of the piece evaporate evenly, so as not to cause the piece bending deformation. After 3-5 days, the dry glue pieces on the bed should be put into the glue box neatly and airtight placed 2-3 days to make the inside water of the piece slowly diffuse to the surface, which called "stuffy glue" or "tile glue". And then open the box, take out the piece and wipe off the water on the surface with cotton cloth, and place in dry glue bed neatly for 2-3 days. Then put it into the glue box according to the previous method, place it airtight place for 2-3 days and take out, and wipe the surface water then put in dry glue bed for 3-5 times to achieve the purpose of drying. Now the process also use microwave drying, which can shorten the drying time.

晾胶过程中要注意控制空气的湿度和环境的温度，湿度过低，则干燥速度太快容易造成胶片碎裂，温度过高，则胶片表面软化，粘连在晾胶床上，影响胶片的外观。

During the drying process, it should be paid attention to control the humidity of the air and the temperature of the environment. If the humidity is too low, the drying speed is too fast, which may cause the piece to crack, if the temperature is too high, then the piece surface become softening and adhere to the drying bed, which affecting the appearance of the piece.

干燥后的胶片用粗棉布蘸取温水擦拭胶片表面，使胶片表面有光泽，出现明显的布纹。

After drying, the piece surface should wipe with cheesecloth dipped in warm water, which makes the surface shiny and appears obvious cloth lines.

擦拭后的胶片用印章、印字机或激光雕刻机在胶片表面印制或雕刻产品名称等信息。印字后的胶片放置在紫外灯下照射30分钟灭菌后分装在塑料袋和铝箔袋中，并装盒。

After wiping off, the piece is printed or engraved the product name and other informations on the surface with a seal, printer or laser engraving machine. The printed piece is irradiated and sterilized under the ultraviolet lamp for 30min and divided into plastic bags and aluminum foil bags, then packed it into boxes.

胶剂应存放在密闭的容器内和阴凉干燥处，要防止受潮、受热、但也不可过分干燥，以免胶片碎裂。

Glues should be stored in closed containers, cool and dry places. It should be protected from moisture and heat, but not be excessively dried to prevent the glue from cracking.

案例导入 ¦ Case example

案例 12-1　阿胶（驴皮胶）

12-1　Donkey-Hide Glue

处方：驴皮 50.0kg　冰糖 3.3kg　豆油 1.7kg　黄酒 1.0kg

Ingredients: Donkey Skin 50.0kg　Rock Sugar 3.3kg　Soybean Oil 1.7kg　Yellow Rice Wine 1.0kg

功能与主治：补血滋阴，润燥，止血。用于血虚萎黄，眩晕心悸，肌痿无力，心烦不眠，虚风内动，肺燥咳嗽，劳嗽咯血，吐血尿血，便血崩漏，妊娠胎漏。

Functions and indications: To nourish blood and Yin, moisten dryness, stop bleeding. Used for blood deficiency and chlorosis, dizziness, palpitations, muscle weakness, upset and insomnia, endogenous deficient wind, pulmonary dryness and cough, hemoptysis, vomit and urine blood, metrorrhagia and metros taxis, fetal leakage in pregnancy.

制法：将驴皮漂泡去毛，切块洗净，分次水煎，滤过，合并煎液，浓缩后分别加入适量的黄酒、冰糖和豆油至稠膏状，冷凝，切块，晾干、即得。

Making Procedure: Donkey skin should bleach to remove hair, cut into pieces, decoct in water for several times, filter, combine with decoction. After concentration, adding appropriate amount of yellow rice wine, rock sugar and soybean oil to the thick paste, condense, cut into pieces, dry, get.

用法与用量：烊化兑服，3~9g。

Usage and dosage: Melting to take,3-9g.

注解：（1）《神农本草经》所载阿胶的原料为牛皮，自宋代起，阿胶全部用驴皮煎煮，而以牛皮煎胶称为“黄明胶”；五代起，牛革皆为制造衣甲军需品之用，可供煎煮阿胶的大牲畜皮张只有驴皮。因此，自宋代起阿胶之名已被驴皮胶所独享，并载于本草，沿用至今。在阿胶原料驴皮紧缺，阿胶产量严重供不应求的时期，以猪皮为原料代替。为了区别于阿胶，而特命名为“新阿胶”。

Notes: ① The raw material of donkey-hide glue was recorded in *shen nong beng cao jing* is cattlehide. Since the Song dynasty, donkey-hide glue has been decocted with donkey hide, while decocted with cattlehide is called “yellow-bright glue”. From the Five dynasty, cattlehide was used to make military supplies for clothing and armour while only donkey skin was used for decocting donkey-hide glue. Therefore, since the Song dynasty, the name of colla corii asini has been exclusively enjoyed by donkey-hide glue and recorded in the herb still in use. During the period when donkey-hide glue raw materials and the production of donkey-hide glue were severely in short supply, with pipskin as raw materials to replace it. In order to distinguish from colla corii asini, and specifically named “new colla corii asini”.

（2）阿胶成品呈黑褐色，有光泽，可能是其含色氨酸，水解时产生腐黑质所致；黄明胶如琥珀色，是因其不含色氨酸，水解时没有腐黑质产生。经分析，阿胶含总蛋白为 91.6%，黄明胶含总蛋白为 93.0%；阿胶含无机磷为 18.6%（mg/g），黄明胶含无机磷为 15.9%（mg/g），两者几乎相同。

② The final product of donkey-hide glue is dark brown and shiny, which may be caused by its containing tryptophan and sapropelic matter produced when hydrolyzed. Yellow-bright glue is like amber because it does not contain tryptophan and no sapropelic matter produced when hydrolyzed. According to the analysis, donkey-hide glue contains 91.6% of total protein and Yellow-bright glue contains 93.0% of total protein. Donkey-hide glue contains 18.6% (mg/g) of inorganic phosphorus, while yellow-bright glue contains 15.9% (mg/g)

of inorganic phosphorus, both of them are almost same.

思考题：制胶时为什么要加入豆油，浓缩至“挂旗”如何判断？

Question: why to add soybean oil when preparing glues, how to judge when condensed to “hang flag”?

第四节 胶剂的质量要求与检查

12.4 Quality Requirements and Inspections of Glues

PPT

一、胶剂的质量要求

12.4.1 Quality Requirements of Glues

胶剂一般应检查总灰分、重金属、砷盐等，除另有规定外，还应进行以下相应检查。

The general inspections of glues should check total ash content, heavy metal, arsenic salt, etc. Unless otherwise specified, the following corresponding inspections should also be carried out.

1. 外观 胶剂应为色泽均匀、无异常臭味的半透明固体。无显著气泡、油泡及其他杂质，质地脆而坚实，平整，拍之即碎裂，碎裂面有光泽，不呈黯浊色。

(1) Appearance Glues should be translucent solid with uniform color and no abnormal odor. No significant bubbles, oil bubbles and other impurities. The texture is brittle, solid, flat, and cracks when it is beat. The cracked surface is shiny and does not appear cloudy.

2. 水分 按现行版《中国药典》水分测定法（第一法）测定，不得过15.0%。

岗位对接

(2) Determination of water Glues should be determined in accordance with the current edition of *Chinese Pharmacopoeia* by the water determination method (first method), and should contain no more than 15.0%.

3. 微生物限度 按现行版《中国药典》微生物限度检查法检查，应符合规定。

(3) Microbial limit Glues should be checked in accordance with the current edition of the *Chinese pharmacopoeia* by the method of microbial limit inspection, and should meet the requirements.

重点小结

二、胶剂的质量检查

12.4.2 Quality Inspection of Glues

题库

性状、水分、总灰分、重金属、砷盐、微生物限度检查等应符合现行版《中国药典》质量要求。

Character, Determination of water, Total ash content, Heavy metal, Arsenic salt, Microbial limit inspection, etc., should meet the quality requirements of the current edition of *Chinese Pharmacopoeia*.

（曾 锐）

第十三章　胶囊剂
Chapter 13　Capsules

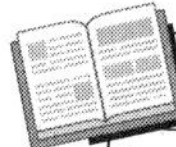

学习目标 ¦ Learning Goals

知识要求：

1. 掌握　硬胶囊、软胶囊的含义、特点与制法。

2. 熟悉　硬胶囊、软胶囊的质量检查，肠溶胶囊的含义、特点与制备，空心胶囊和软质囊材的原料与辅料。

3. 了解　空心胶囊的制法、规格及质量要求。

能力要求：

学会各类胶囊剂的制备与质量检测方法，能制备不同类型的胶囊，并检查和评价产品质量。

Knowledge requirements:

1. To master the definition, characteristics and preparation method of hard capsule and soft capsule.

2. To be familiar with the quality examination of hard capsule and soft capsule, the definition, characteristics and preparation of enteric capsules, the raw material and excipients of hollow capsules and soft capsule wall material.

3. To know the preparation method, specification and quality requirement of hollow capsules.

Ability requirements:

Learn the preparation and quality testing methods of various capsules, be able to prepare different types of capsules, check, and evaluate the product quality of products

第一节　概述
13.1　Overview

PPT

一、胶囊剂的含义
13.1.1　The Definition of Capsules

胶囊剂系指将饮片用适宜方法加工后，加入适宜辅料填充于空心胶囊或密封于软质囊材中的

剂型。胶囊壳通常由明胶、增塑剂和水组成，因各成分比例不尽相同，制备工艺有所差异。近年来，也有应用甲基纤维素（MC）、羟丙甲纤维素（HPMC）、海藻酸钠、聚乙烯醇、变性明胶及其他高分子材料为囊材，以改变胶囊剂的溶解性能或产生肠溶性。

Capsules refers to a kind of dosage form that the decoction pieces are processed by the appropriate method, then be added appropriate additives in before filled in hollow capsules or sealed in soft capsules. Capsule shells are usually composed of gelatin, plasticizer and water. Due to the different proportions of each components, the preparation process is different. In recent years, methylcellulose (MC), hypromellose (HPMC), sodium alginate, polyvinyl alcohol, denatured gelatin, and other high-molecular materials have also been used as capsule wall materials to change the dissolving properties or produce enteric properties of capsules.

胶囊剂是目前临床口服给药最常用的剂型之一。早在明代，我国就已有类似的剂型（面囊，以淀粉或面粉制成）使用。19 世纪中叶，法国和英国的药剂师先后发明了软胶囊和硬胶囊。随着自动胶囊填充机的问世，胶囊剂从理论上和技术上得到了较大的发展，目前，胶囊剂的品种数目仅次于注射剂和片剂，居第三位。2020 年版《中国药典》一部收载有 260 余种胶囊剂。

Capsules are currently one of the most commonly used forms for clinical oral administration. As early as the Ming Dynasty, similar dosage form (flour pouch, made of starch or flour) were already used in China. In the mid-19th century, France and Britain pharmacists have invented soft capsule and hard capsule sequentially. With the advent of automatic capsule filling machines, capsules have gained great development both theoretically and technically. At present, the variety and number of capsules are the third largest only less than injections and tablets. There are more than 260 kinds of capsules in the first part of *Chinese Pharmacopoeia* (2020 Edition).

二、胶囊剂的特点

13.1.2 The Characteristics of Capsules

1. 可掩盖药物不良气味，提高药物稳定性。因药物装在胶囊壳中与外界隔离，保护了药物不受湿气、空气中的氧以及光线的影响，在一定程度上可提高其稳定性。

(1) Mask bad odor of drugs, improve the stability of drugs. Due to the medicine is contained in the capsule shell and isolated from the outside world, it can be protected from the moisture, the oxygen in the air and the light, which improves the stability to some extent.

2. 药物生物利用度高。胶囊剂中的药物在制备时不需添加黏合剂和施加压力，所以在胃肠道中崩解快，一般服后 3~10 分钟即可崩解释放药物，较片剂、丸剂显效快，吸收好。

(2) High bioavailability. The drug in the capsule does not need to be added with adhesive and be pressurized during preparation, which lead to its quick disintegration in the gastrointestinal tract. Generally, drugs in capsules can be disintegrated and released in 3-10min after taking, which works more quickly and absorbed better than tablets and pills.

3. 可定时定位释放药物。可将药物先制成颗粒，然后用不同释放速度的材料包衣（或制成微囊），按所要求的比例混匀，装入空心胶囊中即可达到定时定位释放药物的目的。

(3) Release the drug at a fixed time and location. The drug can be made into granules first, then coated with different release rates of material (or made into microcapsules), and mixed in the required ratio, and put into hollow capsule to achieve the purpose of releasing drugs timely at the targeted position.

4. 可弥补其他剂型的不足。若药物含油量高或呈液态，则不宜制成丸剂、片剂，可制成软胶囊或液体硬胶囊；服用剂量小、难溶于水、消化道内不易吸收的药物，可使其溶于适当的油中，制成软胶囊，或采用液体灌装技术制成硬胶囊。既增加了消化道的吸收，提高疗效，又增强药物稳定性。

(4) Make up for the lack of other dosage forms. If the drug is high in oil or is in liquid state, it is not easy to make pills or tablets. However, it can be made of soft capsules or liquid hard capsules. The pharmaceutical raw materials, which is in small dose, hardly soluble in water and difficult to absorb in the digestive tract, can be dissolved in appropriate oil, and be made into soft capsule; or it can be made into hard capsule using liquid filling technology. Capsules not only increase the absorption of the digestive tract, improve efficacy, but also enhance the stability of the drug.

5. 整洁，美观，容易吞服，便于携带，囊壳上可着色或印字以便识别。

(5) Neat, beautiful, easy to be swallowed, easy to be carried, and the capsule shell can be colored or printed for easily identifying.

但以下几种情况不宜制成胶囊剂：①易溶性药物（如碘化物、溴化物、氯化物等）以及小剂量、刺激性强的药物。因胶囊剂在胃中溶化时，由于局部浓度过高而刺激胃黏膜；②一般情况下，药物的水溶液或醇溶液，可使胶囊壁溶解；③易风化药物，可使胶囊壁软化；④吸湿性药物，可使胶囊壁过分干燥而变脆。

However, capsules are not suitable for the following situations: ① Soluble drugs (such as iodide, bromide, chloride, etc.) and low-dose, highly irritating drugs. Because when capsules dissolve in the stomach, local concentration is too high which can stimulate the gastric mucosa; ② Generally, the capsule wall can be dissolved in their aqueous solution or alcohol solution; ③ The easily weathered drugs, which can soften capsule walls; ④ The hygroscopic drug, which can make the capsule wall excessively dry and become brittle.

三、胶囊剂的分类
13.1.3 The Classifications of Capsules

胶囊剂按胶囊壳的软硬材质不同及溶解部位不同主要分为硬胶囊（通称为胶囊）、软胶囊（胶丸）和肠溶胶囊。

Capsules are mainly divided into hard capsule (commonly known as capsules), soft capsule (gelatin pills) and enteric capsules according to the difference in hard or soft materials of capsule shell and different dissolved sites.

1. 硬胶囊 系指将提取物、提取物加饮片细粉或饮片细粉或与适宜辅料制成的均匀粉末、细小颗粒、小丸、半固体或液体，填充于空心胶囊中的胶囊剂。

(1) Hard capsule refers to a kind of capsules that use the extract, extract with fine powder of decoction pieces, or fine powder of decoction pieces or mixed with appropriate excipients to make uniform powder, fine particles, pellets, semi-solid or liquid and then fill them in hollow capsules.

2. 软胶囊 系指将提取物、液体药物或与适宜的辅料混匀后用滴制法或压制法密封于球形或橄榄形的软质囊材中的胶囊剂。

(2) Soft capsule refers to a kind of capsules in which the extract, liquid medicine is sealed in a spherical or olive-shaped soft capsule using the drop method or pressing method or after be mixed with appropriate excipients.

3. 肠溶胶囊 系指囊壳不溶于胃液，但能在肠液中崩解、溶化或释放的胶囊剂。

(3) Enteric capsules refers to the capsules in which the capsule shell is insoluble in gastric juice but disintegrates, solubilizes or releases in the intestinal juice.

第二节 胶囊剂的制法

13.2 Preparation of Capsules

PPT

一、硬胶囊的制法

13.2.1 Preparation of Hard Capsule

硬胶囊的制备一般分为空心胶囊的制备和填充物料的制备、填充、封口、包装等工艺过程。工艺流程，如图 13-1 所示。

The preparations of hard capsule are generally divided into the preparation of hollow capsules, preparation of filling materials, filling, sealing, packaging and so on. The process flow is shown in Figure 13-1.

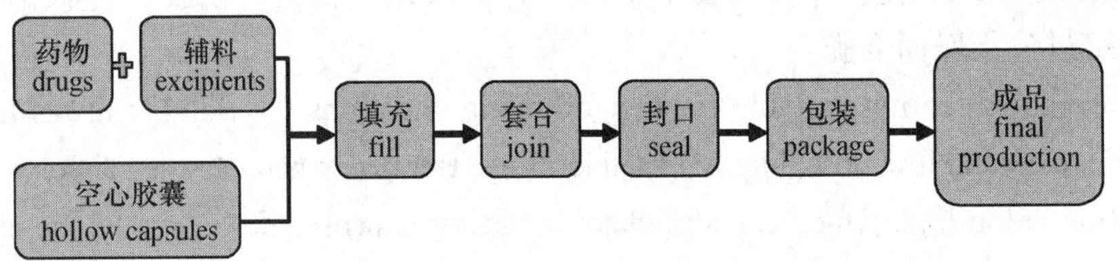

图 13-1 硬胶囊制备的一般工艺流程图

Figure 13-1 Flow Diagram of Preparation Process of Hard Capsule

（一）空心胶囊的制法

(1) Preparation of Hollow Capsule

案例导入

1. 空心胶囊的囊材 空心胶囊的主要原料为明胶。除了符合现行版《中国药典》规定以外，还应具有一定的黏度、胶冻力和 pH 值等。黏度能影响胶囊壁的厚度，胶冻力则决定囊壳的强度。除了明胶以外，制备空心胶囊时还应添加适当的辅料，以保证其质量，如增塑剂、增稠剂、着色剂、遮光剂、防腐剂、增光剂等。

① The wall material of hollow capsules The main raw material for hollow capsules is gelatin. In addition to conform the provisions of current version of *Chinese Pharmacopoeia*, gelatin should also have some viscosity, gel strength and pH value. The viscosity can affect the thickness of the capsule wall, while the gel force determines the strength of the capsule shell. In addition to gelatin, appropriate auxiliary materials should be added to ensure its quality when preparing hollow capsules, such as plasticizers, thickeners, colorants, sunscreens, preservatives, brighteners and so on.

2. 空心胶囊的制法 空心硬胶囊壳分上、下两节，上节粗而短，下节细而长。目前普遍采用的空心硬胶囊制备方法是将不锈钢制的栓模浸入明胶溶液形成囊壳的栓模法。其生产工艺过程如图 13-2 所示。

② Preparation of hollow capsules The hollow hard capsule shell is divided into two sections, the upper section is thick and short, the lower section is thin and long. At present, the commonly used method for preparing hollow hard capsules is to immerse the stainless-steel bolt mold into gelatin solution to form the capsule shell. The production process is shown in Figure 13-2.

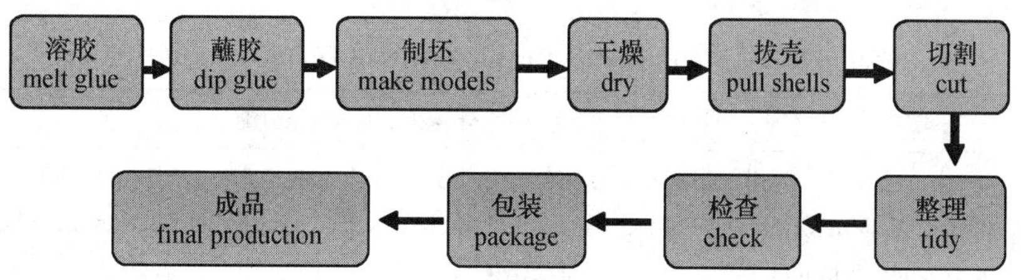

图 13-2 空心胶囊生产工艺过程

Figure 13-2 Preparation Process of Hollow Capsules

3. 空心胶囊的规格和质量要求

③ Specifications and quality requirements of hollow capsules

（1）空心胶囊的规格 空心胶囊的规格由大到小分为 000、00、0、1、2、3、4、5 号共 8 种，一般常用 0~3 号。随着胶囊号数由小到大，其容积则由大到小，如表 13-1 所示。

a. *Specifications of hollow capsules* The specification of hollow capsules is divided into 8 kinds from large to small, 000, 00, 0, 1, 2, 3, 4, 5. 0 to 3 pecifications are most commonly used. As the capsule number from small to large, its volume is from large to small, as shown in Table 13-1.

表 13-1 空心胶囊容积与药物填充的质量

Table 13-1 Hollow Capsules Volume and Drug Filling Quality

规格（specification）/ 号	容积（volume，cm^3）	填充质量*（filling quality，g）
000	1.37	1.096
00	0.95	0.760
0	0.68	0.554
1	0.50	0.400
2	0.37	0.296
3	0.30	0.240
4	0.21	0.168
5	0.13	0.104

注：* 填充物的密度为 0.8g/ cm^3。

Note: * The density of the filler is 0.8g / cm^3.

（2）空心胶囊主要质量要求 见表 13-2。

b. *Main quality requirements of hollow capsules* As shown in Table 13-2.

表 13-2 空心胶囊的质量要求

项目	质量规定
外观	应色泽均匀，囊壳光洁无异物，无纹痕、变性和破损，无砂眼、气泡，切口平整圆滑，无毛缺
干燥失重	在 105℃干燥 6h，减少质量应在 12.5%~17.5%之间
脆碎度	取空心胶囊 50 粒，置（25 ± 1）℃恒温 24h，按现行版《中国药典》操作，破脆数不能超过 15 粒
崩解时限	于 37℃水中振摇，10min 应全部溶化或崩解
炽灼残渣	透明空心胶囊残留残渣不得超过 2.0%，半透明空心胶囊应在 3.0%以下，不透明空心胶囊应在 5.0%以下
重金属	取炽灼残渣项下遗留的残渣，依法检查，含重金属不得超过百万分之四十
铬	照原子吸收分光光度法计算，含铬量不得超过百万分之二
贮藏	置于密闭环境，在温度 10~25℃，相对湿度 35%~65% 条件下贮存

Table 13-2 Main Quality Requirements of Hollow Capsules

Item	Standards of quality
Appearance	Capsule shell should be uniform in color and luster, free of foreign body, no lines marks, degeneration and damage, no sand hole and bubbles, and the incision shall be smooth and has no deficiency
Loss on drying	Drying at 105℃ for 6h, the reduced mass should be between 12.5%-17.5%
Friable degree	Take 50 hollow capsules, set them at (25 ± 1)℃ for 24h. According to the operation of the current version of *Chinese Pharmacopoeia*, the number of crispy capsules cannot exceed 15
Disintegration time limit	Shake in water at 37℃ and the capsules should be dissolved or disintegrated in 10 min
Residue on ignition	The residue of transparent hollow capsules shall not exceed 2.0%, translucent hollow capsules should be below 3.0%, and the opaque hollow capsules should be less than 5.0%
Heavy metal	Take the residue left under the ignition residue, check it according to the law. The content of heavy metals shall not exceed forty parts per million
Chrome	According to calculation of atomic absorption spectrophotometry, the content of chrome should not more than two parts per million
Storage	Stored in airtight condition at temperature 10-25℃ and relative humidity 35%-65%

（二）药物的填充

(2) Drug Filling

1. 空心胶囊的选择 空心胶囊有普通型和锁口型两类。药物填充多用容积控制，而药物的形状、密度、晶态、颗粒大小和剂量不同，所占的容积亦不同，故应按药物剂量所占容积来选用最小的空心胶囊。

① Selection of hollow capsules There are two types of hollow capsules: ordinary type and lock type. Drug filling is usually controlled by volume, while the differences of shape, density, crystalline state, particle size, or dose of the drug also occupied different volumes. Therefore, the smallest hollow capsule should be selected according to the volume of drug dose.

2. 填充药物的处理 一般是固体，如粉末、结晶、细粒、颗粒、微丸、小丸等，也可以是半固体或液体。

② Treatment of filled drug Generally, the filled drug is solid, such as powder, crystals, fine particles, granules, mini-pills, pillers, etc., it can also be semi-solid or liquid.

药物的处理方法有以下几点：

The methods for drug handling are as followings:

（1）剂量小的饮片，可直接粉碎成细粉，过六号筛，混匀后填充。

a. Decoction pieces of small dosage can be directly crushed into fine powder, passed through the No.6 sieve, then mix well and fill.

（2）剂量较大的饮片可先将部分粉碎成细粉，其余饮片经提取浓缩成稠膏后与细粉混匀，干燥，研细，过筛，混匀后填充，也可以将全部饮片经提取浓缩成稠膏后加适当辅料，制成微小颗粒，经干燥混匀后填充。

b. Decoction pieces of larger dosage can be partially crushed into fine powder, the remaining pieces should be extracted and concentrated to thick paste and then mixed with fine powder, dried, finely ground, screened, and mixed for filling. Alternatively, all the decoction pieces may be extracted and concentrated to thick paste and then added appropriate excipients to make fine particles. Then dry, mix them well and then fill.

（3）处方组成中若有结晶性或提取的纯品药物时，应先研成细粉再与群药细粉混匀后填充。

c. If there is crystalline or extracted pure drug in the prescription, it should be made into fine powder and then fill them after being mixed with the other medicine powder.

（4）性质稳定的半固体或液体也可以直接填充，这种液体或半固体药物直接灌装的技术可使硬胶囊具有软胶囊的优点，而且能够改善均匀度，克服粉尘交叉污染，通过固体溶液或缓释技术控制药物释放。

d. Semisolid or liquid with stable properties can also be directly filled. The technology of directly filling the liquid or semi-solid drugs can make the hard capsules have the advantages of soft capsules, and can improve the uniformity, overcome the cross contamination of dust, and can control the drug release through the solid solution or slow-release technology.

（5）麻醉药、毒性药细粉应稀释后填充。

e. The fine powder of anesthetic and toxic drugs should be diluted before filling.

（6）挥发油应先用吸收剂或方中其他药物细粉吸收，或制成包合物或微囊后再填充。

f. Volatile oil should be absorbed by the absorbent or other medicine powder in the prescription, or made into an inclusion compound or microcapsule before filling.

（7）易引湿或混合后发生共熔的药物可酌加适量稀释剂，混匀后填充。

g. Drugs that are easy to be wet or be eutectic after mixing can be added an appropriate amount of diluent, mix them well and then fill.

3. 药物填充的方法 药物的填充方法分手工填充和自动硬胶囊填充机填充。一般小量制备时，可用手工填充法。大量生产时，多采用自动填充机。目前高效胶囊填充机的型号很多，国内外均有生产。其工作原理基本类似，主要流程如图 13-3 所示。

③ Methods of drug filling The filling methods of drugs can be divided into manual filling method and automatic hard capsule filling machine filling method. When the preparation is small, manual filling method can be used. For mass production, most use automatic filling machine. At present, there are many models of high efficiency capsule filling machine, which are produced at home and abroad. The working principle is similar, and the main process is shown in Figure 13-3.

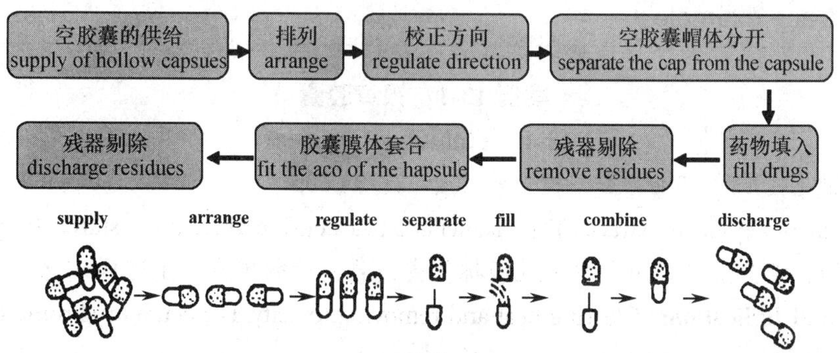

图 13-3 全自动胶囊填充操作流程示意图

Figure 13-3 The Main Process of Automatic Capsule Filling

胶囊的填充方式主要分为以下四种类型，如图 13-4 所示：①由螺旋进料器压进药物（如图 13-4a 所示）；②用柱塞上下往复将药物压进（如图 13-4b 所示）；③药物自由进入（如图 13-4c 所示）；④在填充管内先由捣棒将药物压成一定量后再填充于囊壳中（如图 13-4d 所示）。图 13-4c 所需要物料可自由流动；图 13-4a、图 13-4b 需物料有较好的流动性；图 13-4d 适用于流动性较差

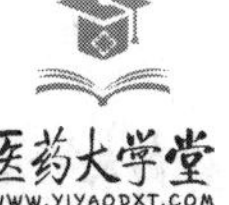

的物料。

The filling methods of the capsule is mainly divided into the following four types, as shown in Figure 13-4: a.Press the medicine by the screw feeder (as shown in Figure 13-4a). b.Press the medicine by the plunger up and down repeatedly (as shown in Figure 13-4b). c.The medicine enters freely (as shown in Figure 13-4c); d.Press the medicine into a certain amount by the tamper in the filling tube and then fill the medicine in the capsule shell (as shown in Figure 13-4d). Figure 13-4c shows that the required materials can flow freely; Figure 13-4a and Figure 13-4b show that the required materials have good fluidity; Figure 13-4d is suitable for materials with poor fluidity.

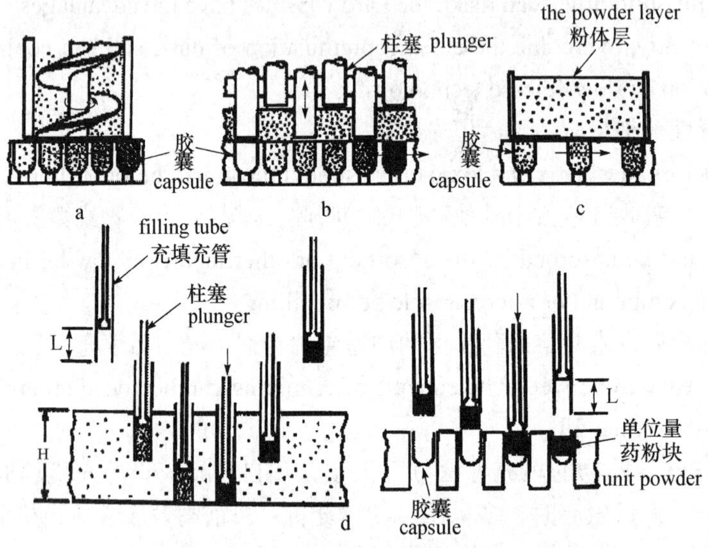

图 13-4 硬胶囊自动填充机的类型

Figure 13-4 The Types of Automatic Filling Machine for Hard Capsule

为防止填充药物后发生泄漏现象，可在胶囊的套合处包封上一层或多层药用包衣材料或采用锁口胶囊。

案例导入 ¦ Case example

案例 13-1 银黄胶囊

13-1 Yinhuang Capsule

处方：金银花提取物 100g 黄芩提取物 40g 淀粉 160g

Prescription: Honeysuckle extract 100g Scutellaria baicalensis extract 40g starch 160g

功能与主治：清热解毒。用于急慢性扁桃体炎，急慢性咽喉炎，上呼吸道感染。

Functions and Indications: Clearing heat and removing toxicity. For acute or chronic tonsillitis, acute or chronic pharyngitis, upper respiratory tract infection.

制法：取金银花提取物、黄芩提取物、淀粉混匀，以 75% 乙醇溶液制软材，挤压过 40 目制湿颗粒，40~50℃干燥，整粒，装胶囊，约制成 1000 粒（0.30g/ 粒），即得。

Making Procedure: Take honeysuckle extract, Scutellaria baicalensis extract and starch, mix well. Make soft material with 75% ethanol solution, then squeezed it through 40 mesh sieve to make wet granules. Dry them at 40-50℃, arrange and fill in capsules, then make about 1000 grains(0.30g / grain).

用法与用量：口服，一次 2~4 粒，一日 4 次。

Usage and dosage：Take orally for 2-4 each time and 4 times a day.

注解：①金银花提取物的制备：取金银花分别加水 10 倍、7 倍煎煮两次，第一次 1 小时，第二次 45 分钟。滤过，滤液加入石灰乳调节 pH 值至 10~12，静置，滤取沉淀，加适量水，加硫酸调节 pH 值至 6~7，搅匀，滤过，滤液浓缩至稠膏状，烘干，即得。②黄芩提取物的制备：取黄芩分别加水 8 倍、6 倍煎煮两次，每次 1 小时，合并煎液，滤过，滤液加硫酸调节 pH 值至 2，静置，滤取沉淀，用乙醇适量洗涤后，干燥，即得。③金银花中的主要有效成分绿原酸对热不稳定，干燥过程中应严格控制温度，一般要求在 60℃以下。黄芩中的主要有效成分为黄芩苷，提取时黄芩苷在一定温度下易被药材中共存酶酶解成苷元而降低疗效，故提取时直接用沸水提取，使酶在高温下变性失活而避免其对黄芩苷的影响。④装胶囊过程中应注意控制适当的温度和湿度。一般温度在 20~25℃，相对湿度以 30%~45% 为宜，以避免胶囊中的药粉或颗粒吸湿。

Notes: ① Preparation of honeysuckle extract: take honeysuckle and cook twice. The first time is 1h with 10 times water, the second time is 45mins with times water. After filtering, then add lime milk to the filtrate to adjust the pH value to 10-12. Leave it still, filter the precipitate, then add an appropriate amount of water before adding sulfuric acid to adjust the pH value to 6-7. Then stir the solution well, filter it, and concentrate the filtrate to a thick paste. At last, dry to obtain.

② Preparation of Scutellaria baicalensis extract: take Scutellaria baicalensis and cook it twice with 8 times and 6 times water, each time for 1hour. Combine the decoction then filter. The filtrate is adjusted to pH 2 with sulfuric acid. Leave it still. Filter the sediment, wash it with appropriate amount of ethanol, and then dry it to obtain.

③ Chlorogenic acid, the main active ingredient in honeysuckle, is unstable to be heated. The drying temperature should be strictly controlled during the drying process, the general requirement is below 60℃. Baicalin is the main active ingredients in Scutellaria. When baicalin is extracted, it is easy to be enzymatically decomposed into aglycone by the co-enzyme in the medicinal material at a certain temperature, which reduces the curative effect. Therefore, using boiling water to extract directly can make enzyme denaturation and inactivation at high temperature, avoiding its impact on baicalin.

④ In the procession of capsule filling, should pay attention to controlling the appropriate temperature and humidity. The general temperature is 20-25℃ and relative humidity in 30%-45% is appropriate, in order to avoid the capsule powder or particles absorbing moisture.

思考题：①空心胶囊规格应该如何选定？②制备过程中哪些是关键步骤？

Questions: ① How to choose specifications of hollow capsule?

② Which steps are the key to the preparation process?

二、软胶囊的制法

13.2.2　Preparation of Soft Capsule

软胶囊的制备过程包括囊材的制备及填充药物的制备、填充与成型等工艺。软胶囊的制备工艺流程如图 13-5 所示。

Soft capsule preparation process includes the preparation of the capsule material and the preparation, filling and molding the filled drug. Soft capsule preparation process is shown in Figure 13-5.

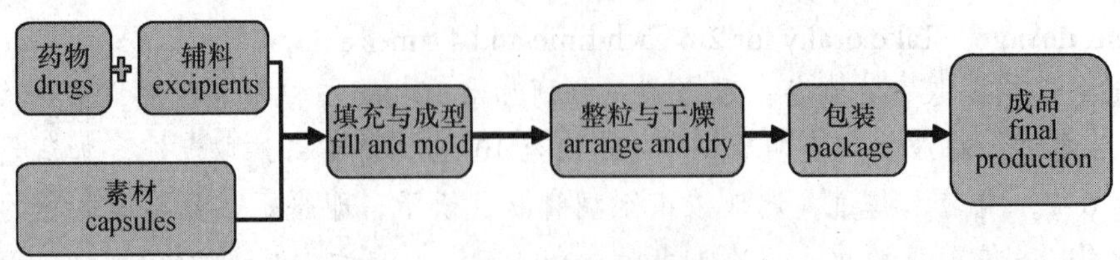

图 13-5 软胶囊制备工艺流程

Figure 13-5 Flow Diagram of Preparation Process of Soft Capsule

(一) 软胶囊的囊材

(1) The Material of Soft Capsules

软胶囊囊材的组成主要是胶料、增塑剂、附加剂和水。胶料一般为明胶或阿拉伯胶；常用的增塑剂有甘油、山梨醇；附加剂包括防腐剂（如对羟基苯甲酸甲酯和对羟基甲酸丙酯的 4：1 混合物，用量一般为明胶的 0.2%~0.3%）、色素（如食用规格的水溶性染料）；香料（如 0.1% 的乙基香兰醛或 2% 的香精）、遮光剂（如二氧化钛，常用量为每 1kg 明胶原料中加入 2~12g），此外加入 1% 的富马酸可增加胶囊的溶解性；加二甲基硅油可改善空心胶囊的机械强度，提高防潮防霉能力等。

The compositions of soft capsule materials are mainly glue, plasticizers, additive and water. Generally glue is gelatin or gum acacia; commonly used plasticizers are glycerol and sorbitol; additives include preservatives (methyl p-hydroxybenzoate and propyl p-hydroxyformate were mixed 4 to 1, and the dosage is generally 0.2%-0.3% of gelatin), pigments (such as water-soluble dyes of food standard), spices (such as 0.1% ethyl vanillin or 2% essence), light-screening agent (such as titanium dioxide, the usual amount is 2-12g per 1kg of gelatin). In addition, adding 1% fumaric acid can increase the solubility of the capsule; adding dimethyl silicone oil can improve the mechanical strength of the hollow capsule and the ability of moisture-proof and mildew proof.

软胶囊的主要特点是可塑性强、弹性大。囊材弹性主要与明胶、增塑剂及水的比例有关。在软胶囊的制备和贮存过程中，囊材中的水分会有所变化，因此，明胶与增塑剂的比例对软胶囊的制备及质量有着十分重要的影响。若增塑剂用量过低，则囊材会过硬，相反，若用量过高，则囊材过软。通常较适宜的重量比为：干明胶与干增塑剂之比为 1.0：(0.4~0.6)，水与干明胶之比为（1.0~1.6）：1.0。选择胶囊硬度时应考虑所填充药物的性质以及药物与软胶囊囊材之间的相互影响。

The main features of soft capsule are high in plasticity and flexibility. The main flexibility of the capsule wall material is related to the ratio of gelatin, plasticizers and water. In the process of preparation and storage of soft capsule, the moisture content in the capsule wall material will change. Therefore, the proportion of gelatin and plasticizer has a very important influence on the preparation and quality of soft capsule. If the plasticizer is of little amount, the capsule wall material will be too hard, on the contrary, if it is vast, the capsule wall material will be too soft. Usually, the suitable weight ratio is: the ratio of dry gelatin to dry plasticizer is 1.0：(0.4-0.6), and the ratio of water to dry gelatin is (1.0-1.6)：1.0. The choice of capsule hardness should take the nature of the filled drug and the interaction between the drug and the material of the soft capsule wall into account.

(二) 软胶囊大小的选择

(2) Selection of Soft Capsule Size

软胶囊的形状有球形、橄榄形等多种形状。在保证填充药物达到治疗量的前提下，为便于成型，软胶囊的容积要求尽可能小。当固体药物颗粒混悬在油性或非油性液体介质中，以混悬剂的形式作为软胶囊的填充物时，所需软胶囊的大小可用“基质吸附率”来决定。基质吸附率是指 1g

固体药物制成填充胶囊的混悬液时所需液体基质的克数，即：

There are spherical shape, olive shape and other shapes of soft capsule. In ensuring the filled drugs achieving the premise of treatment, soft capsule volume is required to be as small as possible in order to facilitate the molding. When the solid drug particles are suspended in an oily or non-oily liquid medium and used as a soft capsule filler in the form of the suspension, the size of the required soft capsule can be determined by the "matrix adsorption rate". The matrix adsorption rate refers to the grams of liquid matrix required when 1g of the solid drug is used to make a capsule-filled suspension, that is:

基质吸附率 = 基质重量 / 固体重量

Matrix adsorption rate = matrix weight / solids weight

固体药物颗粒的大小、形状、物理状态、密度、含水量以及亲油性或亲水性等都对其基质吸附率有一定的影响，从而影响软胶囊的大小。

The size, shape, physical state, density, water content, as well as lipophilicity or hydrophilicity of solid drug particles all have certain influence on the matrix adsorption rate, thus affecting the size of the soft capsule.

（三）软胶囊内填充物的要求

(3) The Requirements of Fillers in Soft Capsule

软胶囊内可填充各种油类或对囊壁无溶解作用的液态药物、溶液、混悬液，甚至是固体药物等。由于囊材以明胶为主，而明胶的本质是蛋白质，因此首先要求填充物对蛋白质性质无影响。填充药物还必须组分稳定、体积适宜、与软质囊材具有良好的相容性、具有良好的流变学性质和适应在 35℃条件下生产的非挥发性物质。在进行处方设计时，软胶囊中往往加入一些辅料。如维生素 A 胶囊中加聚山梨酯 -80，以提高药物的吸收和生物利用度，加入 10%甘油或丙二醇可减少聚乙二醇对囊材壁的硬化作用等。

Soft capsule can be filled with a variety of oils or liquid drugs, solution and suspension which have no dissolution effect on capsule wall, even as to solid drugs. Since the capsule wall material is mainly gelatin, and the essence of gelatin is protein. So, the first requirement is that the filler has no effect on the gelatin properties. Secondly, the filled drug must have stable compositions, suitable volume, good compatibility with the material of soft capsule wall, good rheological properties and be the non-volatile substances which are suitable for producing at 35℃. Some auxiliary materials are often added in soft capsule when designing formulation. For example, adding polysorbate 80 to vitamin A capsules can improve the absorption and bioavailability of the drug, adding 10% glycerol or propylene glycol can reduce the hardening effect of polyethylene glycol on the wall of the capsule.

油是软胶囊中最常用的药物溶剂或混悬介质。如果填充药物具有吸湿性或含有与水混溶的液体时（如聚乙二醇、甘油、丙二醇、聚山梨酯 -80 等），应注意其吸湿性对囊材壁的影响。如果药物是亲水性的，可在药物中保留 3%~5% 的水分。但若药物的含水量超过 5%，或含低分子量水溶性或挥发性有机物（如乙醇、丙酮、羧酸、胺类或酯类等），这些液体则容易透过明胶壁而使囊材软化或溶解；醛类药物也可以使明胶变性，因此上述两类药物均不宜制成软胶囊。

The most commonly used pharmaceutical solvent or suspension medium in soft capsule is oil. If the filled drug is hygroscopic or contains liquid miscible with water (such as polyethylene glycol, glycerin, propylene glycol, polysorbate 80, etc.), attention should be paid to the effect to its hygroscopicity on the capsule wall. If the drug is hydrophilic, it can retain 3% to 5% of the water. However, if the water content of the drug exceeds 5%, or it contains low molecular weight water-soluble or volatile organic compounds (such as ethanol, acetone, carboxylic acid, amines or esters and so on), these liquids can easily pass

through the wall of the gelatin to soften or dissolve the capsule wall material. And the aldehyde drug can also denature gelatin. Thus, the two kinds of drugs above are not suitable to be made into soft capsule.

填充药物的酸碱度也是影响软胶囊质量的重要因素之一。生产中常选用磷酸盐、乳酸盐等缓冲溶液调节填充药物的 pH，使之控制在 4.5~7.5 的范围内，以防止囊材中的明胶在强酸下水解而泄漏，或在强碱下变性而影响崩解和溶出。

The pH value of the filled drug is also one of the important factors affecting the quality of soft capsule. In production, buffer solutions such as phosphate and lactate are often used to adjust the pH value of the filled drug, and control its pH within the range of 4.5 to 7.5. So as to prevent the gelatin capsule wall material from leaking due to hydrolysis under strong acid, or from disintegration and dissolution due to denaturation under strong alkali.

装填混悬液时，还需注意混悬液必须有较好的流动性和微粒混悬稳定性，所含固体药物的粒度应控制在 80 目以下。

When filling the suspension, it should also be noted that the suspension must have good fluidity and particle suspension stability. The particle size of the solid drug should be controlled below 80 mesh.

（四）软胶囊的制法

(4) The Preparation Method of Soft Capsule

案例导入

软胶囊的制备方法可分为压制法（模压法）和滴制法，其中压制法制成的软胶囊称为有缝软胶囊，滴制法制成的软胶囊称为无缝软胶囊。

Soft capsule preparation methods can be divided into pressing method (molding method) and dropping method, the soft capsule made by pressing method known as slit soft capsule, and the soft capsule made by the dropping method is called seamless soft capsule.

1. 压制法 压制法是将胶液制成厚薄均匀的胶片，再将药液置于两个胶片之间，用钢板模或旋转模压制软胶囊的一种方法。压制法制备主要包括配制囊材胶液、制胶片和压制软胶囊三个过程。根据囊材处方，将一定配比的原、辅料配成胶液，制成厚薄均匀的胶片，药液置于两胶片间，用自动旋转轧囊机或钢板压制而成。模的形状决定了软胶囊的形状，多为球状或椭球形。

① **Pressing method** Pressing method is a kind of method that can make the glue into a film of uniform thickness, and then placed the liquid between the two films, using steel plate mold or rotary mold to make soft capsule. Preparation of pressing method mainly includes three processes: the preparation of glue solution of capsule wall material, the preparation of the film and compressing the soft capsule. According to the prescription of the capsule wall material, a certain proportion of the raw and auxiliary materials are mixed into a glue liquid to make a film with uniform thickness. The medicine liquid is placed between the two films and pressed by an automatic rotary roller or steel plate. The shape of the mold determines the shape of the soft capsule, which is mostly spherical or ellipsoidal.

大量生产时，常采用自动旋转轧囊机，在电动机带动下各部分均自动运转，连续操作。本法的特点是连续自动化生产，产量高，成品率高，装量差异小。其工作原理，如图 13-6 所示。

In mass production, often use automatic rotating capsule machines with the motor driving each part to operate automatically and continuously. The method is characterized by continuous automated production, high yield, high rate of finished products and small difference in capacity. Its working principle is shown in Figure 13-6.

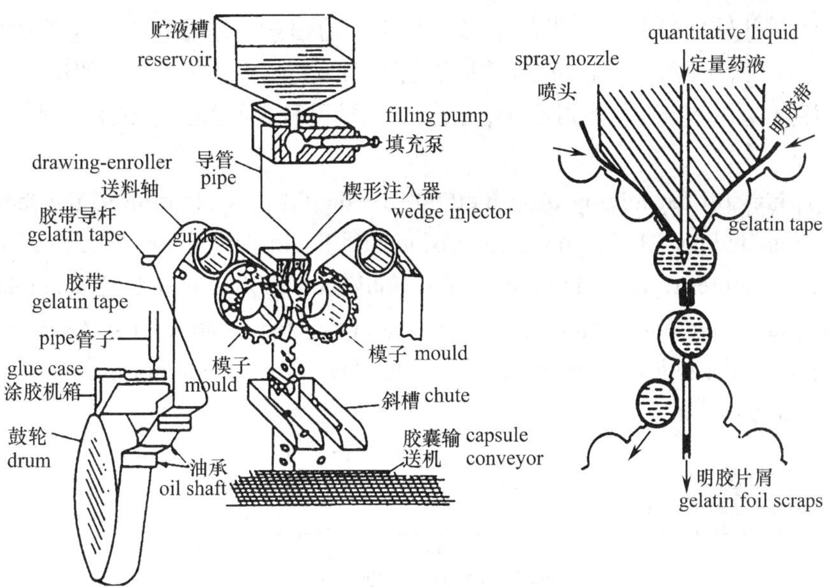

图 13-6 自动旋转轧囊机旋转模压示意图

Figure 13-6 Schematic Diagram of Rotary Die Pressing of Automatic Rotary Roller

2. 滴制法 系指通过滴制机制备软胶囊的方法。即利用明胶液与油状药物为两相，分别盛装于贮液槽中，通过双层喷头（外层通入胶液，内层通入药液）按不同速度喷出，使一定量的明胶液包裹定量的药液后，滴入另一种不相混溶的冷却液中，由于表面张力作用使胶液进入冷却液后呈球形并凝固成软胶囊。滴制法制备示意图，如图 13-7 所示。

② **Dropping method** It is the method that preparing soft capsules by dripping machine. That is to say, the gelatin liquid and the oily medicine are divided in two phases, and are respectively contained in the liquid storage tanks. They are sprayed at different speeds through the double-layer spray head (the outer layer is injected with glue and the inner layer is sprayed with medicine liquid). After a certain amount of gelatin solution is wrapped in a fixed amount of medicine solution, it is dripped into another immiscible coolant. Due to the surface tension, the glue enters the coolant and becomes spherical and solidified into a soft capsule. The schematic diagram of dropping preparation method is shown in Figure 13-7.

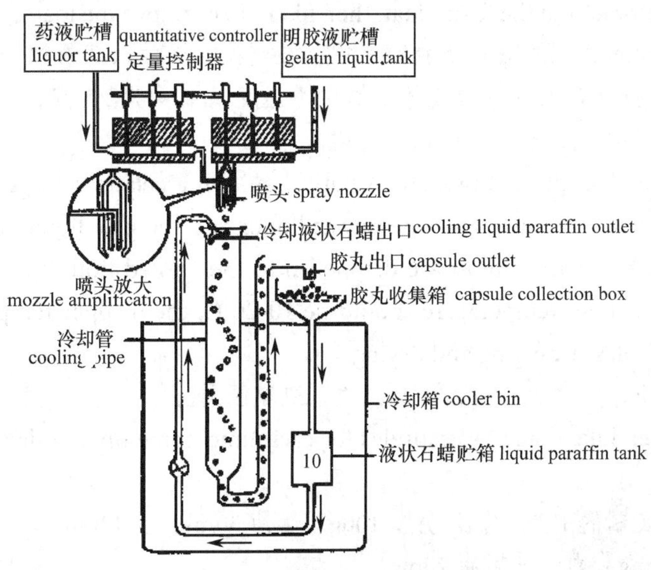

图 13-7 滴制法制备软胶囊示意图

Figure 13-7 Schematic Diagram of Dropping Preparation Method

采用滴制法制备软胶囊时，应当注意影响其质量的因素，主要包括：①明胶液的处方组成比例；②胶液的黏度；③药液、胶液及冷却液的温度；④药液、胶液及冷却液三者的相对密度；⑤软胶囊的干燥温度。在实际生产过程中，根据不同的品种，必须经过试验，才能确定最佳的工艺条件与参数。

When preparing soft capsule by drop method, we should pay attention to the factors that affect its quality, mainly including: ① The proportion of gelatin liquid prescription; ② The viscosity of glue liquid; ③ The temperatures of medicine liquid, glue liquid and cooling liquid; ④ The relative density of medicine liquid, glue liquid and cooling liquid; ⑤ The drying temperature of soft capsule. In the actual production process, according to different varieties, the best process conditions and parameters can be determined only through tests.

案例导入 ¦ Case example

案例 13-2　牡荆油胶丸

13-2　Mujing Oil Soft Capsules

处方：牡荆油（95%）1000ml　食用植物油 3000ml

Prescription: vitex oil (95%) 1000ml; edible vegetable oil 3000ml

功能与主治：祛痰、镇咳、平喘药。用于治疗慢性支气管炎等。

Functions and Indications: expectorant, antitussive and antasthmatic. For the treatment of chronic bronchitis.

制法：取牡荆油与经加热灭菌、澄清的食用植物油充分搅拌，即得透明的淡黄色药液。取明胶加入适量的水使其膨胀，另将甘油及余下的水置胶锅中加热到 70~80℃，混合均匀，加入已膨胀的明胶搅拌，熔化，保温 1~2 小时，静置，使泡沫上浮、除去，滤过，即得。

Making Procedure: Take vitex oil and clarified edible vegetable oil which has been heated and sterilized, and fully mix them to obtain a transparent light-yellow liquid medicine. Adding appropriate amount of water in gelatin and make it expand. The other glycerol and the rest of the water are set in a plastic pot heated to 70-80℃, and mix them well. Then add the expanded gelatin, stir, melt, keep warm for 1-2h, and leave it alone for letting the foam float, then filter after remove the foam.

采用滴制法，将制好的明胶液置明胶贮槽中，牡荆油药液放入药液贮槽内；药液与胶液应保持 60℃；将药液与明胶液滴入冷却的液体石蜡中（温度以 10~17℃为宜，室温为 10~20℃，滴头温度为 40~50℃），制得胶丸，整丸，干燥，即得。

Using dropping method, put the prepared gelatin liquid in a gelatin storage tank, and the vitex oil is placed in the physic liquor storage tank; the physic liquor and the glue liquid should be kept at 60℃; the physic liquor and the gelatin liquid are dripped into the cooled liquid paraffin (the appropriate temperature is 10-17℃, room temperature should be 10-20℃, the dripper temperature should be 40-50℃), to make into capsules, arranging and drying.

用法与用量：口服，一次 1~2 粒，一日三次，或遵医嘱。

Usage and dosage: Take orally 1-2 capsules for each time, three times a day, or follow the doctor's advice.

注解：①明胶液配制的配方一般为明胶 100g、甘油 30ml、水 130ml。

②本品每丸重 80mg，内含牡荆油 20mg。

③牡荆油的提取：取新鲜牡荆叶置提取器中，用水蒸气蒸馏法提取挥发油，再用油水分离器

分出牡荆油，脱水，滤过，即得。

④在胶丸干燥的过程中，滴出的胶丸先均匀摊于纱网上，在10℃以下低温吹风4小时以上，再用擦丸机擦去表面的液状石蜡，然后再低温（10℃以下）吹风20小时以上，取出。用乙醇：丙酮=5：1的混合液或石油醚洗去胶丸表面油层，再吹干残留的溶剂，于40~50℃下干燥约24h。取出干燥的胶丸，用乙醇洗涤，在40~50℃下吹干，即可。

Notes: ① The formulation of gelatin solution is generally gelatin 100g, glycerin 30ml and water 130ml. ② Each pill weighs 80mg and contains 20mg of vitex oil. ③ Extraction of vitex oil: put fresh vitex leaves in extractor, and extract volatile oil by steam distillation, then separate vitex oil by oil-water separator before dehydrate and filter. ④ In the process of drying the capsule, the dripped capsule should be spread evenly on the gauze, with winds blow at temperature below 10℃ for more than 4h. Then the liquid paraffin on the surface of the dripped capsule is rubbed off by the rubbing machine, and then blow the dripped capsule at a low temperature (below 10℃) for more than 20h before remove. Use mixture of ethanol：acetone = 5：1 or petroleum ether to wash away the oil layer of the surface of the capsule, then blow the residual solvent to dry and dry them at 40-50℃ for about 24h. Remove the dried soft capsules, washed with ethanol, drying at 40-50℃ to obtain.

三、肠溶胶囊的制法
13.2.3 Preparation of Enteric Capsule

案例导入

肠溶胶囊可以使药物在肠道定位释放出来，从而在人体肠道发挥局部或全身治疗作用，主要适于一些具有腥臭味、刺激性或遇酸不稳定或需要在肠内溶解后释放药物的制备。肠溶胶囊按种类可分为小肠溶胶囊（即普通肠溶胶囊）和结肠溶胶囊。

Enteric capsule can positioning release the drug in the intestinal tract, which play a local or systemic therapeutic role in the human intestinal tract. It is mainly suitable for the preparation of some drugs with stench or irritation, acid unstable drugs or drugs need to be released after dissolve in the intestines. Enteric capsule can be divided into small intestinal soluble capsule (normal enteric capsules) and colon-soluble capsule.

肠溶胶囊较传统胶囊的优势主要体现在：①药物不溶于胃液，可避免或降低某些药物对胃壁的副作用；②可防止酸不稳定性药物在胃部的降解，提高药物疗效；③可定点释药，提高药物在肠道的局部浓度，充分发挥治疗作用；④使含特殊成分的药物（如蛋白质或肽类）经口服发挥疗效。

The advantages of enteric capsules over traditional capsules are mainly as follows: ① The drug is insoluble in gastric juice, it can avoid or reduce the side effects to the stomach wall. ② It can prevent the degradation of acid unstable drugs in the stomach, and improve its efficacy. ③ Targeted release of drugs to increase the local concentration of the drug in the intestinal tract and give full play to the therapeutic effect. ④ Making drugs containing special ingredients (such as proteins or peptides) play an effect by oral administration.

肠溶胶囊主要有甲醛浸渍法和包衣法两种制备方法。甲醛浸渍法是将明胶与甲醛作用生成甲醛明胶，使囊壳中的明胶无游离氨基存在，失去与酸结合能力，从而只能在肠液中溶解。但该方法受甲醛浓度、浸渍时间、胶囊贮存时间等因素影响较大，因此其肠溶性非常不稳定，现很少应用此法制备肠溶胶囊。

There are two preparation methods for enteric capsules: formaldehyde impregnation method and coating method. Formaldehyde impregnation method is the method that make gelatin reacting with formaldehyde to form formaldehyde gelatin, which losing the capacity to combine with acid because of free of amino in gelatin, and can only be dissolved in intestinal fluid. However, this method is greatly affected by factors such as formaldehyde concentration, immersion time, and storage time of capsule. Therefore, the solubility of enteric is very unstable, and it is rarely used to prepare enteric capsules.

包衣法是指在明胶囊壳表面或胶囊内容物表面包裹肠溶衣料，如用聚乙烯基吡咯烷酮作底衣层，再用蜂蜡等作外层包衣，也可用聚丙烯酸树脂Ⅱ号、邻苯二甲酸醋酸纤维酯等溶液包衣。包衣法制备的肠溶胶囊肠溶性较稳定，因此，该方法是目前制备肠溶胶囊最常用的方法。具体操作步骤如下：①胶囊壳包衣法将囊壳涂上一层肠溶材料，达到肠溶的效果。常用肠溶材料有邻苯二甲酸醋酸纤维酯（CAP）、聚丙烯酸树脂类共聚物等。先将邻苯二甲酸醋酸纤维酯（CAP）、聚乙烯基吡咯烷酮（PVP）溶液喷射于胶囊上，作为底衣层，以增加其黏附性，然后用邻苯二甲酸醋酸纤维酯（CAP）、聚丙烯酸树脂Ⅱ号等进行外层包衣。可将药物直接填充到具有肠溶作用的空心胶囊内。目前，国内已有生产可在不同肠道部位溶解的空心胶囊。②胶囊内容物包衣法将内容物（颗粒、小丸等）包肠溶衣后装入空心胶囊中，此空心胶囊虽在胃中溶解，但内容物只能在肠道中溶解、崩解和溶出。

The coating method is to coat the enteric materials on the surface of the capsule shell or the contents of the capsule. Such as using polyvinylpyrrolidone as the bottom coating, and then use beeswax as the outer coating, or use polyacrylic resin II, phthalate fiber and other solutions for coating. Enteric capsules prepared by the coating method is stable. Therefore, this method is currently the most commonly used method for preparing the enteric capsules. Specific operation steps are as follows: ① The capsule shell coating method is used to coat the capsule shell with an enteric material to achieve an enteric effect. Commonly used enteric materials include cellulose acetate phthalate (CAP), polyacrylic resin copolymers, and so on. Firstly spray CAP solution and polyvinylpyrrolidone (PVP) solution on the capsules as a base coat layer to increase its adhesion. Then CAP, Polyacrylic resin II or other enteric materials are coated as an outer layer. The drug can be directly filled into hollow capsules which is enteric. At present, hollow capsules that can be dissolved in different intestinal parts have been produced in China. ② Capsule content coating method is the method that the contents (particles, pillers, etc.) are enteric-coated and filled into hollow capsules. Although this hollow capsule is dissolved in the stomach, the contents can only be dissolved, disintegrated and dissolved in the intestine.

第三节 胶囊剂的质量检查、包装与贮藏

13.3 Quality Inspection, Packaging and Storage of Capsules

PPT

一、胶囊剂的质量检查

13.3.1 Quality Inspection of Capsules

胶囊剂的质量检查主要包括性状、理化鉴别、含量测定和微生物限度检查等项目。有些在现行

版《中国药典》制剂通则项下有规定，有些则应通过试验和研究，根据具体品种制订相应的标准。

Capsule quality inspection mainly includes traits, physical and chemical identification, determination of content and microbial limit check items. Some have regulations in general provisions of the current version of the *Chinese Pharmacopoeia*, while some should be through trials and researches, according to the specific varieties to develop the appropriate standards.

（一）外观

(1) Appearance

胶囊剂应整洁，不得有黏结、变形、渗漏或囊壳破裂，并应无异臭。

Capsules should be neat, free from adhesion, deformation, leakage or rupture of capsule shell, and free from abnormal smell.

（二）水分

(2) Moisture

硬胶囊的内容物，除另有规定外，水分不得超过 9.0%（硬胶囊内容物为液体或半固体者不检查水分）。

Unless otherwise specified, the moisture content of hard capsule shall not exceed 9.0% (if the content of hard capsule is liquid or semi-solid, water content will not be checked).

（三）装量差异

(3) Loading Differences

现行版《中国药典》规定的检查方法及标准。测定方法是取供试品 10 粒，每粒装量与标示装量相比较（规定含量测定的或无标示装量的胶囊剂，则与平均装量相比较），应当在规定范围以内，超出装量差异限度的胶囊不得多于 2 粒，并不得有 1 粒超出限度 1 倍。

Current version of *Chinese Pharmacopoeia* appendix provides inspection methods and standards of loading differences. Determination of the method is to take 10 test capsules, and compare the loading capacity of each capsule with the marked loading capacity (for the capsule with specified content or without marked loading capacity, compare with the average loading capacity). The number of the capsules that exceed the difference limit of loading capacity should be no more than 2. The number of the capsules that exceed twice of the difference limit of loading capacity should be no more than 1.

（四）崩解时限

(4) Time Limit of Disintegration

硬胶囊和软胶囊，取供试品 6 粒，加挡板进行检查，硬胶囊剂应在 30 分钟内、软胶囊应在 1 小时内全部崩解；肠溶胶囊，取供试品 6 粒，先不加挡板在盐酸溶液中检查 2 小时，每粒囊壳不得有裂缝或崩解现象，然后在人工肠液中进行检查，1 小时内全部崩解。

For hard capsule and soft capsule, take 6 capsules as the test sample and adding baffles for inspection. Hard capsule should be completely disintegrated within 30min, and soft capsules should be within 1h. For enteric capsules, taking 6 capsules to detect, first be checked in hydrochloric acid solution for 2h without baffle, and no cracks or disintegration would occur in each capsule shell. And then be checked in the artificial intestinal juice, all capsules should be disintegrated within 1h.

（五）其他

(5) Others

胶囊剂的含量测定、溶出度、释放度、含量均匀度、微生物限度等均应符合要求。内容物包衣的胶囊剂应检查有机溶剂残留量。

Content determination, dissolution rate, dissolution rate, content uniformity and microbial limits of

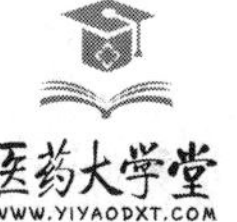

capsules should all meet the requirements. The contents coated capsules should be checked for residual organic solvents.

二、胶囊剂常见质量问题
13.3.2 Common Quality Problems of Capsules

（一）装量差异超限
(1) Loading Differences Out of Limits

导致胶囊剂装量差异超限的原因主要有囊壳因素、药物因素、填充设备因素等。在制备硬胶囊过程中要选用正规厂家的合格空心胶囊，通过加入适宜辅料或者制颗粒等方法改善药物的流动性，使填充准确，同时对填充设备要及时维修保养，确保正常运转。

The main reasons leading to the difference in the amount of capsule are capsule shell factors, drug factors, filling equipment factors and so on. In the process of preparing, the qualified hollow capsules from regular manufacturers should be selected, and the fluidity of drugs should be improved by adding appropriate auxiliary materials or making granules to ensure accurate filling. Meanwhile, the filling equipment should be promptly prepared and maintained to ensure the normal operation.

（二）吸潮
(2) Moisture Absorption

中药胶囊的吸潮问题是制药工作中遇到的较为普遍的难题，因为中药胶囊吸潮后往往会变软、结块，甚至霉变，从而影响药品的质量和疗效。可以通过改进制备工艺（如制粒、防潮包衣），利用玻璃瓶包装、双铝箔包装、铝塑包装等方法解决。

The moisture absorption problem of traditional Chinese medicine capsules is a more common problem encountered in pharmaceutical work. Because traditional Chinese medicine capsules tend to be soft, caking, or mildewed after moisture absorption, thus affecting the quality and efficacy of drugs. It can be solved by improving the preparation process (such as granulation, moisture-proof coating), using glass bottle packaging, double aluminum foil packaging, aluminum-plastic packaging and other methods.

三、胶囊剂的包装、贮藏
13.3.3 Packaging and Storage of Capsules

胶囊剂易受温度与湿度的影响，因此包装材料必须具有良好的密封性能。现常用的有玻璃瓶、塑料瓶和铝塑泡罩式包装。用玻璃瓶和塑料瓶包装时，应将容器洗净、干燥，装入一定数量的胶囊后，容器内间隙处塞入干燥的软纸、脱脂棉或塑料盖内带弹性丝，防止震动。易吸湿变质的胶囊剂，还可在瓶内放一小袋烘干的硅胶作为吸湿剂。

Capsules are susceptible to temperature and humidity, so packaging materials must have good sealing properties. Now glass bottles, plastic bottles and aluminum-plastic blister packaging are commonly used. When packing with glass bottles and plastic bottles, the container shall be cleaned and dried. After a certain number of capsules are filled, the gap in the container shall be filled with dry soft paper, absorbent cotton or plastic cover with elastic wire to prevent vibration. Capsules are easy to absorb moisture and deteriorate, so can also put a small bag of dried silica gel in the bottle as a hygroscopic agent.

胶囊剂宜在阴凉干燥处贮藏。一般来说，高湿度（相对湿度≥ 60%，室温）易使胶囊剂吸湿、软化、变黏、膨胀、内容物结团，并会造成微生物滋生。因此，须选择适当的贮藏条件，一般而言，应在小于 25℃、相对湿度不超过 45% 的干燥阴凉处密闭贮藏。

Capsules should be stored in a cool dry place. Generally speaking, high humidity (relative humidity ≥60%, at room temperature) is easy to make the capsule absorb moisture, soften, become sticky, expand, content agglomerate, and cause microbial growth. Therefore, it is necessary to select appropriate storage conditions. In general, it should be hermetically stored in a dry and cool place below 25℃ and with a relative humidity of less than 45%.

（张　臻）

岗位对接

重点小结

题库

第十四章 丸剂
Chapter 14 Pills

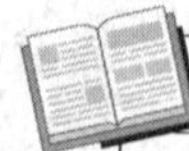

学习目标 | Learning Goals

知识要求：

1. **掌握** 水丸、蜜丸、水蜜丸、浓缩丸、滴丸的含义、特点；泛制法、塑制法、滴制法制备丸剂的基本原理和方法。

2. **熟悉** 糊丸、蜡丸的含义、特点与制法；滴丸成型原理、过程及影响因素；各类丸剂的质量检查方法；丸剂常见质量问题与解决措施。

3. **了解** 丸剂的常见包衣种类与方法。

能力要求：

学会水丸、蜜丸、水蜜丸、浓缩丸、滴丸的制备与质量检查方法。

Knowledge requirements:

1. To master the definition and characteristics of water-bindered pills, honeyed pills, water-honeyed pills, condensed pills and dripping pills. To master the basic principle and preparation process of pills by generic method, molding method and dropping method.

2. To be familiar with the definition, characteristic and preparation process of pasted pills and waxed pills, as well as the forming principle, preparation process and quality influencing factors of dripping pills. To be familiar with the quality inspection methods of all types of pills, as well as the common quality problems of pills and the related resolutions.

3. To know the common types and methods for coating pills.

Ability requirements:

Learn the preparation and quality inspection methods of water-bindered pills, honeyed pills, water- honeyed pills, condensed pills and dripping pills.

第一节 概述
14.1 Overview

PPT

一、丸剂的含义
14.1.1 The Definition of Pills

丸剂系指饮片细粉或（和）饮片提取物加适宜的黏合剂或其他辅料制成的球形或类球形剂型，主要供内服。作为中药传统剂型之一，丸剂最早记载于《五十二病方》，在《神农本草经》《太平惠民和剂局方》等古典医籍中均有记载。剂型与疗效存在紧密联系，临床应用中常选择水丸取其易化、蜜丸取其缓化、糊丸取其迟化，蜡丸取其难化。丸剂作为中药制剂主要剂型之一，2020 年版《中国药典》（一部）中收载品种超过达 300 个。

Pills is one kind of solid preparation dosage forms with the spherical or near spherical shape, made of the uniform mixture of the powder and/or extraction of decoction pieces with the suitable excipients. Pills are mainly for internal administration. As one of the traditional dosage forms of TCM, most of the classical medical books had recorded this dosage form such as *Recipes for fifty-two ailments*, *Shen Nong's Herbal Classic* and *Prescriptions of Peaceful Benevolent Dispensary*. The dosage form is closely related to the curative effect. Based on the relationship between dosage form and therapeutic effect, different kind of pills were employed for different diseases in clinics, given their respective characters. Commonly, water-bindered pills are thought to disintegrate easily and release drugs rapidly. Honeyed pills are thought to melt slowly. Drug-release of pasted pills and waxed pills are thought to be very gradual and lagging behind. Nowadays, pill is still one of the main dosage forms of TCM preparations. According to the statistics, there are total over 300 types of pills recorded in the 2020 edition of *Chinese Pharmacopoeia* (Part Ⅰ).

二、丸剂的特点
14.1.2 The Characteristics of Pills

丸剂的优点：①不同类型的丸剂，释药与作用速度不同。传统丸剂溶散、释药缓慢，可延长药效，适用于慢性病的治疗或病后调和气血；新型水溶性基质滴丸奏效迅速，可用于急救；②固体、半固体药物以及黏稠性的液体药物均可制成丸剂；③提高药物稳定性，减少刺激性、降低毒性或不良反应；④制法简便，既可小量制备，也适于工业生产。

Pills have the following advantages: Ⅰ. Different types of pills have different rates of drug releasing and biological effect. For example, the traditional pill types like honeyed pills commonly dissolves and releases drugs slowly, which is suitable for chronic diseases treatment or tonifying *Qi* and *Blood* after illness. Nevertheless, dripping pills made by water-soluble matrix which can release drugs and produce curative effects quickly, and could be used for first aid; Ⅱ. A variety of drugs including solid, semi-solid and viscous liquid drugs can be encapsulated into pills; Ⅲ. Pills could improve drug stability, reduce gastrointestinal irritation, and decrease toxicity or adverse reactions; Ⅳ. The preparation approach of pills is simple, so that both small-scale preparation and industrial manufacture are suitable.

丸剂的缺点：①某些传统品种剂量大，服用不便，尤其是儿童患者；②制备时控制不当易致溶散迟缓；③以原粉入药，微生物易超标。

Moreover, there are also some drawbacks for pills, such as the large dosage of some traditional pill types. It could result into inconvenient administration, especially for children. Secondly, because of the improper technological parameter, the prepared pills would exhibit over-slow dissolution. Additionally, pills containing raw herbal powder are apt to excessive amounts of microorganisms, even to exceed the limit.

三、丸剂的分类及制法

14.1.3 The Classification and Preparation of Pills

丸剂根据赋形剂种类分为水丸、蜜丸、水蜜丸、浓缩丸、糊丸、蜡丸等。根据制法分为泛制丸、塑制丸和滴制丸。

According to the types of excipients, pills can be divided into water-bindered pills, honeyed pills, water-honeyed pills, condensed pills, pasted pills, waxed pills and so on. According to the preparation method, they could be divided into pills made by generic-method, pills made by molding method and pills made by dropping method.

1. 泛制法 系指在转动的适宜设备中，将饮片细粉与赋形剂交替润湿、撒布、不断翻滚，黏结成粒，逐渐增大的制丸方法。主要用于水丸、水蜜丸、糊丸、浓缩丸的制备。

(1) Generic method This method indicates to produce pills by wetting, spreading and rolling the mixture of herbal fine powder and excipient alternately in the suitable rotating equipment. By this method, powder will bond into particles, and gradually increase to form pills. It is mainly used for the preparation of water-bindered pills, water-honeyed pills, pasted pills and condensed pills.

2. 塑制法 系指饮片细粉加适宜的黏合剂或润湿剂，混合均匀，制成软硬适宜、可塑性好的丸块，再依次制丸条、分粒、搓圆而成丸粒的一种制丸方法。多用于蜜丸、水蜜丸、浓缩丸、糊丸和蜡丸的制备。

(2) Molding method This method indicates to produce pills by mixing herbal fine powder with suitable adhesive or wetting agent evenly, and then make it rod-like, particle-like, and pellet-like mixture. It is mainly used in the preparation of honeyed pills, water-honeyed pills, condensed pills, pasted pills and waxed pills.

3. 滴制法 系指药物与基质制成溶液或混悬液，滴入另一种与之不相混溶的液体冷凝液中，冷凝成丸粒的制丸方法，主要用于滴丸剂的制备。

(3) Dropping method This method indicates to produce pills by dropping the mixture solution or suspension containing drugs and pill substrates into another cold liquid condensate, which cannot be miscible each other. And then the liquid drop can be shrinking into pills. It is mainly used in the preparation of dripping pills.

第二节 水丸
14.2 Water-bindered Pills

一、水丸的含义与特点
14.2.1 Definition and Characteristics

水丸系指饮片细粉以水（或黄酒、醋、稀药液、糖液等）为黏合剂或润湿剂制成的球形或类球形制剂。

Water-bindered pill is one kind of solid dosage forms with spherical or near spherical shape, made of herbal fine powder and adhesive or wetting agents using water, yellow rice wine, vinegar, diluted medicinal juice, syrup, etc.

水丸的特点：①服用后在体内易溶散和吸收，显效快；②一般不另加其他固体赋形剂，实际含药量高；③在制备时可将一些易挥发、有刺激性气味、性质不稳定的药物泛入内层，可防止挥散或变质；或可根据泛制时药物的加入顺序和包衣手段来控制药物释放的速度和部位。④丸粒小、表面致密光滑，便于服用和贮藏；⑤生产设备简单，但制备工序复杂，易引起微生物污染，溶散时限较难控制。

Water-bindered pill exhibited the following characteristics: Ⅰ. It is easy to dissolve in vivo. Drugs in water-bindered pills could be absorbed rapidly, so that it can produce rapid therapeutic effect; Ⅱ. Generally, it contains high drug content because of its few solid excipients; Ⅲ. The volatile or instable drugs, or drugs with pungent smell could be encapsulated into the inner layer of pills, to prevent the volatilization. Additionally, the drug release rate and location could be controlled mediated by the sequence of drug adding and the means of coating; Ⅳ. Due to its small volume and compact smooth surface, it is easy to take and store; Ⅴ. Although the production equipment for water-bindered pill is simple, the preparation process is complex. Owing to the complex preparation process, water-bindered pills are liable to suffer microbial contamination, and uncontrollable dissolution time limit.

二、水丸的赋形剂
14.2.2 Excipients

水丸的赋形剂主要有润湿剂和黏合剂。前者的作用在于润湿药物细粉，诱导其黏性，后者的主要作用在于增强药物细粉的黏性，旨在利于成型。有的赋形剂如酒、醋等，还能利用自身性能起到协同或改变处方药物性能的作用。常用赋形剂有以下几种：

The excipients of water-bindered pills mainly include wetting agents and adhesive agents. The role of wetting agents is to moisten the powder and induce its viscosity, while the main function of adhesive agents is to enhance the viscosity of herbal powder and facilitate the formation of pills. Some excipients, such as wine and vinegar, can play a synergistic role on the therapeutic effect or change the medicinal properties of drugs. The commonly used excipients are listed as following.

1. 水 是最常用的润湿剂，常采用蒸馏水、冷沸水或离子交换水，主要起润湿物料、诱发黏

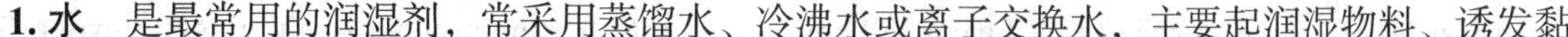

性的作用。

(1) Water It's the most commonly wetting agent, distilled water, cold boiling water or ion exchange water are most commonly used. It mainly plays the role of wetting and inducing the viscosity of raw material.

2. 酒 常用白酒和黄酒，借“酒力”发挥引药上行、祛风散寒、活血通络、矫腥除臭等作用。酒中含有的乙醇能溶解药粉中的树脂、油脂等成分，增加药粉黏性，但其诱导黏性能力不如水。

(2) Wine Wine and yellow rice wine are commonly used. Mediated by the “wine power”, it benefits to leads drugs upward, dispels wind and dissipates cold, promotes blood circulation and dredges collaterals, and eliminates stinking smell. Alcohol in wine can dissolve the resin, grease and other liposoluble components in herbal powder. Although alcohol could increase the viscosity of herbal powder, its ability is weaker than water.

3. 醋 常用米醋，含醋酸为3%~5%，既能润湿，又能使药物中的碱性成分成盐而增加溶解度，还具有引药入肝、理气止痛等作用。

(3) Vinegar Rice vinegar is commonly used, which contains the concentration of acetic acid ranging from 3% to 5%. It can not only moisten powders, but also increase solubility of alkaline components in the raw materials by salifying. Moreover, it also benefits to introduce drugs into liver meridian, regulate *Qi* and relieve pain.

4. 药汁 若处方中含不易粉碎的饮片或鲜药材时，可将其提取或压榨制成药汁，既可发挥自身黏性作用或诱导其他药粉的黏性制丸，又可减少服用体积，使其药性存留。

(4) Herbal juice or extracting solution Fresh herbal materials are commonly pressed into juice, while the herbal decoction pieces uneasy to crush are commonly extracted primarily. Either herbal juice or extracting solution can play its own viscosity role or induce the viscosity of other herbal powder. Meanwhile, the pretreatment approaches could reduce the volume of pills.

三、水丸的制法
14.2.3 Preparation of Water-bindered Pills

泛制法制备水丸的工艺流程如图14-1所示。

The preparation process of water-bindered pills by generic method is shown in Figure 14-1.

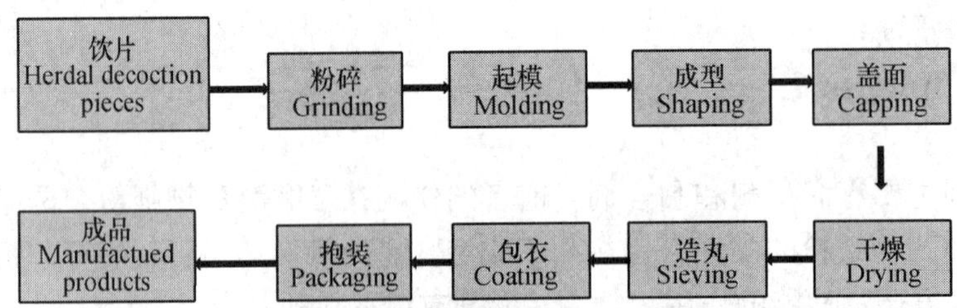

图14-1 泛制法制备水丸工艺流程图

Figure 14-1 Flow Diagram of Preparation Process of Water-bindered Pills by Generic Method

1. 原料准备 泛丸用药粉一般应为细粉或最细粉，起模、盖面或包衣用粉应为最细粉（选用黏性适中的饮片粉碎制得）。部分饮片经提取、浓缩后制成的药汁可作为赋形剂。

(1) Raw materials preparation Herbal powder used for molding, capping or coating should be at the finest level. The powder added during pill shaping should be fine powder or the finest powder. Some herbal pieces could be extracted into herbal extraction solution with concentrated as excipients.

2. 起模 系利用赋形剂的润湿作用诱导出药粉的黏性，使药粉相互黏着成细小的颗粒，并层层增大使成丸模的操作过程。起模是泛制法制备水丸的关键操作，也是丸剂成型的基础。起模的方法主要有粉末直接起模和湿颗粒起模。

(2) Molding During this process, the viscosity of herbal powder is induced by the wetting property of the added excipients, so that the powder could stick together to form the tiny particles. Along with the increased herbal powder added gradually, the particles will enlarge layer by layer to form the pill mold. This process is the key operation to prepare water-bindered pills by generic method and also the basis for pill shaping. The pill molding could be generated by herbal powder directly and wet particles, respectively.

（1）粉末直接起模 在泛丸锅内喷少量水使其润湿，撒布少量药粉，转动泛丸锅，刷下锅壁黏附的粉末，再喷水、撒粉，反复循环多次，粉粒逐渐增大至直径约 1mm 的球形颗粒状，筛取 1 号筛和 2 号筛之间的颗粒，即得模子。

Method Ⅰ is to generate pill mold using herbal powders directly. Briefly, spray a small amount of water was splashed on the surface of pan. And then, a small amount of herbal fine powder was sprinkled into the wet pan. Along with the pan rotating, the adhesive powder on the wall of the pan was brushed down. To splash water and sprinkle herbal powder repeatedly for several times, powder particles gradually increase to about 1mm in diameter. The pill molds were obtained by sieving the particles between no.1 sieve and no.2 sieve.

（2）湿颗粒起模 将药粉以水混匀，按照制粒工艺制成软材，将软材挤压通过 2 号筛制得颗粒，将颗粒置泛丸锅中经旋转、碰撞、摩擦成球状，过筛分等即得模子。

Method Ⅱ is to generate pill mold using the tiny wet particles. Briefly, the herbal powder was mixed with water and generated wet particles according to the granulation process, in which the wet mixed herbal powder mixture is extruded through no.2 sieve. The obtained wet particles were put into the pan, and then continue to rotate pan, so that particles could collide, rub and polish into spheres. Finally, the pill molds were obtained by sieving the spheres between no.1 sieve and no.2 sieve.

3. 成型 系指将经筛选合格的丸模逐渐加大至接近成品的操作。加大成型的方法和起模相同。

(3) Shaping This process is to increase the size of obtained pill molds till it is close to the final manufactured product, using the same procedures as Molding Process.

4. 盖面 将已经成型、筛选合格的丸粒，用药材细粉或水继续在泛丸锅内滚动操作，使达到成品规定的大小标准，丸粒表面致密、光洁，色泽一致。

(4) Capping After sieving, the shaped pills were capped using the fine herbal powder in the rolling pan to achieve the required size of the final manufactured product. After that, the surface of pills should be dense and smooth, with the uniform color.

5. 干燥 盖面后的丸粒应及时干燥，温度一般控制在 80℃以下，含挥发性成分的水丸控制在 60℃以下。多采用烘房、烘箱进行，还可采用沸腾干燥、微波干燥、远红外线干燥等方法。

(5) Drying After capping, the pills should be dried in time. Commonly, the temperature should be below 80℃, while the dried temperature should be set below 60℃ when pills contain volatile components. During this process, besides the conventional heating in drying room or drying oven, fluidized drying, microwave drying and far infra-red drying method also can be used.

6. 选丸 为保证水丸的外观、重量差异等质量要求，干燥后应采用手摇筛、振动筛、滚筒筛、检丸器或连续成丸机组等进行筛选。

(6) Pill sieving In order to ensure the quality requirements of water-bindered pills including appearance, weight difference and others, pills should be sieved by hand shaking sieve, vibrating sieve, rotary sieve, pill detector or continuous pill forming machine set after drying.

7. 包衣 根据医疗需要，将水丸表面包裹衣层的操作称为包衣或上衣，包衣后的丸剂称为“包衣丸剂”。

(7) Coating Sometimes, according to requires of treatment, the surface of water-bindered pills should be coated with some materials.

8. 质检包装 按照水丸的质量标准对成品进行检验，质量检查合格后即可包装。

(8) Quality inspection and Packaging The finished pill products shall be inspected according to the quality standard. The qualified pills can be then packed.

案例导入 ¦ Case example

案例 14-1 防风通圣丸

14-1 Fangfeng Tongsheng Pills

处方： 防风 50g 荆芥穗 25g 薄荷 50g 麻黄 50g 大黄 50g 芒硝 50g 栀子 25g 滑石 300g 桔梗 100g 石膏 100g 川芎 50g 当归 50g 白芍 50g 黄芩 100g 连翘 50g 甘草 200g 白术（炒）25g

Ingredients Saposhnikoviae Radix 50g; Schizonepetae Spica 25g; Menthae Haplocalycis Herba 50g; Ephedrae herba 50g; Rhei Radix et Rhizoma 50g; Natrii Sulfas 50g; Gardeniae Fructus 25g; Talcum 300g; Platycodonis Radix 100g; Gypsum Fibrosum 100g; Chuanxiong Rhizoma 50g; Angelicae Sinensis Radix 50g; Paeoniae Radix Alba 50g; Scutellariae Radix 100g; Forsythiae Fructus 50g; Glycyrrhizae Radix rt Rhizoma 200g; Atractylodis Macrocephalae Rhizoma (stir-baked) 25g.

功能与主治： 解表通里，清热解毒。用于外寒内热，表里俱实，恶寒壮热，头痛咽干，小便短赤，大便秘结，瘰疬初起，风疹湿疮。

Functions and indications To release the exterior, unblock the interior, clear heat and remove toxin. Used for external cold and interior heat, excess in dual exterior and interior, evil cold and strong heat, headache and dry throat, scanty dark urine, constipation, beginning of scrofula, rubella wet sores.

制法： 以上十七味，滑石粉粉碎成极细粉；其余防风等十六味粉碎成细粉、过筛、混匀，用水制丸，干燥，用滑石粉包衣，打光，干燥，即得。

Making Procedure Pulverize the above ingredients except Talcum into a fine powder, sift and mix well. Add an appropriate quantity of water, make pills, and dry. Pulverize Talcum into a very fine powder, coat the pills, polish and dry. Alternatively, pulverize the above seventeen ingredients into a fine powder, sift and mix well, add an appropriate quantity of water, make pills, and dry.

用法用量： 口服。一次 6g，一日 2 次。

Usage and dosage For oral administration, 6g per time, twice a day.

注解： ①芒硝主要成分为 $Na_2SO_4 \cdot 10H_2O$，极易溶于水。以芒硝水溶液泛丸，既能使之成形，又能起治疗作用。

②滑石粉既是药物，又用作包衣剂，节省了辅料，同时也可防止薄荷、荆芥中挥发性成分的散失。

③在滑石粉中加入 10% 的 $MgCO_3$，可增加洁白度，并增强其附着力。

④包衣前丸粒应充分干燥，包衣时撒粉用量要均匀，黏合剂浓度要适量，否则易造成花斑。

Notes: ① $Na_2SO_4 \cdot 10H_2O$ is the main component of Natrii Sulfas, which is easy to dissolve in

water. With the aqueous solution of Natrii Sulfas preparing water-bindered pills, it not only can facilitate the formation of pills, but also can exert therapeutic effects. ② The role of talcum powder is not only a drug but also a coating agent. So that can reduce the usage of excipients and prevent the loss of volatile components in Menthae Haplocalycis Herbaa and Schizonepetae Spica. ③ Note Ⅲ. Talcum powders contained the concentration of $MgCO_3$ reaching 10%, that can increase its whiteness and enhance its adhesion. ④ Pills should be fully dried before coating. The dosage of coating powders should be uniform. The concentration of adhesive agent should be appropriate. Otherwise it is easy to cause spots.

思考题：丸剂包衣的目的以及其操作注意事项是什么？

Question：What are the purpose of pills coating and what are the attention of preparation?

第三节 蜜丸

14.3 Honeyed Pills

PPT

一、蜜丸的含义与特点

14.3.1 Definition and Characteristics

蜜丸系指饮片细粉以蜂蜜为黏合剂制成的丸剂。以蜂蜜和水为黏合剂制成的丸剂称水蜜丸。传统蜜丸分为大蜜丸和小蜜丸，每丸重量在 0.5g（含 0.5g）以上的称大蜜丸，0.5g 以下的称小蜜丸。

Honeyed pills are made of herbal fine powder using honey as adhesives. Among them, the pill using the mixture of honey and water as adhesives is called as water-honeyed pills. Based on the weight of honeyed pills, they could be divided into large honeyed pills and small honeyed pills, in which over 0.5g (also including 0.5g) for each pill is big honeyed pills, while those weighing less than 0.5g per pill are small honeyed pills.

二、蜂蜜的炼制

14.3.2 Refining of Honey

蜂蜜的炼制系指将蜂蜜加热熬炼至规定程度的操作。炼蜜的目的是为了除去杂质、降低水分含量、破坏酶类、杀死微生物、增加蜂蜜黏性等。在制备蜜丸时，应根据物料特性对蜂蜜进行适当炼制。炼制的蜂蜜分为嫩蜜、中蜜、老蜜 3 种规格，应根据药材性质选择，详细规格见表 14-1。

As the adhesives of honeyed pills, commercial honey in market should be refined by heating, in order to remove impurities, reduce water content, destroy enzymes, kill microorganisms, and increase the viscosity of honey. During the honeyed pills preparation, honey should be refined to the certain extent according to the characteristics of raw materials. The refined honey can be divided into three specifications, i.e. tender honey, medium honey and mature honey. The properties and the suitable raw material of different specifications of refined honey are listed in Table 14-1.

表 14-1　蜂蜜的炼制规格及适用性

规格	炼蜜温度（℃）	含水量（%）	相对密度	适用物料
嫩蜜	105~115	17~20	1.35	含有较多油脂、黏液质、胶质、糖、淀粉、动物组织等黏性较强物料
中蜜	116~118	14~16	1.37	黏性中等的物料
老蜜	119~122	10 以下	1.40	黏性差的矿物质或纤维质物料

Table 14-1　Refining Specifications and Applicability of Honey

Specifications	Temperature (℃)	Water content (%)	Relative density	Suitable raw materials
Tender honey	105~115	17~20	1.35	Raw material with strong viscosity contains oil, slime, gum, polysaccharide, starch, animal tissue, etc.
Medium honey	116~118	14~16	1.37	Raw material with moderate viscosity
Mature honey	119~122	<10	1.40	Raw material with poor viscosity like mineral or fibrous material

嫩蜜的色泽与生蜜比无明显变化，略有黏性；中蜜是将嫩蜜继续加热炼制，手捻有一定黏性，两手指分开无白丝出现时为度，是用途最广泛的炼蜜规格，现行版《中国药典》中多采用中蜜规格为用；将中蜜继续加热，呈红棕色，手捻之甚黏，两手指分开出现长白丝，呈“滴水成珠”时即为老蜜。

Specifically, tender honey exhibits the similar color and lustre as raw honey, with the slight stickiness. Medium honey could be obtained by the continued heating and refining with the increased stickiness, compared to that of tender honey. The viscosity limitation of medium honey is no white silk between the separated two fingers appear when it is twisted with fingers. Medium honey is the most widely used specification used for honey pills in the current 2020 edition of *Chinese Pharmacopoeia*. Furthermore, mature honey could be obtained by the continued heating and refining of medium honey, showing reddish brown appearance. Compared to medium honey, mature honey exhibits stickier. Long white silk between two separated fingers could be observed when it was twisted with fingers. Besides, it will exhibit as beads when it was dropped on papers.

三、蜜丸的制法

14.3.3　Preparation of Honeyed Pills

蜜丸主要采用塑制法制备，工艺流程，如图 14-2 所示。

Honeyed pills are mainly prepared by molding method. The process flow chart is shown in Figure 14-2.

1. 物料准备　采用适宜方法对饮片进行粉碎，过筛，制备得到细粉或最细粉；按照物料性质选择蜂蜜炼制规格；将制丸工具清洁后用 70% 乙醇擦拭备用。

(1) Raw materials preparation　The fine or finest herbal powder are prepared by crushing the herbal decoction pieces using a suitable method and then sieving. Meanwhile, honey is refined into the suitable specification according to the property of herbal powder. Additionally, all tools to prepare pills are cleaned and wiped with 70% ethanol.

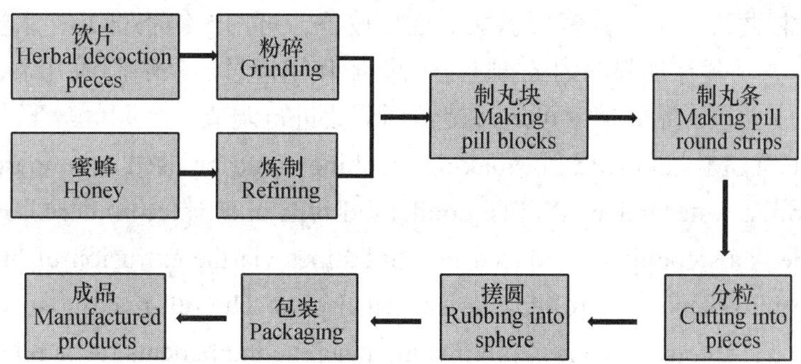

图 14-2　蜜丸塑制法制备工艺流程图

Figure 14-2　Flow Diagram of Preparation Process of Honeyed Pills by Molding Method

2. 制丸块　是塑制法的关键工序。在药粉中加入适量的蜂蜜，充分混匀，制成软硬及黏稠度适宜的丸块，并具有一定的可塑性。

(2) Making pill blocks　It is the key process in molding method. Briefly, a certain amount of refined honey is added into herbal powder and mixed into pill blocks with suitable hardness, viscosity, and plasticity. There are some notes need to notice.

（1）炼蜜规格　炼蜜规格应根据药粉性质、粒度、含水量、温度和湿度来选择。

① The honey refining specifications should be selected according to property, particles size and water content of herbal powder, operation temperature and humidity.

（2）和药时的蜜温　处方中含有树脂、胶质、糖等成分的中药，和药蜜温应低于 80℃。当处方中含有冰片、麝香等芳香挥发性药物时，应采用温蜜和药，处方药物黏性较差时以老蜜趁热加入和药。

② The honey temperature to mix with herbal powder should be selected according to the property of herbal powder. To mix with herbal powder containing resin, gum and polysaccharide, the honey temperature should be lower than 80℃, while the honey temperature should be lower than 60℃ when there are some aromatic volatile drugs such as Bornrolum, Moschus in the prescription. Additionally, the herbal powder with poor viscosity should be mixed with the heating mature honey.

（3）蜂蜜用量　一般用量为 1 ∶ 1~1 ∶ 1.5。如药粉自身黏性强，则用蜜量少，黏性差者用蜜量多；冬季用蜜量多，夏季少；手工和药比机械和药用蜜量大。

③ Generally, the dosage ratio of honey and herbal powder is 1 ∶ 1~1 ∶ 1.5. If the material powder has good viscosity, the use dosage of honey could be reduced, while more honey should be used for the herbal powder with poor viscosity. Additionally, using much more honey when the process is implemented in winter than that in summer. The dosage of honey in hand-made process will be more than that by machine.

3. 制丸条、分粒与搓圆　将上述丸块采用一定方法制成条状，再进行分割搓圆的操作。随着制药设备的不断发展，在大生产中多采用机器制丸，生产中常见的生产设备有中药自动制丸机和光电自控制丸机。

(3) Making pill round strips, Cutting into pieces and Rubbing into sphere　The prepared pill blocks will be shaped into strips, and then cut into pieces, following with rubbing these pieces into small spheres. With the development of pharmaceutical equipment, these processes could be finished in pill making machines such as TCM automatic pill making machine and photoelectric automatic control pill making machine in industrial production.

（1）中药自动制丸机　是一种多用途丸剂成型设备，可用于制备蜜丸、水蜜丸、浓缩丸、水丸，如图 14-3 所示。药料在加料斗内经推进器的挤压作用通过出条嘴制成丸条，丸条经导轮被传递至刀具切、搓而成丸粒，制丸速度可通过旋转调节钮进行调节。

Specifically, the TCM automatic pill making machine could be used to prepare multiple types of pills like honeyed pills, water-honeyed pills, condensed pills and water-bindered pills. As shown, the mixture in the hopper pills could be produced into pill stipes via the extrusion of propeller, which will be subsequently cut into pieces and rolled into spherical pills. The pill-making speed can be adjusted. Otherwise, photoelectric automatic control pill making machine implements the similar procedures, while it is controlled by photoelectric signal system.

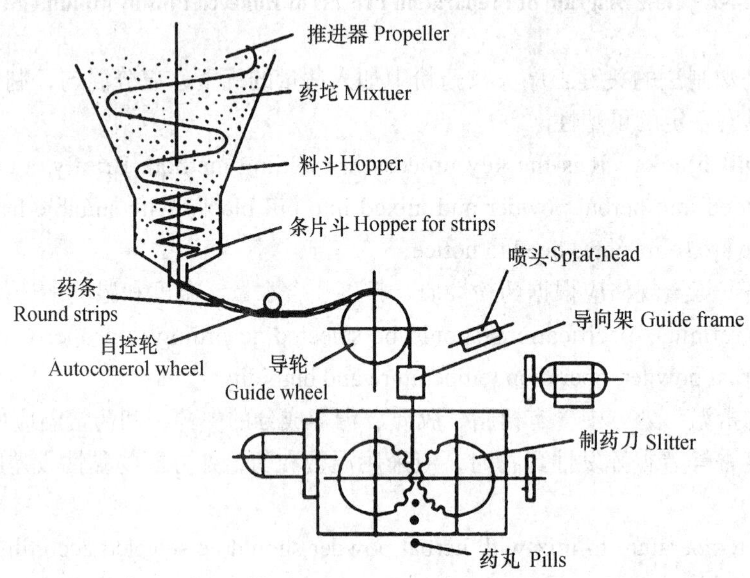

图 14-3　中药自动制丸机示意图

Figure 14-3　Automatic Pelletizing Machine of TCM Pills

（2）光电自控制丸机　采用光电讯号系统控制制丸条、切丸等工序。

Photoelectric automatic control pill machine using photoelectric signal control the process of strip making and cutting pills, etc..

4. 干燥、质检、包装　为了保证蜜丸的滋润状态，成丸后应立即分装。为防止蜜丸霉变，成品可采用微波干燥、远红外辐射干燥等方法进行干燥，同时有一定的灭菌效果。干燥后的丸剂，质量检查合格后即可包装。

(4) Drying, Quality inspection and Packaging　In order to ensure the moist state of honeyed pills, they should be subpackaged after preparation immediately. In order to prevent mildew, these finished products can be dried by microwave drying, far-infrared radiation drying, etc. During the drying process, it also has certainly sterilization outcome. The dried pills can be packaged after quality inspection.

四、蜜丸常见质量问题与解决措施
14.3.4　Common Quality Problems and Solutions

1. 表面粗糙　主要原因有：①药粉过粗；②蜜量过少且混合不均匀；③润滑剂用量不足；④药料含纤维多；⑤矿物类或贝壳类药量过大等。可采用提高药材的粉碎度；加大用蜜量或用较老的蜂蜜；制丸机传送带与切刀部位涂足润滑剂；将富含纤维类药材或矿物类药材提取浓缩成稠

膏兑入炼蜜中等方法解决。

(1) One of the common quality problems is rough surface. It could be caused by some main reasons, including the oversize particle of herbal powder, insufficient honey, uneven mixing with herbal materials, less lubricant, too much fiber in herbal materials, too many minerals or shellfish, etc. In order to solve these problems, some solutions could be implemented to reduce the particle size of herbal materials, increase the amount of honey or use the mature honey specification, smear sufficient lubricant in the conveyor belt and cutting knife of pill-making machine, prepare the concentrated extraction solution derived from herbal materials rich in fiber or mineral materials, and mix it with the refined honey.

2. 空心 主要原因是丸块揉搓不够。在生产中应注意控制好和药及制丸操作；有时是因药材油性过大，蜂蜜难以黏合所致，可用嫩蜜和药。

(2) Hollow pill is another quality problem, mainly caused by the insufficient kneading during the preparation of pill blocks. Sometimes, the oily herbal materials are difficult to stick together. The tender honey can be used as the adhesives to mix with herbal materials.

3. 丸粒过硬 蜜丸在存放过程中变得坚硬。其原因有：①炼蜜过老；②和药蜜温低；③用蜜量不足；④含胶类药材比例大，和药时蜜温过高使其烊化后又凝固；⑤蜂蜜质量差或不合格。可采取控制好炼蜜程度或和药蜜温、调整用蜜量、使用合格蜂蜜等措施解决。

(3) In addition, some pills will become too flinty during storage. This problem would be caused by the excessive heating and refining of honey, the excessively low honey temperature, the insufficient honey, the caused gelatinization of gel-based medicinal materials on the extra-high honey temperature, or the unqualified honey. Therefore, measures can be taken to regulate the honey refining degree, mixing temperature, the amount of honey, or use the qualified honey, etc.

4. 皱皮 蜜丸贮存一定时间后，在其表面呈现皱褶现象。主要原因有：①炼蜜较嫩，含水量过多，水分蒸发后导致蜜丸萎缩；②包装不严，蜜丸湿热季节吸湿而干燥季节失水；③润滑剂使用不当。可针对原因采取相应措施解决。

(4) The surface of some pill would appear wrinkles after they are stored for a certain period. The main reasons are ascribed to the high water content in the tender honey, inadequate packing and improper use of lubricant. Specifically, the water evaporation will lead to the shrinkage of honeyed pills. The untight packaging would result in the moisture absorption in humid season, while water loss in dry season. Corresponding measures can be taken to solve the causes.

5. 微生物限度超标 采用热蜜和药，缩短制丸操作时间，可以有效降低微生物数量。

(5) The application of the hot honey benefit to shorten the preparation time, so that to reduce the microbial population.

五、水蜜丸
14.3.5 Water-Honeyed Pills

案例导入

水蜜丸可采用塑制法（方法同蜜丸）和泛制法（方法同水丸）制备。

Water-honeyed pills can be prepared by molding method and by generic method, which are similar as honeyed pills and water-bindered pills, respectively.

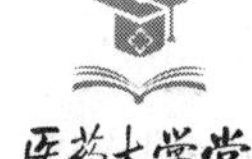

采用塑制法制备水蜜丸时，应注意药粉的性质与蜜水的浓度和用量，一般情况下，黏性适中的药料每100g用炼蜜40g，含纤维和矿物药较多的药料每100g用炼蜜50g左右，含黏液质、糖、胶类等较多的药料每100g用炼蜜10~50g，按炼蜜：水=1：（2.5~3.0）制备蜜水，搅匀后、煮沸、

滤过备用。

During the preparation of water-honeyed pills by molding method, both the concentration and dosage of honey water solution should be evaluated according to the properties of the herbal powder. In general, 100g of herbal materials with moderate viscosity need to mix with 40g of refined honey. 100g of herbal materials containing fiber and minerals should be mixed with about 50g of refined honey. To mix with 100g of herbal materials rich in mucilage, polysaccharide and gels needs about 10-50g of refined honey. Nevertheless, the honey water solution could be prepared using the refining honey, with the ratio of refining honey and water at 1：(2.5-3.0), by stirring, boiling, and filtering.

采用泛制法制备时，炼蜜应以沸水稀释后使用。在起模阶段必须以水起模，以免黏结。在加大成型阶段，先用低浓度的蜜水加大丸粒，待逐步成型时用浓度稍高的蜜水，成型后再改用低浓度蜜水撞光即可。水蜜丸中含水量较高，成丸后应及时干燥，以防霉变。

Moreover, when using the generic method, the refined honey should be diluted with boiled water aforehand. The wetting agent used to produce the molds should be water, instead of honey water. Different concentration of honey water could be used in the different preparation stages. During the shaping process, the low concentration of honey water can be used to increase the size of pill molds. A slightly higher concentration of honey water can be used till pills are basically shaped. However, it will be changed into a low concentration of honey water during the polishing process. In view of the high water content in water-honeyed pills, after produced it should be dried in time to prevent mildew.

第四节 浓缩丸

14.4 Condensed Pills

PPT

一、概述

14.4.1 Overview

浓缩丸系指饮片或部分饮片提取浓缩后，与适宜的辅料或其余饮片细粉以水、蜂蜜或蜂蜜和水为黏合剂制成的丸剂。根据使用黏合剂的不同，分为浓缩水丸、浓缩蜜丸和浓缩水蜜丸。浓缩丸服用、携带及贮藏均较方便，但浓缩丸在提取浓缩过程中受热时间较长，可能会影响部分有效成分的稳定性。

Condensed pills are made of the mixture of condensed extraction solution of entire or partial herbal decoction pieces in prescription, and appropriate excipients or fine herbal powder of residual pieces in prescription, with the assistance of adhesives including water, honey or honey water solution. Based on the varieties of adhesives, condensed pills could be divided into condensed water-bindered pill, condensed honeyed pills, and condensed water-honeyed pills. They may be classified into concentrated water-bindered pills, concentrated honeyed pills and concentrated water-honeyed pills based upon the different binders used in the production. Condensed pills are convenient to take, carry and store. However, because of the prolonged heating during extraction and concentration, some effective components in condensed pills would be instable.

二、浓缩丸的制法
14.4.2　Preparation of Condensed Pills

1. 药物处理原则　处理原则一般为：贵重细料药、含淀粉较多的药料，宜粉碎成细粉；质地坚硬、富含纤维、体积大、黏性大的药料，宜提取制膏。有效成分（或有效部位）明确且含量较高的药料，可提取有效成分或有效部位，缩小体积。

(1) Pretreatment principle of raw materials　Commonly, these herbs with high price or rich in starch should be smashed into fine powder. Nevertheless, the texture-hard, fiber-rich, bulky or viscous herbs should be extracted in advance. These definite bioactive components or fraction with high content in herbs could be obtained by specific extraction and isolation, to reduce the herbal volume.

2. 制备工艺　主要有泛制法和塑制法，近年来，还出现了压制法制备技术用于浓缩丸的制备。

(2) Preparation process of condensed pills　The preparation methods of condensed pills mainly include generic method and molding method for the different types of condensed pills. In recent years, press forming method also has been employed to prepare condensed pills.

（1）泛制法　主要用于水丸型浓缩丸的制备。以饮片提取液浓缩成清膏作为黏合剂，其余饮片粉碎成细粉用于泛丸；或将稠膏与细粉混合，干燥，再粉碎成细粉，以用水或不同浓度乙醇为润湿剂泛制成丸。

Specifically, the generic method is mainly used to prepare the concentrated water-bindered pills. Firstly, part of herbal decoction pieces is extracted. The concentrated extraction solution with a low concentration is subsequently used as adhesive to mix with fine powder obtained from the smashed residual herbal decoction pieces. Pills could be prepared by the generic method using the mixture as materials directly. Additionally, there is another preparation process approach. The high concentration herbal extraction could mix with herbal fine powder firstly. After drying and smashing, the obtained fine mixture powder is used to produce pills by generic method using water or ethanol solution as wetting agents.

（2）塑制法　用于蜜丸型浓缩丸的制备。取部分饮片提取浓缩成膏作为黏合剂，其余饮片粉碎成细粉，再加适量炼蜜，混合均匀，制丸块、丸条，分粒，搓圆，即得。

Otherwise, the molding method is mainly used to prepare the concentrated honeyed pills. Similarly, part of herbal decoction pieces is extracted and concentrated into paste as adhesive. The herbal fine powder of residual decoction pieces will mix with the herbal extraction paste and some refined honey, to make the pill block, pill round strips, cut them into pieces and rub them into spherical pills.

（3）压制法　该法将部分浸膏和饮片细粉制成颗粒（多采用流化床制粒），利用压片机压制成丸模，将剩余提取物、药粉及适量赋形剂在丸模基础上增圆成型。

In the press forming method, part of herbal extract and fine powder of herbal pieces are made into granules, mostly mediated by fluidized bed granulation approach. The herbal granules could be pressed into pill molds by tablet press machine. Pills could generate by adding the remaining extract, herbal powder and appropriate excipients on the surface of pill molds gradually.

浓缩水蜜丸、浓缩水丸成丸后应及时干燥（80℃以下），含挥发性成分的丸剂干燥温度应保持在60℃以下，不宜加热者采用其他适宜方法干燥。

Concentrated water-honeyed pills and concentrated water-bindered pills should be dried in time (normally at below 80℃) after preparation. While pills containing volatile ingredients should be dried at

below 60℃. The drying of pills containing thermo-labile ingredients should be cautious.

案例导入 | Case example

案例 14-2　黄连上清丸

14-2　Huanglian Shangqing Pills

处方： 黄连 15g　栀子（姜制）120g　连翘 120g　蔓荆子（炒）120g　防风 60g　荆芥穗 120g　白芷 120g　黄芩 120g　菊花 240g　薄荷 60g　大黄（酒炙）480g　黄柏（酒炒）60g　桔梗 120g　川芎 60g　石膏 60g　旋覆花 30g　甘草 60g

Ingredients: Coptidis Rhizoma 15g; Gardeniae Fructus (processed with ginger) 120g; Forsythiae Fructus 120g; Viticis Fructus (stir-baked) 120g; Saposhnikoviae Radix 60g; Schizonepetae Spica 120g; Angelicae Dahuricae Radix 120g; Scutellariae Radix 120g; Chrysanthemi Flos 240g; Menthae Herba 60g; Rhei Radix et Rhizoma (stir-baked with with) 480g; Phellodendri Cortex (stir-baked with wine) 60g; Platycodonis Radix 120g; Chuanxiong Rhizoma 60g; Gypsum Fibrosum 60g; Inulae Flos 30g; Glycyrrhizae Radix et Rhizoma 60g

功能与主治： 清热通便，散风止痛。用于上焦风热，头晕脑胀，牙龈肿痛，口舌生疮，咽喉红肿，耳痛耳鸣，暴发火眼，大便干燥，小便黄赤。

Functions and indications: This pill have the therapeutic effects of clearing heat, relaxing constipation, dispelling wind and relieving pain. It is used for wind-heat attacking upward and exuberant heat, dizziness and vertigo, toothache, mouth and tongue sores, swollen sore throats, ear pain and tinnitus, constipation, deep-coloured urine due to in lung and stomach.

制法： 以上十七味，黄连、大黄、白芷、桔梗、旋覆花、黄柏、防风、栀子、石膏中部分粉碎成细粉，过筛，备用；连翘、川芎、荆芥穗、薄荷用水蒸气蒸馏提取挥发油，蒸馏后的水溶液另器保存；药渣加入其余菊花等，加水煎煮两次，第一次 2 小时，第二次 1.5 小时，合并煎液，滤过，滤液加入蒸馏后的水溶液浓缩至相对密度为 1.03~1.05（70℃）的清膏，与上述细粉泛丸，干燥，放冷，加入挥发油，混匀，共制成 1000g，即得。

Making Procedure: Firstly, Above 17 ingredients, Coptidis Rhizoma, Rhei Radix et Rhizoma, Angelicae Dahuricae Radix, Platycodonis Radix, Inulae Flos, Phellodendri Cortex, Saposhnikoviae Radix, Gardeniae Fructus, Gypsum Fibrosum in part crushed into fine powder. Next, Forsythiae Fructus, Chuanxiong Rhizoma, Schizonepetae Spica and Menthae Herba use steam distillation to extract volatile oil, and the distilled aqueous solution is stored in another vessel. The residue was added to other Chrysanthemi Flos, Fried twice in water, the first 2h, the second 1.5h, combined with decoction, filtered. The filtrate was added to distilled aqueous solution and concentrated to a paste with a relative concentration of 1.03-1.05 (70℃). Pills could be prepared by the generic method using the mixture of the paste and fine powder. After drying and cooling, pills was added volatile oil, and made into 1000g.

用法与用量： 口服，一次 3g，一日 2 次。

Usage and dosage: For oral administration，3g per time, twice a day.

注解： ①本制剂根据饮片性质及所含有效成分，对含挥发油较多的连翘等四味饮片采用双提法进行提取，其余饮片粉碎所得细粉与上述提取所的清膏以泛制法制备成浓缩丸。

②本制剂挥发油可采用喷加的方式使其均匀分布于丸粒表面，密闭放置一定时间使其充分吸收，也可采用 β- 环糊精包合后再与其他物料混合泛丸成型。

③在干燥时应充分考虑温度对丸剂稳定性的影响，应保持低温干燥或其他干燥方式；还可采

用包衣手段以进一步增强制剂的稳定性。

Notes: ① According to the properties of the prepared pieces and the effective ingredients, the four-flavor prepared pieces containing more volatile oil, such as Forsythiae Fructus, were extracted by double extraction method. Pills could be prepared by the generic method using the mixture of the paste and fine powder obtained from the pulverization of the remaining prepared pieces. ② The volatile oil of this preparation can be sprayed to make it evenly distributed on the surface of the pill, sealed and placed for a certain time to make it fully absorbed, or it can be mixed with other materials after the inclusion of β-cyclodextrin to prepared make into pills. ③ During drying, the influence of temperature on the stability of pill should be fully taken into account.Low-temperature drying or other drying methods should be maintained. Coating can also be used to further enhance the stability of the preparation.

思考题：①本制剂能否采用塑制法制备？

②本制剂可采用哪些干燥方法？

Questions: Firstly, Can the preparation be prepared by the Molding method? Secondly, what drying methods can be used for this preparation?

第五节　糊丸与蜡丸

14.5　Pasted Pills and Waxed Pills

PPT

一、糊丸

14.5.1　Pasted Pills

案例导入

1. 糊丸的含义与特点

(1) Definition and characteristics

糊丸系指饮片细粉以米糊或面糊等为黏合剂制成的丸剂。糊丸历史悠久，始见于汉代《伤寒论》方中，在宋代广泛使用。传统糊丸以米糊、面糊作为黏合剂，质地坚硬，在胃内溶散迟缓，释药缓慢，可延长药效发挥，且能减少药物对胃肠道的刺激，一般含有剧毒或刺激性较强的药物的处方多制成糊丸。

Pasted pills are made of herbal fine powder using rice paste or flour paste as adhesives. The application of pasted pills has a long history, which was first recorded in *Treatise on Febrile Diseases* in Han dynasty and widely used in the Song dynasty. Pasted pills exhibit hard texture and slow dissolution in gastrointestinal tract, because of the strong viscidity of rice paste and flour paste. Therefore, pasted pills display slow drug release, prolonged therapeutic efficacy and reduced the gastrointestinal irritation. The prescriptions containing extremely toxic or strong irritant drugs are apt to be made as paste pills.

2. 糊丸的制法

(2) Preparation of pasted pills

（1）泛制法　以水起模，用稀糊（经滤过除去块状物）作为黏合剂泛丸，操作方法同水丸。

糊丸干燥宜置于通风处阴干或低温干燥，切忌高温烘烤或曝晒。

（2）塑制法　与蜜丸制法相似，只是以糊代替炼蜜。应尽量缩短制丸时间，以免丸粒表面粗糙、裂缝。

The preparation of pasted pills mainly adopts generic method and molding method. The operational approach of pasted pills by generic method is similar as that of water-bindered pills, while using water for molding and dilute paste as adhesives. However, the pasted pills only should be dried by air dry in the ventilated and shade place or heated at low temperature. They must avoid heating at high temperature or exposure under strong sunlight. The operational approach of pasted pills by generic method is similar as that of honeyed pills, while using paste as adhesives instead of refined honey. In this process, the pill preparation time should be shortened as far as possible to avoid the occurrence of rough or crack surface of pills.

二、蜡丸
14.5.2 Waxed Pills

1. 蜡丸的含义与特点　蜡丸系指饮片细粉以蜂蜡为黏合剂制成的丸剂。蜡丸在体内不溶散，缓慢持久释放药物，与现代骨架型缓释、控释释药系统相似。毒性或刺激性强的药物，制成蜡丸可减轻毒性和刺激性，但其释药速度的控制难度大，目前蜡丸品种较少。

(1) Definition and characteristics　Waxed pills are made of herbal fine powder using beeswax as adhesives. Waxed pills exhibit much slower drug release in vivo, compared to pasted pills. They are commonly deemed as the rudiment of the modern sustained drug release and controlled drug release systems. In clinics, drugs with extremely strong toxicity or irritation could be loaded in wax pills to reduce toxicity and irritation. However, it is difficult to control the drug release rate of wax pills in practice. Therefore, only few wax pill products retain in market at present.

2. 蜡丸的制法　蜡丸多采用塑制法制备。将精制的处方量蜂蜡，加热熔化，冷却至60℃左右，待蜡液开始凝固，表面有结膜时，加入药粉，迅速搅拌至混合均匀，趁热制丸条，分粒，搓圆。

(2) Preparation of Waxed pills　Wax pills are mostly prepared by molding method. Briefly, the purified beeswax is weighted for its prescription dosage and primarily melt by heating. When the melt beeswax cools down to about 60℃, the wax began to solidify with surface film appearing. Herbal powder is quickly added and mixed with melt beeswax thoroughly. The mixture will be made into round strips, cut into pieces and rub them into spherical pills

第六节　滴丸
14.6 Dripping Pills

一、滴丸的含义与特点
14.6.1 Definition and Characteristics

滴丸系指饮片提取物与适宜的基质加热熔融混匀，滴入不相混溶的冷凝介质中制成的球形或类球形制剂，一般采用滴制法制备。滴丸是基于固体分散技术制成的丸剂，中药滴丸的研制始于20

世纪70年代末，1977年版《中国药典》开始收载滴丸剂，目前已上市的中药滴丸有20多种。

TCM dripping pills are the solid preparations made by dripping the uniformly heated melted mixture of herbal extraction and appropriate matrix excipients into the immiscible and non-interacting cooling medium. The dropped mixture will generate into spherical or near spherical pill in the cooling medium. This preparation method is called as dropping method, based on the solid dispersion technology. The development of TCM dripping pills began in the late 1970s, and the TCM dripping pill products were recorded in the 1977 edition of *Chinese Pharmacopoeia*. Right now, over 20 types of TCM dripping pill products could be found in domestic market.

滴丸主要特点有：①药物在基质中呈分子、胶体或微粉状态高度分散；②生产工艺简单，周期短，效率高；③滴丸中药物被基质包裹，增加了药物的稳定性；④滴丸可使液态药物固体化；⑤用药部位多，既可以口服，也适于耳、鼻、口腔等局部用药；⑥滴丸载药量较小，服用剂量大，因此对药物的前处理要求较高。

Totally, dripping pills have the following characters. Firstly, drugs are highly dispersed in the matrix excipients with the molecular, colloidal or micro-powder state, so that they could be released and absorbed rapidly in vivo. Secondly, dripping pills have the simple preparation process, short preparation period and high preparation efficiency. Thirdly, the stability of drugs in dripping pills could be enhanced because of the coat of matrix excipients. The fourth property is that liquid drugs in dripping pills could be solidified. Additionally, dripping pills could be administered in many application sites, including gastrointestinal tract for systemic administration, and local application sites such as ears, nose and mouth. However, being limited to the small volume, dripping pills only can load a few drugs, so that a large dosage of dripping pills needs in clinics. Therefore, the pretreatment of drugs in dripping pills is demanding.

二、滴丸的制法

14.6.2 Preparation of Dripping Pills

案例导入

1. 滴丸基质要求与选用 滴丸中除药物以外的赋形剂称为基质。滴丸基质应具备以下条件：①不与药物发生任何化学反应，不影响主药的疗效和检测；②熔点较低或加一定量热水（60℃以上）能溶化成液体，遇骤冷又能凝固，室温下保持固体状态；③对人体安全无害。

(1) Requirements and selection principle of matrix excipients in dripping pills Matrix excipients are important for dripping pills shaping. Matrix excipients in dropping pill cannot interact with drugs or influence the therapeutic efficacy and detection of drugs. Also, matrix excipients should have a low melting point. It could be melted into liquid state at over 60℃, while transform into solid when shock cooling. More importantly, it should be safe and harmless to human health.

滴丸基质分为水溶性和非水溶性两大类。水溶性基质有聚乙二醇类、明胶、聚氧乙烯单硬脂酸酯（S-40）、硬脂酸钠等，用于速释滴丸的制备；非水溶性基质有硬脂酸、单硬脂酸甘油酯、虫蜡、蜂蜡、石蜡、氢化植物油等。

Matrix excipients in dripping pills be classified as the water-soluble and water-insoluble type. The water-soluble matrixes, such as polyethylene glycols, gelatin, polyoxyethylene monostearate (s-40), and sodium stearate, could be employed to prepare the rapid-release dripping pills. Nevertheless, the water-insoluble matrixes, such as stearic acid, monostearate glyceride, insect wax, beeswax, paraffin, and hydrogenated plant oil, are commonly used for sustained-release dripping pills.

2. 冷凝液的要求与选用 在滴丸成型过程中，使液滴冷凝成为固体药丸的液体称为冷凝液。冷凝液与药丸直接接触，并影响液滴最终成型，应符合下列要求：①不溶解药物与基质，也不与主药或基质发生化学反应；②密度与液滴密度接近，可使滴丸在冷凝液中缓缓下沉或上浮，使其能够充分凝固，丸形圆整；③使用安全。

(2) Requirements and selection principle of cooling medium for dripping pills During the shaping of dropping pills, the liquid droplet of melted mixture could transform the solid pills by the condensation of cooling medium. For the cooling medium, it should have no influence on the quality of both drug and matrix. It cannot neither dissolve nor interact with both drug and matrix. The density of cooling medium should be close to that of liquid droplet, so that the liquid droplets can sink or float up in cooling medium slowly, to benefit the complete condensation and facilitate pills rounding. Meanwhile, the cooling medium also should be safe and harmless to human health.

常用的冷凝液分两类：①水溶性基质常选用液状石蜡、甲基硅油、植物油、煤油等液体油类冷凝液；②非水溶性基质常用水、不同浓度乙醇等作为冷凝液。

Similarly, the commonly used cooling medium can be divided into two types, i.e. water-soluble and water-insoluble medium. The selection of cooling medium type should depend on the property of matrix excipients. The water-insoluble cooling mediums such as liquid paraffin, methyl silicone oil, plant oil, kerosene and so on fit for the water-soluble matrixes. Nevertheless, the water-soluble cooling mediums like water and ethanol solution fit for the water-insoluble matrixes.

3. 药物的前处理 滴丸载药量小，一般要求对处方药物要采用适宜的方法进行提取精制，将有效部位或有效成分投料制丸，一些贵重药物也可直接粉碎投料。

(3) Pretreatment of drugs Herbs for dripping pills should be extracted and purified into bioactive fraction or components in advance, owing to the small drug loading capacity of dripping pills. Some expensive herbs also can be smashed into fine powder and prepare for dripping pills directly.

4. 制备工艺 主要采用滴制法，工艺流程如图 14-4 所示。

(4) The preparation of dripping pills The preparation of dripping pill is mediated by dropping method, whose process flow chart is shown in the Figure 14-4.

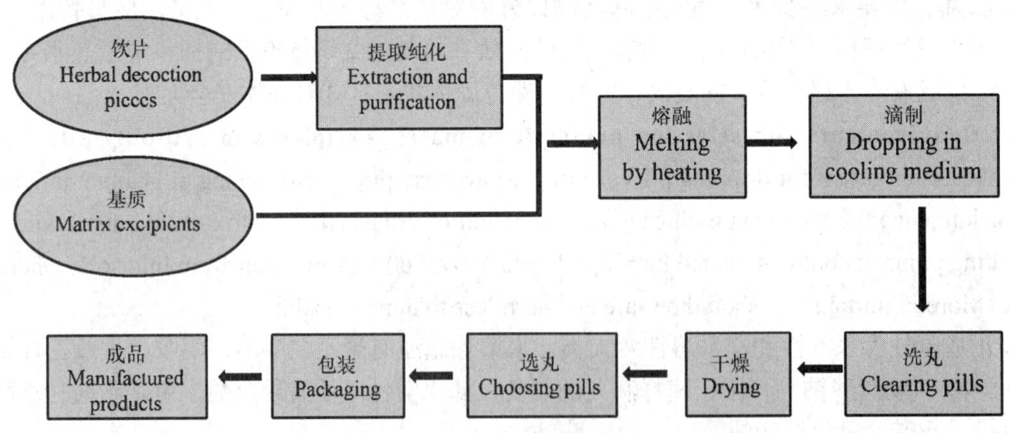

图 14-4 滴丸的制备工艺流程图

Figure 14-4 Preparation Process Flow Chart of Dripping Pills by Dropping Method

将处理好的药物溶解、乳化或混悬于适宜的已熔融基质中，保持恒定温度（80~100℃），经一定大小管径的滴头，匀速滴入冷凝液中，凝固形成的丸粒徐徐沉于器底或浮于冷凝液的表面，取出，擦拭冷凝液，干燥，即得。干燥后的滴丸质量检查合格后即可包装。

Briefly, the pretreated drugs are dissolved, emulsified, or suspended in the selected melted matrixes, maintaining a constant temperature (80-100℃). The mixture is dropped via a dropper with a certain diameter into the cooling medium at a constant speed. The droplet in cooling medium will solidify into pills, which will slowly sink to the bottom of condenser pipe or float on the upper cooling medium. The generated pills can be collected, wiped off the residual cooling medium and dried. After qualified, the produced dripping pills can be packaged.

目前，生产上采用的滴丸自动化生产线由滴丸机、集丸离心机和筛选干燥机三部分组成，其中滴丸机由药物调制供应系统、冷却收集系统、循环制冷系统组成。滴丸机示意图见 14-5，药物与基质的熔融液由贮液罐经泵进入药液滴罐，经滴头滴入冷凝液，药滴在冷凝液中收缩冷凝成球状，丸球沉落后由螺旋循环接收系统进入集丸抽斗，实现连续生产。

At present, the automatic production line of dropping pill is composed of three parts: dripping pill machine, collecting pill machine by centrifugation and screening & drying machine. Particularly, dripping pill machine consists of drug modulation supply system, cooling collection system and circulating refrigeration system, as shown in Figure 14-5. The mixture of drugs and melted matrixes stored in liquid tank could enter into medicine droplet tank, and drop into cooling medium via a dropper. The droplets in cooling medium will congeal into spherical pills. After pills fall down, they will be collected by spiral loop collecting system and enter the pill collecting drawer. In that way, pills in this machine could be continuously produced.

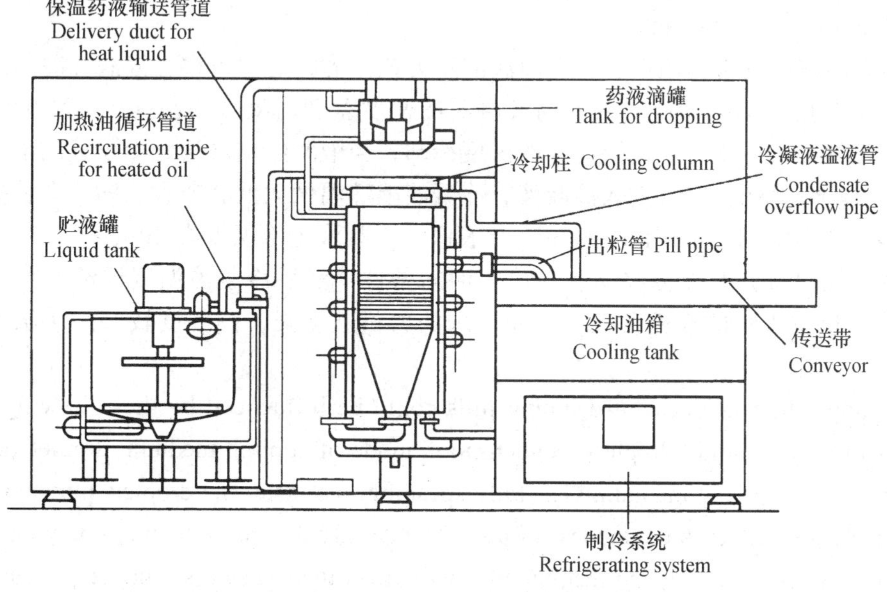

图 14-5 滴丸机结构示意图

Figure 14-5 The Structure of Dropping Pill Machine

三、滴丸的质量评价与影响滴丸质量的因素

14.6.3 Quality Evaluation of Dripping Pills and Its Quality Influence Factors

滴丸的质量评价目前多以丸重差异系数、丸型圆整度、溶散时限与滴制难易程度等多个指标进行综合评分评定。

At present, the quality of dripping pills is generally evaluated by multiple indexes such as variation

coefficient of pills' weight, roundness of pills, dissolution time limitation and difficult degree of pill dripping.

影响滴丸丸重的重要因素有：①滴头大小。在一定范围内滴头口径越大，滴制的丸粒越大；②滴制温度。滴制物料的温度升高，表面张力下降，丸重减少；温度降低，丸重增大。滴制的温度在整个制备过程中应当恒定；③滴距（滴头与冷凝液液面的距离，通常在10cm以内）。滴距过大易使滴出的液滴因重力作用被跌碎，从而影响丸重的一致性；④料液空气。熔料和冷凝工艺使料液中引入了空气又未排除，导致丸粒中空洞而致丸重差异；⑤其他因素。滴速变化、储存液内因料液液位改变导致静压改变等可导致滴丸丸重差异。

There are several factors would influence the weight of dripping pills: droplet head size, droplet temperature, the distance between the droplet head and cooling medium, the residual air in droplet, and other factors. Specifically, the larger droplet head will result in the larger pills within a range. The raised temperature of droplet will result in the declined surface tension and decreased pill weight. Therefore, the temperature of droplet mixture shall be constant throughout the preparation process. Commonly, the distance between the droplet head and the liquid level of cooling medium should keep within 10cm. If the dripping distance is too long, the droplet would be easily broken due to the gravity action. It will influence the consistency of pills' weight. The unremoved bubble would be incorporated into the material mixture during the melting and condensation process, which will result in the hollow pills and non-uniform pill weight. Otherwise, there are some other factors influence the weight of dripping pills such as the change of dripping speed, and the static pressure change caused by the liquid level change in storage liquid tank.

影响滴丸圆整度的重要因素有：①液滴的重力或浮力，一般来讲，液滴在冷凝液中的移动速度越快，圆整度越易受影响。液滴与冷凝液的密度差和冷凝液的黏度也会对圆整度产生影响；②冷凝液的冷凝方式。应保持适当的梯度冷却，当液滴经空气达到冷凝液的液面时，被碰撞成扁形，并携带有部分空气进入冷凝液，冷凝液上部温度太低会导致收缩成丸前凝固，使得滴丸不圆整，产生空洞、带尾巴等现象。一般保持冷凝液上部温度在40~60℃，下部温度控制在10~15℃，使得滴丸有充分收缩和释放气泡的条件，然后冷凝液温度逐渐下降。③液滴大小。液滴小，单位重量的表面积大，收缩成球的力量就愈强，圆整度较好。④滴丸处方和冷凝液。

Furthermore, the roundness of dripping pills could be influenced by the following influences: gravity or buoyancy of liquid droplets, condensation mode of cooling medium, droplet size, dripping pill prescription and cooling medium. Generally speaking, the faster the droplets move in the cooling medium, the easier to affect the roundness of pills. The density difference between droplets and cooling medium and the viscosity of cooling medium also will affect the roundness. The temperature of cooling medium should keep appropriate gradient, in which the upper and lower temperature should keep at 40-60℃ and 10-15℃, respectively. The temperature gradient benefits droplet contraction fully and to release the residual bubbles. If the upper temperature of cooling medium is too low, the residual air in droplet would retain in pills, resulting in the aspheric pills such as hollow pills and pills with a tail. Additionally, the small droplet commonly produces into a round pill, because the large surface area per unit weight will result in the strong force to shrink as a sphere.

第七节 丸剂的包衣

14.7 Pill Coating

一、包衣目的

14.7.1 Purpose of Pill Coating

在丸剂的表面上包裹一层物质，使之与外界隔绝的操作称为包衣。丸剂包衣的主要目的包括：①可以掩盖药丸自身的恶臭、异味，增强患者的顺应性；②可以使丸剂表面平滑、美观，便于吞服；③可以防止丸剂所含主药氧化、变质或挥发，防止吸潮及虫蛀；④根据临床治疗需要，将处方中部分药物作为包衣材料，使其在服用后首先发挥药效；⑤通过包肠溶衣，发挥定向治疗作用或减少药物在胃液中的损失。

Pill coating is to cover a layer of substance on the surface of pill, to isolate it from outside.

The main purposes of pill coating include several items. ① It could cover stink or unpleasant odor of pill core and improve the patient's compliance. ② It could make pills smooth surface, nice appearance and easy to swallow. ③ It could avoid drugs in pills oxidation, deterioration or volatilization, and to prevent moisture absorption and moth damage. ④ According to the clinical treatment need, some drugs in prescription could be coated on the surface of pills to make them play the therapeutic role faster. ⑤ Pills with enteric coating could take a targeting therapeutic effect in intestinal tract, or avoid drugs to be damaged by gastric juice.

二、包衣种类

14.7.2 Types of Pill Coating

丸剂包衣的种类根据包衣材料，主要分为药物衣、保护衣和肠溶衣。

Based on the coating substance, the types of pill coating are mainly divided into drug coating, protective substance coating and enteric coating.

1. 药物衣 是指将制剂处方中的药物作为包衣材料，该药物有明显的药理作用，用于包衣既可发挥药效，又可保护丸粒、增加丸剂美观。常见的药物衣主要有朱砂衣、甘草衣、黄柏衣、雄黄衣、青黛衣、百草霜衣、滑石衣、礞石衣、牡蛎衣、金箔衣等。

(1) Drug coating is to coat the drugs in prescription on the surface of pills. In that way, drugs could not only take the faster bioactivity, but also protect the pills and improve the pills' appearance. Commonly, several drugs could be used as coating substances, such as cinnabar, liquorice, Cortex Phellodendri Chinensis, Realgar, indigo naturalis, plant soot, french chalk, chlorite schist, concha ostreae, gold foil, and so on.

2. 保护衣 选取处方以外，无明显药理作用而性质稳定的物质作为包衣材料，为使丸粒与外界隔离而起保护作用，主要包括糖衣和薄膜衣。

(2) Protective substance coating is to coat the chemical stable substance but without Obvious pharmacological action on the surface of pills, to isolate it from outside. It mainly includes sugar-coating and film-coating.

3. 肠溶衣 选用适宜的肠溶性材料将丸剂包衣后使其在胃液中不溶散而在肠液中溶散，使药物在特定部位释放。主要材料有丙烯酸树脂类、纤维醋酸酯等。

(3) Enteric coating is to coat the enteric materials on the surface of pills, to prevent pills disintegration in stomach, while disintegrate in intestines. In that way, drugs could be specifically delivered into intestines, and be absorbed in the targeted site. The main enteric materials are acrylic resin, fiber acetate and so on.

三、丸剂包衣的方法
14.7.3 Method of Pill Coating

1. 包衣原材料的准备 将选择的包衣材料粉碎成极细粉，可以保证包衣丸的表面光滑。除蜜丸外，其他丸剂在包衣时通常需要外加适宜的黏合剂，以保证包衣材料能够在包衣过程中黏着于丸粒表面，常用的黏合剂主要有 10% 阿拉伯胶浆等。

① The selected coating material should be crushed into the finest powder, which can ensure the smooth surface of pills. Except honeyed pills, other types of pills usually need to some suitable adhesives, commonly like acacia mucilage, added during the coating process, to ensure the coating materials can stick on the surface of pills.

2. 包衣方法 丸剂包衣方法主要有滚转包衣法、流化包衣法等。

丸剂包糖衣、薄膜衣及肠溶衣的包衣方法与片剂相同，可参考片剂章节。

② The mainly used methods for pill coating include trundle pan coating, fluidized bed coating and so on. The specific process of pill coating with sugar, polymer film and enteric materials is similar as that of tablet coating, which will be introduced in *Chapter 16 Tablet*.

第八节　丸剂的质量检查、包装与贮藏
14.8 Quality Inspection, Packaging and Storage of Pills

PPT

一、质量检查
14.8.1 Quality Inspection

（一）外观检查
(1) Appearance Inspection

丸剂外观应圆整均匀、色泽一致。蜜丸应细腻滋润，软硬适中。蜡丸表面应光滑无裂纹，丸内不得有蜡点和颗粒。滴丸应大小均匀，色泽一致，无粘连现象，表面不应残留冷凝液。

Pills should have the round and uniform appearance with the consistent color and lustre. Particularly, the appearance of honeyed pills should be delicate and moist, neither too hard nor too soft. The surface of waxed pills should be smooth without cracks, waxy points or coarse particles. Dropping pills should have no adhesion each other, and no cooling medium is allowed to retain on its surface.

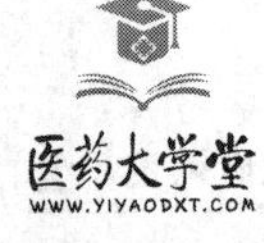

（二）水分

(2) Moisture Content Limitation

取供试品照现行版《中国药典》中水分测定法测定。除另有规定外，蜜丸、浓缩蜜丸中所含水分不得过15.0%；水蜜丸、浓缩水蜜丸不得过12.0%；水丸、糊丸和浓缩水丸不得过9.0%；蜡丸不检查水分。

Moisture content of pill samples should be determined according to the moisture measurement method recorded in the current edition of *Chinese Pharmacopoeia.* Unless there is otherwise specified, the moisture content in both honeyed pills and concentrated honeyed pills cannot exceed 15%. The moisture content in water-honeyed pills and concentrated water-honeyed pills cannot exceed 12%. The moisture content in water-binded pills, pasted pills and concentrated water-binded pills cannot exceed 9%. Nevertheless, waxed pills need not to inspect moisture content.

（三）重量差异

(3) Weight Variation

按丸数服用的丸剂照现行版《中国药典》中第一法检查，按重量服用的丸剂照第二法检查。

The inspection methods for weight variation of types of pills are different. The inspection method for pills including dripping pills taken by numbers is based on the first method of *weight variation section* recorded in the current edition of *Chinese Pharmacopoeia.* The inspection method for pills taken by weights is based on the second method of *weight variation section* recorded in the current edition of *Chinese Pharmacopoeia.*

包糖衣丸剂应检查丸芯的重量差异并符合规定，包糖衣后不再检查重量差异，其他包衣丸剂应在包衣后检查重量差异并符合规定；凡进行装量差异检查的单剂量包装丸剂，不再进行重量差异检查。

Notably, only the pills with sugar-coating should be inspected for the weight variation of pill cores, instead of the whole sugar-coating pills. Pills with other kind of coating substances should be inspected for the weight variation of the whole pills coated. The single-dose packaged pill will be inspected for the filling variation, instead of weight variation.

（四）装量差异

(4) Filling Variation

单剂量分装的丸剂，照现行版《中国药典》检查，装量差异限度应符合规定。

The filling variation of pills with single-dose packages should be inspected according to the method recorded in the current edition of *Chinese Pharmacopoeia*.

（五）溶散时限

(5) Disintegration Time

按现行版《中国药典》中崩解时限检查法片剂项下的方法加挡板进行检查。除另有规定外，小蜜丸、水蜜丸和水丸应在1小时内全部溶散；浓缩丸和糊丸应在2小时内全部溶散。滴丸应在30分钟内溶散，包衣滴丸应在1小时内溶散，以明胶为基质的滴丸，可在人工胃液中进行检查。

The disintegration time of pills should be inspected according to the method for tablets recorded in the current edition of *Chinese Pharmacopoeia.* Unless there is otherwise specified, small honeyed pills, water-honeyed pills and water-binded pills should disintegrate completely within 1h. The concentrated pills and pasted pills should disintegrate completely within 2h. Dripping pills with or without coating should disintegrate completely within 1h or 30min, respectively.

蜡丸按现行版《中国药典》崩解时限检查法项下的肠溶衣片检查法检查，应符合规定。除另

有规定外，大蜜丸及研碎、嚼碎等或用开水、黄酒等分散后服用的丸剂不检查溶散时限。

Waxed pills should be inspected for the method of "General rule 0921" in the current edition of *Chinese Pharmacopoeia.* Unless there is otherwise specified, big honeyed pills, pills which are administrated by the pretreatment of trituration, chewing, or dispersion in water/yellow rice wine need no disintegration time inspection.

（六）微生物限度

(6) Microbial Limit

照现行版《中国药典》微生物限度检查法检查，应符合规定。

The number of total microorganisms in pills should be inspected according to the *Microbial limit test* method in the current edition of *Chinese Pharmacopoeia.* It must meet the corresponding requirements.

二、丸剂的包装与贮藏

14.8.2 Package and Storage of Pills

岗位对接

重点小结

题库

包装材料的选择应根据各类丸剂的性质来确定。小丸常用玻璃瓶、塑料瓶或瓷瓶等包装。为防止运输时对丸粒的撞击，可采用棉花、纸填充瓶内空隙，并以软木塞浸蜡或塑料内衬浸蜡为内盖再加外盖密封。大、小蜜丸和浓缩丸多用纸盒、蜡壳、塑料小圆盒、铝塑泡罩等材料包装。目前生产中已实现机械化包装。除另有规定外，丸剂应密封贮藏，蜡丸应密封并置阴凉干燥处贮藏。

The selected package material should depend on the property of kinds of pills. Commonly, the small pills could be packaged in glass, plastic or porcelain bottles, in which cotton or paper can fill the space inside the bottle. The bottles could be sealed by cork or plastic lining impregnated wax as the inner cap, with an additional outer cover. Both honeyed pills and condensed pills could be packaged in paper box, wax shell, plastic small round box, aluminum plastic blister packaging container. At present, pills are commonly packaged by a mechanization machine. Unless otherwise specified, pills should be stored in sealed container. Waxed pills sealed should be placed in a cool dry place.

（章津铭）

第十五章　颗粒剂
Chapter 15　Granules

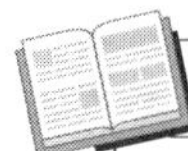

学习目标 | Learning Goals

知识要求：

1. **掌握**　颗粒剂的含义、特点与制法。
2. **熟悉**　颗粒剂的质量检查。
3. **了解**　混悬性颗粒的制法。

能力要求：

学会颗粒剂的制备与质量检测方法，能制备颗粒剂，并检查和评价产品质量。

Knowledge requirements:

1. **To master** the definition, characteristics and preparation of granules.
2. **To be familiar with** the quality inspection of granules.
3. **To know** the preparation methods of suspended granules.

Ability requirements:

To learn the preparation and quality inspection methods of granules, be able to prepare granules, inspect and evaluate the quality of granules products.

第一节　概述
15.1　Overview

PPT

一、颗粒剂的含义与特点
15.1.1　The Definition and Characteristics of Granules

颗粒剂系指原料药物与适宜的辅料制成具有一定粒度的干燥颗粒状制剂。颗粒剂是在汤剂、散剂、糖浆剂、药酒等剂型的基础上发展起来的新剂型。具有以下特点：①吸收快，起效迅速。②剂量小，口感好，适合儿童用药。③生产工艺适于工业化生产。④服用、携带、贮藏和运输方便。不足之处：①成本相对较高。②含有中药浸膏或以糖为主要赋形剂的颗粒剂容易吸潮结块、潮解，从而发生微生物繁殖、药物降解等变化，故应注意选择密封防潮的包装材料和干燥条件贮存。

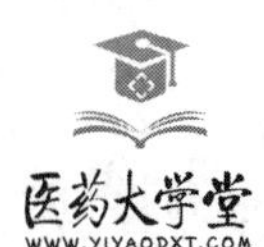

Granules are dry granular preparations with appropriate particle size made of drug substances and suitable excipients. Granules are new dosage forms developed on the basis of decoction, powders, syrups, medicinal wines and other dosage forms. Granules have the following characteristics: Rapid absorption and quick effect. Small dosage, tasty, be suitable for children. The production process is suitable for industrial production. Easy to take, carry, store and transport. Disadvantages: High cost. Because of containing Chinese medicine extract or sugar as the main excipient, granules are easy to absorb moisture, agglomerate and deliquesce, which will cause changes in microbial reproduction and drug degradation. Therefore, it is necessary to select sealed and moisture-proof packaging materials and dry conditions for storage.

二、颗粒剂的分类
15.1.2 The Classification of Granules

颗粒剂可分为可溶颗粒（通称为颗粒）、混悬颗粒、泡腾颗粒、肠溶颗粒、缓释颗粒和控释颗粒等。按溶解性能和溶解状态，颗粒剂分为可溶颗粒、混悬颗粒和泡腾颗粒三类。可溶颗粒可分为水溶颗粒和酒溶颗粒。水溶颗粒加水冲溶，药液澄清，中药颗粒剂大多为此类；酒溶颗粒溶于白酒，服用前加一定量的饮用酒溶解饮用。混悬颗粒系难溶性原料药物与适宜辅料混合制成的颗粒剂。临用前加水或其他适宜的液体振摇即可分散成混悬液。泡腾颗粒系指含有碳酸氢钠和有机酸，遇水可放出大量气体而呈泡腾状的颗粒剂。本章主要介绍这三类中药颗粒。

Granules may be classified as soluble granules (usually as known as granules), suspended granules, effervescent granules, enteric-coated granules, sustained-release granules and controlled-release granules. According to the dissolution performance and dissolution state, granules are divided into three types: soluble granules, suspended granules and effervescent granules. Soluble granules can also be divided into water-soluble granules and alcohol-soluble granules. Water-soluble granules are dissolved by adding water, and the solution is clarified. Most of Chinese medicinal granules belong to water-soluble granules. Alcohol-soluble granules could be dissolved in white wine, and a certain amount of drinking wine is added before drinking. Suspended granules are dry granules appropriate particle size made of insoluble solid drug substances and suitable excipients. Water or other suitable liquid is added with shaking before use to distribute the contents and form a suspension. Effervescent granules are granules containing sodium bicarbonate and organic acids, which release a quantity of effervescent gas when water is added. This chapter mainly introduces these three types of Chinese medicinal granules.

PPT

第二节　颗粒剂的制法

15.2　Preparation of Granules

一、颗粒剂的制备工艺流程

15.2.1　The Preparation Process of the Granules

颗粒剂的制备工艺流程见图 15-1。

The preparation process of the granules as shown in Figure 15-1.

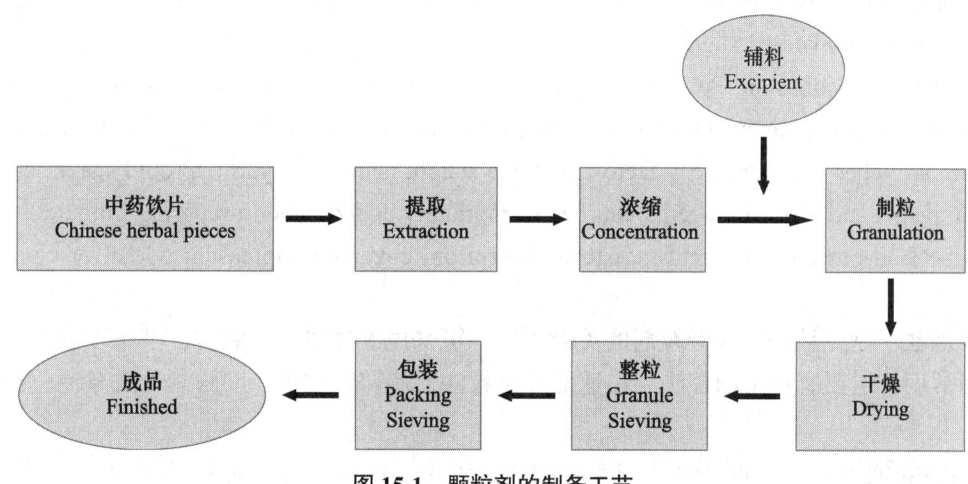

图 15-1　颗粒剂的制备工艺

Figure 15-1　The Preparation Process of the Granules

二、水溶性颗粒的制法

15.2.2　Preparation of Water-Soluble Granules

1. 饮片的提取　制备水溶性颗粒时饮片多采用煎煮法提取，也可根据饮片中有效物质的性质采用渗漉、浸渍或回流等提取方法。含芳香挥发性成分的饮片一般以水蒸气蒸馏法提取挥发性成分，药渣再加水煎煮提取。对于热敏性物料及挥发油为主要成分的药材，应采用超临界流体提取法、连续逆流提取法等低温动态浸提新工艺。

(1) Extraction of decoction pieces　When preparing water-soluble granules, the decoction pieces are mostly extracted by water decoction method. The extraction methods (infiltration, dipping, reflux, etc.) can also be used, according to the properties of the active ingredients in the decoction pieces. The decoction pieces containing aromatic volatile ingredients are generally extracted by steam distillation, and the residues are extracted by water decoction method. For the manufacture of volatile or heat-labile drug substances, new low-temperature dynamic extraction methods, e.g. supercritical fluid extraction, continuous countercurrent extraction, should be used.

2. 提取液的精制　提取液的精制方法以往多采用乙醇沉淀法，目前也有采用高速离心、大孔树脂吸附、絮凝沉淀、膜分离等方法。精制液可浓缩成适宜密度的稠浸膏，也可进一步干燥成干浸膏；或将精制液直接喷雾干燥后用湿法或干法制粒。

(2) Purification of extract The purification of extract used ethanol precipitation method in the past. At present, there are also methods, such as high-speed centrifugation, macroporous resin adsorption, flocculation precipitation, and membrane separation, etc. The extract solution can be concentrated into a thick extract with a suitable density, or further dried into a dry extract. In addition, the extract solution can be directly spray-dried and then granulated by wet or dry methods.

3. 辅料的选用 水溶性颗粒剂常用的辅料为糖粉和糊精。糖粉是可溶性颗粒的优良赋形剂，并有矫味及黏合作用。糖粉易吸湿结块，应注意密闭保存。糊精系淀粉的水解产物，宜选用可溶性糊精。其他赋形剂还有乳糖、可溶性淀粉、甘露醇、羟丙基淀粉等。制备颗粒剂时可适当添加矫味剂和芳香剂。为防潮、掩盖药物的不良气味或控制药物释放速度，颗粒剂也可进行薄膜包衣。

(3) Selection of excipients The excipients for water-soluble granules are generally powdered sugar and dextrin. Powdered sugar is an excellent excipient of soluble granules and has the effects of taste correction and adhesion. Powdered sugar is easy to absorb moisture and agglomerate, should be stored in well closed containers. Dextrin is the hydrolysis product of starch, and soluble dextrin should be used. There are other excipients, e.g. lactose, soluble starch, mannitol, hydroxypropyl starch, etc. Flavor correction agents and aromatic agents can be appropriately added, when preparing granules. Granules may also be film-coated to prevent moisture absorption, cover up unpleasant odour, or control drug release.

4. 制颗粒 制颗粒是制备颗粒剂的关键工序，可采用湿法或干法制粒，其中以湿法制粒在生产中最为常用，主要有挤出制粒法、快速搅拌制粒法、旋转制粒法、沸腾制粒法及流化喷雾制粒法等。

(4) Granulation Granulation is the key process for preparing granules. Wet or dry granulation can be used, among which wet granulation is the most commonly used in production, i.e. extrusion granulation, rapid stirring granulation, rotating granulation, boiling granulation and fluidized spray granulation, etc.

制软材是湿法制粒的关键工序，即将赋形剂置适宜的设备内混合均匀，加入药物清膏（或干膏粉）搅拌混匀，加适量一定浓度的乙醇调整湿度，制成“手握成团、轻压即散”的软材的过程。软材黏性太强制得的颗粒坚硬，软材黏度太弱制得的颗粒松散，细粉多。

Making soft material is the key process of wet granulation. It is a process in which the excipients are mixed well in a suitable equipment, and the thin extracts (or dried extract powder) are added to stir and mix. A suitable amount of ethanol is added to adjust the humidity to make the process of holding the soft material into a ball and pressing it lightly into friability. The particles made of soft material with too strong viscosity are hard, and the particles made of soft material with too weak viscosity are loose and have more fine powder.

（1）挤出制粒 将辅料置适宜的容器内，加入药物稠膏（或干浸膏粉）混合均匀，必要时加适量一定浓度的乙醇调整湿度，制成软材。再以挤压方式通过筛网（板）（10~14 目）制成均匀的颗粒。

a. Extruded granulation Put excipients in a suitable container, add the thick extracts (or dried extract powder) and mix well. If necessary, add a suitable amount of ethanol to adjust the humidity to make a soft material, then extrude through a sieve (plate) (10-14 mesh) to make uniform particles.

辅料的用量，可根据清膏的相对密度、黏性强弱等适当调整，但辅料总用量不宜超过清膏量的 5 倍。以干浸膏细粉为原料制粒时，辅料的用量不宜超过其重量的 2 倍。

According to the relative density and viscosity of the thin extracts, the amount of excipients added should be controlled, which is not more than 5 times of that of the thin extracts in general. When granulating with dried extract powder as crude drug, the amount of excipients added is not more than 2 times of that of dried extract powder.

小量制备可用手工制粒筛，大生产多用摇摆式制粒机，而黏性较差的药料宜选用旋转式制粒机制粒。

For small-scale preparation, manual granulation sieves can be used. For large-scale production, swing granulators are used. For medicines with poor viscosity, rotary granulators should be used.

（2）快速搅拌制粒　将适量适宜固体辅料与清膏置快速搅拌制粒机的盛器内，密闭。开动机器，搅拌桨以一定的转速转动，使物料形成从盛器底部沿器壁抛起旋转的波浪，波峰正好通过高速旋转的制粒刀，使均匀混合的物料被切割成带有一定棱角的小块，小块间互相摩擦形成球状颗粒。通过调整搅拌桨叶和制粒刀的转速可控制粒度的大小。

b. Quickly stirring granulation　The appropriate amount of suitable solid excipients and the thin extracts are placed in the closed container of rapid mixing granulator. Start the machine, the stirring paddle rotates at a certain speed, so that the materials form a rotating wave that is thrown from the bottom of the container along the wall. The crest just passes the high-speed rotating granulating knife, so that the uniformly mixed materials are cut into small angled pieces. Small pieces rub against each other to form spherical particles. The particle size can be controlled by adjusting the rotation speed of the stirring blade and the granulating knife.

（3）流化喷雾制粒　又称“一步制粒”或沸腾制粒。目前多用于无糖型或低糖型颗粒剂的制备。该法系将一定粒度的制粒用辅料（一般粒度为40~60目）置于流化喷雾制粒设备的流化室内，通入滤过的加热空气，使粉末预热干燥并处于沸腾状态，再将预处理的药液以雾状间歇喷入，使粉粒被润湿而黏结成多孔状颗粒，继续流化干燥至颗粒中含水量适宜，即得。制成的颗粒呈多孔状，大小均匀，外形圆整，流动性好。

c. Fluidized spray granulation　It is also known as “one-step granulation” or boiling granulation, which is mostly used for the preparation of sugar-free or low-sugar granules. In this method, granulating excipients with a certain particle size (generally with a particle size of 40 to 60 mesh) are placed in the fluidization chamber of a fluidized spray granulation equipment, and filtered heated air is introduced to preheat and dry the powder and bring it to a boiling state. Then, the pre-treatment medicinal solution is sprayed intermittently in the form of a mist, so that the powder particles are wetted and adhered into porous particles, and then fluidized and dried until the water content in the particles is suitable. The granules are porous, uniform in size, round in shape, and good in fluidity.

（4）干法制粒　将喷雾干燥等方法制得的干膏细粉，加入适宜的干燥黏合剂等辅料，用干燥制粒机压成薄片，再粉碎成颗粒。这种制粒工艺，辅料用量少，有利于进一步减小剂量，并可避免湿热条件下有效成分的损失，并能提高颗粒的稳定性和溶化性。

d. Dry granulation　The dried fine powder obtained by spray drying method and appropriate excipients such as drying adhesive, etc., are pressed into thin slices with a dry granulator, and then pulverized into particles. In this granulation process, the amount of excipients is small, which is beneficial to further reducing the dosage, avoiding the loss of active ingredients under humid and hot conditions, and improving the stability and solubility of the particles.

5. 干燥　湿颗粒应及时干燥，以免久置黏结变形。干燥温度一般以60~80℃为宜，干燥时温度应逐渐上升，以免颗粒表面干燥过快而结壳，影响颗粒内部水分的蒸发；且颗粒中的糖粉骤遇

高温时会熔化，使颗粒变得坚硬；尤其是糖粉与柠檬酸共存时，温度稍高更易黏结成块。

(5) Drying The wet particles should be dried in time to avoid long-term bonding deformation. Generally, the drying temperature is preferably 60-80℃. The temperature should be gradually increased during drying to prevent the surface of the granules from drying too fast and crusting, which will affect the evaporation of the water inside the granules; and the powdered sugar in the granules will melt when it is exposed to high temperatures. It becomes hard; especially when the powdered sugar and citric acid coexist, the temperature is slightly higher and it is easier to stick into agglomerates.

颗粒的干燥程度应适宜，含水量一般控制在 2% 以内。

Drying should be conducted appropriately, water content is generally controlled within 2%.

6. 整粒 干燥的颗粒一般先经一号筛筛除粗大颗粒，再经五号筛筛除细粉，使颗粒均匀。粗大颗粒可适当破碎后再次整粒，筛下的细粉可重新制粒，或并入下次同一批号药粉中，混匀制粒。

(6) Granule Sieving The dried granules are generally sieved through a No. 1 sieve to remove coarse granules, and then filtered through a No. 5 sieve to remove fine powder, make the granules uniform. Coarse granules can be appropriately broken and re-granulated, and the fine powder under the sieve can be re-granulated or incorporated into the next batch of medicinal powder, mixed well and granulated.

处方中的芳香挥发性成分，一般宜溶于适量乙醇中，雾化喷洒于干燥的颗粒上，密闭至规定时间，待闷吸均匀后包装，或用 β- 环糊精包合后混入。

The volatile components in the prescription should generally be dissolved in an appropriate amount of ethanol, atomized and sprayed on the dried granules, sealed for a required time, packaged after being smeared or mixed, or mixed with β-cyclodextrin inclusion.

7. 包装 整粒后的干燥颗粒应及时密封包装。生产上一般采用自动颗粒包装机进行分装。为防止颗粒吸湿软化，以至结块霉变，应选用不易透气、透湿的包装材料，如复合铝塑袋、铝箔袋或不透气的塑料瓶等，并于阴凉干燥处贮存。

(7) Packaging The dried granules should be preserved in tightly closed containers in time. Generally, automatic granule packaging machines are used for packaging. In order to prevent the granules from absorbing moisture and softening, and even the agglomeration of mold, packaging materials that are not easily breathable and moisture-permeable, such as composite aluminum plastic bags, aluminum foil bags, or air-proof plastic bottles, should be used and stored in a cool and dry place.

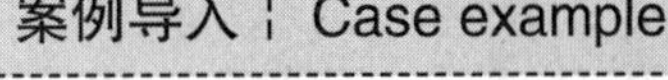

案例导入

案例 15-1 正柴胡饮颗粒

15-1 Zhengchaihuyin Granules

处方：柴胡 100g 陈皮 100g 防风 80g 甘草 40g 赤芍 150g 生姜 70g 糊精适量

Formula: Bupleuri Radix 100g; Citri Reticulatae Pericarpium 100g; Saposhnikoviae Radix 80g; Glycyrrhizae Radix et Rhizoma 40g; Radix Paeoniae Rubra 150g; Zingiberis Rhizoma Recens 70g; Dextrin Q.S.

功能与主治：发散风寒，解热止痛。用于外感风寒所致的发热恶寒、无汗、头痛、鼻塞、喷嚏、咽痒咳嗽、四肢酸痛；流感初起、轻度上呼吸道感染见上述证候者。

Functions and Indications: To disperse wind-cold, clear heat and relieve pain. Fever and chills,

absence of sweating, headache, stuffy nose, sneezing, itchy throat, cough, soreness and weakness of the limbs due to externally contracted wind-cold; early stage of influenza and low-grade upper respiratory tract infection with the symptoms described above.

制法： 以上六味，加水煎煮二次，每次1.5小时，合并煎液。滤过，滤液浓缩至相对密度为1.10~1.20（50℃）的清膏，加乙醇使含醇量达50%，搅拌，静置过夜。滤过，滤液回收乙醇，浓缩至相对密度为1.35~1.40（50℃）的清膏，减压干燥后粉碎。取干浸膏粉1份、糊精1.5份，以适量乙醇润湿制粒。80℃以下干燥后整粒，即得。

Making Preparation: Decoct the above six ingredients with water for 2 times, 1.5hours for each, and combine the decoctions. Filter, concentrate the filtrate to a thin extract with the density index of 1.10-1.20 (50℃). Add ethanol to 50% content, stir well, stand over night, and filter. Recover ethanol and concentrate to a thick extract with a density index of 1.35-1.40 (50℃). Dry in vacuum to dry extract, grind, to 1 portion of the dry extract, add 1.5 portions of dextrin, make granules with ethanol, dry below 80℃, and prepare granules.

用法与用量： 开水冲服，一次3g，一日3次，小儿酌减或遵医嘱。

Usage and Dosage: Take the medicine orally after mixing it with hot water, 3g per time, three times a day. Reduce the dosage in children or as advised by health professionals.

注解： ①本品为黄棕色至红棕色的颗粒；味微苦。

②本品制粒时选用乙醇作润湿剂，可以避免浸膏粉遇水后黏性过强而不易制粒。

③该制剂为无蔗糖颗粒，2020年版《中国药典》一部中还收载了含蔗糖的正柴胡饮颗粒，系将浓缩的清膏1份与蔗糖2份、糊精1.5份混匀制粒，干燥后整粒即得。

Notes: ① The product is yellowish brown to reddish brown granules with slight bitter taste. ② Ethanol is used as a wetting agent in granulation, which can prevent the extract powder from being too sticky after being exposed to water and difficult to granulate. ③ The preparation is sucrose-free granules. The sucrose-containing Zhengchaihuyin granules are also included in the 2020 edition of the *Chinese Pharmacopoeia*, 1 portion of the dry extract, 2 portions of sucrose and 1.5 portions of dextrin mix well, dry, and prepare granules.

思考题： 浸膏粉制粒与稠浸膏制粒相比有什么优势？颗粒的质量与哪些因素相关？

Questions: What are the advantages of extract powder granulation compared with thick extract granulation? What factors are related to the quality of particles?

三、酒溶性颗粒的制法

15.2.3 Preparation of Alcohol-Soluble Granules

酒溶性颗粒所含有效部位（成分）及所用辅料应能溶于白酒，通常可酌加糖或其他可溶矫味剂。应用时加入一定量的饮用白酒即溶解成为澄清的药酒，可替代药酒服用。处方中饮片的提取，以60%左右（以欲制药酒的含醇量为准）的乙醇为溶剂，一般采用渗漉法、浸渍法或回流法等方法，提取液回收乙醇后，浓缩至稠膏状，备用。制粒、干燥、整粒、包装等制备工艺同水溶性颗粒。

The effective parts (ingredients) and excipients in the alcohol-soluble granules should be soluble in liquor, and usually sugar or other soluble flavoring agents can be added as appropriate. When applied, an appropriate amount of drinking liquor is added to dissolve into a clear medicinal liquor, which can

be taken instead of medicinal liquor. The extraction of the decoction pieces in the prescription uses about 60% ethanol (based on the alcohol content of medicinal liquor to be prepared) as the solvent, and extraction methods such as the infiltration method, the dipping method, the reflux method, etc. After the ethanol is recovered, the solution is concentrated to a thick extract. Granulation, drying, breaking, pack and other preparation processes are the same as water-soluble granules.

案例导入

四、混悬颗粒的制法
15.2.4 Preparation of Suspended Granules

混悬颗粒中粉碎成细粉的药物兼有赋形剂作用。制备时通常将含热敏性、挥发性成分或淀粉较多的饮片以及贵重细料药等粉碎成细粉，过六号筛备用；一般性饮片参照可溶颗粒制备要求制成提取物，将提取物与饮片细粉及适量辅料混匀，采用适宜方法制粒，干燥后整粒，即得。

The drug crushed into fine powder in suspended granules has the function of excipient. During preparation, the decoction pieces containing heat-labile, volatile components or more starch and precious fine drug are usually crushed into fine powder, passed through No. 6 sieve. According to the preparation requirements of soluble granules, the extracts are prepared from the general decoction pieces. The extracts, the fine powder, and the appropriate amount of excipients are mixed, granulated by an appropriate method, and dried to form granules.

五、泡腾颗粒的制法
15.2.5 Preparation of Effervescent Granules

泡腾颗粒是由药物和泡腾崩解剂等辅料组成，遇水后迅速产生二氧化碳，使药液呈泡腾状态，使颗粒快速崩解，具速溶性。常用作泡腾崩解剂的有机酸为枸橼酸或酒石酸等，弱碱常用碳酸钠或碳酸氢钠。

Effervescent granules are composed of drugs and excipients (effervescent disintegrants, etc.). When water is added, it release carbon dioxide rapidly, which makes the liquid form a state of effervescence, and the granules rapidly disintegrate with instant solubility. The organic acids commonly used as the effervescent disintegrants are citric acid, tartaric acid, etc., the weak Bases such as sodium carbonate or sodium bicarbonate are usually used.

制法为将处方药料提取、纯化得清膏或干膏细粉，分成两份，一份中加入有机酸及其他适量辅料制成酸性颗粒，干燥备用；另一份中加入弱碱及其他适量辅料制成碱性颗粒，干燥备用。两种颗粒混合均匀，整粒，包装即得。应严格控制干燥颗粒中的水分，以免服用前酸碱发生反应。应严格控制干燥颗粒中的水分，以免服用前酸碱发生反应。可用 PEG6000 等对碳酸氢钠进行混合分散和表面包裹，可有效隔离碳酸氢钠与柠檬酸的直接接触，增加泡腾颗粒的贮存稳定性。

The preparation method should be processed by extraction, purification and concentration of the prescription crude drug to form a thin extract or dried extract powder, and divided into two parts. One part is added with an organic acid and other appropriate amounts of excipients to form acid granules, which are dried for use; the other part is added with weak base and other appropriate amounts of excipients to form alkaline granules, which are dried for use. The two kinds of granules are mixed well, granulated and packaged. The moisture in the dried granules should be strictly controlled to avoid acid-base reactions before taking. PEG6000 can be used for mixing and dispersing sodium bicarbonate and surface coating,

which can effectively isolate the direct contact between sodium bicarbonate and citric acid, and increase the storage stability of effervescent granules.

第三节 颗粒剂的质量检查
15.3 Quality Inspection of Granules

PPT

一、外观性状
15.3.1 Appearance

颗粒剂应干燥，颗粒均匀，色泽一致，无吸潮、结块、潮解等现象。

Granules should be dry, uniform in particle size and color, and show no evidence of moisture absorption, agglomeration and deliquescence.

二、粒度
15.3.2 Particle Size

除另有规定外，按现行版《中国药典》制剂通则颗粒剂项下粒度要求检查，不能通过一号筛与能通过五号筛的总和，不得过 15%。

Unless otherwise specified, carry out the method for Particle size for Granules in the General Requirements for Preparations of the *Chinese Pharmacopoeia*. The total weight of granules which cannot pass through No.1 sieve and can pass through No.5 sieve should not be more than 15% of the test sample.

三、水分
15.3.3 Determination of Water

颗粒剂按现行版《中国药典》中水分测定法测定，除另有规定外，水分不得过 8.0%。

To carry out the method for Determination of water for Granules in the General Requirements for Preparations of the *Chinese Pharmacopoeia*. The granules should contain no more than 8.0% of water, unless otherwise specified.

四、溶化性
15.3.4 Dispersion

可溶颗粒、泡腾颗粒按现行版《中国药典》制剂通则颗粒剂项下要求进行溶化性检查，应符合规定。混悬颗粒以及规定检查溶出度或释放度的颗粒剂可不进行溶化性检查。

To carry out the method for Dispersion for Granules in the General Requirements for Preparations of the *Chinese Pharmacopoeia*, soluble granules and effervescent granules should comply with the requirements. Dispersion test may not be required for suspended granules or granules that comply with Dissolution or Drug Release Test.

五、装量差异
15.3.5 Weight Variation

单剂量包装的颗粒剂，应符合现行版《中国药典》制剂通则颗粒剂项下装量差异检查的规定。凡规定检查含量均匀度的颗粒剂，不再进行装量差异检查。

To carry out the method for Weight variation for Granules in the General Requirements for Preparations of the *Chinese Pharmacopoeia*, single-dose granules should comply with the requirements. The test of weight variation may not be required for granules where the Test for Content Uniformity is specified.

岗位对接

六、装量
15.3.6 Filling

多剂量包装的颗粒剂，应符合现行版《中国药典》中最低装量检查法检查的规定。

Multi-dose granules should comply with the test of Minimum Fill of the *Chinese Pharmacopoeia*.

重点小结

七、微生物限度
15.3.7 Microbial Limit

题库

按现行版《中国药典》制剂通则颗粒剂项下要求进行微生物限度检查，应符合规定。

To carry out the method for Microbial limit for Granules in the General Requirements for Preparations of the *Chinese Pharmacopoeia*, granules should comply with the requirements.

（贾永艳）

第十六章 片剂
Chapter 16 Tablets

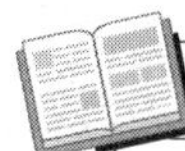

学习目标 | Learning Goals

知识要求：

1. 掌握 片剂的含义、特点、种类与应用；片剂常用辅料的种类、性质和应用；中药片剂的一般制法。

2. 熟悉 压片机的构造、性能及其使用保养；压片过程中可能发生的问题和解决方法；片剂包衣的目的、种类、素片的要求与包衣工艺；片剂的质量检查。

3. 了解 中药片剂新产品设计中应注意的主要问题。

能力要求：

1. 能够使用相应的设备，制备合格的片剂。

2. 能够解决片剂制备过程中出现的问题。

Knowledge requirements:

1. To master the definition, characteristics, types and applications of tablets; the types, properties and applications of common excipients for tablets; the general operations of the manufacture of traditional Chinese medicinal tablets.

2. To be familiar with the structure, performance and maintenance of tablet press; possible problems associated with tableting process and their solutions; the purpose and types of tablet coating, the requirements of tablet core, and the coating technology; quality control of tablets.

3. To know the main problems in the design of new products of traditional Chinese medicinal tablets.

Ability requirements:

1. To be able to use appropriate equipment for the manufacture of qualified tablets.

2. Have the ability to solve the problems in the manufacture of tablets.

第一节　概述

16.1　Overview

PPT

一、中药片剂的含义与特点

16.1.1　The Definition and Characteristics of Traditional Chinese Medicinal Tablets

中药片剂系指提取物、提取物加饮片细粉或饮片细粉与适宜辅料混匀压制或用其他适宜方法制成的圆片状或异形片状的制剂，分为提纯片、浸膏片、半浸膏片和全粉片。片剂是目前临床应用最广泛的剂型之一，主要供内服，亦可外用。

Traditional Chinese medicinal tablets refer to solid preparations of various shapes, round or heteromorphic, prepared by compression or other appropriate methods using the mixture of extract, extract and fine powder of decoction pieces, or fine powder of decoction pieces with suitable excipients. Traditional Chinese medicinal tablets can be divided into purified tablets, extract tablets, semi-extract tablets and powdered crude drug tablets. Tablet is one of the most widely used clinical dosage forms, which is mainly for internal use but can also be administered externally.

片剂始创于 19 世纪 40 年代，随着科学的进步，片剂的生产技术、机械设备和质量控制等方面有了巨大的发展。流化喷雾技术、全粉末直接压片、全自动程序控制包衣，以及生产工序联动化和新型辅料的研究开发等，对改善生产条件和提高片剂质量起到了重要的作用。中药片剂的研究和生产始于 20 世纪 50 年代，它是对汤剂、丸剂等传统剂型的改进。随着中药现代化研究及现代工业药剂学的发展，逐步摸索出一套适合于中药片剂生产的工艺条件，如对含脂肪油、挥发油片剂的制备，提高中药片剂的硬度、改善崩解度的方法，适合中药片剂的包衣工艺等，中药片剂的类型和品种不断增加，质量迅速提高，成为主要的中药剂型。

Tablets were founded in 1840’s. With the science development, the manufacturing technology and equipment of tablets, and the tests for their quality control have made great progress. Development of new technologies such as fluidization spray, powder direct compression and automatic coating, as well as novel excipients have played an important role in improving the manufacturing conditions and the quality of tablets. The research and production of traditional Chinese medicinal tablets began in the 1950s, which is an improvement of traditional dosage forms such as decoction, pill, etc. With the development of traditional Chinese medicine modernization and modern industrial pharmaceutics, technologies suitable for the manufacture of traditional Chinese medicinal tablets have been gradually explored, such as the preparation technology of tablets containing fatty oil and volatile oil, methods for improving the hardness and disintegration of traditional Chinese medicinal tablets, and technologies suitable for the coating of traditional Chinese medicinal tablets. As a result, the types of traditional Chinese medicinal tablets are increasing and their qualities are improving rapidly, becoming the main dosage forms of traditional Chinese medicine.

片剂有如下优点：①通常片剂的溶出度及生物利用度较丸剂好。②含量均匀、剂量准确。③质量稳定。片剂为干燥固体，受外界水分、空气、光线等因素的影响较少，并且可通过包衣提

高其稳定性。④体积小，携带、运输和服用方便。⑤生产成本低。生产的机械化、自动化程度较高、产量大。

Tablets have the following advantages: ① The dissolution and bioavailability of tablets are generally better than that of pills; ② Having uniform content and accurate dosage; ③ Having stable quality. Tablets are in solid state and less affected by external moisture, air or light, and their stability can be further improved by coating. ④ Packed in small size, and easy to carry, transport and administer. ⑤ Low-cost of manufacture. The mechanization and automation of manufacturing process are high and the output is large.

片剂也存在一些缺点：①婴幼儿和昏迷患者不宜吞服；②易引湿受潮、含挥发性成分的片剂久贮含量下降；③因辅料不当、压力不当等常出现崩解度、溶出度和生物利用度等问题。

There are also some disadvantages of tablets: ① Not suitable for infants and patients in coma; ② Absorbing moisture easily and losing volatile components during long-term storage; ③ Problems associated with tablet disintegration, dissolution and bioavailability often occur due to improper excipients and compression pressure.

二、片剂的分类
16.1.2 The Classification of Tablets

依据临床需求、药物的理化性质、胃肠道吸收部位及程度、湿热稳定性等，可以制备不同类型的片剂。按照给药途径和作用特点，片剂归纳起来可以分为三大类，即口服用片剂、口腔用片剂和外用片剂。

Different types of tablets can be manufactured according to clinical needs, physicochemical properties of drugs, the site and degree of absorption in gastrointestinal tract, moisture and heat stability, etc. According to the administration route and the action properties, tablets can be generally divided into three categories: oral tablets, tablets for oral cavity use and tablets for external use.

（一）口服用片剂
(1) Oral Tablets

口服用片剂是指供口服的片剂。大多数口服片剂经胃肠道吸收而发挥作用，但也有部分口服片剂在胃肠道发挥局部作用。口服片剂又分为以下若干种。

Oral tablets refer to the tablets for oral administration. Most of the oral tablets exert their actions by absorption into systemic circulation in gastrointestinal tract, but some produces local effect in gastrointestinal tract. Oral tablets are further divided into the following categories.

1. 普通压制片 又称为素片，系指药物与辅料混合后，经压制而成的片剂。

① **Simple uncoated tablets**, also known as plain tablets, refer to tablets compressed directly by the mixture of drugs and excipients.

2. 包衣片 系指在压制片（片芯）外包衣膜的片剂。按照包衣材料的不同，又可以分为糖衣片、薄膜衣片、肠溶衣片等。

② **Coated tablets** refer to tablets (core tablets) covered with a layer. According to different coating materials, coated tablets can be divided into sugar coated tablets, film coated tablets, enteric coated tablets, etc.

3. 咀嚼片 系指口腔中咀嚼后吞服的片剂。咀嚼片硬度应适宜，常选用蔗糖、甘露醇、山梨醇等水溶性辅料做填充剂和黏合剂。

③ **Chewable tablets** refer to tablets intended to be chewed and then swallowed. Chewable tablets

should have suitable hardness. Sucrose, mannitol, or sorbitol, which are excipients freely soluble in water, are usually utilized as fillers and binders.

4. 分散片 系指在水中能迅速崩解并均匀分散的片剂。分散片适用于难溶性药物，在21℃±1℃的水中3分钟应能崩解分散，并通过二号筛。

④ **Dispersible tablets** refer to tablets that are intended to be disintegrated rapidly and dispersed uniformly in water. Dispersible tablets are suitable for insoluble drugs, and should be disintegrated and dispersed in 21℃ ± 1℃ water within 3 minutes to give a uniform dispersion that can pass through No.2 sieve.

5. 泡腾片 系指含有碳酸氢钠和有机酸，遇水可产生气体而呈泡腾状的片剂。该片剂中的药物应是易溶性的。常用的有机酸有酒石酸、枸橼酸、富马酸等。适用于老人、儿童及吞咽困难的患者。

⑤ **Effervescent tablets** refer to tablets containing sodium bicarbonate and organic acid, which can release carbon dioxide and become effervescent when encountering water. The drug substances in effervescent tablets should be freely soluble in water. Organic acids such as tartaric acid, citric acid and fumaric acid are usually used. Effervescent tablets are suitable for the elderly, children and patients with dysphagia.

6. 口崩片 系指在口腔中可快速崩解或溶解的片剂。这类片剂的特点是服用时不用水，特别适合于老人、儿童及吞咽困难的患者。常采用水溶性好的山梨醇、木糖醇、赤藓醇等作为填充剂和矫味剂，以及强效崩解剂。

⑥ **Orally disintegrating tablets** refer to tablets that are intended to be disintegrated or dissolved rapidly in the mouth without given additional water, especially suitable for the elderly, children and patients with dysphagia. Excipients of good aqueous solubility like sorbitol, xylitol and erythritol are often used as fillers, binders and flavoring agents. In addition, super disintegrants are often applied.

7. 多层片 系指由两层或多层组成的片剂。可分为上下或内外两层或多层，每层可含有不同的药物或辅料，这样可以避免复方制剂中不同药物之间的配伍变化，或者达到缓控释的效果。

⑦ **Multilayered tablets** refer to tablets composed of two or more layers. Tablets can be designed and manufactured to have separate layers or a core tablet inside a tablet. In this way, two or more drugs can be kept separate in a single tablet to avoid changes in drug compatibility or realize sustained and controlled drug release.

8. 缓释片 系指在规定的释放介质中缓慢地非恒速释放药物的片剂。具有服药次数少、作用时间长等优点。

⑧ **Sustained-release tablets** refer to tablets that release drug substances in a gradual, non-constant rate way in a specified release medium. They have the advantages of less dosing frequency and prolonged effect.

9. 控释片 系指在规定的释放介质中缓慢地恒速释放药物的片剂。具有血药浓度平稳、服药次数少、作用时间长等优点。

⑨ **Controlled-release tablets** refer to tablets that release drug substances in a gradual, constant rate way in a prescriptive release medium. They have the advantages of stable blood concentration, less dosing frequency and prolonged effect.

（二）口腔用片剂
(2) Tablets for Oral Cavity Use

1. 含片 系指含于口腔中缓缓溶化产生局部或全身作用的片剂，常用于口腔及咽喉疾病的治疗。

① **Lozenges** refer to tablets that are intended to be slowly dissolved in the oral cavity to exert local or systemic action. Lozenges are intended mainly for oral and throat diseases.

2. 舌下片 系指置于舌下能迅速溶化，药物经舌下黏膜吸收发挥全身作用的片剂。舌下片可避免肝脏对药物的首过作用，主要适用于急症的治疗。

② **Sublingual tablets** refer to tablets that are intended to be inserted beneath the tongue, where they are dissolved rapidly and the drug substances are absorbed directly through mucosa to obtain a systemic effect. As a result, the first pass effect may be avoided. Sublingual tablets are intended mainly for treatment of emergencies.

3. 口腔贴片 系指黏贴于口腔，经黏膜吸收后起局部或全身作用的片剂。可在口腔内缓慢释放药物，常用于口腔及咽喉疾病的治疗。

③ **Dental patches** refer to preparations that are intended for adhesion to the mucous membrane of the mouth for local or systemic effect. Dental patches can slowly release drug substances in the oral cavity and are intended mainly for treatment of oral and throat diseases.

（三）外用片剂
(3) Tablets for External Use

1. 阴道片 系指置于阴道内使用的片剂。阴道片在阴道内应易溶化、溶散、融化或崩解并易释放药物，主要起局部消炎、杀菌及收敛或避孕等作用。

① **Vaginal tablets** refer to tablets that are made to be used for insertion into the vagina. Vaginal tablets may be rapidly dissolved, dispersed, melted, or disintegrated in vagina, and the drug substances are released to obtain a local antiphlogistic, antimicrobial, astringent or contraceptive effect.

2. 外用溶液片 系指临用前加适量水或缓冲液溶解制成溶液而供外用的片剂，一般用于消毒、洗涤伤口、漱口等。

② **Soluble tablets for external use** refer to tablets that are dissolved in water or buffer solution before administration and used externally. They are mainly intended for disinfection, wound washing, gargling, etc.

三、中药片剂的类型
16.1.3 The Classification of Traditional Chinese Medicinal Tablets

中药片剂按饮片的加工处理方法不同，可分为四种类型，即提纯片、全粉片、全浸膏片和半浸膏片。

According to different processing methods of decoction pieces, traditional Chinese medicinal tablets can be divided into four types: purified tablets, powdered crude drug tablets, extract tablets and semi-extract tablets.

1. 提纯片 系指将处方饮片经过提取获得有效成分或有效部位的细粉，加适宜辅料制成的片剂。如银杏叶片、北豆根片、益心酮片等。

(1) Purified tablets refer to tablets that are manufactured by the mixture of fine powder of effective ingredients or decoction pieces-extracted parts and excipients, such as Ginkgo leaves tablet, Beidougen tablet, Yixintong tablet, etc.

2. 全粉片 系指将饮片粉碎制得细粉，加适宜辅料制成的片剂。如参茸片、安胃片等。

(2) Powdered crude drug tablets refer to tablets manufactured by the mixture of fine powder of pulverized decoction pieces and excipients, such as Shenrong tablet, Anwei tablet, etc.

3. 全浸膏片 系指将饮片全部提取制得浸膏，以全量浸膏制成的片剂。如穿心莲片、复方丹参片等。

(3) Extract tablets refer to tablets manufactured solely by extract of decoction pieces, such as Chuanxinlian tablet, Fufang Danshen tablet, etc.

4. 半浸膏片 系指将部分饮片粉碎为细粉与部分饮片提取制得的稠浸膏混合制成的片剂。如藿香正气片、银翘解毒片等。

(4) Semi-extract tablets refer to tablets manufactured by the mixture of fine powder of some pulverized decoction pieces and thick paste extracted from the other part of decoction pieces, such as Huoxiang Zhengqi tablet, Yinqiao Jiedu tablet, etc.

英文翻译

PPT

第二节 片剂的辅料

片剂的辅料是指片剂中除主药以外所有附加物料的总称，亦称赋形剂。片剂的辅料是一些生理惰性的物质，加入的目的在于确保压片过程中物料的流动性和可压性，制得的成品有良好的崩解性等。片剂的辅料应对人体无毒、无害，性质稳定，不与主药发生反应，不影响主药的溶出、吸收和含量测定等，且价廉易得。若辅料选择不当，不仅会影响压片过程，还对片剂的质量、稳定性及疗效的发挥均有一定程度的影响。

按照用途，辅料可分为稀释剂与吸收剂、润湿剂和黏合剂、崩解剂、润滑剂四大类。

一、稀释剂与吸收剂

二者统称为填充剂。当处方中主药含量太少（小于100mg）或中药片剂中含浸膏量多或浸膏黏性太大，给制片带来困难时，需加入稀释剂；当原料药（含中间体）中含有较多挥发油、脂肪油或其他液体时，需加入吸收剂吸收后，再进行制片。常用稀释剂或吸收剂有以下品种：

1. 淀粉 本品为白色细腻的粉末，是葡萄糖分子聚合而成的直链或支链高聚物，属多糖类。淀粉在水或乙醇中均不溶解，但在水中加热到62~72℃可糊化。淀粉性质稳定，可与大多数药物配伍；但淀粉的流动性与可压性较差，常与黏合力较强的糊精、糖粉等混合使用，以改善其可压性。淀粉是最常用的稀释剂和吸收剂。天花粉、山药、贝母等含淀粉较多的中药材，粉碎成细粉后可作为稀释剂，兼有吸收剂和崩解剂的作用。

2. 糊精 本品为白色或类白色的无定形粉末，是由淀粉或部分水解的淀粉，在干燥状态下经加热改性而制得的聚合物。本品在沸水中易溶，在乙醇或乙醚中不溶。其水溶液呈弱酸性，具有较强的黏性。糊精具有较强的聚集、结块趋势，作为片剂的稀释剂，应控制其用量，以防止片剂表面出现水印、麻点，以及崩解或溶出迟缓；用量超过50%时，可用乙醇作为润湿剂，制得硬度适宜的颗粒。常与淀粉、蔗糖配合使用。但应注意糊精对某些药物的含量测定有干扰。

3. 糖粉 本品为无色结晶或白色结晶性松散粉末，味甜，为蔗糖粉碎而成。本品在水中极易溶解，在乙醇中微溶，在无水乙醇中几乎不溶。糖粉为片剂优良的稀释剂，兼有矫味和黏合作用，多用于含片、咀嚼片及纤维性较强或质地疏松的中药制片。糖粉黏合性强，可增加片剂的硬度，使片剂表面光洁；但因其具有较强的引湿性，久贮会使片剂硬度增大，导致崩解或溶出困难。除可溶片及含片外，一般不单独使用，常与糊精、淀粉配合使用。

4. 乳糖 本品为白色结晶性颗粒或粉末，从牛乳中提取，是由一分子葡萄糖和一分子半乳糖缩合而成，略带甜味，在水中易溶。乳糖无引湿性，性质稳定，可与大多数药物配伍；具有良好的流动性和可压性，制成的片剂光洁、美观，不影响药物的溶出，对主药的含量测定影响较小，是优良的片剂稀释剂。由喷雾干燥法制得的球形乳糖，可供粉末直接压片。

5. 预胶化淀粉 也称可压性淀粉，为白色或类白色粉末，本品系淀粉经物理或化学改性（淀粉部分或全部胶化）的产物。预胶化淀粉微溶于冷水（在冷水中可溶 10%~20%），不溶于乙醇。其具有良好的流动性、可压性和自身润滑性，兼具黏合和崩解性能，常用于粉末直接压片。

6. 微晶纤维素 本品为白色或类白色粉末或颗粒状粉末，由多孔微粒组成，是一种以 β-1，4 葡萄糖苷键结合的直链式多糖，系含纤维素植物的纤维浆制得的 α- 纤维素，在无机酸的作用下部分解聚、纯化而得。根据粒度大小和含水量的不同，有若干规格，如 PH101、PH102、PH200、PH301 等。MCC 除作为稀释剂外，兼具黏合、助流、崩解等作用，素有“干黏合剂”之称，可用于粉末直接压片。

7. 糖醇类 主要包括甘露醇和山梨醇，为白色结晶性粉末，味甜，溶解时吸热，有凉爽感，常用于咀嚼片、口崩片，但价格稍贵，常与蔗糖配合使用。近年来开发的赤藓糖醇，甜度只有蔗糖的 60%~70%，在口中溶解时有温和的凉爽感，且不会产生酸性物质对牙齿造成伤害，是制备口崩片的最佳辅料，但价格较贵。

8. 无机盐类 主要包括硫酸钙、磷酸氢钙及磷酸钙等无机钙盐。其性质稳定，微溶于水，可与多种药物配伍，制成的片剂外观光洁、硬度适宜、崩解度较好。常用于含挥发油和脂肪油较多的中药制片，为中药浸出物、油类及含油浸膏的良好吸收剂。

二、润湿剂与黏合剂

润湿剂与黏合剂在制片中具有使固体粉末黏结成型的作用。本身无黏性，但可润湿物料，诱发其自身黏性的液体称为润湿剂，适用于有一定黏性的药料，如中药浸膏粉及含有黏性成分的中药细粉等。本身有黏性，能使药粉黏结成颗粒便于制粒和压片的辅料称为黏合剂。无黏性或黏性不足的药料，需加入黏合剂，以利于制粒和压片。黏合剂有液体和固体两种类型，一般来说，液体的黏合剂黏性较大，容易混匀；而固体的黏合剂（也称“干燥黏合剂”）往往兼具稀释剂和崩解剂的作用。黏合剂用量不足或黏性不够，则制得的片剂疏松易脆；若黏合剂用量过大或黏性过强，则片剂过于坚硬，不易崩解。因此，黏合剂的选择和用量要合适。常用的润湿剂和黏合剂有如下几种。

1. 水 水是常用的润湿剂，凡药料本身具有一定黏性，如中药半浸膏粉或其他黏性物质，用水润湿即能黏结制粒。遇水稳定的药物，水是首选的润湿剂。但当处方中含水溶性成分较多或中药浸膏黏性较强时，有润湿不均匀、结块、颗粒干燥后发硬等现象，可用低浓度的淀粉浆或适宜浓度的乙醇溶液代替。不适用遇水敏感和不耐热的药物。

2. 乙醇 乙醇是润湿剂，用于遇水易分解、在水中溶解度大或遇水黏性太大的药物。中药浸膏制粒常用不同浓度的乙醇 - 水溶液作润湿剂，常用浓度为 30%~70%。乙醇浓度越高，物料被润湿后的黏性越小。用乙醇作润湿剂时应迅速搅拌、立即制粒，以免乙醇挥发。

3. 淀粉浆 是片剂中最常用的黏合剂。俗称淀粉糊，系由淀粉加水在 70℃左右糊化而得的稠厚胶体。常用 8%~15% 的浓度，并以 10% 淀粉浆最为常用。若物料可压性较差，可再适当提高淀粉浆的浓度到 20%，相反，也可适当降低淀粉浆的浓度。淀粉浆的制法有两种：①冲浆法，

系将淀粉混悬于少量（1~1.5倍）水中，然后根据浓度要求冲入一定量的沸水，不断搅拌糊化而成。②煮浆法，系将淀粉混悬于全量水中，在夹层容器中边加热边搅拌（不宜用直火加热，以免焦化），直至糊化。淀粉浆价廉易得且黏合性良好，是制粒首选的黏合剂。

4. 聚维酮（PVP） 本品系乙烯基吡咯烷酮的聚合物，为白色至乳白色的粉末。根据分子量不同有多种规格，其中用作黏合剂最常用的型号是K30。聚维酮可溶于水和乙醇。常用10%水溶液作黏合剂，3%~15%的乙醇溶液用于对水敏感的药物。亦可用作直接压片的干黏合剂。聚维酮常用于溶液片、泡腾片、咀嚼片等的制粒。缺点是引湿性强。

5. 纤维素衍生物 系天然纤维素的衍生物。甲基纤维素、羧甲基纤维素钠、羟丙基纤维素、羟丙基甲基纤维素等均可用作黏合剂，常用浓度为5%左右。这类聚合物的聚合度和取代度不同，其黏度等性质亦不同。其中乙基纤维素不溶于水而溶于乙醇，可作为水敏感药物的黏合剂。乙基纤维素黏性较强，会对片剂的崩解和药物的释放产生阻滞作用，常用于缓控释制剂的制备。

6. 糖浆 本品为蔗糖的水溶液，其黏合力强，适用于中药纤维性强、质地疏松或弹性较大的药物，常用浓度为50%~70%。不宜用于酸性或碱性较强的药物，以免产生转化糖而增加引湿性。饴糖、炼蜜和液状葡萄糖与糖浆类似，黏合性较强，但均具引湿性。因此，用作黏合剂时，制得的颗粒不易干燥，片剂易吸潮。

7. 阿拉伯胶浆、明胶浆 两者的黏合力均较大，适用于松散不易制粒的药物，或硬度要求大的片剂，如含片。常用浓度为10%~20%。使用时必须注意浓度与用量，若浓度过高、用量过大，将影响片剂的崩解。

8. 其他 海藻酸钠、聚乙二醇及硅酸铝镁等也常用作黏合剂。

中药稠膏，既是药物原料，又兼具黏合剂的作用。

三、崩解剂

崩解剂系指能促使片剂在胃肠液中迅速崩解成细小颗粒，有利于药物溶出的辅料。崩解剂的主要作用是瓦解因黏合剂或高度压缩而产生的结合力。除含片、舌下片、植入片、长效片、咀嚼片等，一般片剂均需加崩解剂。此外，中药半浸膏片因含有中药细粉，其本身遇水后能缓缓崩解，故一般不另加崩解剂。

（一）片剂的崩解机理

片剂的崩解过程经历润湿、吸水膨胀、瓦解过程。崩解剂的作用机制主要有如下几种：

1. 毛细管作用 崩解剂能保持压制片的孔隙结构，形成易于润湿的毛细管道。当片剂置于水中时，水能迅速地随毛细管进入片剂内部，使整个片剂被水浸润而促进崩解。如淀粉及其衍生物和纤维素类衍生物等。

2. 膨胀作用 崩解剂自身具有很强的吸水膨胀性，吸水后，体积显著增大，促使片剂的内部结合力瓦解而崩散。如羧甲基淀粉钠、低取代羟丙基纤维素。

3. 润湿热作用 有些药物溶解时产热，致使片剂内部残存的空气膨胀，促使片剂崩解。

4. 产气作用 崩解剂能产生气体，借气体膨胀而使片剂崩解。如泡腾崩解剂。

（二）常用的崩解剂

1. 干淀粉 系指在100~105℃干燥1小时左右，含水量在8%以下的淀粉。干燥淀粉是毛细管形成剂，为亲水性物质，可增加孔隙率而改善片剂的渗水性。通常适用于不溶性或微溶性药物，但对易溶性药物作用较差。淀粉的流动性与可压性较差，用量过多会使颗粒的流动性降低并且影响片剂的硬度。其用量一般为干颗粒的5%~20%。

2. 羧甲基淀粉钠 本品为无臭、无味的白色无定形粉末。羧甲基淀粉钠具有较强的吸水性和膨胀性，能吸收其干燥体积30倍的水，吸水膨胀后体积可增大至原体积的200~300倍。羧甲基淀粉钠具有良好的流动性及可压性，制得的片剂有适宜的硬度和较快的溶出速度。常用作不溶性药物和可溶性药物的崩解剂，既可用于直接压片，又可用于湿法制颗粒压片，其用量一般为干颗粒的4%~8%。

3. 低取代羟丙基纤维素 本品为白色或类白色结晶性粉末，不溶于水，但有良好的吸水性，由于低取代羟丙基纤维素的比表面积和孔隙率都很大，故具有较大的吸水速度和吸水量，是一种良好的膨胀剂。另外，低取代羟丙基纤维素的毛糙结构与药粉和颗粒之间有较大的镶嵌作用，使黏度增强，可提高片剂的硬度和光洁度。

4. 交联羧甲基纤维素钠 本品为无臭、无味的白色细颗粒状粉末，是由羧甲基纤维素钠交联而成的聚合物。能吸收数倍于本身重量的水而膨胀，膨胀至原体积的4~8倍。

5. 交联聚维酮 本品为白色粉末，流动性好，不溶于水、乙醇、乙醚等溶剂。在水中能迅速吸水膨胀，无胶凝倾向，崩解性能优越。

6. 泡腾崩解剂 系指遇水能产生二氧化碳气体从而达到崩解作用的酸碱系统，由碳酸盐（常用碳酸钠或碳酸氢钠）和有机酸（常用枸橼酸或酒石酸）组成，是专属于泡腾片的特殊崩解剂。因此，泡腾片应妥善包装，避免受潮造成崩解剂失效。

（三）崩解剂的加入方法

崩解剂的加入方法有外加法、内加法和内外加法。①外加法是将崩解剂加入压片前的干颗粒中，崩解作用起自颗粒之间。片剂崩解迅速，但因颗粒内无崩解剂，故片剂不易崩解成细粉，药物溶出稍差。②内加法是指将崩解剂与处方物料混合一起制粒。崩解作用起自颗粒内部，颗粒崩解较完全。但崩解剂与水接触较为迟缓，崩解作用较弱。③内外加法是将崩解剂的一部分与处方物料混合一起制粒，另一部分加在已干燥的颗粒中，混匀压片。此法集中了前两种方法的优点，是崩解剂较为理想的加入方法。

四、润滑剂

为了能顺利加料和出片，减少黏冲，降低颗粒与颗粒、药片与模孔壁间的摩擦力，使药片光滑美观，在压片前均需在颗粒（或结晶）中加入适宜的润滑剂。润滑剂是一个广义的概念，是助流剂、抗黏剂和润滑剂（狭义）的总称。其中：①助流剂：降低颗粒之间的摩擦力，增加颗粒的流动性，改善颗粒的填充状态；②抗黏剂：减轻原辅料对冲模的黏附性，使压片顺利进行，还可使片剂表面光滑；③润滑剂：降低压片和推片时药片与冲头或模孔壁之间的摩擦力，保证压片时应力分布均匀，防止裂片。常用的润滑剂有以下几种。

1. 硬脂酸镁 本品为白色细腻的粉末，有良好的附着性，所制得片剂光滑美观，为常用的润滑剂。此类润滑剂为疏水性物质，用量过大会影响片剂崩解且容易造成裂片，一般用量为0.3%~1%。

2. 滑石粉 本品为白色结晶粉末，用后可均匀分布在颗粒表面，改善颗粒表面的粗糙性，增加颗粒的润滑性和流动性。不溶于水，但有亲水性，常与硬脂酸镁联用改善硬脂酸镁对片剂崩解的不良影响。本品颗粒细而比重大，附着力较差，在压片过程中可因振动易与颗粒分离并沉在颗粒底部，造成上冲黏冲、片面色泽不均等问题。

3. 氢化植物油 本品系由精制植物油催化氢化，经喷雾干燥而制得的粉末。使用时将其溶解于轻质液体石蜡或己烷中，再喷洒于干颗粒上，以利于其均匀分布。

4. 聚乙二醇 常用聚乙二醇4000或聚乙二醇6000，具有良好的润滑作用。水溶性较好，不

影响片剂的崩解和溶出。

5. 十二烷基硫酸钠 本品系阴离子型表面活性剂，具有良好的润滑作用，能增强片剂的机械强度，并能促进片剂崩解和溶出。

6. 微粉硅胶 本品为白色的轻质粉末，化学性质稳定，流动性好。比表面积大，对药物有较强的吸附力，特别适用于油类和浸膏类药物。微粉硅胶有较强的亲水性，是常用的助流剂，可用于粉末直接压片，一般用量为 0.15%~3%。

第三节 中药片剂的制法

16.3 Manufacturing Operations of Traditional Chinese Medicinal Tablets

PPT

片剂制备的过程中，应根据药物的性质和临床需要确定处方，选择适宜的辅料和制备方法。压片方法包括制粒压片法和粉末直接压片法，根据不同的制粒方法，制粒压片法又分为湿法制粒压片法和干法制粒压片法，其中湿法制粒压片法应用更为广泛。

In the manufacturing process of tablets, tablet formulation should be firstly determined according to drug properties and clinical requirements, and then suitable excipients and preparation method are selected. In general terms, there are two tableting methods: granulation and direct compression method. According to different granulating processes, the granulation method is also divided into wet granulation and dry granulation, among which the wet granulation is more widely used.

一、湿法制粒压片法

16.3.1 Wet Granulation

本法适用于药物不能直接压片，且遇湿、热稳定的片剂的制备，一般工艺流程见图 16-1。

Wet granulation is applicable to drug substances that cannot be compressed directly into tablets but are stable to moisture and heat as shown in Figure 16-1.

（一）原、辅料的处理

(1) Treatment of Raw Materials

1. 选用合格的原料，进行洁净、灭菌、炮制和干燥处理，制成饮片。

① Selecting qualified raw materials and preparing decoction pieces through cleaning, sterilizing, processing and drying.

2. 中药饮片须经过浸提、分离、精制处理，尽量除去无效物质，保留有效成分，以缩小体积，减少服用量。

② The decoction pieces of traditional Chinese medicines are extracted, separated and refined to remove ineffective substances as much as possible and retain the effective ones, in order to reduce their volume and dosing amount.

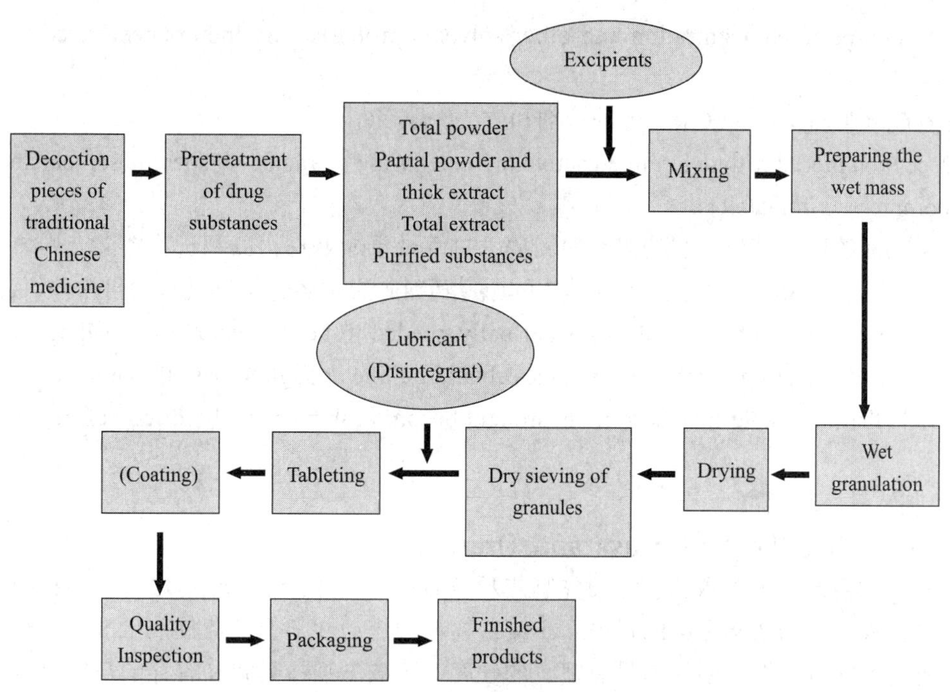

图 16-1 湿法制粒压片工艺流程

Figure 16-1 Preparation Process of Wet Granulation

3. 含水溶性有效成分，或含纤维较多、黏性较大、质地泡松或坚硬的饮片，以水煎煮，浓缩成稠膏。必要时采用高速离心或加乙醇处理等纯化方法去除杂质，再制成稠膏或干浸膏，或经喷雾干燥制成细粉。

③ Decoction pieces containing water soluble active ingredients or high amount of fibers, or decoction pieces of great viscosity, or of loose or hard texture, are decocted with water and concentrated to a thick extract. If necessary, high speed centrifugation or treatment by ethanol are applied to remove impurities, and then the decoction pieces are processed into thick extract or dry extract, or spray-dried fine power.

4. 含淀粉较多的饮片、贵重药、毒性药、树脂类药及受热有效成分易破坏的饮片等，一般粉碎成 100 目左右细粉，用适当方法灭菌后备用。

④ Decoction pieces containing high amount of starch, valuable drugs, toxic drugs, resin drugs, or decoction pieces containing active ingredients that are sensitive to heat, are usually pulverized into fine powder that can pass through a 100 mesh sieve, and then preserved for future use after sterilization by appropriate method.

5. 含挥发性成分较多的饮片宜用双提法，先提取挥发性成分备用，药渣再与余药加水煎煮，并与蒸馏后药液共制成稠膏或干浸膏粉。

⑤ For decoction pieces containing high amount of volatile ingredients, a dual extraction method should be employed. The volatile ingredients are firstly extracted by distillation, the drug residuals and the remaining drug substances are then decocted with water, and finally the decoctions are combined with the distilled substances and subsequently processed into thick extract or dry extract powder.

6. 含脂溶性有效部位的饮片，可用适宜浓度的乙醇或其他溶剂以适当的方法提取，再浓缩成稠膏。

⑥ Decoction pieces containing active ingredients that are lipid soluble can be extracted by alcoholic

solution of appropriate concentration and other solvents properly, and then concentrated to the thick extract.

7. 有效成分明确的饮片采用特定的溶剂和方法提取后制片。

⑦ Decoction pieces with determined active ingredients are extracted by specific solvent and method, and then compressed into tablets.

8. 化学药品的原、辅料一般均需经过粉碎、过筛及干燥处理，以利于物料混合均匀，颗粒细度以通过五至六号筛为宜。对于易受潮结块的原、辅料，必须经过干燥处理后再粉碎、过筛。

⑧ Raw materials of chemical drugs are usually needed to be pretreated by crushing, sieving and drying to facilitate uniform mixing. The particles should be fine enough to pass through No. 5 to 6 sieve. Raw materials that are liable to absorb moisture and become caking must be dried before crushing and sieving.

（二）制软材、制颗粒

(2) Preparing the Wet Mass and Granules

1. 制颗粒的目的 大多数药物需要先制成颗粒后进行压片，制颗粒可以增加物料的流动性和可压性，具体来说，药物制颗粒的目的：①改善物料的流动性，保证片剂剂量准确，减小片重差异；②改善物料的可压性，使片剂具有适宜的硬度；③减少细粉吸附和容存的空气以减少药片的松裂；④避免粉末分层，使片剂中药物含量均匀；⑤避免粉尘飞扬、黏冲、拉模等现象。

① **The purpose of granulation** Most drugs need to be granulated before tableting. The purpose of granulation is to increase the flowability and compressibility of materials, which is specifically described as: a. Improving the flowability of materials, assuring the accuracy of tablet dosage units, and reducing the variation of tablet weight. b. Improving the compressibility of materials to prepare tablets with suitable hardness. c. Reducing the absorption of fine powder and the volume of entrapped air to protect the tablets from cracking. d. Protecting the powder from delamination to assure the content uniformity of tablets. e. Preventing phenomenon like dust flying, tablet sticking to punch faces or picking.

2. 制颗粒的方法

② **The methods of granulation**

（1）饮片细粉制粒法 系指将全部饮片细粉混匀，加入适量黏合剂或润湿剂制成适宜的软材，挤压过筛制粒的方法。若处方中含有较多矿物性、纤维性药料，应选用黏性较强的黏合剂；若处方中含有较多黏性成分，则选用水或乙醇作为润湿剂即可。此法适用于小剂量的贵重药、毒性药及几乎不具有纤维性的饮片，如参茸片、安胃片等。

a. Granulation of fine powder of decoction pieces Firstly, premix all the fine powder of decoction pieces, and then add appropriate amount of binder or wetting agent to form the damp mass. Finally, wet-screen the damp mass into granules. If mineral or fibrous drug substances represent a majority of tablet formulation, a binder with strong cohesiveness should be selected; if there are more viscous components in the formulation, wetting agent like water or ethanol should be used. This method is applicable to small doses of valuable drugs, toxic drugs, and decoction pieces almost with no fibrous property, such as Anrong tablet and Anwei tablet.

案例导入 ¦ Case example

案例 16-1 新清宁片

16-1 Xinqingning Tablets

处方：熟大黄 300g

Ingredients: Rhei Radix et Rhizoma (prepared) 300g

功能与主治：清热解毒，泻火通便。用于内结实热所致的喉肿、牙痛、目赤、便秘、下痢、发热；感染性炎症见上述证候者。

Functions and indications: To clear heat, remove toxin, purge fire and open the bowels. Pattern of interior excess heat bind, manifested as swollen throat, toothache, red eyes, constipation, diarrhea and fever; Infectious inflammation with the symptoms described above.

制法：取熟大黄粉碎成细粉，加乙醇适量，制成颗粒，干燥，加淀粉及硬脂酸镁适量，混匀，压制成 1000 片，包糖衣，即得。

Making Procedure: Pulverize Rhei Radix et Rhizoma (prepared) to fine powder, add a quantity of ethanol, make granules, dry, add a quantity of starch and magnesium stearate, mix thoroughly, compress into 1000 tablets and coat with sugar or film.

用法与用量：口服。一次 3~5 片，一日 3 次；必要时可适当增量；学龄前儿童酌减或遵医嘱；用于便秘，临睡前服 5 片。

Usage and dosage: For oral administration, 3-5 tablets per time, three times a day. Increase the dosage if necessary. Reduce the dosage in pre-school children or as advised by health professionals. 5 tablets before sleep for constipation treatment.

注解：（1）本品为单味制剂，系将熟大黄粉碎为细粉，加适量辅料混匀制软材，制颗粒，压片而成。

Notes: ① This product is a single component preparation, which is prepared by pulverizing Rhei Radix et Rhizoma (prepared) to fine powder, mixing with a quantity of excipients thoroughly to form the damp mass, then granulating, and finally compressing into tablets.

（2）硬脂酸镁起润滑作用，为润滑剂，其润滑性强，附着性好；具疏水性，用量大会影响片剂崩解，或产生裂片。用量一般为干颗粒的 0.3%~1%。

② Magnesium stearate serves as the lubricant of good lubricity and adhesion. It is a hydrophobic material. Too much magnesium stearate in the formulation will negatively affect the disintegration of tablets or lead to tablet cracking. Its usual concentration range is between 0.3% and 1% of dry granules.

思考题：熟地黄黏性较强，选用乙醇作其润湿剂，浓度应该如何控制？

Questions: Rhei Radix et Rhizoma (prepared) has strong viscosity. When ethanol is used as the wetting agent, how to control its concentration?

案例导入

（2）饮片细粉与稠浸膏混合制粒法　系指将处方中部分饮片制成稠浸膏，另一部分饮片粉碎成细粉，两者混合后制颗粒的方法。此法应根据饮片性质及出膏率决定磨粉的饮片量，还应考虑片剂的崩解度，力求使稠浸膏与饮片细粉混合后恰可制成适宜的软材。此法的优点在于稠浸膏与中药细粉除具有治疗作用外，稠浸膏还有黏合作用，饮片细粉可促进片剂崩解，充分利用中药饮片，体现中药制剂“药辅合一”的原则。

b. Granulation of the mixture of fine powder and thick extract　Firstly, process some part of decoction pieces into thick extract, and then pulverize the remaining part into fine powder. Finally mix the above two for granulation. In this method, the amount of decoction pieces that are pulverized should be determined by the properties of the pieces and the extraction ratio of the thick extract, as well as the disintegration of the tablet, so as to prepare appropriate damp mass after mixing thick extract with the fine powder of decoction pieces. The advantage of this method is that in addition to the therapeutic effect exerted by the thick extract and the fine powder, the thick extract can also act as a binder, and the powder of decoration pieces can promote tablet disintegration, taking full advantage of the traditional Chinese medicinal pieces and embodying the principle of "integration of drug and excipients" for traditional Chinese medicines.

案例导入

（3）全浸膏制粒法　用全浸膏制粒法制颗粒有三种情况：一是将干浸膏直接粉碎成颗粒。应选用黏性适中、吸湿性不强的干浸膏，粉碎成颗粒后通过 2~3 号筛，制成的颗粒应较细小，以防压片时产生花斑、麻点。二是干浸膏粉制粒。将干浸膏粉碎成细粉，加润湿剂后制软材制颗粒。三是稠浸膏制粒，将药物提取物浓缩至一定相对密度，加入辅料后制颗粒。全浸膏片因不含中药细粉，服用量少，易达到卫生标准，尤其适用于有效成分含量较低的药物，但所制得的片剂有易吸湿、黏性大等缺点。

c. Granulation of whole extract　There are three ways for the granulation of the whole extract: The first one is to directly pulverize the dry extract into granules. Dry extract with suitable viscosity and little hygroscopicity shall be firstly selected, and then pulverized into granules and sifted through No. 2 to 3 sieve. The granules should be fine enough to prevent speckles and pockmarks on the surface of the tablet. The second one is to granulate with dry extract powder. Firstly, pulverize the dry extract into fine powder, and then add the wetting agent into it to form damp mass for granulation. The third one is to make granules by thick extract. Concentrate the drug extract to a relative density and add a quantity of excipients to make granules. The extract tablet is easy to meet the hygienic standards because it doesn't contain fine powder of traditional Chinese medicine and has low administration dose, especially suitable for drugs with low content of active ingredients. However, the extract tablet is hygroscopic and very viscous.

（4）提纯物制粒法　系指将提纯物细粉与适宜的稀释剂、崩解剂等混匀后，加入黏合剂或润湿剂制成合适的软材，制颗粒的方法。

d. Granulation of purified drugs　Mix the fine powder of purified drugs with a quantity of diluent and disintegrant, and then add the binder or wetting agent to form suitable wet mass for granulation.

案例导入 | Case example

案例 16-2　益心酮片

16-2　Yixintong Tablets

处方：山楂叶提取物 32g

Ingredients: Hawthorn Leaves Extract 32g

功能与主治：活血化瘀，宣通血脉。用于瘀血阻脉所致的胸痹，症见胸闷憋气、心前区刺痛、心悸健忘、眩晕耳鸣；冠心病心绞痛、高脂血症、脑动脉供血不足见上述证候者。

Functions and indications: To activate blood, resolve stasis, and promote blood circulation. Used for chest *bi* disorder due to static blood obstructing collaterals, manifested as chest oppression, labored breathing, stabbing pain in the precordium, palpitations, forgetfulness, dizziness and tinnitus; Angina pectoris in coronary heart disease, hyperlipemia or cerebral blood insufficiency with the symptoms

described above.

制法： 取山楂叶提取物，与淀粉 32g、糊精 25g、蔗糖 5g 混匀，制成颗粒，在 60℃以下干燥，加入适量滑石粉、硬脂酸镁，混匀，压制成 1000 片，包糖衣或薄膜衣，即得。

Making Procedure: Hawthorn Leaves Extract, starch 32g, dextrin 25g, sucrose 5g, mix thoroughly, make granules, dry below 60℃. Add a quantity of talcum and magnesium stearate, mix thoroughly, compress into 1000 tablets, coat with sugar or film.

用法与用量： 口服，一次 2~3 片，一日 3 次。

Usage and dosage: For oral administration, 2-3 tablets per time, three times a day.

注解：（1）淀粉的可压性差，作稀释剂时用量不宜过多，必要时与糊精、蔗糖等混合使用，改善其可压性。

Notes: ① Starch has poor compressibility, so too much starch as diluent in the formulation should be avoided. Starch can be used along with dextrin and sucrose to improve its compressibility, if necessary.

（2）滑石粉不溶于水，但具亲水性；助流性、抗黏着性良好，但附着性较差。多与硬脂酸镁等联合应用，用量一般为 2%~3%。

② Talc is insoluble in water, but is hydrophilic. It is an excellent glidant and antiadherent, but of poor adhesion. It is often used along with magnesium stearate at a usual concentration range between 2% and 3%.

思考题： 山楂叶提取物应该采用何种方法制得？

Questions: How to prepare the extract of hawthorn leaves?

（三）湿颗粒的干燥

(3) The Drying of Moist Granules

湿颗粒应及时干燥，温度一般为 60~80℃。干燥温度过高会使颗粒中的淀粉粒糊化，影响片剂崩解，还可能引起含浸膏的颗粒软化结块。对于含挥发性成分及苷类成分的颗粒，干燥温度应控制在 60℃以下，避免有效成分散失或被破坏；对热稳定的药物，干燥温度可提高至 80~100℃。湿颗粒的含水量在 3%~5% 之间为宜，含水量过高会产生黏冲现象，过低则易出现顶裂现象。

The moist granules should be dried immediately after preparation, at a temperature of 60 to 80℃. Excessive drying may cause the gelatinization of starch in the granules, negatively affecting the disintegration of tablets, or softening the granules containing extract, or leading to the caking of granules. For granules containing volatile ingredients and glycosides, the drying temperature should not exceed 60℃ to avoid the loss or decomposition of active ingredients. For thermostable drugs, the drying temperature can be increased up to 80 to 100℃. The moisture content of wet granules is preferably between 3% and 5%. Too high moisture content will cause the granules to stick to the punch faces, while too low moisture content will lead to the capping of tablets.

（四）干颗粒的质量要求

(4) Quality Requirements for Dry Granules

干颗粒应具有适宜的流动性和可压性，同时还应符合以下要求。

The dry granules should have suitable flowability and compressibility, and meanwhile meet the following requirements.

1. 主药含量 应符合规定。

A. Drug content should comply with the requirements.

2. 含水量 中药片剂品种不同，颗粒含水量要求不同，一般为 3%~5%。化学药干颗粒的含

水量一般为 1%~3%。干颗粒含水量对中药片剂成型及片剂质量影响很大。

B. Moisture content The requirement for the moisture content of granules is varied depending on the types of traditional Chinese medicinal tablets, which is usually between 3% and 5%. The moisture content of dry granules of chemical drugs is usually between 1% and 3%. The moisture content of dry granules significantly affects the formation and quality of traditional Chinese medicinal tablets.

3. 颗粒的大小、松紧及粒度 颗粒大小应根据片重及药片直径选择，制备中药片剂一般选用能通过二号筛或更细的颗粒；干颗粒的松紧度影响片剂的外观，硬颗粒在压片时易产生麻面，松颗粒则易产生松片。干颗粒中粗细颗粒的比例应适宜，细颗粒填充于大颗粒间，使片剂中药物含量准确，片重差异小。通常以含有能通过二号筛的颗粒占总量的 20%~40% 为宜，且无通过六号筛的细粉。

C. The size, hardness and size distribution of granules The size of the granules should be determined by the weight and diameter of the tablet. Granules for the preparation of traditional Chinese medicinal tablets should be small enough to pass through No. 2 sieve or even smaller. The hardness of dry granules affects the appearance of tablets. Hard granules are prone to cause pockmarked tablet face, and loose granules are easy to produce fragile tablets. The proportion of the coarse and fine granules in the total should be appropriate with fine granules filled between the large ones, so as to ensure an accurate drug content of the tablet and a small tablet weight variation. Generally, the proportion of the granules that can pass through No. 2 sieve is preferably between 20% and 40%, and very fine particles that can pass through No. 6 sieve should be removed.

（五）压片前干颗粒的处理

(5) Treatment of Dry Granules before Tableting

1. 整粒 系指颗粒干燥后再通过一次筛网，使其中结块、粘连的颗粒重新分散成均匀的干颗粒，以利于压片。整粒所用筛网的规格一般与制湿颗粒时相同，通常选用二号筛。

A. Dry sieving of granules refers to the process that the granules are sieved again through the screen after drying to break the agglomerates and cakes into granules of desired particle size and distribution, so as to facilitate tableting. The size of the screen for dry sieving is usually the same as that for wet sieving, and No. 2 sieve is often used.

2. 加挥发油或挥发性药物 处方中若含有挥发油，或制备时提取的挥发油成分，可加入干颗粒混匀后筛出的部分细粒中，再与全部干颗粒混匀。若挥发性药物为固体，如薄荷脑，可先用少量乙醇溶解后或与其他成分研磨共熔后均匀地喷洒在颗粒上。所有方法最后均应密闭贮放数小时，使挥发性成分在颗粒中渗透均匀，以免压片时产生裂片等现象。若挥发油含量超过 0.6% 时，常需要加适量吸收剂将挥发油吸收后，再混合压片；亦可将挥发油微囊化或制成环糊精包合物后加入干颗粒中，此法既便于压片又可以减少挥发性成分的损失。

B. Adding volatile oil or drugs If volatile oil or extracted volatile oil is included in the formulation, it can be firstly mixed with the fine particles separated after dry sieving, and then blended with the remaining dry granules. If the volatile drug is in the solid state, such as menthol, it can be dissolved with a small amount of ethanol or co-grounded with other ingredients to form a eutectic mixture, and then sprayed evenly over the spread-out granules. Whatever method is employed, the granules should be kept tightly sealed for several hours to make the volatile components permeate evenly into the granules, so as to avoid tablet cracking during compression. If the content of volatile oil exceeds 0.6%, it often needs to be absorbed by a quantity of absorbent and then blended with other ingredients for tableting. Or the volatile oil can be encapsulated into microcapsules or cyclodextrin inclusions, and

then mixed with the dry granules, so as to facilitate the tableting process and reduce the loss of volatile components as well.

3. 加润滑剂或崩解剂 润滑剂通常在整粒后用细筛筛入干颗粒中混合均匀。崩解剂应先干燥、过筛，再加入干颗粒中混合均匀。

C. Adding lubricant or disintegrant After dry sieving, the lubricant is usually sifted into dry granules by a small-size sieve and then mixed thoroughly with them. The disintegrant should be dried and sieved first, and then blended with the dry granules.

（六）压片

(6) Compressing the Granules into Tablets

1. 片重的计算 若已知每批药料应制的片数及每片重量，所制的干颗粒重应等于片数乘片重，片重可按下式计算。

A. Calculation of tablet weight If the number of tablets to be prepared of each batch and the weight of each tablet are determined, the weight of dry granules should be equal to the number of tablets multiplied by the tablet weight. The tablet weight can be calculated according to the equation below.

$$\text{片重}=\frac{\text{干颗粒重量}+\text{压片前加入的辅料重}}{\text{理论片数}}$$

若药料的片数与片重未定时，可先称出颗粒总重量相当于若干单服重量，再根据单服重量的颗粒重来决定每服的片数，片重可按下式计算。

Otherwise, the total granules can be weighed out first, whose weight is equal to the weight of several dose units. The number of tablets for each dose can be determined by the weight of granules for each dose. Then, the tablet weight can be calculated according to the following equation.

$$\text{单服颗粒重量}=\frac{\text{干颗粒总重量}}{\text{单服次数}}$$

$$\text{片重}=\frac{\text{单服颗粒重量}}{\text{单服片数}}$$

若生产中部分饮片提取浓缩成膏，另一部分饮片粉碎成细粉混合制成半浸膏片，片重可用下式计算。

For semi-extract tablets which are prepared by the mixture of thick extract and fine powder, the tablet weight can be calculated according to the following equation. The thick extract is obtained by the extraction and concentration of some decoction pieces, while the fine powder is obtained by the pulverization of the other part of decoction pieces.

$$\begin{aligned}\text{片重}&=\frac{\text{干颗粒重量}+\text{压片前加入的辅料重量}}{\text{理论片数}}\\&=\frac{(\text{成膏固体重量}+\text{原粉重量})+\text{压片前加入的辅料重量}}{\text{原药材总重量}/\text{每片原药材重量}}\\&=\frac{(\text{药材重量}\times\text{收膏率}\times\text{膏中总固体百分含量}+\text{原粉重量})+\text{压片前加入的辅料重量}}{\text{原药材总重量}/\text{每片原药材重量}}\end{aligned}$$

若已知每片主药的含量时，可通过测定颗粒中主药含量再确定片重。

If the drug content in each tablet is known, the tablet weight can be determined by analysis of the drug content in the granules.

$$片重=\frac{每片含主药量}{干颗粒测得的主药百分含量}$$

2. 压片机及压片过程 常用的压片机主要有单冲压片机和旋转式压片机两种。单冲压片机的产量一般用于小量生产，目前生产上主要使用旋转式压片机。

B. Tablet presses and tableting process The common tablet presses can be divided into two classes: single-station reciprocating presses and multi-station rotary presses. The single-station press is usually used for the production of tablets of small batch size, while the rotary press for large-scale manufacture.

（1）单冲压片机 单冲压片机的主要构造见图 16-2，其主要构造为：①加料器：加料斗、饲粉器。②压缩部件：上、下冲和模圈。③调节器：包括出片调节器、片重调节器和压力调节器。出片调节器调节下冲在模孔内上升的高度，使下冲冲头恰与模圈上缘相平，使压成的片剂便于推出；片重调节器调节下冲在模孔内下降的深度，通过调节模孔的填充量而调节片重；压力调节器与上冲的冲杆相连接，当上冲下降深度大时，上、下冲头在冲模内的距离小，颗粒所受的压力大，压出的片剂薄而硬，反之，则受压小，压出的片剂厚而松。

a. Single-station press The schematic structure of the single-station press is depicted in figure 16-2, which comprises: ① A feeding device: a hopper and a feed shoe. ② The compression unit: upper and lower punches, and a die. ③ The regulation unit: an ejection regulator, a weight regulator, and a hardness control. The ejection regulator is to adjust the raising position of the lower punch, so that its highest position is at par with the surface of the die, so as to facilitate the ejection of finished tablets. The weight regulator is to adjust the depth of the lower punch to accommodate the required quantity of granules/powder for each fill. The hardness control is connected with the holder of the upper punch. As the lowering distance of the upper punch is increased, the upper punch penetrates further into the die cavity, shortening the distance between upper and lower punches. Thus, for a given fill, the granules/powder are more highly consolidated and a harder and thinner tablet is formed. On the contrary, the granules/powder are lightly compacted and a softer and thicker tablet is formed.

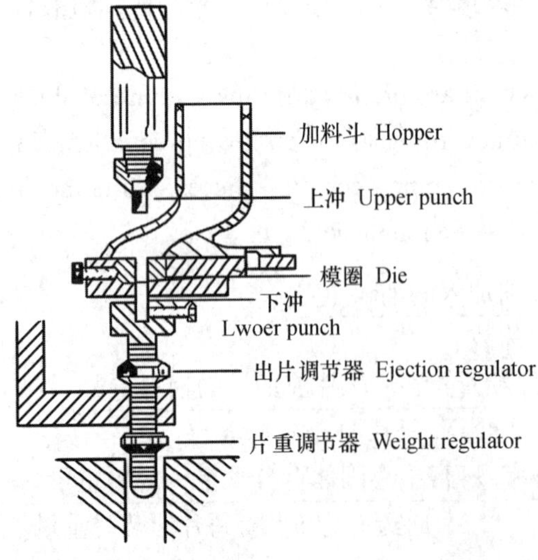

图 16-2 单冲压片机主要构造示意图

Figure 16-2 Schematic Structure of the Single-Station Press

单冲压片机的压片过程见图 16-3：①上冲抬起，饲料器移动到模孔之上；②下冲下降到适宜的深度（根据片重调节，使模孔容纳的颗粒重恰等于片重），摆动饲料器，使颗粒填满模孔；③饲料器由模孔上移开，使模孔中的颗粒与模孔的上缘相平；④上冲下降使颗粒压成片剂；⑤上冲抬起，下冲随之上升到与模孔上缘相平时，饲料器再移到模孔之上，将药片推开进入接收器中，同时进行第二次饲料，如此反复进行压片。

A single-station press produces tablets through a number of steps that can be described as figure 16-3: ① The upper punch is withdrawn and the feed shoe moves forward over the die. ② The lower punch is forced downward to an appropriate depth (adjusted by the tablet weight to ensure that the weight of the accommodated granules/powder in the die cavity is just equal to that of the tablet) and the granules/powder are allowed to fall from the hopper to fill the die. ③ The excess material is swept from the die table by the feed shoe. ④ The lower punch remains stationary and the upper punch lowers into the die to compress the granules/powder into a tablet. ⑤ The upper punch is then withdrawn while the lower punch pushes upwards to expel the tablet. The tablet is then removed from the die surface by the discharge chute, while the hopper shoe moves forward over the die again for the next feeding. The tableting cycle is repeated for the next batch.

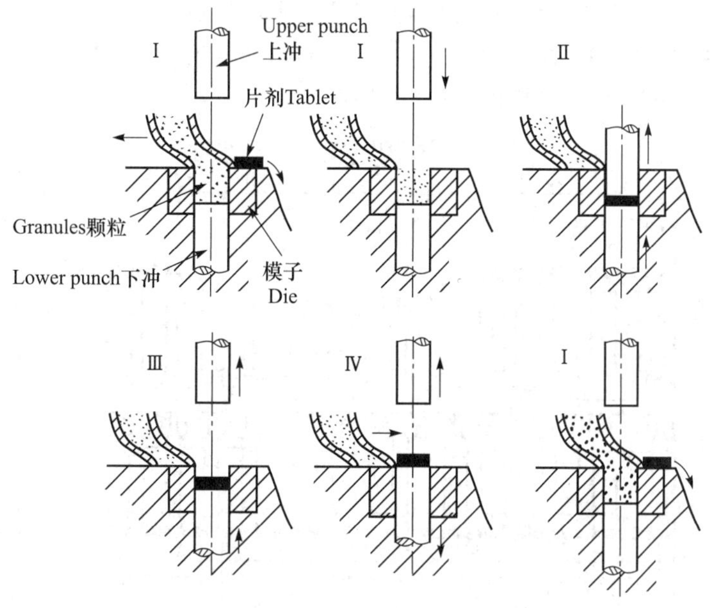

图 16-3 单冲压片机的压片过程

Figure 16-3 The Tableting Process of A Single-Station Press

单冲压片机的产量一般为 80~100 片 / 分钟，适用于新产品的试制或小量生产；单冲压片机为上冲加压，压力分布不均匀，易出现裂片，且噪音较大。

Single-station presses usually produce 80 to 100 tablets per minute, suitable for trial manufacturing or batch production in small size. During the compression stage, the compaction force on the filled material is exerted only by the upper punch while the lower punch is static. This may cause the cracking of tablet due to uneven distribution of compression force. Besides, single-punch tablet press also has the disadvantage of loud noise.

（2）旋转压片机 旋转式压片机的结构示意图和工作原理如图 16-4，其主要工作部件有：机台、压轮、片重调节器、压力调节器、加料斗、刮粉器、吸尘器和保护装置。机台分为三层，机台的上层装有若干上冲，在中层的对应位置装有模圈，在下层的对应位置装有下冲。上冲与下冲

各自随机台转动并沿着固定的轨道有规律地上、下运动。当上、下冲分别经过上、下压轮时，上冲向下、下冲向上运动，并对模孔中的物料加压；机台中层的固定位置装有刮粉器，片重调节器装于下冲轨道的刮粉器对应的位置，用以调节下冲经过刮粉器时的高度，以调节模孔的容积，即片重；用上下压轮的上下移动位置调节压缩压力。

b. Multi-station rotary press The schematic structure and working principle of rotary tablet press is depicted in figure 16-4. The basic components of a rotary tablet press consist of a turret, compression rollers, a weight control unit, a hardness control, a feeding device, a swipe blade, a vacuum cleaner and a protective unit. The turret is divided into three portions with the upper and lower turrets holding a number of upper and lower punches, respectively, and several dies mounted in a circle in the middle die table. A set of tooling consists of an upper punch, a lower punch and a die, and each punch is matched top and bottom. As the head of the machine rotates, the punches move up and down as guided by the fixed cam tracks. When passing between the compression rollers, the vertical movement of both upper and lower punch (the upper punch moves downward and lower punch upward) compresses the powder or granular material in the die bore into a tablet. The swipe blade is fixed in the die table, and a weight control unit is installed in the lower cam track corresponding to the position of the swipe blade. The weight control unit is used to lower the lower punch to a required height when it passes by the swipe blade, so as to adjust the capacity of the die cavity, i.e. the tablet weight. The compression force is adjusted by the distance of the vertical motion of upper and lower compression rollers.

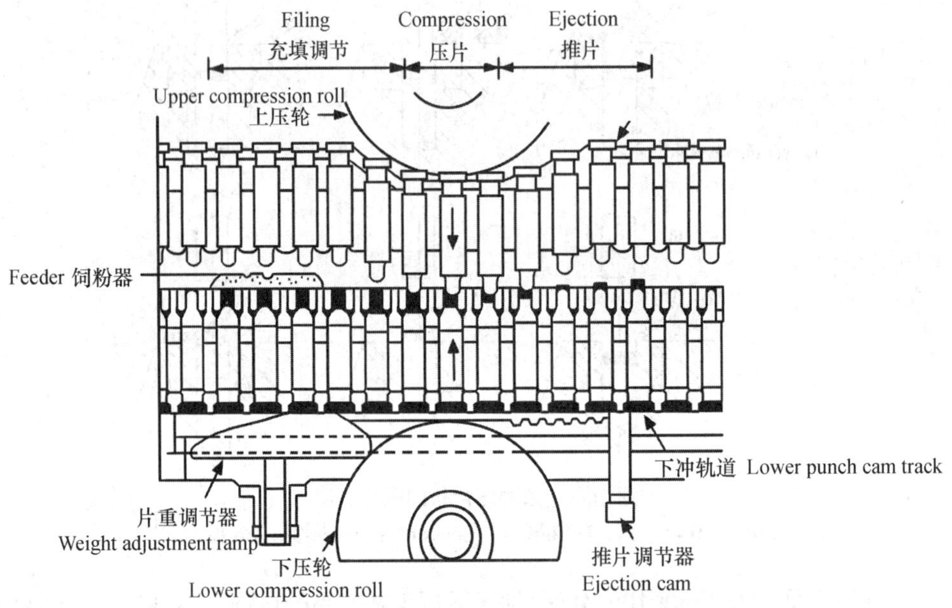

图 16-4 旋转压片机的结构与工作原理

Figure 16-4 The Schematic Structure and Working Principles of A Multi-Station Rotary Press

旋转式多冲压片机的饲料方式合理，片重差异较小，双侧加压，压力分布均匀，生产效率高，是目前生产中广泛使用的压片机。旋转压片机有多种型号，按冲头数分有 16 冲、19 冲、27 冲、33 冲、55 冲、75 冲等，按流程分有单流程和双流程两种。单流程仅有一套上、下压轮，旋转一周每个模孔仅压出一个药片；双流程有两套压轮、饲粉器、刮粉器、片重调节器和压力调节器等，均装于对称位置，中盘转动一周，每副冲压制两个药片。目前产量最大的压片机可达 80 万片/h。

The rotary tablet press is widely used for the manufacture of tablets due to the following advantages:

a reasonable feeding system, small tablet weight variation, the two punches contributing equally to the compaction pressure, resulting in tablets with similar hardness on both sides, and high production efficiency. Many models of rotary tablet press are available. According to the number of stations, there are rotary press with 16, 19, 27, 33, 55 and 75 stations. Also, there are single sided and double-sided rotary press. A single sided rotary press consists of one set of upper and lower compression rollers, and produces single tablet per station for each revolution. A double-sided rotary press consists of a rotating multi station die table equipped with two sets of compression rollers, feeding devices, swipe blades, weight control units, and hardness control units, all installed in the symmetrical position, producing two tablets per station for each revolution. Currently, the maximum output of the rotary press is up to 800,000 per hour.

二、干法制粒压片法
16.3.2 Dry Granulation

干法制粒压片法系指不用润湿剂或液态黏合剂而制成颗粒进行压片的方法。主要适用于热敏性物料、遇水易分解的药物，其特点是方法简单、省工省时。采用干法制粒时，应注意由于高压引起的晶型转变和活性降低等问题。常用的干法制粒压片主要有滚压法和重压法。

Dry granulation is the method of producing granules without any wetting agent or liquid binder prior to tablet manufacture, especially suitable for drugs that are sensitive to heat or moisture. It is a simple and low-cost method. However, when dry granulation is applied, attention should be paid to the problems like polymorphic transformations and decreased activity of active ingredients triggered by high compression pressure. There are two widely used dry granulation methods: slugging and roll compaction.

1. 滚压法　滚压法是将药物和辅料均匀混合后，利用转速相同的两个滚动圆筒之间的缝隙，将药物粉末滚压成板状物，再粉碎成颗粒的方法。

(1) Roll compaction　This process consists of compressing the well mixed powder of drug and excipients between two counter-rotating rolls to produce ribbons that will be subsequently milled into granules.

2. 重压法　重压法是将药物与辅料均匀混合后，利用重型压片机压成直径为 20~25mm 大片，再粉碎成适宜大小的颗粒的方法。

(2) Slugging　is a method that a heavy-duty tablet press is employed to compact the well mixed powder of drug and excipients for the formation of extra-large tablets (slugs), typically 20 to 25 mm in diameter, which are subsequently broken down into granules of appropriate size.

三、粉末直接压片法
16.3.3 Direct Compression

粉末直接压片法系指将药物的粉末与适宜的辅料混合后，不经过制颗粒而直接进行压片的方法。粉末直接压片法的优点是工艺过程较简单，省去制粒、干燥等工序，省时，节能；不加水，不受热，有利于药物的稳定性；片剂崩解后成为药物的原始粒子，比表面积大，有利于药物的溶出。其不足之处是辅料的价格昂贵，生产过程中粉尘较多，片剂的外观较差，且易裂片。

Direct compression is a process by which tablets are compressed directly from powered active drug substance and suitable excipients into a firm compact without employing the process of granulation. The advantages of direct compression include simpler process without involvement of the unit operations of granulation and drying, time and energy saving; better stability for drugs sensitive to moisture and heat; tablet breaking into original powder particles with large specific surface area, facilitating drug dissolution. However, direct compression is limited by its need to use expensive excipients, the problem of more dust generation, and the likelihood to produce tablets with poorer appearance or prone to cracking.

进行粉末直接压片时，药物需要有适当的粒度、结晶形态、可压性及流动性。但大多数药物并不具有以上特点，故在一定程度上限制了粉末直接压片的发展。 目前解决的措施主要有以下两方面。

Therefore, the drug substances must have suitable particle size distribution, crystalline form, compressibility and flowability for direct compression. However, most of the drugs do not have the above characteristics, limiting the development of direct compression to some extent. Currently, there are two ways to solve these problems.

1. 改善压片原料的性能 若粉末流动性差，会造成片重差异大、易裂片等问题，可加入优良的辅料以改善压片原料的性能。可用于粉末直接压片的优良辅料有：微晶纤维素、可压性淀粉、喷雾干燥乳糖、微粉硅胶及磷酸氢钙二水合物等。

(1) Improving the properties of tableting raw materials Insufficient flowability of powder will lead to problems of wide variations in tablet weight and tablet cracking, which could be remedied by the incorporation of excellent excipients to improve the properties of raw materials. Advanced excipients for direct compression include MCC, directly compressible starch, spray-dried lactose, colloidal silicone dioxide, and calcium hydrophosphate dihydrate.

2. 改进压片机械的性能 粉末直接压片时，加料斗内粉末常出现空洞或流动速度不均的现象，以致片重差异较大，一般采用振荡器或电磁振荡器来克服，即利用上冲转动时产生的动能来撞击物料，使粉末均匀流入模孔。此外，还可改进设备，增加预压过程，减慢车速，克服粉末中容存空气较多的问题；也可以安装自动密闭加料设备以克服药粉加入漏斗时飞扬。

(2) Improving the performance of tableting machine When direct compression is employed, flow problems such as ratholing (when the powder empties through a central flow channel, the material at the hopper walls remains stagnant, leaving an empty hole through the material) and erratic flow rate often occur, leading to wide variations in tablet weight. This could be overcome by the use of rotating agitator or electromagnetic oscillator, that is, use the kinetic energy created by the rotation of the upper punch to impact over the falling material, helping in uniform powder flow into the die cavity. In addition, problem of more air entrapment can be overcome by innovation of the tableting machine, incorporation of the pre-compression stage, and reducing the rotation speed. Or an automatic sealed feeding device is equipped to realize dust-proof loading.

四、压片时可能发生的问题与解决办法
16.3.4 Compression Issues: Causes and Remedies

（一）片剂成型机制
(1) Mechanisms of Tablet Formation

片剂的成型是药物的颗粒或粉末在压力作用下产生足够的内聚力以及辅料的黏合作用而紧密结合的结果。为了改善药物的流动性，同时克服压片时成分的分离，常需要将药物制成颗粒后压片。因此颗粒的压制、固结是片剂成型的主要过程。片剂的成型机制及影响因素如下：

The formation of tablet is the result of the closely combination of drug granules or powder driven by the sufficient interior cohesiveness generated under compression pressure or the binding effect of excipients. To improve the flowability of drugs, and meanwhile overcome the separation or segregation of the primary ingredients during compression, the materials usually need to be granulated before tableting. Therefore, the compression and consolidation of granules are the main process of tablet forming. The mechanism and influencing factors of tablet formation are as follows:

1. 机械力的作用 颗粒形态不规则，表面粗糙或因压缩而变形等，使被压缩的粒子间相互嵌合，从而使片剂成型。

① **Effect of mechanical force** Due to the irregular shape and surface roughness of granules or their deformation under compression, the compressed particles fit between each other to form the tablet.

2. 粒子间力的作用 压缩时因颗粒破碎或塑性形变等，使粒子间的距离高度接近而接触面积增大，通过颗粒间范德华力等发挥作用，同时因粒子破碎而产生大量的新界面，有较大的界面自由能，使粒子结合力增强。在压力继续作用下，颗粒黏结，比表面积减少，颗粒产生塑性变形，变形的颗粒则借助于分子间力、静电力等而结合成较坚实的片剂。

② **Effect of the force between particles** Due to the breakage or plastic deformation of granules during compression, the particles are highly approached to each other to increase the contact area, so that the Van der Waals force between particles can exert its effect. Meanwhile, a large number of new interfaces are formed due to particle breakage, generating larger interfacial free energy to enhance the adhesive and cohesive forces between particles. Under the continuing effect of compression pressure, the particles are bonded to each other, resulting in decreased specific surface area and plastic deformation. The deformed particles are combined with each other through intermolecular force and electrostatic force to form a more solid tablet.

3. 组分熔融形成"固体桥" 颗粒压缩时可产生热量，产生热量的大小与压力大小等有关。药物及辅料的熔点低，有利于"固体桥"的形成，使片剂成型。

③ **Formation of "solid bridge" by melting of the components** Heat is generated during the compression of granules, the magnitude of which is positively correlated to the compression force. The low melting point of drugs and excipients is beneficial to the formation of "solid bridge" and the subsequent formation of tablets.

4. 可溶性成分重结晶形成固体桥 压片时颗粒中一般均含有适量水分，水溶性成分溶于这些水中成饱和溶液。压制时，可溶性成分失水重结晶形成固体桥，而有利于颗粒的固结成型。

④ **Formation of "solid bridge" by recrystallization of soluble components** Granules for tableting usually contain a certain amount of water, and the water-soluble components will dissolve in this water to form a saturated solution. During compression, those components loose water and recrystallize to form a solid bridge, which is beneficial to the consolidation of particles and formation of tablets.

5. 片剂的弹性复原 固体颗粒被压缩时，既发生塑性变形，又发生一定程度的弹性变形，因此在压制的片剂内聚集一定的弹性内应力，其方向与压缩力相反。当外力解除后弹性内应力趋向松弛和颗粒恢复原来形状，使体积增大 2%~10%，片剂的这种膨胀现象称为弹性复原。当黏合剂用量不当或黏结力不足时，片剂出片后就可能引起表面一层出现裂痕，所以片剂的弹性复原及压力分布不均匀是裂片的主要原因。

⑤ **The elastic recovery of tablets** When the solid particles are compressed, both plastic and elastic deformation occur to some extent. Therefore, a certain elastic internal stress accumulates in the compressed tablet, whose direction is opposite to the compression force. When the external force is relieved, the elastic internal stress tends to relax and the particles return to their original shape, increasing the volume of tablet by about 2%-10%. This expansion of tablet is called elastic recovery, which may cause tablet capping, if binder with insufficient amount or cohesiveness is applied, after ejection of the tablet. Therefore, the elastic recovery and uneven pressure distribution are the main causes of tablet cracking.

（二）压片时可能发生的问题与解决的办法

(2) Compression Issues: Causes and Remedies

1. 裂片 片剂受到振动或经放置后，从顶部或腰间开裂，分别称为顶裂或腰裂。产生裂片的原因有：①制粒时黏合剂或润湿剂选择不当，或用量不足，或细粉过多，或颗粒过粗过细。②颗粒含油类成分较多，减弱了颗粒间的黏合力；或含纤维性成分过多，富有弹性而引起裂变。③颗粒干燥过度引起裂片。④颗粒中容存的空气来不及逸出而引起裂片。⑤冲模不符合要求，上冲与模圈不吻合，冲头向内卷以及模孔口径改变，均可导致裂片。

① **Capping** The upper (capping) or lower part (lamination) of the tablet separates horizontally either partially away from the main body or completely to form a cap when the tablet is vibrated or during the handling process. Causes for tablet capping include: Improper or insufficient amount of binder or wetting agent for granulation, or the existence of large amount of fines, or too coarse or too fine particles. The existence of large amount of oil components in the particles, weakening the cohesiveness between particles, or too many elastic fibrous components. Excessive drying of granules. The entrapped air in the granules during decompression. Poor finished dies, unmatching of the upper punch with the die hole, upper punch cup edges curling inward, and change of die hole diameter, all leading to tablet capping.

解决裂片的主要措施是选用弹性小、塑性大的辅料；选用适宜制粒方法；选用适宜压片机，调节压片机的压力或减慢车速，整体上提高物料的压缩成形性，降低弹性复原率。

The major solutions of the capping of tablets are given here: application of pharmaceutical excipients with small elasticity and large plasticity; selection of proper granulation method as well as tablet press; adjustment of the compression force and reducing the turret speed; increasing the entire compressibility of the material and reducing the degree of elastic recovery.

2. 松片 片剂硬度不够，稍加触动即散碎的现象称为松片。造成松片的原因主要有：①物料质地的影响：原料中含有较多的挥发油、脂肪油等，或含动物胶质类、动物皮类量较大，缺乏黏性，又有弹性；原料中含矿石类药量较多，黏性差，颗粒质地疏松。解决的措施有更换黏性较强的黏合剂或加大其用量。②含水量的影响：过分干燥的颗粒受压时弹性较大，压成的片剂硬度较差。制粒过程中应控制颗粒含水量。③压缩条件不当：主要是压缩压力不足等，可适当增加压力，减慢车速，增加受压时间。④制剂工艺的影响：制粒时乙醇浓度过高；润滑剂和黏合剂不适；熬制浸膏时温度控制不当造成部分浸膏炭化，使浸膏黏性降低；浸膏粉碎不细，表面积小等。除应根据实际情况予以解决外，稠膏、黏合剂应趁热与粉料混合，并充分混合均匀以增加软材的黏性。

② **Loose tablets** Tablet with insufficient mechanical strength will fracture during handling process. Causes for loose tablets mainly include: Influence of material texture: raw materials containing high amount of volatile oil, fat oil, or animal gelatin, and animal skin, which are elastic and lack of viscosity. Or raw materials containing a lot of mineral drugs, which are of poor viscosity, resulting in granules of loose texture. The remedy is to use binder with stronger cohesiveness or higher amount. The influence of moisture content: too dry granules exhibit a strong elastic deformation during compression, resulting in tablets with insufficient hardness. This can be avoided by controlling the moisture content of

granules during granulation. Improper compression conditions: mainly include insufficient compression force. This can be resolved by increasing appropriately the compression force, reducing the turret speed or prolonging the dwell time. Influence of manufacturing process: mainly include application of ethanol with too high concentration for granulation; incorporation of improper lubricant and binder; decocting the extract under improper temperature, resulting in carbonization of part of the extract and decrease of its viscosity; insufficient pulverization of the extract, resulting in particles with small specific surface area. In addition to remedies specific to actual causes, the thick extract and binder should be mixed thoroughly with powder material while they are hot to increase the cohesiveness of the damp mass.

3. 黏冲 片剂的表面被冲头黏去一薄层或一小部分，造成片面粗糙不平或有凹痕的现象称为黏冲。颗粒湿度大或含有引湿性成分、冲模表面粗糙或刻字太深或润滑剂用量不足或分布不均匀都可能造成黏冲。中药片剂尤其是浸膏片，由于浸膏中含有易引湿成分，要特别注意颗粒的防潮，压片环境保持干燥，或适当增加润滑剂。

③ **Sticking** It occurs when a thin layer or a small portion of the tablet surface attaches or sticks to the faces of the punches, resulting in rough or dented surface of the tablet. Granules of high moisture content or containing hygroscopic ingredients, punches with rough surface or having deeply engraved letters, insufficient amount or uneven distribution of lubricant are all causes of tablet sticking to the punch faces. For traditional Chinese medicinal tablets, especially extract tablets, special attention should be paid to the protection of granules from moisture, the maintenance of a dry manufacturing environment, or incorporation of higher amount of lubricant, due to the highly hygroscopic ingredients contained in the extract.

4. 片重差异超限 片重差异超出规定的范围，即为片重差异超限。产生严重片重差异的主要原因有：①颗粒的流动性差。②颗粒中细粉太多或颗粒大小相差悬殊。③加料斗内的颗粒时多时少。④冲头与冲模吻合性不好。具体解决办法有减小颗粒大小差异、筛去过多细粉、适量增加润滑剂，或停机检查，调整后再压片。

④ **Out-of-limit in tablet weight variation** refers to the tablet weight variation exceeding an acceptable range. Causes of wide variations in tablet weight mainly include: Poor flowability of granules. Large amount of fines in the granules or a wide particle size distribution. Erratic amount of granules in the hopper. Unmatching of the punches with the die hole. Specific resolutions include: narrowing the size distribution of granules, removing excessive fines through sifting, increasing appropriately the amount of lubricant, or checking and adjusting the machine before restart of tableting.

5. 崩解迟缓 片剂崩解时间超过《中国药典》规定的时限，即为崩解迟缓。造成崩解迟缓的原因主要有：①崩解剂的品种、用量或加入方法不当，或干燥不足。②黏合剂黏性太强、用量过多，或疏水性黏合剂用量过大。③颗粒过硬或压力过大。④含胶、糖或浸膏的片剂引湿后，崩解时间可能会延长。应根据不同情况加以解决，如选择合适的崩解剂、选用黏性小的黏合剂或降低其用量，减小压片压力或注意防潮等。

⑤ **Delayed disintegration** The tablet disintegrates exceeding the required time limits of the current edition of *Chinese Pharmacopeia* is called delayed disintegration. Causes of delayed disintegration mainly include: Improper type, amount or addition mode of disintegrant is selected, or insufficient drying. Binders with strong cohesiveness or large amount are used, or incorporation of more hydrophobic binders. Very hard granules or too high compression force are employed for tablet preparation. Moisture absorption of tablet containing gelatin, sugar or extract. Different resolutions should be applied according to different causes, such as selection of proper disintegrants, use of binders of smaller cohesiveness or amount, decrease of compression force, or protection against moisture.

6. 变色与斑点 产生的原因及解决方法：①中药浸膏制成的颗粒硬度过大，或润湿剂未经过筛混匀，可能会发生花斑现象，需返工处理。所用润滑剂需经研细过筛，与颗粒充分混匀即可改善；②压片时，上冲涂抹的润滑油过多，滴入颗粒中产生油点。可在上冲头上装橡皮圈以防油垢滴入颗粒中，并应经常擦拭冲头和橡皮圈。

⑥ **Mottling** Causes and remedies are: Very hard granules prepared from traditional Chinese medicinal extract, or lubricant that is not sieved and mixed well with other tableting materials. In that case, the tablets need to be reprocessed. A mottled appearance could be remedied by grinding the lubricant to fines, sieving, and then mixing it thoroughly with granules. The oil spots may stem from the oily lubricant which is applied on the upper punch with an excessive amount and drops into the granules. A rubber band can be installed on the upper punch to prevent oil dirt from dripping into the particles, and the punches and rubber band should be wiped frequently.

7. 引湿受潮 中药片剂（尤其是浸膏片）中含有多种容易引湿的成分如糖类、树胶、蛋白质、鞣质、无机盐等。在制备过程及压成片剂后，如果包装不严，容易引湿受潮和黏结，甚至霉变。解决方法：①在干浸膏中加入适量辅料，如磷酸氢钙、氢氧化铝凝胶粉、淀粉、糊精、活性炭等；②加入部分中药细粉，用量通常为原药总量的 10%~20%；③优化提取、分离、纯化工艺，除去部分水性杂质；④将 5%~15% 的玉米朊乙醇溶液、聚乙烯醇溶液喷雾或混匀于浸膏颗粒中，待颗粒干燥后进行压片；⑤对片剂包衣，可减少片剂的引湿性；⑥改善包装材料，加强包装材料的防潮性。

⑦ **Hygroscopicity and moisture absorption** Traditional Chinese medicinal tablets (especially extract tablets) contain a variety of hygroscopic components, such as sugar, gum, protein, tannin and inorganic salt. Tablets of this kind are easy to absorb moisture and agglomerate, or even become mildewy due to improper packaging of in-process or finished products. It could be remedied by Adding a quantity of excipients to the dry extract, such as calcium hydrogen phosphate, gel powder of aluminium hydroxide, starch, dextrin and activated carbon. Adding some fine powder of traditional Chinese medicine, usually at a concentration range between 10% and 20% of the total raw materials. Optimizing the extraction, separation and purification processes to remove some water-soluble impurities. Spraying 5%-10% alcoholic solution of zein or PVA solution over or mixing it with the granules of extract, and then performing tablet compression after drying of the granules. Coating the tablet to reduce its hygroscopicity. Enhancing the water-proof properties of the packaging materials.

第四节　片剂的包衣

16.4　Tablets Coating

PPT

片剂包衣是指在片剂表面包裹上适宜材料的衣层的操作。被包的片剂称“片芯”，包衣的材料称“衣料”，包成的片剂称“包衣片”。

Tablet coating refers to the operation of coating a suitable material on the tablet surface. The coated tablet is called “tablet core”, the coating material is called “cloth material”, and the coated tablet is called “coating tablet”.

一、片剂包衣的目的、种类与要求
16.4.1 Purpose, Types and Requirements of Tablet Coating

（一）片剂包衣的目的
(1) Purpose of Tablet Coating

1. 隔绝空气，避光，防潮，提高药物的稳定性。

① Isolate the air, protect from light and moisture, and improve the stability of the drug.

2. 掩盖药物的不良气味，增加患者的顺应性。

② Mask the bad smell of the drug and increase patient compliance.

3. 包肠溶衣，避免药物对胃的刺激，防止胃酸或胃酶对药物的破坏。

③ Enteric coating could avoid the irritation of the stomach by the drug and prevent the destruction of the drug by gastric acid or enzymes.

4. 包缓释或控释衣；改变药物释放速度，减少服药次数，降低不良反应。

④ Coating slow-release or controlled-release clothing can change the drug release rate, reduce the times of taking medications, and reduce adverse reactions.

5. 隔离有配伍禁忌的成分，避免相互作用，有助复方配伍。

⑤ Isolate ingredients that are incompatible with each other and avoid interactions, which helps compound compatibility.

6. 改善外观，使片剂美观，且便于识别。

⑥ Improve appearance, make tablets beautiful and easy to identify.

（二）包衣片的种类和质量要求
(2) Types and Quality Requirements of Coated Tablets

1. 包衣片的种类糖衣片、（半）薄膜衣片、肠溶衣片以及缓释衣片、控释衣片。

① The types of coated tablets include sugar-coated tablets, (semi) film-coated tablets, enteric-coated tablets, and sustained-release coated tablets, controlled-release coated tablets.

2. 片芯的质量要求除符合一般片剂质量要求外，应为片面呈弧形而棱角小的双凸片或拱形片，以利包衣完整严密；硬度较大、脆性较小，且应干燥，保证包衣过程反复滚动时不破碎。包衣前应筛去片粉及碎片。

② The quality requirements for tablet cores, in addition to meeting the general tablet quality requirements, should be arcuate or arched tablets with small edges and corners to facilitate complete and tight coating. It should be greater hardness and less brittleness, and be dry to ensure that the coating process does not break when repeatedly rolled. Sieve powder and debris before coating.

3. 衣层的质量要求应均匀牢固；与片芯成分不起作用；崩解度符合规定；在有效期限内保持光亮美观，颜色一致，无裂片、脱壳现象，不影响药物的溶出和吸收。

③ The quality requirements of the coating layer should be uniform and firm. It has no effect on the core composition of the tablet. The degree of disintegration meets the requirements. It remains bright and beautiful during the expiration date, and has the same color, without cracks and shelling, and does not affect the dissolution and absorb.

二、片剂包衣的方法与设备
16.4.2 Methods and Equipments for Tablet Coating

（一）片剂包衣的方法
(1) Tablet Coating Method

1. 滚转包衣法 系将筛去浮粉的片芯置于包衣锅中，在锅不断转动的条件下，逐渐包裹上各种适宜包衣材料的包衣方法，为片剂包衣最常用的方法。可用于包糖衣、薄膜衣和肠溶衣等。

① **Rolling coating method** It is the most commonly used method for tablet coating by placing the center of the sieve to remove the floating powder in the coating pot and gradually wrapping various suitable coating materials under the condition of continuous rotation of the pot. It can be used for sugar coating, film coating and enteric coating.

2. 流化包衣法（悬浮包衣法） 系依靠气流的作用，使片剂悬浮于包衣室中且上下翻动，同时均匀喷入包衣材料溶液，因溶剂迅即挥发而包上衣料的方法。本法包衣时间短、速度快，适用于小片和颗粒包衣，尤适用于包薄膜衣。

② **Fluid coating method (suspension coating method)** Relying on the action of airflow, the tablets are suspended in the coating room and turned upside down, and the coating material solution is evenly sprayed into the coating material. This method has short coating time and fast speed, and is suitable for small tablets and granule coating, especially for film coating.

3. 压制包衣法（干压包衣法） 系利用干压包衣机将包衣材料制成的干颗粒压在片芯外层的包衣方法。该法可避免水分、高温对药物的不良影响，适用于包糖衣、肠溶衣或药物衣，可用于长效多层片的制备，或有配伍禁忌药物的包衣。但对机械精密度要求高，且易出现偏心等质量问题。

③ **Compression coating method (dry pressing coating method)** The coating method is to press the dry particles made of coating material into the outer layer of the core by using the dry pressing machine. This method can avoid the adverse effects of water and high temperature on drugs. It is suitable for sugar-coating, enteric coating or drug coating. It can be used for the preparation of long-acting multi-layer tablets or coating with contraindicated drugs. However, the requirements for mechanical precision are high, and prone to eccentricity and other quality problems.

（二）片剂包衣设备
(2) Tablet Coating Equipment

1. 包衣锅 有倾斜包衣锅、埋管包衣锅（在包衣锅内部装上特殊档板或在锅内采用埋管装置的改进型包衣机）及高效水平包衣锅等。由包衣锅、加热装置（起加速挥散包衣溶剂的作用）、鼓风设备（起调节温度和吹去多余细粉的作用）、除尘设备（排除包衣时的粉尘及湿热空气）和动力部分等组成。全自动包衣机，则由电脑程序控制包衣全过程。

① **Coating pans** There are inclined coating pot, buried pipe coating pot (in the interior of the coating pot with a special baffle plate or an improved coating machine with buried pipe device) and efficient level coating pot. It consists by the coating pot, heating device (to accelerate the role of dispersing coating solvent), blowing equipment (to adjust the temperature and blow away the role of excess fine powder), dust removal equipment (to remove the dust and hot and humid air) and power parts. Automatic coating machine controls the whole process of coating by the computer program.

2. 悬浮包衣机 由包衣室、喷嘴、衣料盛装器、加热滤过器及鼓风设备等组成。有流化型、喷流型和流化转动型等不同类型装置。

② **Suspension coating machine** It is composed of coating room, nozzle, material holder, heating filter and blast equipment. There are fluidized type, jet type and fluidized rotary type and other different types of devices.

3. 干压包衣机 一般采用两台压片机联合起来实施压制包衣，两台压片机以特制的传动器连接配套使用。一台压片机专门用于压制片芯，然后由传动器将压成的片芯输送至包衣转台的模孔中（此模孔内已填入包衣材料作为底层），随着转台的转动，片芯的上面又被加入大约等量的包衣材料，然后加压，使片芯压入包衣材料中间而形成压制包衣片。

③ Dry compression coating machine Generally, use two tablet presses to implement compression coating. The two tablet presses are connected and matched with a special drive. One tablet press is used to press the tablet core, and then driven by the drive. The device sends the pressed tablet core to the die hole of the coating turntable (the die hole has been filled with the coating material as the bottom layer). As the turntable rotates, about the same amount of coating material is added to the top of the tablet core, and then pressurizing the tablet core into the middle of the coating material to form a compressed coated tablet.

三、片剂包衣物料与工序
16.4.3 Tablet Coating Materials and Coating Operations

（一）糖衣物料及其包衣操作
(1) Sugar Coating Materials and Coating Operations

糖衣片为应用最早也是中药包衣片目前仍广泛应用的片剂主要类型之一。糖衣片包衣物料以蔗糖、滑石粉为主，价廉、易得、无毒，但辅料用量较多，包衣时间较长，近年来随着高分子分散体乳胶包衣技术的发展，出现了薄膜包衣取代糖包衣的趋势。

Sugar-coated tablets are one of the main types of tablets that are the earliest and also widely used in traditional Chinese medicine coating tablets. The coating materials of sugar-coated tablets are mainly sucrose and talc, which are cheap, readily available, and non-toxic, but the amount of auxiliary materials is relatively large. The coating time is relatively long. In recent years, with the development of polymer dispersion latex coating technology, it has been a trend of film coating instead of sugar coating.

1. 糖衣物料

① Sugar-coated material

（1）糖浆 采用含转化糖较少的干燥粒状蔗糖制成，浓度为 65%~75%（g/g），用于粉衣层与糖衣层。高浓度有利于包衣迅速干燥析晶；保温使用有利于均匀分布。应新鲜配制，久贮因转化糖含量增高，衣层不易干燥。

a. Syrup The syrup is made of dry granular sucrose with less invert sugar, with a concentration of 65% to 75% (g / g), which is used for the powder coating layer and the sugar coating layer. The high concentration is beneficial for the coating to quickly dry and crystallize. The use of heat preservation is favorable for uniform distribution. It should be freshly prepared, and the coating layer is not easy to dry due to the increased invert sugar content in long-term storage.

（2）有色糖浆 为含可溶性食用色素的糖浆，用于有色糖衣层。常用色素有苋菜红、柠檬黄、胭脂红、亮蓝等，用量一般为 0.03% 左右，可单独或配合应用。一般先配成浓色糖浆，用时以糖浆稀释至所需浓度。二氧化钛可作避光剂。

b. Colored syrup It is a syrup containing soluble food coloring, used for colored sugar coatings. Commonly used pigments are garden red, lemon yellow, carmine, bright blue, etc.. The dosage is generally about 0.03%, which can be used alone or in combination. In general, prepare a thick-colored

syrup and dilute it to the required concentration with syrup. Titanium dioxide can be used as a light-shielding agent.

（3）胶浆　常用作黏结剂，可增加衣层黏性、塑性和牢固性，并对片芯起保护作用。常用品种有 10%~15% 明胶浆、35% 阿拉伯胶浆、4% 白及胶浆或一定浓度的聚乙烯醇（PVA）、聚维酮（PVP）、苯二甲酸醋酸纤维素（CAP）溶液等。多用于包隔离层。

c. Glue　It is often used as a bonding agent, which can increase the viscosity, plasticity and firmness of the coating, and protect the core. The commonly used varieties are 10%-15% gelatin glue, 35% arabic glue, 4% rhizoma bletillae glue or a certain concentration of polyvinyl alcohol (PVA), povidone (PVP), cellulose acetate phthalate (CAP) solution, etc.. It is mostly used for coating insulation layer.

（4）滑石粉　包衣应选用白色滑石粉细粉，用前过 100 目筛。用于包粉衣层（粉底层）。为了增白和对油类的吸收，可在滑石粉中加入 10%~20% 碳酸钙（或碳酸镁）（酸性药物不能用）或适量淀粉。

d. The talc powder　Coating should be made of white talc powder and passed through a 100 mesh sieve before using. It is used to coat the powder coating layer (bottom layer). In order to whiten and absorb oils, calcium carbonate (or magnesium carbonate) can be added to talc powder (acid drugs cannot be used) or an appropriate amount of starch. The concentration ranges of calcium carbonate (or magnesium carbonate) are between 10% and 20%.

（5）川蜡（虫蜡）　作为糖衣片打光剂，用前应精制处理。即以 80~100℃加热使熔化后过 100 目筛，去除悬浮杂质，并兑加 2% 硅油混匀，冷却后制成 80 目细粉备用。

e. Sichuan wax (insect wax)　As a sugar-coated tablet polishing agent, it should be refined before using. Heat it at 80~100℃ to melt it and then through a 100 mesh sieve, remove suspended impurities, and mix with 2% silicone oil. After cooling, make 80 mesh fine powder for future use.

2. 包糖衣工序　用包衣机包糖衣的工序，按先后依次为：隔离层→粉衣层→糖衣层→有色糖衣层→打光。根据不同品种需要，有的工序可以省略。

② **Sugar coating process**　The process of sugar coating with coating machine is as follows: isolation layer → powder coating layer → sugar coating layer → colored coating layer → polishing. According to the needs of different varieties, some processes can be omitted.

（1）隔离层　系指包在片芯外起隔离作用的胶状物衣层。凡含引湿性、易溶性或酸性药物的片剂，包隔离层将片芯与糖衣隔离，可防止药物吸潮变质或防止糖衣被破坏。

a. Isolation layer　Refers to a gelatinous coating layer that is wrapped around the core of the tablet and acts as a barrier. For tablets containing hygroscopic, soluble or acidic drugs, the barrier layer isolates the tablet core from the sugar coating to prevent drug from absorbing moisture and deterioration or prevent the sugar coating from being damaged.

操作时，将片芯置包衣锅中滚动，加入胶浆或胶糖浆，使之均匀黏附于片芯上。为防止片芯相互粘连或黏附于锅壁可加少量滑石粉。吹热风（30~50℃）使衣层充分干燥。一般包 4~5 层。酸性药物的片剂从第一层即应包隔离层，如只为防潮或增加片剂硬度而包隔离层，可先包 4~5 层粉衣层后再包隔离层。

During operation, roll the tablet core in a coating pan, add glue or gum syrup to make it adhere to the tablet core evenly. To prevent the tablet cores from sticking to each other or sticking to the pot wall, a small amount of talcum powder can be added. Blow hot air (30-50℃) to fully dry the coating layer. Generally, four or five layers are covered. The tablets of the acidic drug should be covered with an isolation layer from the first layer. If the isolation layer is only used to prevent moisture or increase the

hardness of the tablet, it can be coated 4-5 layers of powder coating, then wrapped the isolation layer.

（2）粉衣层（粉底层）　包粉衣层的目的在于消除片芯原有棱角，为包好糖衣层打基础。包衣物料为糖浆与滑石粉。无需包隔离层的片剂可直接包粉衣层。

b. Powder coating layer (powder layer)　The purpose of the powder coating layer is to eliminate the original edges and corners of the tablet core and to lay the foundation for the sugar coating layer. The coating material include syrup and the talc powder. The tablets without the isolation layer can be directly wrapped powder coating layer.

包粉衣层，操作时药片在包衣锅中滚转，加入适量温热糖浆使表面均匀润湿后，加入适量滑石粉，使之均匀黏着在片剂表面，继续滚转加热并吹风干燥。重复操作，至片芯的核角全部消失，使圆整、平滑为止。一般包 15~18 层可达到要求。

The powder coating layer is rolled in a coating pan during operation. After adding an appropriate amount of warm syrup to make the surface evenly wet, a suitable amount of talcum powder is applied to make it evenly adhere to the tablet surface. Continue to roll and heat and blow dry. Repeat the operation until all the core angles of the tablet core disappear, so that it is round and smooth. Generally, layers between 15 and 18 can meet the requirements.

采用混浆包衣新工艺，可缩短工时，减少粉尘飞扬，使衣层牢固。操作时将片芯投入包衣锅内滚动，吹热风使温度达 40~45℃，加入一定量的混合浆（由单糖浆、滑石粉、胶浆等制成的混悬液，根据需要可加入适量着色剂），使均匀吸附于药片表面，吹热风使充分干燥后再包第二层。若操作不当，易致片面不均匀不平滑。

The new technology of coating with mixed slurry can shorten working hours, reduce dust flying and make the coating firm. During operation, put the tablet core into the coating pot to roll, blow hot air to make the temperature reach 40-45℃, add a certain amount of mixed slurry (suspension made of single syrup, talc, colloidal slurry, etc., according to the need to add an appropriate amount of colorant), make uniform adsorption on the surface of the tablet, blow hot air to make full drying and then wrap the second layer. If the operation is improper, it is easy to cause uneven and not smooth surface.

（3）糖衣层　是由糖浆在片面缓缓干燥形成的蔗糖结晶体联结而成的薄膜层。其目的是增加衣层的牢固性和甜味，使片面坚实、平滑。包衣材料只用糖浆而不用滑石粉，操作与包粉衣层相似。应注意每次加入糖浆后，待片面略干后再加热吹风（约 40℃）。一般包 10~15 层。

c. The sugar coating layer　It is a thin film layer of sucrose crystals formed by the syrup drying slowly on the surface. It could increase the firmness and sweetness of the coating layer and make the surface firm and smooth. The coating material is only syrup and no talcum powder is used. The operation is similar to the powder coating layer. It should be noted that after the syrup is added each time, the tablet surface is slightly dried and then heating and blowing (about 40℃). Generally, the layers are between 10 and 15.

（4）有色糖衣层（亦称色衣或色层）　包衣物料为有色糖浆。其目的是增加美观，便于区别不同品种。光敏性药物的片剂包深色糖衣层具有保护作用，含较多挥发油的片剂或片芯颜色较深的片剂也应包深色衣。

d. Colored sugar-coating layer (also known as colored coat or color layer)　The coating material is colored syrup. The purpose is to increase the beauty and facilitate the differentiation of different varieties. Photosensitive drugs with the dark sugar-coated layer has a protective effect. Tablets with more volatile oils or tablets with darker cores should also be coated in dark-colored clothes.

包有色糖衣层，要配制不同浓度的有色热糖浆。操作与包糖衣层相似，应先用浅色糖浆，并

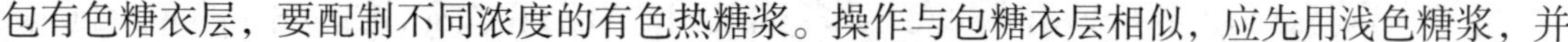

由浅渐深，有利色泽均匀。有色糖衣层一般要包 8~15 层。

The colored sugar-coated layer should be prepared with different concentrations of colored hot syrup. The operation is similar to the sugar-coated layer, and the light-colored syrup should be used first, and it should be gradually darkened to form uniform color. The colored sugar-coated layer should generally be covered with 8-15 layers.

（5）打光　是在包衣片表面擦上一薄层虫蜡的操作。其目的是使片衣表面光亮美观，且有防潮作用。打光时，片剂含水量应适中。多采用“闷锅打光”，即在加完最后一次有色糖浆接近干燥时，锅体停止转动，锅口加盖并定时转动数，使剩余水分慢慢散去而析出微小结晶。转动锅体，同时撒入 2/3 量所需蜡粉，转动摩擦至有光泽时，再加入剩余蜡粉，继续转动锅体直至片面极为光亮。将片子移入石灰干燥橱或硅胶干燥器内，吸湿干燥 10 小时左右，即可包装。蜡粉的用量一般为每 1 万片以不超过 3~5g 为宜。

e. Polishing　It is the operation of rubbing a thin layer of insect wax on the surface of the coated tablet. The purpose is to make the surface of the tablet bright and beautiful, and have moisture-proof effect. When polishing, the moisture content of the tablet should be moderate. “Stuff pot polishing” is often used. When the last colored syrup is nearly dry, the pot body stops rotating, the pot mouth is capped and the number of rotations is made regularly, so that the remaining moisture is slowly dispersed and tiny crystals are precipitated. Rotate the pot body and sprinkle 2/3 of the required wax powder at the same time. Rotating and rubbing until it is shiny and then adding the remaining wax powder, and continue to rotate the pot until the surface is extremely bright. Move the tablets into a lime drying cabinet or a silica gel dryer, and absorb and dry for about 10hours. It can be packed. The amount of wax powder is generally not more than 3-5g per 10,000 tablets.

3. 包糖衣操作要点　①必须层层充分干燥。②浆粉用量适当。如包粉衣层时，糖浆和滑石粉的用量，开始时逐层增加，片芯原有棱角基本包圆滑后，糖浆量相对稳定，滑石粉量逐层减少。③干燥温度符合各工序要求。如包粉衣层温度一般控制在 35~55℃，且应逐渐升高，片芯基本包平时温度升至最高，以后开始下降。而包糖衣层，锅温一般控制在 40℃左右，以免糖浆中水分蒸发过快使片面粗糙；且每次加入糖浆后，应待片面略干后再吹风（约 35℃）至干。包有色糖衣层，温度应逐渐下降至室温，以免温度过高水分蒸发过快，致片面粗糙，产生花斑且不易打光。④浆、粉加入时间掌握得当。如包粉衣层前 3 层时，糖浆加入拌匀后，滑石粉应立即加入搅匀，以免水分渗入片芯，而后续层数滑石粉的加入时间可适当推迟。

③ The main points of sugar coating operation　Ⅰ. The layers must be fully dried. Ⅱ. The amount of syrup powder is appropriate. For example, when coating the powder coating layer, the amount of syrup and talc powder is increased layer by layer at the beginning. After the original edges and corners of the tablet core are basically rounded, the amount of syrup is relatively stable, and the amount of talcum powder is reduced layer by layer. Ⅲ. The drying temperature meets the requirements of each process. For example, the temperature of the powder coating layer is generally controlled at 35-55℃, and it should be gradually increased. The temperature rises to the highest when the tablet core is basically flat and then begins to drop. For sugar coating layer, the temperature is generally controlled at about 40℃, so as to prevent the water in the syrup from evaporating too quickly to make the surface rough. And after adding the syrup each time, the surface should be slightly dry before blowing (about 35℃) to dry. The temperature should be gradually lowered to room temperature when coating colored sugar-coating layer. The moisture will evaporate too quickly when the temperature is too high, which will cause the surface to be rough, cause variegated spots and not easy to polish. Ⅳ. The time for adding the pulp and powder is

properly controlled. For example, for the first 3 layers of powder coating, after the syrup is added, the talc powder should be added and stirred immediately to prevent moisture from penetrating into the tablet core, and the time for adding the subsequent layers of talc can be appropriately delayed.

4. 包糖衣过程中可能发生的问题与处理办法

④ Problems and treatments that may occur during the sugar coating process

（1）色泽不匀或花斑 原因在于有色糖浆用量过少或未混匀；包衣时干燥温度过高，糖晶析出过快致片面粗糙不平；衣层未干即打光；中药片受潮变色。处理方法："加厚衣层"或"加深颜色"。操作时注意控制温度，多搅拌，勤加少上。必要时先用适当溶剂洗除部分或全部片衣，干燥后重新包衣。

a. The color unevenness or variegation The reason is that the amount of colored syrup is too little or not mixed well. When coating, the drying temperature is too high and the sugar crystal precipitates out too fast, resulting in tablet surface roughness. Polishing before drying. Chinese medicine tablets discolor with moisture. The solution are "thicken" or "darken". When operating, pay attention to controlling the temperature, stir more, add less frequently. If necessary, wash off some or all of the clothes with proper solvent, and then recoat after drying.

（2）脱壳 原因在于片芯本身不干；包衣时未及时充分干燥，水分进入片芯；衣层与片芯膨胀系数不同。处理方法：选用符合干燥要求的片芯；包衣时严格控制胶浆、糖浆用量以及滑石粉加入速度；注意层层干燥及干燥温度和程度；发现轻微脱壳，应洗除衣层重新包衣。

b. Decladding The reason for decladding is that the tablet core itself is not dry. The coating core is not fully dried in time, and moisture enters the core of the tablet. The coating layer and the tablet core have different expansion coefficients. The treatment method is to select tablet cores that meet the requirements for drying. When coating, strictly control the amount of glue, syrup and the speed of talcum powder adding. Pay attention to the layer drying and drying temperature and degree. If find that the shells are slightly hulled, and the layers should be washed and recoated.

（3）片面裂纹 原因在于糖浆与滑石粉的用量不当，尤其是粉衣层过渡到糖衣层过程中滑石粉用量减得太快；温度太高干燥过快，析出粗糖晶使片面留有裂缝；酸性药物与滑石粉中的碳酸盐反应生成二氧化碳或糖衣片过分干燥。处理方法：包衣时控制糖浆与滑石粉用量、干燥温度与干燥程度，使用不含碳酸盐的滑石粉，并注意贮藏温度。

c. Partial crack The reason is that the dosage of syrup and talc powder is improper, especially the dosage of talc powder is reduced too fast from the powder coating layer to the sugar coating layer. The temperature is too high and the drying is too fast, so the precipitation of crude sugar crystals left partial cracks. The acid reacts with the carbonates in talc to form carbon dioxide or sugar coated tablets that are excessively dried. The treatments include when coating, control syrup and talc dosage, drying temperature and drying degree, use talc powder with carbonate-free, and pay attention to the storage temperature.

（4）露边和高低不平 原因在于包衣物料用量不当，温度过高或吹风过早；片芯形状不好，边缘太厚；包衣锅角度太小，片子在锅内下降速度太快，碰撞滚动使棱角部分糖浆、滑石粉分布少。处理方法：调整用量，糖浆以均匀润湿片面为度，粉料以能在片面均匀黏附一层为宜；在片剂表面不见水分时再吹风，以免干燥过快，甚至产生皱皮现象；调整衣锅至最佳角度；露边不严重继续包数层粉衣层，以包严为止。

d. Exposed and uneven The reason is that the coating material dosage is improper. The temperature is too high or the blowing is too early. The shape of tablet core is not good and the edge is too thick. The

angle of the coating pan is too small, and the tablet is falling too quickly in the pan. Collision and rolling make the distribution of syrup and talcum powder at the corners less. The treatment method is to adjust the amount, the syrup should be uniformly wetted to the surface, and the powder should be able to adhere to the layer evenly on the surface. Blow again when no water appears on the tablet surface, so as not to dry too fast or even wrinkle. Adjust the pan to the best angle. Continue to cover several layers of powder coating if the exposed is not serious, until it is tight.

（5）糖浆不沾锅　原因在于锅壁上蜡未除尽；操作时电炉使用过早；包衣锅安装角度太小。处理办法：洗净锅壁蜡粉；采用吹热风、电炉低温等方法，使片子和锅壁均匀升温；适当调试包衣锅角度。

e. The syrup will not stick to the pan　The reason is that the wax on the wall is not removed. Electric furnace is used too early in operation. Installation angle of coating pot is too small. The solution is to wash the pot wall. By means of blowing hot air and low temperature of electric furnace, the plate and the wall of the pot are heated evenly. Adjust the angle of coating pot properly.

（6）打不光擦不亮　原因在于片面糖晶大而粗糙；打光的片剂过干或太湿；蜡粉受潮、用量过多。处理方法：控制好包衣条件，调整衣片干湿度和蜡粉用量。

f. Polishing problem　The reason is that the sugar crystal of tablet surface is large and rough. Polishing tablets that are too dry or too wet. The wax powder is affected with moisture and overdosage. The solution is to control the coating condition, adjust the drying humidity and amount of wax powder.

（二）薄膜衣物料及其包衣操作

(2) Film Coating Materials and Coating Operations

薄膜衣系指在片芯外包上以高分子材料为主的薄层衣膜。与糖衣相比，薄膜衣具有衣层薄增重少（仅增重 2%~4%）、生产周期短、效率高、对片剂崩解影响小等优点，但也存在不能完全掩盖片芯原有色泽及有机溶剂残留等缺点。如片芯色深可先包粉衣层掩盖，待其棱角消失、色泽均匀后再包薄膜衣，称为包“半薄膜衣”。目前多采用不溶性聚合物的水分散体作为包衣材料，已逐步取代了有机溶剂薄膜包衣。

Film coating refers to a thin layer coating film mainly composed of polymer materials on the core of the film. Compared with sugar coating, film coating has the advantages of a thin coating layer with less weight increase (only 2% to 4% weight increase), short production cycle, high efficiency and little impact on tablet disintegration, but it also has the disadvantages that it cannot completely cover the original color and core of the tablet and the residual organic solvents. If the color of tablet core is deep, the coating can be covered by the powder layer first, and then the edges and corners disappear, the color is uniform, and then the film coating, known as the “semi-film coating”. At present, aqueous dispersions of insoluble polymers are mostly used as coating materials, which have gradually replaced organic solvent film coating.

1. 薄膜衣物料　薄膜衣物料主要由高分子材料及增塑剂、增光剂、着色剂等附加材料组成。高分子包衣材料为成膜材料，按衣层的作用可分为普通型、缓释型和肠溶型。应具有可塑性，能形成牢固的薄膜。

① **Film-coating materials**　Film-coating materials are mainly composed of polymer materials and additional materials such as plasticizers, brighteners, colorants, etc. Polymer coating materials are film-forming materials, which can be divided into ordinary type, slow-release type and enteric type according to the role of the coating layer. It should be plastic and can form a firm film.

（1）成膜材料　普通型薄膜包衣材料主要在于避免或降低片芯吸湿和防止粉尘污染等，缓释型薄膜包衣材料能调控释药速度，肠溶型薄膜包衣材料有耐酸性，仅在肠液中溶解。除成膜性

外，高分子成膜材料应能溶解或均匀分散于乙醇、丙酮等有机溶剂中，易于包衣操作；无毒、无不良气味；对光、热、湿性质稳定；在消化道中能迅速溶解或崩解等。为满足包衣要求，两种以上薄膜衣料可配合应用。成膜性、溶解性和稳定性与其分子结构、相对分子质量等有关。常用品种多属于纤维素类及丙烯酸树 脂类。

a. Film-forming materials The common film coating materials are mainly used to avoid or reduce the moisture absorption of the core and prevent dust pollution. Slow-release film coating materials can regulate the drug release rate, and enteric film coating materials have the ability of acid resistance and only soluble in intestinal fluid. In addition to film-forming properties, high-molecular film-forming materials should be able to dissolve or evenly disperse in organic solvents such as ethanol and acetone, and be easy to coat, and non-toxic, no bad odor, stable to light, heat and humidity in nature. It can quickly dissolve or disintegrate in the digestive tract. In order to meet the coating requirements, more than two types of film coatings can be used in conjunction. Film-forming, solubility and stability are related to its molecular structure, relative molecular mass, etc. Common varieties mostly belong to cellulose and acrylic resins.

①羟丙基甲基纤维素（HPMC） 应用广泛的薄膜包衣材料，成膜性优良，膜坚韧透明，不易粘连与破碎，对片剂崩解度影响小。本品有多种黏度等级，浓度在 2%~10% 不等。低黏度级高浓度作水性薄膜包衣溶液，高黏度级用有机溶剂溶液。欧巴代（Opachy）即为含有 HPMC 的包衣材料，有胃溶、肠溶、中药防潮及抛光用等不同类型。

Hydroxypropyl methylcellulose (HPMC) It is widely used as a film coating material. It has excellent film-forming properties, and the film is tough and transparent, is not easy to stick and break, and has a small effect on tablet disintegration. This product has a variety of viscosity grades. The concentration ranges from 2% to 10%. Low-viscosity grades and high-concentrations are used as aqueous film coating solutions, and high-viscosity grades are used as organic solvent solutions. Opachy is the coating material containing HPMC, there are different types including stomach solution, enteric solution, Chinese medicine moisture-proof and polishing.

②羟丙基纤维素（HPC） 可溶于胃肠液中；黏性较大，多与其他薄膜衣料混合使用。常用浓度为 5% 乙醇溶液。羟丙甲纤维素酞酸酯（HPMCP）、乙基纤维素（EC）等也可选作肠溶薄膜衣物料。

Hydroxypropyl cellulose (HPC) It is soluble in gastric and intestinal fluid, and greater viscosity. It is often mixed used along with other film coating materials. The usual concentration is 5% ethanol solution. Hydroxypropyl cellulose alanine ester (HPMCP), ethyl cellulose (EC) can also be selected as enteric film clothing materials.

③Ⅳ号丙烯酸树脂国产胃溶型薄膜衣材料 其成膜性、防水性优异；无需加增塑剂，不易粘连。与适量玉米朊合用可提高抗湿性，与羟丙基甲基纤维素合用可改进外观并降低成本。商品名为“Eud- ragit”的薄膜衣材料有胃溶型、肠溶型、不溶型等多种型号，其中 Eudragit E 属于胃溶型薄膜衣材料。

No. Ⅳ acrylic resin The domestically produced gastric-soluble film-coating material of No. Ⅳ acrylic resin has excellent film-forming properties and water resistance. There is no plasticizer needed, and it is not easy to stick together. It can improve moisture resistance when used with a suitable amount of corn, and It can improve the appearance and reduce the cost using with HPMC. The film coating material with the trade name “Eudragit” has many types such as stomach-soluble, enteric-soluble, and insoluble, among which Eudragit E is a gas-soluble film-coating material.

④苯乙烯-乙烯共聚物　为良好的薄膜衣料，成膜性与防潮性好，衣膜高温时不黏，低温时不裂。此膜不溶于水，但在胃液中迅速溶解。尤其适用于引湿性强的中药片。

Styrene-ethylene peyanyan copolymer　Its film formation and moisture-proof property are good. The film is not sticky at high temperature and not crack at low temperature. This film is insoluble in water, but rapidly dissolves in gastric juice. It is especially suitable for Chinese medicine tablets with strong moisture-inducing properties.

其他如70%乙醇配成的5%聚维酮溶液等也可选作薄膜包衣材料。

Others such as 5% povidone solution made up of 70% ethanol can also be used as film coating materials.

（2）附加材料

b. Additional materials

①增塑剂　系指能改变高分子薄膜的物理机械性质，使薄膜衣更具柔韧性的材料。增塑剂与高分子材料要具有化学相似性，如甘油、聚乙二醇、丙二醇等带有羟基，可作为某些纤维素衣料的增塑剂；蓖麻油、甘油（单）三醋酸酯、邻苯二甲酸二乙（或二丁）酯等可作为脂肪族非极性聚合物的增塑剂。

Plasticizer　It refers to materials that can change the physical and mechanical properties of polymer films and makes film coatings more flexible. Plasticizers and polymer materials must have chemical similarities, such as glycerin, PEG, propylene glycol, and other with hydroxyl groups. They can be used as a plasticizer for certain cellulose coatings. Onion sesame oil, glycerin (mono) triacetate, diethyl (or dibutyl) phthalate, etc. can be used as a plasticizer for aliphatic non-polar polymers.

②着色剂与避光剂　为掩盖片心色泽，便于识别或增加避光稳定性，常加用食用色素及二氧化钛等，应严格控制用量。

Colorant and light repellent　In order to cover the color of the tablet core, easy to identify or increase the stability of avoiding light, often add food coloring and titanium dioxide. Their dosage should be strictly controlled.

③释药速度调节剂　又称释药速度促进剂或致孔剂。高分子薄膜材料不同，调节剂的选择也不同。如吐温、司盘、HPMC可作为乙基纤维素薄膜衣的致孔剂。

Release rate regulator　It is also called drug release speed enhancer or porogen. Different polymer film materials have different choices of modifiers. For example, Tween, Span, HPMC can be used as the pore-forming agent of EC film coating.

2. 薄膜衣的包衣操作　薄膜包衣，可采用滚转包衣法或流化包衣法（悬浮包衣法）。其操作与包糖衣基本相同。当片剂在锅内转动或在包衣室悬浮运动时，使包衣溶液均匀分散于片芯（或已先包几层粉衣层的片剂）表面，溶剂挥发干燥后再包第二层，直至需要厚度，加蜡打光即成。

② Film coating operation　Film coating can be applied by roll coating or fluid coating (suspension coating method). Its operation is basically the same as that of sugar coating. When the tablet in the pan or in the coating room suspension movement, make the coating solution evenly dispersed in the surface of tablet core (or has been coated with several layers of powder coating tablets). After the solvent evaporation and drying, coating the second layer, until the required thickness, adding wax and polishing.

为安全使用和回收有机溶剂，包衣机应有良好的排气和回收装置。

For the safe use and recovery of organic solvents, the coating machine should have good exhaust and recovery devices.

（三）肠溶衣物料及其包衣操作

（3）Enteric Coating Materials and Coating Operations

肠溶衣片系指在37℃的人工胃液中2小时内保持完整，而在人工肠液中1小时内崩解或溶解，并释放出药物的包衣片。凡药物易被胃液（酶）破坏或对胃有较强刺激性，或作用于肠道发挥特定疗效的驱虫药、消毒药，或在肠道吸收有部位特性者，均宜包肠溶衣，以使片剂安全通过胃到达肠内崩解或溶解而发挥药效。

Enteric-coated tablets refer to coated tablets that remain intact in artificial gastric juice within 2hours at 37℃, and disintegrate or dissolve within 1hour in artificial intestinal juice, and release the drug. Drugs are easily destroyed by gastric juice (enzymes) or have strong irritant to the stomach, or act as an insect repellent or disinfectant to exert a specific effect in the intestine, or have local characteristics absorbed in the intestine, can be coated with an enteric coating. So that the tablet can safely reach the intestine through the stomach and then disintegrate or dissolve to exert its effect.

1. 肠溶衣物料 肠溶衣物料的溶解度随pH而不同，应在胃液（酸性）中不溶，而在肠液（中性、偏碱性）中能迅速崩解或溶解。常用肠溶衣物料主要有以下品种：

a. Enteric coating materials The solubility of enteric coating materials varies with pH, and should be insoluble in gastric juice (acidic), but can quickly disintegrate or dissolve in intestinal juice (neutral, slightly alkaline). Commonly used enteric clothing materials mainly include the following varieties.

（1）丙烯酸树脂Ⅰ号、Ⅱ号、Ⅲ号 丙烯酸树脂Ⅱ号和Ⅲ号溶于乙醇、甲醇，不溶于水和酸，Ⅱ号在pH6以上、Ⅲ号在PH7以上成盐溶解。生产上常用Ⅱ号和Ⅲ号混合液包衣，调整二者用量比例，可得到不同溶解性能的衣料。本品成膜致密有韧性，具耐酶性，渗透性低，在肠中溶解速度快于邻苯二甲酸纤维素。

Acrylic resins No. Ⅰ*,* Ⅱ*, and* Ⅲ Acrylic resins No. Ⅱ and Ⅲ are soluble in ethanol and methanol, but insoluble in water and acids. No. Ⅱ change into salt at pH 6 or above, and No. Ⅲ change into salt at pH 7 or above. The production is commonly used No. Ⅱ and No. Ⅲ mixture on the coating, with adjusting the dosage ratio of the two to obtain clothing with different dissolution properties. The film of the product is dense and flexible, enzyme resistance, low permeability, and dissolves faster in the intestine than phthalate cellulose.

丙烯酸树脂Ⅰ号为乳胶液，在pH6.5以上时溶解，可用水为分散媒，多作肠溶外层薄膜衣而内层包丙烯酸树脂Ⅱ号使片芯不接触水。

Acrylic resin No. Ⅰ is a latex solution that dissolves at pH 6.5 or more. Water can be used as a dispersing medium. It is usually used as an enteric outer film coat and the inner layer is coated with acrylic resin No. Ⅱ to prevent the core of the tablet from contacting water.

（2）纤维醋法酯（CAP） 又称醋酸纤维素酯，为白色易流动有潮解性的粉末，不溶于水和乙醇，可溶于丙酮或乙醇与丙酮的混合液。包衣时一般用8%~12%的乙醇丙酮混合液。成膜性好，性质稳定，是一种较好的肠溶衣料和防水隔离层衣料。该衣膜在pH≥6时溶解，胰酶能促进其消化。应注意CAP具有吸湿性，在贮藏期中衣膜的网状结构孔隙能让少量水分渗入，使崩解剂吸水失去崩解作用。加用适量虫胶、邻苯二甲酸二乙酯可增加衣层的韧性和抗透湿性。CAP的肠溶包衣水分散体已用于大生产。

Cellulose acetate (CAP) Also known as cellulose acetate, it is a white, easy-flowing, deliquescent powder, insoluble in water and ethanol, and soluble in acetone or a mixed solution of ethanol and acetone. Generally, 8%-12% ethanol and acetone mixture is often used when coating. It has good film formation and stable properties, and is a good enteric coating and waterproof insulation coating. The coating film

is dissolved at pH≥6, and pancreatin can promote its digestion. Attention should be paid to CAP is hygroscopic, and the pores of the mesh structure of the coating film can allow a small amount of water to penetrate during the storage period, so that the disintegrant loses its disintegration when it absorbs water. Adding an appropriate amount of shellac and diethyl phthalate can increase the toughness of the coating and the moisture permeability resistance. The enteric-coated aqueous dispersions of CAP have been used in large-scale production.

此外，羟丙基甲基纤维素邻苯二甲酸酯（HPMCP）也是良好的肠溶衣物料，其衣膜在pH5~6之间（十二指肠上端）即能溶解，性质稳定，贮藏期不会游离出醋酸而引起药物变质。其他可选用的还有聚乙烯醇醋酸酯（PVAP）、醋酸纤维素苯三酸酯（CAT）、丙烯酸树脂EuSlOO、EullOO等。虫胶是昆虫分泌的一种天然树脂，不溶于胃液，在pH 6.4以上的溶液中溶解。20世纪30年代曾被广泛用于包肠溶衣，因其包衣厚度不易控制而影响产品质量，现已少用。

In addition, hydroxypropyl methylcellulose gallate (HPMCP) is also a good enteric coating material. Its coating film can be dissolved between pH 5 to 6 (the upper end of the duodenum), which is stable in nature and acetic acid is not released to cause drug deterioration during storage. Other options include polyvinyl alcohol acetate (PVAP), cellulose acetate trimellitate (CAT), acrylic resin EuSlOO, EullOO, etc. Shellac is a kind of natural resin secreted by insects, which is insoluble in gastric juice and soluble in solutions with a pH above 6.4. In the 1930s, it was widely used for enteric coating, because the thickness of the coating is not easy to control and affects the quality of the product, it uses less nowadays.

2. 肠溶衣的包衣操作 包肠溶衣可用流化包衣法、滚转包衣法或压制包衣法。滚转包衣法包肠溶衣，可在片芯上直接包肠溶性全薄膜衣。也可在片芯包粉衣层至无棱角时，再用肠溶衣液包肠溶衣到适宜厚度，或最后再包数层粉衣层及糖衣层。流化包衣法系将肠溶衣液喷包于悬浮的片剂表面，成品光滑，包衣速度快。压制包衣法系利用压制包衣机将肠溶衣物料的干颗粒压在片芯外而成干燥衣层。

b. Coating operation of enteric coating The enteric coating can be applied by fluid coating, roll coating or compression coating. The roll coating can be used for enteric coating, which can be directly enteric full film coated on the tablet core. When the powder coating layer of tablet core is not edged, enteric coating solution can be used to enteric coating to the appropriate thickness, or several powder coating layers and sugar coating layers can be finally coated. Fluidized coating method refers to the enteric coating solution is spray-coated on the surface of the suspended tablet. The finished product is smooth, and the coating speed is fast. The compression coating method refers to using a compression coater to press the dry particles of the enteric coating material outside the tablet core to form a dry coating layer.

第五节 片剂的质量要求与检查

16.5 Quality Requirements and Inspection of Tablets

PPT

一、片剂的质量要求

16.5.1 Quality Requirements of Tablets

片剂外观应完整光洁、色泽均匀［80~100目色点应 <5%（中药粉末片 <10%）；麻面 <5%，

并不得有严重花斑及异物；包衣片有畸形者不得超过 0.3%]；有适宜的硬度，以免在包装、贮运过程中发生磨损或破坏。

The appearance of the tablet should be complete, bright and clean, and the color should be uniform [80-100 mesh color points should be < 5% (Chinese medicine powder tablets < 10%); the hemp surface should be < 5%, and there should be no serious spots or foreign bodies; the coating tablets with deformity should not exceed 0.3%]. It has suitable hardness to avoid wear and tear during packing, storage and transportation.

重量差异：每片重量与标示片重（或平均片重）相比较，超出重量差异限度的不得多于 2 片，并不得有 1 片超出限度 1 倍。糖衣片的片芯应检查重量差异并符合规定，包糖衣后不再检查重量差异。除另有规定外，其他包衣片应在包衣后检查重量差异并符合规定。

Weight difference Compare the weight of each tablet with the indicated tablet weight (or average tablet weight), no more than 2 tablets exceed the weight difference limit, and no one tablet exceeds the limit by one time. The core of the sugar-coated tablet should check the weight difference and in accordance with the regulations, the weight difference will not be checked after sugar coating. Unless otherwise specified, other coated tablets should be checked for weight difference after coating and meet the requirements.

崩解时限：除另有规定外，药材原粉片 6 片均应在 30 分钟内全部崩解；浸膏（半浸膏）片、糖衣片、薄膜衣片各片均应在 1 小时内全部崩解。肠溶衣片先在盐酸溶液（9→1000）中检查 2 小时，每片均不得有裂缝、崩解或软化现象；再在磷酸盐缓冲液（pH6.8）中进行检查，1 小时内应全部崩解。泡腾片分别置盛有 200ml 水（水温为 15~25℃）的烧杯中，有许多气泡放出，当片剂或碎片周围的气体停止逸出时，片剂应溶解或分散在水中，无集聚的颗粒剩留，除另规定外，各片均应在 5 分钟内崩解。

Disintegration time limit Unless otherwise specified, all 6 original medicinal powder tablets should disintegrate within 30min; each of the extract (semi-extract) tablets, sugar-coated tablets, and film-coated tablets should disintegrate within 1h. Enteric-coated tablets are first inspected in a hydrochloric acid solution (9→1000) for 2h, and each tablet must be free from cracks, disintegration or softening; and then inspected in phosphate buffer solution (pH6.8). All should disintegrate within 1hour. Effervescent tablets are placed in beakers containing 200ml of water (water temperature 15-25℃), and many bubbles are released. When the gas around the tablet or debris stops escaping, the tablet should dissolve or dispersed in water, no agglomerated particles remain, and unless otherwise specified, each tablet should disintegrate within 5 minutes.

凡含有药材浸膏、树脂、油脂或大量糊化淀粉的片剂，如有小部分颗粒状物未通过筛网，但已软化无硬芯者，可作符合规定论。含片、咀嚼片以及规定检查溶出度、释放度、融变时限或分散均匀性的片剂不检查崩解时限。

Tablets containing medicinal extracts, resins, fats or a large amount of gelatinized starch, if a small part of the granules have not passed through the screen, but have been softened without hard core, can be regarded as complying with the regulations. Tablets that are prescribed for dissolution, release, melting time or uniformity of dispersion are not checked for disintegration time.

融变时限：阴道片应检查融变时限。除另有规定外，阴道片 3 片，均应在 30 分钟内全部溶化或崩解溶散并通过开孔金属圆盘，或仅残留少量无硬芯的软性团块。

Melting time limit The vaginal tablet should be checked for melting time limit. Unless otherwise specified, all 3 vaginal tablets should all dissolve or disintegrate and dissolve within 30 minutes and pass through the open-hole metal disc, or only a small amount of non-hard soft mass of the core.

发泡量：阴道泡腾片应检查发泡量。除另有规定外，供试品 10 片，依法检查，平均发泡体积应不少于 6ml，且少于 4ml 的不得超过 2 片。

Foaming volume The amount of foaming of vaginal effervescent tablets should be checked. Unless otherwise specified, there are 10 test samples for inspection. According to law, the average foaming volume should be not less than 6ml, and no more than 2 pieces less than 4ml.

硬度（抗张强度）：中药压制片一般 2~3kg；化学药物压制片一般小片 2~3kg，大片 3~10kg。

Hardness (tensile strength) Chinese medicine pressed tablets are generally 2~3kg. The small tablets of chemical medicine pressed tablets are generally 2~3kg and large tablets are 3~10kg.

脆碎度：一般应低于 1.0%。

Friability It is generally less than 1.0%.

此外，片剂的鉴别、检查、含量测定、溶出度以及微生物限度、小剂量药物片剂的含量均匀度均应符合各品种项下的有关规定。

In addition, the identification, inspection, content determination, dissolution rate, and microbial limit of tablets, and the uniformity of the content of small-dose drug tablets should meet the relevant regulations under each variety.

二、片剂的质量检查

16.5.2 Quality Inspection of Tablets

1. 外观 取样品 100 片平铺白底板上，置于 75W 白炽灯的光源下 60cm 处，在距离片剂 30cm 处用肉眼观察 30 秒，结果应色泽一致。

(1) Appearance Take 100 pieces of samples on a flat white floor, place them 60cm under the light source of a 75W incandescent lamp, and observe them with the naked eye for 30s at a distance of 30cm from the tablet. The results should be consistent in color.

2. 重量差异 取供试品 20 片，精密称定总重量，求得平均片重后，再分别精密称定每片的重量，每片重量与标示片重（无标示片重与平均片重）相比较（片重 0.30g 以下重量差异限度 ±7.5%，片重 0.30g 或 0.30g 以上重量限度差异 ±5.0%），应符合规定。

(2) Weight difference Take 20 pieces of the sample, measure the total weight accurately, calculate the average weight, and then measure the weight of each piece accurately, the weight of each piece was accurately weighed. Each piece with marked weight (not marked weight and average pills weight) to compare (weight difference limit ±7.5% of the weight of the piece below 0.30g, weight difference limit ±5.0% of the weight of the piece above 0.30g or 0.30g) and it shall comply with the provisions.

3. 崩解时限 除另有规定外，取药材原粉片（或浸膏、半浸膏片）供试品 6 片，以水（37℃±1℃）为介质，分别置已调试好的片剂崩解仪吊篮的玻璃管中（每管各加 1 片），加挡板，启动崩解仪进行检查，应符合规定。如果供试品黏附挡板，应另取 6 片，不加挡板按法检查，应符合上述规定。

(3) Disintegration time limit Except as otherwise stipulated, 6 samples of raw powder tablets (or extract and semi-extract tablets) of medicinal materials were taken, and water (37℃±1℃) was used as the medium. The glass tubes in the hanging basket of the debugged tablet disintegrating instrument were placed respectively (one piece for each tube). The disintegrating instrument was started for inspection by adding baffle. If the test product adheres to the baffle, another 6 tablets should be taken. Inspection without the baffle shall comply with the above provisions.

薄膜包衣片，按上述装置与方法，改在盐酸溶液（9 → 1000）中进行检查，应在 1 小时内全部崩解。 如有 1 片不能完全崩解，应另取 6 片复试，均应符合规定。必要时，薄膜包衣片应检查残留溶剂。

For film-coated tablets, according to the above-mentioned device and method, change the test in hydrochloric acid solution (9 → 1000), and all of them should disintegrate within 1hour. If 1 tablet cannot be completely disintegrated, take another 6 tablets and try again. Should comply with the regulations. If necessary, film-coated tablets should be checked for residual solvents.

肠溶衣片，按上述装置与方法不加挡板，先在盐酸溶液（9→1000）中检查 2 小时，应符合上述规定，继将吊篮取出，用少量水洗涤后，每管加入挡板，再按上述方法在磷酸盐缓冲液（pH6.8）中进行检查，1 小时内应全部崩解。如有 1 片不能完全崩解，应另取 6 片复试，均应符合规定。

Enteric-coated tablets, without the baffle according to the above-mentioned device and method, first check in the hydrochloric acid solution (9→1000) for 2hours, which should meet the above requirements. After taking out the hanging basket and washing with a small amount of water, add a baffle to each tube. Then, check in phosphate buffer solution (pH6.8) according to the above method, and all disintegration should be performed within 1 hour. If one tablet cannot be completely disintegrated, another 6 tablets should be taken for retesting, all of which should meet the requirements.

泡腾片，取供试品 6 片，分别置 250ml 烧杯中，烧杯内盛有 200ml 水，水温为 15~25℃，应符合上述要求与规定。如有 1 片不能完全崩解，应另取 6 片复试，均应符合规定。

Effervescent tablets, take 6 tablets for testing, and place them in 250ml beakers. The beaker contains 200ml of water and the water temperature is 15-25℃, which should meet the above requirements and regulations. If 1 tablet cannot be completely disintegrated, another 6 retests should all meet the requirements.

4. 融变时限 阴道片融变时限照《中国药典》中融变时限检查法检查。如有 1 片不符合规定，应另取 3 片复试，均应符合规定。

(4) Melting time limit The melting time limit of vaginal tablets should be checked according to the fusion time limit inspection method of *Chinese Pharmacopoeia*. If one tablet does not meet the requirements, another three tablets should be taken for re-tests, and all should meet the requirements.

5. 发泡量 取 25ml 具塞刻度试管（内径 1.5cm）10 支，各精密加水 2ml，置 37℃ ± 1℃水浴中 5 分钟后，各管中分别投入阴道泡腾片供试品 1 片，密塞 20 分钟内观察最大发泡量的体积，应符合规定。

(5) Foaming volume Take 10 25ml stoppered test tubes (inner diameter 1.5cm), add 2ml of each precision water, and place them in a water bath of 37℃±1℃ for 5 minutes. Put 1 vaginal effervescent tablet in each tube for the test. Observe the volume of the maximum foaming volume within 20min of the plug, which should meet the requirements.

6. 硬度 一般用硬度测定器或片剂四用仪测定。将药片立于两个压板之间，沿片剂直径的方向徐徐加压，直至破碎，测得使其破碎所需之力。

(6) Hardness It is generally determined by a hardness tester or a four-way tablet tester. Place the tablet between two platters and slowly press along the diameter of the tablet until it breaks. Measure the force required to break it.

7. 脆碎度 将片剂（至少 20 片）刷去表面吸附的细粉，称重，放入脆碎度测定仪转鼓内，

以 25r/min 的速度转动 10 分钟，取出观察，如无碎裂、缺角、松片等现象，精密称定，将损失重量与原重量相比，其百分比即为脆碎度。

(7) Brittleness Brush the tablet (at least 20 pieces) to remove the fine powder adsorbed on the surface, weigh it, put it into the drum of the brittle degree tester, rotate it at the speed of 25r/min for 10min, take it out and observe it, if there is no fracture, missing angle, loose pieces and other phenomena, measure it precisely, and compare the lost weight with the original weight, the percentage is the brittle degree.

8. 微生物限度 照《中国药典》中微生物限度检查法检查，应符合规定。

(8) Microbial limit According to Microbial Limit Inspection Method of *Chinese Pharmacopoeia*, should comply with the rules.

第六节 片剂的包装与贮存

16.6 Packaging and Storage of Tablets

PPT

一、片剂的包装

16.6.1 Packaging of Tablets

片剂的包装不仅直接关系成品的外观，对成品的内在质量也有重要影响，而且与其应用和贮藏密切相关。优质的包装材料和包装容器，往往可以提高片剂的物理和化学稳定性。

The packaging of tablets is not only directly related to the appearance of the finished product, but also has an important impact on the intrinsic quality of the finished product, and is closely related to its application and storage. High-quality packaging materials and packaging containers can often improve the physical and chemical stability of the tablet.

常用的片剂包装容器多由塑料、纸塑、铝塑、铝箔或玻璃等材料制成，应根据药物的性质，结合给药剂量、途径和方法选择与应用。片剂包装按剂量可分为单剂量（每片单个密封包装）和多剂量（数片乃至几百片合装于一个容器内）包装；而按容器有玻璃（塑料）瓶（管）包装、泡罩式包装（以无毒铝箔为底层材料，无毒聚氯乙烯为泡罩，中间放入片剂经热压而成）或窄条式带状包装［由两层膜片（铝塑或纸塑复合膜等）经黏合或热压而成］等。片剂包装生产上多采用机械数片机或自动铝塑包装机等。

The commonly used tablet packaging containers are mostly made of plastic, paper plastic, aluminum plastic, aluminum foil or glass and other materials. Selected and applied according to the property of the drug, the dosage, route and method of administration. Tablet packaging can be divided into single dose (a single sealed package for each tablet) and multi-dose (several or even several hundred tablets packed in a container). And according to the container has glass (plastic) bottle (tube) packaging, blister type packaging (with non-toxic aluminum foil as the bottom material, non-toxic PVC as the bubble cover, the middle into tablets by hot pressure) or narrow strip packaging [made of two layers of film (aluminum-plastic or paper-plastic composite film, etc.) by bonding or hot pressing] etc. Tablet packaging production often use mechanical number of tablets or automatic aluminum-plastic packaging machine.

片剂包装应有标签，详细记载通用的名称、主药或有效成分的含量、规格数量、作用与用途、用法与用量、生产批号、有效期及厂名等。对于毒剧药片剂须特别标记，以策安全。

There should be a label on the tablet package, including the general name, the content of the main drug or active ingredient, the specifications, the quantity, the function and purpose, the usage and dosage, the production batch number, the expiry date and the name of the manufacturer, etc. The toxic tablets must be specially marked for safety.

岗位对接

二、片剂的贮存
16.6.2 Storage of Tablets

重点小结

除另有规定外，片剂应密封贮存，并置于干燥、通风处。对光敏感的片剂应避光贮存，受潮易变质的片剂，包装容器内可放入干燥剂。

题库

Unless otherwise specified, tablets should be stored in a sealed, dry, ventilated place. Light-sensitive tablets should be stored away from the light. If the tablets are moist and volatile, packaging containers can be put into the desiccant.

（兰 卫 庄 婕 王 莹）

第十七章　气体药剂
Chapter 17　Gas Potion

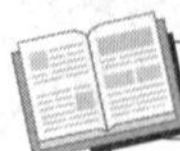

学习目标 | Learning Goals

知识要求：

1. **掌握**　气雾剂和喷雾剂的含义、特点与制法。
2. **熟悉**　气雾剂和喷雾剂的质量检查；气雾剂的组成；影响吸入气雾剂吸收的因素。
3. **了解**　粉雾剂的含义、分类和制法。

能力要求：

学会气雾剂和喷雾剂的制备与质量检测方法，能制备气雾剂和喷雾剂，并检查和评价产品质量。

Knowledge requirements:

1. **To master** the definitions, characteristics and preparations of aerosols and sprays.
2. **To be familiar with** the quality inspections of aerosols and sprays; composition of aerosols; factors affecting the absorption of inhaled aerosols.
3. **To know** the definition, classification and preparation of powder aerosols.

Capacity requirements:

To be able to prepare aerosols and sprays and inspect and evaluate the quality of product.

第一节　气雾剂
17.1　Aerosols

PPT

一、概述
17.1.1　Overview

（一）气雾剂的含义
(1) The Definition of Aerosols

气雾剂系指原料药物或原料药物和附加剂与适宜的抛射剂共同装封于具有特制阀门系统的耐压容器中，使用时借助抛射剂的压力将内容物呈雾状物喷出，用于肺部吸入或直接喷至腔道黏

膜、皮肤的制剂。内容物喷出后呈泡沫状或半固体状，则称之为泡沫剂或凝胶剂 / 乳膏剂。

Aerosols are preparations of active ingredients together with or without additives sealed in containers equipped with a specified valve and which are held under pressure with (a) suitable propellant(s). Upon actuation of propellants, the preparations are released from the container and the vapour generated is inhaled into the lungs, on mucosa of the respiratory tract or skin. Preparations of which contents sprayed out in foamy or semi-solid forms are called foams or gels/creams.

（二）气雾剂的特点

(2) The Characteristics of Aerosols

气雾剂具有以下特点：①具有速效和定位作用。药物呈细小雾滴直达作用部位或吸收部位，局部浓度高，奏效迅速。②密封于容器中，制剂的稳定性高。③给药方便，剂量准确。④刺激性与副作用小。气雾剂也存在一些缺陷，如制备时需要耐压容器、阀门系统和特殊生产设备，成本较高；具有一定的内压，储存和使用不当时易发生爆炸；抛射剂挥发时具有制冷作用，多次使用易刺激皮肤。

Aerosols have the following characteristics: ① Able to work quickly and in specific areas. The drug in small droplets directly arrive the action site or absorption site, with high local concentration and quick effect. ② Sealed in the container, and the stability of the preparation is high. ③ Administration is convenient, dosage is accurate. ④ Little irritation and side effects. There are also some defects, such as high production cost due to the use of pressure container, valve system and special production equipment in preparation; Due to certain internal pressure, it is easy to explode when it is not properly stored or used; The volatilization of propellant has refrigeration effect, so it is easy to stimulate the skin when it is repeatedly used.

（三）气雾剂的分类

(3) The Classification of Aerosols

按用药途径可分为吸入气雾剂、非吸入气雾剂。按处方组成可分为二相气雾剂（气相与液相）和三相气雾剂（气相、液相、固相或液相）。按给药定量与否，可分为定量气雾剂和非定量气雾剂。

Aerosols may be inhalation aerosols and non-inhalation aerosols according to the route of administration. Aerosols may be two phase aerosols (gas and liquid) or three phase aerosols (gas, liquid, solid or liquid) according to the formulation. Aerosols may be metered-dose aerosols and non-metered dose aerosols according to the dosage.

（四）影响吸入气雾剂吸收的因素

(4) Factors Affecting the Absorption of Inhaled Aerosols

药物性质、气雾剂性能、呼吸系统生理因素，以及患者使用方式等因素均会影响气雾剂中药物的吸收。其中主要因素有：①药物的脂溶性与分子量大小。脂溶性药物主要经脂质双分子膜扩散吸收，吸收速率较快；分子量小的药物易通过肺泡表面细胞壁小孔，较高分子化合物吸收快。②雾滴粒径大小。雾滴过粗易沉降在上呼吸道黏膜上，吸收较慢，雾滴过细易由呼气排出，肺部沉积率较低。

Drug properties, aerosols performance, physiological factors of respiratory system and the usage modes of patients all affect the absorption of drug in aerosols. The main factors include: ① Lipid solubility and molecular weight of drug. Lipid soluble drugs are mainly diffused and absorbed by the lipid bimolecular membrane, and the absorption rate is relative fast; drugs with small molecular weight can easily pass through the pores of cell wall on the surface of alveoli, and can be absorbed faster than

the high molecular compounds. ② Droplet size. Too large droplets are easier to settle on the mucous membrane of the upper respiratory tract, the absorption rate is relative slow. Too small droplets are easier to be exhaled, the deposition rate of lung is relative low.

二、气雾剂的组成
17.1.2 The Composition of Aerosols

气雾剂由药物与附加剂、抛射剂、耐压容器和阀门系统四部分组成。

The aerosols consist of four parts: drug and additive, propellant, pressure-resistant container and valve system.

（一）药物与附加剂
(1) Drug and Additive

1. 药物 中药气雾剂中的药物一般为中药饮片经提取、纯化后得到的提取物、有效成分或有效部位。

① The drug The drugs in aerosols of traditional Chinese medicine are generally the extracts, active components or active fractions that extracted and purified from Chinese herbal pieces.

2. 附加剂 根据气雾剂类型和药物理化性质选择合适的附加剂，且所选附加剂应对用药部位无刺激。气雾剂中常用的附加剂有：潜溶剂、乳化剂、助悬剂、抗氧剂、防腐剂等。

② The additive Appropriate additives should be selected according to the type of aerosols and physicochemical properties of the drug, also the selected additives should not stimulate the application site. The commonly used additives in aerosols include: cosolvent, emulsifying agent, suspending agent, antioxidant, preservative, etc.

（二）抛射剂
(2) Propellant

抛射剂一般是一些低沸点的液化气体，在常温下其蒸气压大于大气压。抛射剂既是喷射药物的动力物质，同时也兼作药物的溶剂或稀释剂。常用的抛射剂有丙烷、异丁烷、正丁烷等碳氢化合物，目前氢氟烷烃最为常用。

The propellant is a liquefied gas with low boiling point, its vapor pressure is greater than the atmospheric pressure at normal temperature. The propellant is not only the power substance for spraying drugs, but also the solvent or diluter of drugs. The commonly used propellants include propane, isobutane, N-butane and other hydrocarbons. At present, hydrofluoroalkane is the most commonly used propellant.

（三）耐压容器
(3) Pressure-resistant Container

常用的耐压容器有金属容器、玻璃容器（外面搪有塑料防护层）和塑料容器。

Metal containers, glass containers (with plastic protective coating on the outside) and plastic containers are the commonly used pressure-resistant containers.

（四）阀门系统
(4) Valve System

阀门系统是调节药物和抛射剂从容器中流出量及速度的重要组成部分，其精密程度直接影响气雾剂的剂量准确性。

Valve system is an important component that regulates the amount of sprays and delivery rate of drugs and propellant from the container, the precision of valve system directly affects the dose accuracy

of aerosols.

1. 普通阀门 由封帽、阀门杆、橡胶封圈、弹簧、浸入管、推动钮组成。其中，阀门杆是关键部位，上端有内孔和膨胀室，下端有引液槽供药液进入定量室，内孔是阀门沟通容器内外的孔道，关闭时被弹性橡胶封圈封住，容器内外不通，当揿下推动钮时，内孔与药液相通，容器内容物通过内孔进入膨胀室而喷射出来。

① **General valve** The general valve is composed of sealing cap, valve rod, rubber sealing ring, spring, immersion tube and push button. Valve rod is the key part, its upper end has an inner hole and an expansion chamber, its lower end has a liquid guide tank to supply the liquid medicine into the quantitative chamber. The inner hole is the channel between the inside and outside of the container. It is sealed by an elastic rubber sealing ring in closed state, and the inside and outside of the container are not connected. When the push button is pressed, the inner hole is connected with the liquid medicine, so the liquid medicine could enter the expansion chamber through the inner hole and spray out.

2. 定量阀门 定量阀门系统构造如图 17-1 和图 17-2 所示，除具有一般阀门各部件外，还有一个 0.05~0.2ml 的定量室，其容积决定了每次用药剂量。

② **Quantitative valve** The structure of quantitative valve system is shown in Figure 17-1 and Figure 17-2. In addition to the components of general valve, there is also a quantitative chamber (0.05~0.2ml) whose volume determines the dosage of each application.

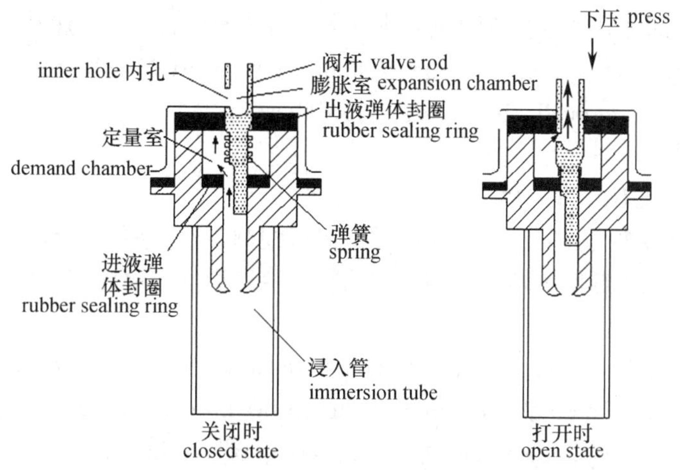

图 17-1 具有浸入管的定量阀门系统构造示意图

Figure 17-1 Structural Diagram of Quantitative Valve System with Immersed Tube

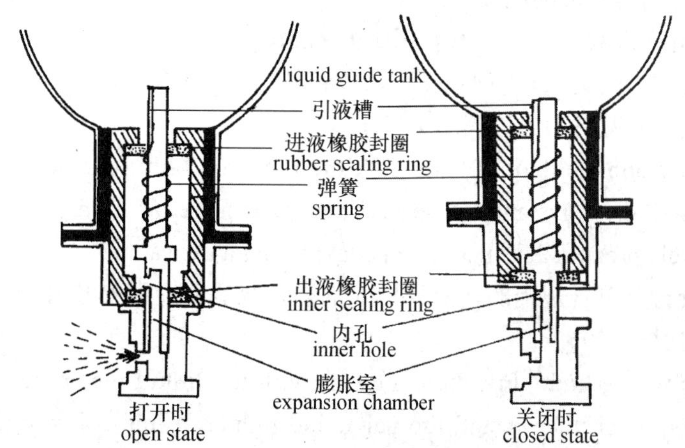

图 17-2 无浸入管的定量阀门系统构造示意图

Figure 17-2 Structural Diagram of Quantitative Valve System Without Immersed Tube

三、气雾剂的制法

17.1.3 The Preparation of Aerosols

气雾剂的制备工艺流程如图 17-3 所示。

The preparation process of aerosol is showed in Figure 17-3.

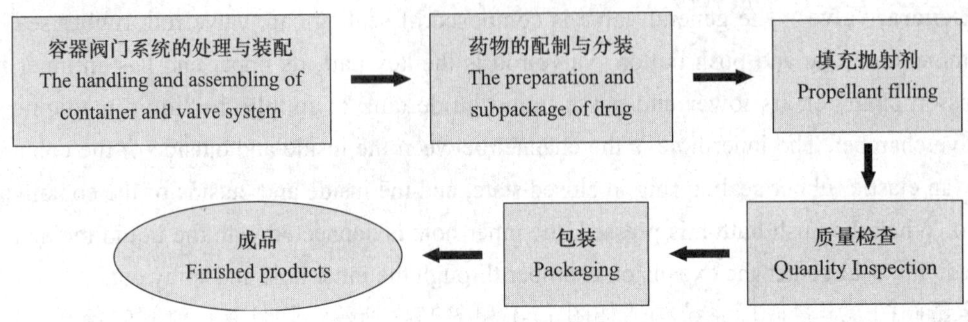

图 17-3 气雾剂制备工艺流程

Figure 17-3 Preparation Process of Aerosols

（一）容器与阀门系统的处理与装配

(1) The Handling and Assembling of Container and Valve System

对容器和阀门各部件分别进行乙醇浸泡或煮沸等清洁处理后，经干燥和灭菌即可进行装配。

The container and components of valve system are respectively cleaned by ethanol soaking or boiling, and then can be assembled after drying and sterilization.

（二）药物的配制

(2) The Preparation of Drug

饮片提取物或细粉按处方要求的气雾剂类型进行配制。溶液型气雾剂的药液应澄清；乳剂型气雾剂应借助适宜的乳化剂使其均匀、细腻、柔软；混悬型气雾剂应将药物粉碎成适宜粒径的微粉，制成稳定的混悬液。

The extract of pieces or powder should be prepared according to the type of aerosols. The solution aerosols should be clear; the emulsion aerosols should be uniform, delicate and soft with the aid of suitable emulsifier; In suspension aerosols, the drug should be crushed into a fine powder with suitable particle size, so as to make a stable suspension.

（三）药物的分装与抛射剂的填充

(3) Drug Subpackage and Propellant Filling

1. 压灌法 先将配好的药液在室温下灌入容器，安装阀门并轧紧，再抽去容器内的空气，然后使用压装机将滤过后的抛射剂通过阀门定量压入。

① **Pressure irrigation method** Firstly, fill the prepared liquid medicine into the container at room temperature, install the valve and tighten it. Then, extract the air from container and use the press machine to quantitatively press in the filtered propellant through the valve.

2. 冷灌法 将冷却至符合规定的药液和抛射剂灌入容器并立即安装阀门、扎紧，此过程必须操作迅速，以减少抛射剂损失。

② **Cold irrigation method** Fill the container with the liquid medicine and propellant which cooled to the specified level, then install the valve and tighten it immediately. This process must be operated quickly to reduce the loss of propellant.

案例导入 ¦ Case example

案例 17-1 麝香祛痛气雾剂

17-1 Shexiang Qutong Qiwuji

处方： 人工麝香 0.33g，红花 1g，樟脑 30g，独活 1g，冰片 20g，龙血竭 0.33g，薄荷脑 10g，地黄 20g，三七 0.33g，乙醇适量，抛射剂适量

Ingredients: Moschus Artifactus 0.33g; Carthami Flos 1g; Camphora 30g: Angelicae Pubescentis Radix 1g: Borneolum Synthe-ticum 20g: Dracaenae Combodianae Resina 0.33g; hexahydrothymol 10g; Rehmanniae Radix 20g; Notoginseng Radix et Rhizoma 0.33g; The amount of ethanol, the amount of propellant.

功能与主治： 活血祛瘀，舒经活络，消肿止痛。用于跌打损伤，瘀血肿痛，风湿瘀阻，关节疼痛。

Functions and indications: To activate blood, resolve stasis, soothe meridians, harmonize collaterals, alleviate swelling and relieve pain. For all kinds of traumatic injuries and swelling pain due to static blood, and joints pain due to wind-dampness obstruction.

制法： 以上九味，取人工麝香、红花、三七分别用 50% 乙醇 10ml 分三次浸渍，每次 7 天，合并浸渍液，滤过，滤液备用；地黄用 50% 乙醇 100ml 分三次浸渍，每次 7 天，合并浸渍液，滤过，滤液备用；龙血竭、独活分别用乙醇 10ml 分三次浸渍，每次 7 天，合并浸渍液，滤过，滤液备用；冰片、樟脑加乙醇 100ml，搅拌使溶解，再加入 50% 乙醇 700ml，混匀；加入上述各浸渍液，混匀；将薄荷脑用适量 50% 乙醇溶解，加入上述药液中，加 50% 乙醇至总量为 1000ml，混匀，静置，滤过，灌装，封口，充入抛射剂适量，即得。

Making Procedure: Macerate separately Moschus Artifactus, Notoginseng Radix et Rhizoma and Carthami Flos with 10ml of 50% ethanol in 3 portions, respectively, 7 days for each times, combine the extracts and filter. Macerate Rehmanniae Radix with 100ml of 50% ethanol in 3 portions, 7 days for each time, combine the extract and filter. Macerate separately Dracaenae Combodianae Resina and Angelicae Pubescentis Radix with 10ml of ethanol in 3 portions, 7 days for each time, combine the extracts and filter. Dissolve Borneolum Syntheticum and Camphora in 100ml of ethanol by stirring, add 700ml of 50% ethanol, stir well, add the above extracts, mix well. Dissolve hexahydrothymol with a quantity of 50% ethanol, add into the above drug liquid, adjust the total volume to 1000ml with 50% ethanol, mix well, stand and filter, pack, seal and add a quantity of the propellant.

用法与用量： 外用。喷涂患处，按摩 5~10 分钟至患处发热，一日 2~3 次；软组织扭伤严重或有出血者，将药液喷湿的棉垫敷于患处。

Usage and dosage: For topical application, apply it to the *pars affecta*. Rub the area for 5-10 minutes until the *pars affecta* feels warm, twice or three times a day. For patients with soft tissue injury or bleeding, soak a cotton pad with the medicine before applying to the *pars affecta*.

注解： 提取工艺采用乙醇长时间连续、多次浸泡，既保证了有效成分充分浸出，又保证了有效成分不因高温被破坏、损失；挥发性成分和溶剂乙醇还兼有促透剂的作用，有利于药物迅速起效。

Notes: The long-term continuous and repeated ethanol immersion not only ensures the full leaching of the effective components, but also ensures that the effective components are not damaged or lost due to high temperature; the volatile components and solvent ethanol also have the role of penetration promoter,

which is conducive to the rapid effectiveness of the drug.

思考题：麝香祛痛气雾剂与麝香祛痛搽剂相比，各有哪些优缺点？

Questions: Compared the Shexiang Qutong Qiwuji with Shexiang Qutong Chaji, what are the advantages and disadvantages of each?

四、气雾剂的质量要求与检查

17.1.4 The Quality Requirements and Inspections of the Aerosols

每瓶总揿次、递送剂量均一性、每揿主药含量、喷射速率、喷出总量、每揿喷量、粒度、装量、无菌、微生物限度检查等项目应符合现行版《中国药典》质量要求。

Number of deliveries per inhaler, uniformity of delivered dose, content of active ingredient delivered by actuation of the vale, delivery rate, total amount of spray, delivered amount in a dose, particle size, filling, sterility and microbial limit, etc., should meet the quality requirements of the current edition of *Chinese Pharmacopoeia*.

五、气雾剂的贮存

17.1.5 Aerosol Storage

除另有规定外，气雾剂应置凉暗处贮存，并避免曝晒、受热、敲打、撞击。

Unless otherwise specified, the aerosol should be stored in a cool and dark place, and avoid violent sun, heating, knocking and impacting.

第二节 喷雾剂与粉雾剂

17.2 Sprays and Powder Aerosols

PPT

一、喷雾剂

17.2.1 Sprays

（一）喷雾剂的含义

(1) The Definition of Sprays

喷雾剂系指原料药物或与适宜辅料填充于特制的装置中，使用时借助手动泵的压力、高压气体、超声振动或其他方法将内容物呈雾状物释出，用于肺部吸入或直接喷至腔道黏膜及皮肤等的制剂。

Sprays are preparations of solutions, emulsions or suspensions of one or more active substances in a suitable vehicle (and/or excipients), filled in special devices, which are delivered from the container in the form of an aerosol with pressure of hand pump, high pressure of gas, ultrasonic vibration and others, to the deep respiratory tract, mucosa of various body cavities or the skin.

（二）喷雾剂的特点

(2) The Characteristics of Sprays

喷雾剂具有以下特点：①可采用压缩的惰性气体为喷雾动力，提高药物稳定性。②与气雾剂相比，喷雾剂设备较简单、制备方便、成本低。③以手动泵为喷雾动力的喷雾剂，雾滴较气雾剂粗，以局部应用为主。④采用压缩气体为喷雾动力，喷射雾滴与喷射量无法维持恒定。

Sprays have the following characteristics: ① Using compressed inert gas as spray power, the stability of drug can be improved. ② Compared with aerosols, the sprays is simpler in equipment, easier to prepare and lower in cost. ③ Using manual pump as sprayer, the spray droplets are larger than aerosol droplets and mainly used in local applications. ④ Using compressed gas as spray power, the spray droplet and volume can not be maintained constant.

（三）喷雾剂的分类

(3) The Classification of Sprays

按内容物组成分为溶液型、乳状液型或混悬型喷雾剂。按用药途径可分为吸入喷雾剂、鼻用喷雾剂及用于皮肤、黏膜的非吸入喷雾剂。按给药定量与否，可分为定量喷雾剂和非定量喷雾剂。

They may be classified as sprays for inhalation, nasal sprays, sprays for non-inhalation intended for topical or mucosal use according to the route of administration. They are presented as metered dose and non-metered dose sprays. Metered dose sprays for inhalation are preparations of solutions, suspensions or emulsions, which release aerosols intended for inhalation by metered-dose atomizing devices.

（四）喷雾剂的制法

(4) The Preparation of Sprays

1. 原料药的准备　中药喷雾剂中的药物一般为中药饮片经提取、纯化后得到的有效成分单体或有效部位。

① **The preparation of raw drug**　The drugs in sprays of traditional Chinese medicine are generally the active component monomer compound or active fractions that extracted and purified from Chinese herbal pieces.

2. 压缩气体的选择　以压缩气体为动力的喷雾剂常用的气体有空气、氮气、二氧化碳、一氧化二氮，其中氮气和二氧化碳最为常用，且压缩气体在使用前必须经过净化处理。

② **The selection of compressed gas**　When compressed gas is used as spray power, the commonly used gas include air, nitrogen, carbon dioxide and two nitrogen oxide. Nitrogen and carbon dioxide are the most commonly used gas and the compressed gas must be purified before use.

3. 附加剂　根据喷雾剂类型和药物理化性质选择合适的附加剂。喷雾剂的常用附加剂有：增溶剂、潜溶剂、乳化剂、助悬剂、防腐剂、pH 值调节剂、润湿剂等。

③ **The additive**　Appropriate additives should be selected according to the type of sprays and physicochemical properties of the drug. The commonly used additives in sprays include: solubilizer, cosolvent, emulsifying agent, suspending agent, preservative, pH regulator, wetting agent, etc.

4. 容器与阀门系统或喷雾装置

④ **The container and valve system or spray device**

（1）金属容器与阀门系统　以压缩气体为动力的喷雾剂，常采用耐压性能较高的金属容器。喷雾剂的阀门系统与气雾剂相似，但阀杆内孔较大，以便于物质的流动。

a. Metal containers and valve system　when compressed gas is used as spray power, metal containers with high pressure resistance are often adopted. Compared with aerosols, the spray valve system is similar, but inner hole is larger so as to facilitate the flow of material.

（2）容器与喷雾装置　常用容器有塑料瓶和玻璃瓶。喷雾装置常采用电子或机械装置制备的手动泵。临床常用超声雾化器或蒸汽雾化器将药液雾化后，供患者吸入治疗（图 17-4）。

b. Containers and spray device　plastic bottles and glass bottles are the commonly used containers. The manual pump in electronic or mechanical mode is often used as the spray device. Ultrasonic atomizer and steam atomizer are often used to atomize the medicinal liquid in clinical inhalation therapy (Figure 17-4).

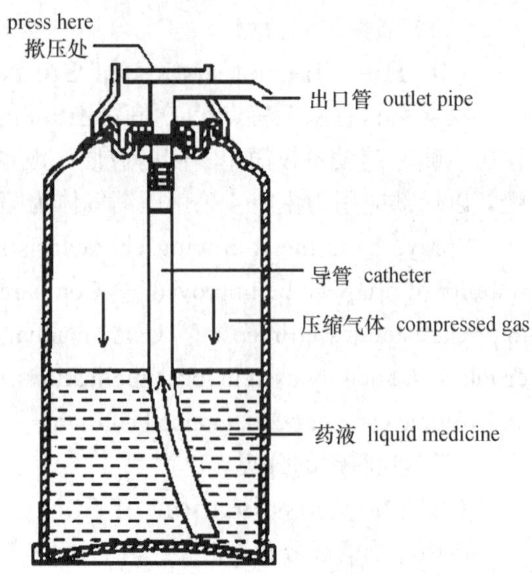

图 17-4　喷雾剂示意图

Figure 17-4　Sketch Map of Sprays

5. 药液的配制与灌装　喷雾剂应在符合洁净度要求的环境中，按处方要求的喷雾剂类型配制。配制完成后，将符合要求的药液分装在合格容器内，装上手动泵即得。采用压缩气体为喷雾动力的喷雾剂药液分装后还应安装阀门，扎紧封帽，压入压缩气体。

⑤ **The preparation and filling of medicinal liquid**　Sprays should be prepared in accordance with spray type, and the environment should meet cleanliness requirements. After preparation, the medicinal liquid is sub-packed in qualified containers, then loaded with manual pump. When compressed gas is used as spray power, the valve should be installed and tightly sealed cap after the sub-packing of medicinal liquid, then compressed gas is pressed in.

二、粉雾剂

17.2.2　Powder Aerosols

（一）粉雾剂的含义与分类

(1) The Definition and Classification of Powder Aerosols

粉雾剂系指微粉化的药物与附加剂及载体采用特制的干粉给药装置，由患者主动吸入雾化药物至肺部或喷至腔道黏膜的剂型。粉雾剂可分为吸入型粉雾剂和非吸入型粉雾剂。

Powder aerosols refers to the dosage forms of micronized drugs, additives and carriers using special dry powder delivery devices, which are inhaled by the patients to the lungs or sprayed into the mucosa of the lumen. According to the route of administration, it can be divided into inhaled powder aerosols, non inhaled powder aerosols.

（二）粉雾剂的特点

(2) The Characteristics of Powder Aerosols

粉雾剂具有以下特点：①用药时不需同步吸气与揿压阀门，病人顺应性更好。②载药量高且不受定量阀门的限制。③患者吸入的是微粉化药物或微粉化药物与载体的均匀混合物，较其他剂型吸收迅速、起效快。④对药物的微粉化技术和给药装置要求较高。

Powder aerosols have the following characteristics: ① It is not necessary to simultaneously inhale and press the valve during medication, so the patient's compliance is better. ② The loading capacity is high and not limited by the quantitative valve. ③ Patients inhale micronized drugs or mixture of micronized drugs and carriers, which absorb more rapidly and take effect faster than other dosage forms.

④ The requirements of micronization technology and drug delivery device are high.

（三）粉雾剂的制法

(3) The Preparation of Powder Aerosols

粉雾剂的制备工艺流程如图 17-5 所示。

The preparation process of powder aerosols is shown in Figure 17-5.

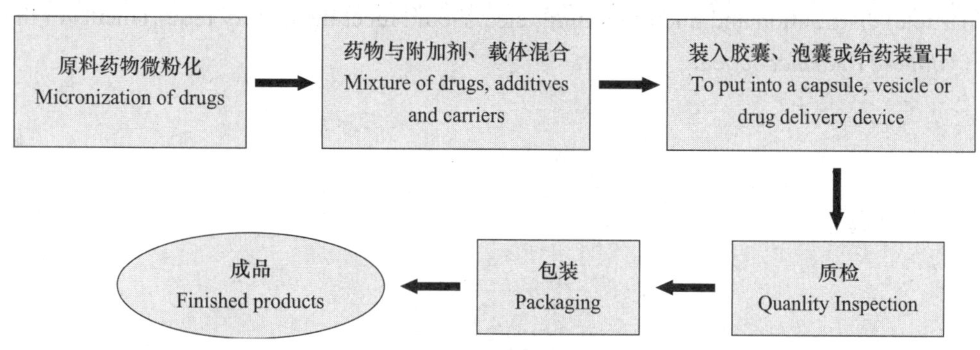

图 17-5 粉雾剂制备工艺流程

Figure 17-5 Preparation Process of Powder Aerosols

（四）吸入粉雾剂的给药装置

(4) Dosing Device for the Inhaled Powder Aerosols

粉雾剂吸入装置可分为：①胶囊型吸入装置：刺破硬胶囊，吸气时药粉从胶囊壁上的孔中释放出来。②泡囊型吸入装置：药物分装于铝箔上的水泡眼中，使用时针刺破铝箔，吸气时药粉即可释出。③贮库型吸入装置：将多个剂量药物分别装入同一装置中，用时只需旋转装置，单剂量的药物即可释出。④粉末雾化吸入装置：将药物贮存于特殊装置中，使用时将定量药物雾化成气溶胶，由患者吸入。

The inhalation device can be divided into: ① capsule type inhalation device: puncture the hard capsule, release the powder from the hole on the capsule wall during inhalation. ② vesicle type inhalation device: the medicine is divided into vesicle eyes on the aluminum foil, puncture the aluminum foil and the powder can be released when inhaled. ③ storage type inhalation device: multiple doses of drugs are respectively loaded into the same device, and only need to rotate the device when using, the single dose of drugs can be released. ④ powder atomization type inhalation device: store the medicine in a special device, atomize the quantitative medicine into aerosol when used, and inhale by the patient.

三、喷雾剂与粉雾剂的质量要求与检查

17.2.3 Quality Requirements and Inspections of Sprays and Powder Aerosols

（一）喷雾剂的质量要求与检查

(1) Quality Requirements and Inspections of Sprays

每瓶总喷次、每喷喷量、每喷主药含量、递送剂量均一性、微细粒子剂量、装量差异检查等项目应符合现行版《中国药典》质量要求。

Total number of deliveries per container, delivery amount in a dose, content of active ingredient in a unit spray, uniformity of delivered dose, fine particle dose, weight variation, etc., should meet the quality requirements of the current edition of *Chinese Pharmacopoeia*.

岗位对接

重点小结

题库

（二）粉雾剂的质量要求与检查

(2) Quality Requirements and Inspections of Powder Aerosols

含量均匀度、装量差异、排空率、每瓶总吸次、每吸主药含量、雾滴（粒）分布、微生物限度检查等项目应符合现行版《中国药典》质量要求。

Uniformity of content, filling, emptying rate, total suction times per bottle, drug content per suction, droplet (particle) distribution and microbial limit, etc., should meet the quality requirements of the current edition of *Chinese Pharmacopoeia*.

（周　宁）

第十八章　其他剂型
Chapter 18　Some Other Dosage Forms

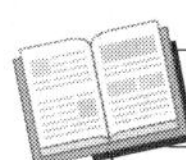

学习目标 ¦ Learning Goals

知识要求：

1．**掌握**　膜剂的含义、处方组成及制备方法。

2．**熟悉**　膜剂的特点、分类、成膜材料及质量检查。

3．**了解**　海绵剂的含义、分类及制法；丹药的含义、特点、分类、制备及生产过程中的防护措施；烟剂、烟熏剂、香囊（袋）剂、离子导入剂与沐浴剂的含义；锭剂、糕剂、钉剂、线剂、条剂、灸剂、熨剂与棒剂的含义和应用特点。

能力要求：

学会膜剂的制备与质量检测方法，能制备不同类型的膜剂，并检查和评价膜剂的产品质量。

Knowledge requirements:

1. **To master** the definition, composition of prescription and preparation method of pellicles.

2. **To be familiar with** the characteristics, classification, film-forming materials and quality inspection of pellicles.

3. **To konw** the the definition, characteristics and preparation method of spongia agent; the definition, characteristics, classification, preparation method and protective methods during production of Dan Yao; the definition of smoke agent, smoke fumigant, aromatic bag agent, penetration of ions and bath agent; the definition and usage of pastille, cake agent, nail agent, thread agent, strip agent, moxibustion agent, compression agent and club agent.

Ability requirements:

To be able to use various preparation methods to manufacture different pellicles, and quality testing methods to evaluate and control the quality of pellicles.

PPT

第一节 膜剂
18.1 Pellicles

一、概述
18.1.1 Overview

（一）膜剂的含义
(1) The Definition of the Pellicles

膜剂系指将饮片用适宜方法加工后与适宜的成膜材料制成的膜状剂型。

The pellicles refer to process medicinal slices and suitable film-forming materials with appropriate method and make them into filmy dosage form.

膜剂适于多种给药途径，可以发挥局部或全身作用。

Pelliclesare suitable for multiple administration ways, and can play a local or systemic therapeutic role.

（二）膜剂的特点
(2) The Characteristics of the Pellicles

1. 生产工艺简单，易于自动化和无菌生产。

① The production process is simple and easy to be automatic and aseptic.

2. 药物含量准确、质量稳定。

② Drug content is accurate and quality is stable.

3. 使用方便，适于多种给药途径。

③ Easy to use, and suitable for a variety of drug delivery routes.

4. 可制成不同释药速度的制剂。

④ Preparations with different release-speed can be made.

5. 多层膜剂可避免配伍禁忌和各成分间的相互干扰。

⑤ Multiple pellicles could avoid drug incompatibility as well as mutual interference among various components.

6. 体积小，重量轻，便于携带、运输和贮存。

⑥ It is handy to be carried, transported and stored due to the small volume and light weight.

但膜剂载药量小，不适用于药物剂量较大的制剂。

But, pellicles drug loading quantity is small leading to this pellicle not suitable for high-dose drugs.

（三）膜剂的分类
(3) The Classification of the Pellicles

膜剂通常厚度为 0.2mm 左右，不超过 1mm，外观有透明的和不透明的，面积按临床应用部位不同而有差别，膜剂常用分类方法有以下两种。

The thickness of a pellicle is usually about 0.2 mm and less than 1mm, the appearance can be transparent or opaque, its area vary according to the clinical application site. There are two classification methods of pellicles.

1. 按组成结构分类 可分为单层膜剂、多层膜剂、夹心膜剂等。

① **Classified by structure** such as single-layer pellicle, multi-layer pellicle and sandwich pellicle, etc.

2. 按给药途径分类 可分为口服膜剂、口腔用膜剂、眼用膜剂、耳鼻喉用膜剂、阴道用膜剂、植入膜剂、皮肤用膜剂等。

② **Classified by administration** such as oral pellicle, way ophthalmic pellicle, ENT pellicle, vaginal pellicle, implanted pellicle and skin pellicle, etc.

二、膜剂常用的成膜材料与辅料

18.1.2 The Commonly Film-Forming and Auxiliary Materials of Pellicles

（一）成膜材料

(1) Film-Forming Materials

成膜材料既是药物的载体，又可以控制药物的释放速度，是膜剂重要的组成部分。理想的成膜材料应符合以下要求：①生理惰性，无毒、无刺激，不与药物发生作用，能被机体代谢或排泄，外用应不妨碍组织的愈合过程，不过敏，长期使用应无致畸、致癌等不良反应；②无不适臭味，性能稳定，不降低主药药效，不干扰含量测定；③成膜、脱膜性能好，成膜后有足够的机械强度和柔韧性；④用于口服、腔道、眼用膜剂的成膜材料应具有良好的水溶性，能逐渐降解、吸收或排泄；外用膜剂应能按照设计要求完全释放药物；⑤价格低廉，来源丰富。

The film-forming material can not only be the carrier of drug, but also can control the release speed of drug, so it's an important part of pellicles. The ideal film-forming material should meet certain requirements: a.physiological inertia, non-toxic, no stimulation, no drug effect, can be metabolized or excreted by the body, external use should not interfere with the healing process of the tissue, not allergic, long-term use should be no teratogenic, carcinogenic and other adverse reactions;b.No unpleasant odor, stable performance, do not reduce the main drug efficacy, do not interfere with the determination of content; c.film-forming, film-stripping is good, enough mechanical strength and flexibility after filmed;d. The film-forming material used for oral, lumen and ophthalmic film agent should have good water solubility and can be gradually degraded, absorbed or excreted; The external film agent should be able to release the drug completely according to the design requirements; ⑤ The price is low, the source is abundant.

常用的成膜材料有天然和合成的高分子化合物。

The commonly used film-forming materials can be classified into natural and synthetic polymer compounds.

1. 天然的高分子成膜材料 常用的天然成膜材料有明胶、虫胶、阿拉伯胶、琼脂、白及胶、海藻酸、玉米朊、纤维素等，常需加入适量防腐剂并常与其他成膜材料合用。

① **Natural film-forming materials** The commonly used are gelatin, shell-lac, Arabic gum, agar, gum Bletilla, alginic acid, zein and cellulose etc. Meanwhile, suitable amount of preservatives should be added and several kinds of film-forming materials should be used at the same time.

2. 合成的高分子成膜材料 常用的合成高分子成膜材料有聚乙烯醇、纤维素衍生物类、聚乙烯氨基缩醛衍生物、聚乙烯胺类、聚乙烯吡咯烷酮、丙烯酸共聚物等。均成膜性能优良，成膜后的抗拉强度和柔韧性较好。

② **Synthetic film-forming materials** The commonly used are polyvinyl alcohol, cellulose derivatives, polyvinyl aminoacetal derivatives, polyvinyl amine, polyvinyl pyrrolidone, acrylic acid copolymer, etc. Those materials have good film-forming ability and have good tensile strength as well as flexibility after film forming.

（二）其他辅料

(2) Auxiliary Materials

1. 增塑剂 增塑剂能使膜剂柔韧性增强，并有一定的抗拉强度。常用的增塑剂有甘油、三醋酸甘油酯、乙二醇、山梨醇等。

① **Plasticizer** Plasticizer can make pellicles more flexible, and has a certain tensile strength. Commonly used plasticizer are glycerol, glycerol triacetate, ethylene glycol and sorbitol, etc.

2. 着色剂、遮光剂和填充剂 常用着色剂为食用色素；遮光剂常用二氧化钛（TiO_2）；制不透明膜剂时常需加入碳酸钙（$CaCO_3$）、二氧化硅（SiO_2）、淀粉、糊精、滑石粉等作为填充剂。

② **Colorant, opacifier and filler** The commonly used colorant is food coloring, the opacifier is titanium dioxide（TiO_2）, and when opaque films is made, some fillers should be added, such as calcium carbonate ($CaCO_3$), silica (SiO_2), starch, dextrin, talcum powder, etc.

3. 矫味剂 蔗糖、甘露醇、甜蜜素等常用作口服型膜剂的矫味剂。

③ **Corrigent** Sucrose, mannitol and sodium cyclamate are commonly used as corrigents of oral pellicles.

4. 表面活性剂 常用聚山梨酯-80、十二烷基硫酸钠、豆磷脂等，在处方中起润湿剂的作用。

④ **Surfactant** Such as polysorbate - 80, sodium dodecyl sulfate and bean lecithin, etc. acts as a wetting agent in the prescription.

案例导入

三、膜剂的制备

18.1.3 Preparation of Pellicles

（一）膜剂的处方组成（表 18-1）

(1) The Prescription of Pellicles（Table 18-1）

表 18-1 膜剂的处方组成

成分	含量
主药	0~70%（g/g）
成膜材料（PVA 等）	30%~100%
着色剂（色素）	0~2%
遮光剂（二氧化钛）	0~2%
增塑剂（甘油等）	0~20%
表面活性剂（吐温-80、豆磷脂等）	1%~2%
填充剂（$CaCO_3$、SiO_2 等）	0~20%
矫味剂（蔗糖等）	适量
脱膜剂（液体石蜡、甘油、硬脂酸）	适量

Table 18-1　The Prescription of Pellicles

Component	Content
Main drug	0-70%（g/g）
Film-forming material（PVA etc.）	30%-100%
Colorant（pigment）	0-2%
Opacifier（TiO_2）	0-2%
Plasticizer（glycerol etc.）	0%-20%
Surfactant（Tween-80, soybean phospholipid, etc.）	1%-2%
Filler（$CaCO_3$, SiO_2 etc.）	0%-20%
Corrigent（sucrose etc.）	Suitable amount
De-film agent（liquid paraffin, glycerol, stearic acid）	Suitable amount

（二）膜剂的制法

(2) The Preparation Method of Pellicles

膜剂的制备方法主要有：涂膜法、挤压法、延压法、热塑法等，目前国内制备中药膜剂多采用涂膜法。涂膜法制备工艺流程如图 18-1 所示。

The preparation methods of pellicles mainly include: coating method, extrusion method, rolling method, thermoplastic method, etc. At present, coating method is widely used in the preparation of traditional Chinese medicine pellicles in China. Coating method's progress is shown in Figure 18-1.

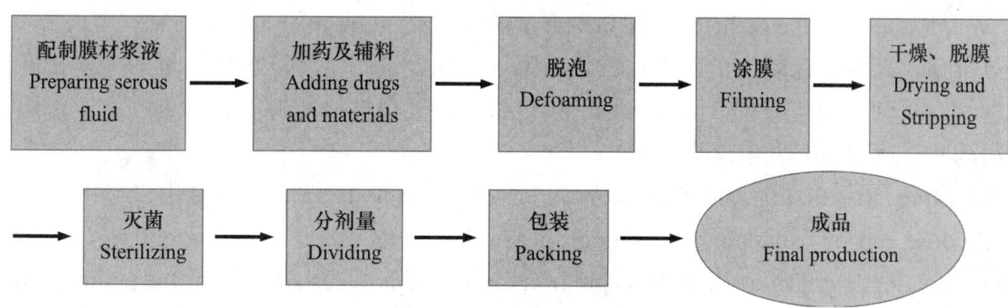

图 18-1　膜剂制备工艺流程

Figure 18-1　Preparation Process of Pellicle

1. 配制膜材浆液　取成膜材料加适宜的溶剂浸泡，使其充分溶胀，可于水浴上加热，溶解、滤过，即得均匀的浆液。

① **Preparing serous fluid**　Soaking film-forming materials with suitable solvent, make the materials full swelling which can be heated on the water bath, then dissolving, filtrating, finally, we get the homogeneous serous fluid.

2. 加药及辅料　可分为：①药物如为亲水性者，可直接与辅料加入浆液中，搅拌使溶解；②药物如为疏水性者，需研成极细粉末再与甘油、聚山梨酯 -80 等润湿剂研匀，再混悬于浆液中；③对于含药的乳浊液，应在其他药物、附加剂与胶浆混匀后，再加入胶浆中，以免不易分散均匀；④挥发性药物应待胶浆温度降至 50~60℃时加入，以免受热损失。

② **Adding drugs and auxiliary materials**　Can be divided into four situations which are as follow: a.If the drug is hydrophilicity, it can be directly added into the serous fluid with materials, and then stir to dissolve;b.If the drug is hydrophobic, it is necessary to grind the drug into impalpable powder,

then mix with wetting agents, such as glycerinum, tween-80, etc.then suspending into the serous fluid;c. For emulsion which contains drug, should be added into serous fluid after other drugs and materials has been added and mixed, in order to make them disperse uniformly;d.Volatile drug should join into serous fluid when the slurry temperature drops to 50-60℃ to avoid heat loss.

3. 脱泡 脱泡的目的是提高膜剂的外观质量，可采取保温法、热匀法、减压法三种方法脱泡。

③ **Defoaming** The purpose of defoaming is to improve the appearance quality of the pellicles. Three methods of defoaming can be adopted normally, such as the ways of heat preservation heat evenly and reduced pressure.

4. 涂膜 将加入药液的膜浆，倾倒在涂有脱膜剂的平板上，用固定厚度的推杆涂铺成膜，大量生产可用涂膜机进行，将脱泡后的药物浆液置于涂膜机如图 18-2 所示的料斗中，浆液经流液嘴流出，涂布在预先涂有脱膜剂的循环带上，使成厚度与宽度一致的涂层。

④ **Filming** Pour the drug-contained serous fluid onto the plate coated with the de-film agent, and apply the fixed thickness push rod to form the membrane, the mass production can be carried out by the coating machine. The serous fluid after defoaming is placed in the hopper of the coating machine as shown in Figure 18-2. The serous fluid flows out through the flow nozzle and is coated on the circulating belt precoated with the de-film agent to form a coating with the same thickness and width.

5. 干燥、脱膜 经自然干燥或低温加热除去溶剂，脱膜即得。脱膜直接影响到药膜的外观质量。膜脱得好，可得到一张完整的药膜；反之，则膜容易被撕裂或外观不规则。

⑤ **Drying and Stripping** The solvent can be removed by natural drying or low temperature heating. This step affect the appearance quality of pellicles directly.A complete pellicle can be obtained if striping well, conversely, the pellicle could be tear easily or has a irregular appearance.

6. 分剂量、灭菌、包装 干燥、脱膜后的膜剂，经含量测定计算出单剂量的分格长度，热烫划痕或剪切，灭菌，包装即得。膜剂所用的包装材料应无毒性、能够防止污染、方便使用，并不能与原料药物、成膜材料发生理化作用。

⑥ **Dividing, Sterilizing and Packing** After drying and stripping the pellicles, the cell length of a single dose can be calculated by content measurement, and then it can be obtained by scalding, scratching, shearing, sterilization and packaging. The packaging materials used in the pellicles should be non-toxic, non-pollution, convenient to use, and can not produce physical and chemical effects with drugs and film-forming materials.

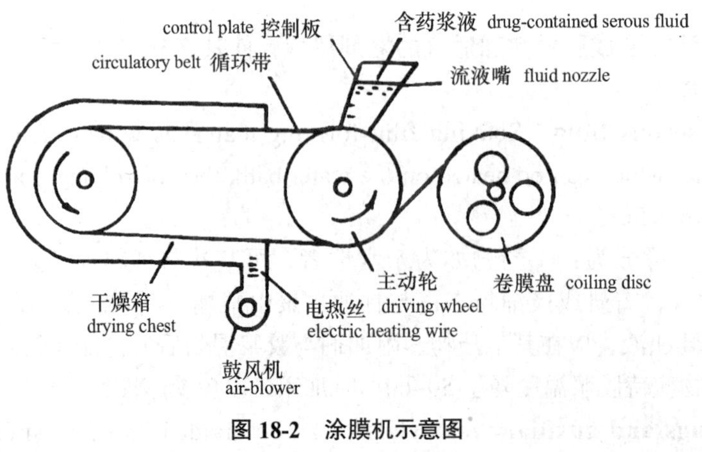

图 18-2 涂膜机示意图

Figure 18-2 Filming Machine

四、膜剂的质量检查

18.1.4 Quality Inspection of Pellicles

膜剂的质量检查除现行版《中国药典》膜剂项下的规定，有些应根据具体品种制订相应的标准。

Besides provisions of the current edition of *Chinese Pharmacopoeia*, The quality inspection of some pellicles should be based on specific varieties of the corresponding standards.

1. 外观 膜剂应完整光洁，厚度一致，色泽均匀，无明显气泡。多剂量的膜剂，分格压痕应均匀清晰，并能按压痕撕开。

(1) Appearance The appearance should be complete, the thickness should keep consistent, and color uniformed without obvious bubbles. For multidose film agent, the indentation shall be uniform and clear, and the indentation can be torn.

2. 重量差异 膜剂应按照现行版《中国药典》膜剂项下进行重量差异检查，除另有规定外，按照表 18-2，每片重量与平均重量相比较，超出重量差异限度的膜片不得多于 2 片，并不得有 1 片超出限度的 1 倍。

(2)Weight variation The pellicles should be inspected for weight variation according to the current edition of *Chinese Pharmacopoeia*, Unless other specified, accroding to Table18-2, compare to the average weight the pieces which over weight variation limit must be no more than 2 slices and should not have 1 piece that beyond the limit of 1 times.

表 18-2 膜剂的重量差异限度

膜剂的平均重量	重量差异限度
0.02g 及以下	± 15%
0.02~0.20g	± 10%
0.20g 以上	± 7.5%

Table18-2 Pellicles Weight Variation Limit

The average weight of the pellicles	Weight variation limit
<0.02g	± 15%
0.02-0.20g	± 10%
>0.20g	± 7.5%

3. 含量测定 取规定量的药膜，剪碎，按现行版《中国药典》规定的方法进行含量测定，应符合规定。

(3) Content determination Cutting up the specified drug pellicle, determining the content according to the regulated method of the current edition of *Chinese Pharmacopoeia*, and it should comply with the stipulations.

4. 微生物限度 除另有规定外，按现行版《中国药典》规定的非无菌产品微生物限度检查法检查，应符合标准。

(4) Microbial limit Unless otherwise specified, according to the current edition of *Chinese Pharmacopoeia* stipulated in the non-sterile product microbial limit test method inspection, should meet the standard.

5. 定性检查 取规定量的药膜，剪碎，按现行版《中国药典》规定方法对有关药物进行定性

鉴别，应符合规定。

(5) Qualitative examination Cutting up the specified drug pellicle, exam the pellicle according to the regulated method of the current edition of *Chinese Pharmacopoeia*, should comply with the stipulations.

6. 稳定性实验 经光照、高温、高湿加速实验或在室温下留样观察一段时间，其含量、外观、微生物检查等均应符合规定。

(6) Stability test Through light, high temperature, high humidity accelerated experiment or retention samples at room temperature to observe for a period of time, the content, appearance, microbiological examination and etc. should conform to the stipulations.

第二节 海绵剂

18.2 Spongia Agent

PPT

一、海绵剂的含义

18.2.1 The Definition of Spongia Agent

海绵剂系由亲水性胶体溶液经发泡、固化、冷冻、干燥后灭菌而制成的一种海绵状固体剂型，常用作创面或外科手术的辅助止血剂。

Spongia agent is a kind of sponge-solid dosage, which is made of hydrophilic colloid solution after foaming, curing, freeze, drying and sterilization, and it is a auxiliary hemostatic agent for wounds or surgeries.

二、海绵剂的分类

18.2.2 The Classifications of Spongia Agent

海绵剂根据原料的不同可分为蛋白质胶原类海绵，如明胶海绵、血浆海绵、纤维蛋白海绵，多糖类海绵，如淀粉海绵、海藻酸钠海绵等。根据含药与否可分为吸收性海绵、含药海绵。

According to the differences of raw materials, spongia agent can be divided into various kinds, and the classifications are as follow:Protein collagen sponge, Such as gelfoam sponge, plasma sponge, fibrin sponge, and polysaccharide sponge, such as starch sponge, sodium alginate sponge. According to contain drug state can be divided into absorptive sponge, drugs-contain sponge.

三、海绵剂的制法

18.2.3 The Preparation of Spongia Agent

由于海绵剂所用高分子材料的不同，制备过程略有差异。一般制备工艺流程如图 18-3 所示。

The preparation process of spongia agent is slightly different due to different polymer materials. The general preparation process is shown in Figure 18-3.

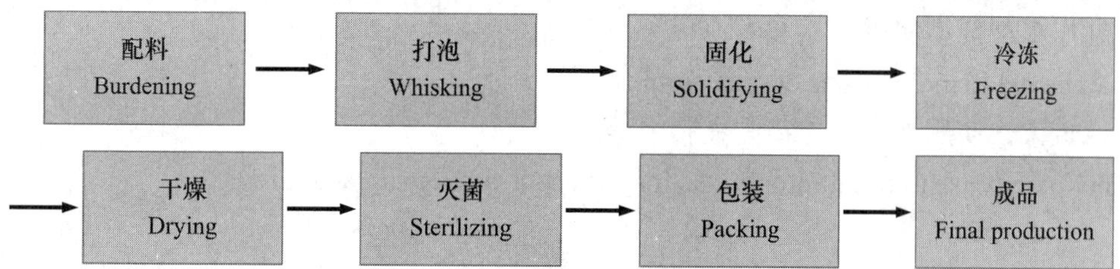

图 18-3 海绵剂制备工艺流程

Figure 18-3 Spongiaes Preparation Process

第三节 丹药

18.3 Dan Yao

一、丹药的含义

18.3.1 The Definition of Dan Yao

丹药系指用汞及某些矿物类药物，在高温条件下经过烧炼而制成的不同形状的含汞无机化合物。一般用于外科及皮肤科。

Dan Yao refers to a kind of mercury and some mineral drugs, which has various shapes and can be made through clinkering mercury and some other mineral drugs under the condition of high temperature. Usually used in surgery and dermatology.

目前临床常用的有红升丹、白降丹等。它们的毒性都很强，只能外用，使用不当会导致中毒或死亡。

丹药在中国已有两千多年的历史，它是我国劳动人民长期与疾病作斗争中，以及在冶炼技术的基础上发展起来的。中医古籍中也有将疗效显著或颜色红的制剂冠以“丹”字的记载，如大活络丹（丸剂）、王枢丹（锭剂）及化癣丹（液体制剂）等。

At present, the commonly used clinical Dan Yaos are hongshengdan, baijiangdan, etc. They are very toxic and can only be used externally. Improper use can lead to poisoning or death.

Dan Yao in China has a history of more than two thousand years, it is developed through Chinese long struggle against disease, and on the basis of smelting technology.In the ancient TCM books, some records that some agent dubbed the “Dan” can be found because it has distinct curative effect or red color, such as Da Huo Luo Dan (pills), Wang Shu Dan (pastille)and Hua Xuan Dan (liquid agent), etc.

二、丹药的特点

18.3.2 The Characteristics of Dan Yao

1. 药效剧烈，用量少。

(1) Having intensive effect and the dosage is small.

2. 药效确切，用法多样化。

(2) Pesticide effect is exact, and Usages are various.

3. 可制作多种剂型使用。

(3) Can be made into various dosage form.

4. 毒性较大，使用不当易导致重金属中毒。

(4) The toxicity is strong, improper use may cause heavy metal poisoning.

三、丹药的分类
18.3.3 The Classification of Dan Yao

丹药可根据制备方法及色泽进行分类。按制备方法可分为升丹和降丹，按色泽可分为红丹与白丹。升丹及红丹的典型代表是红升丹（HgO），降丹及白丹的典型代表是白降丹（$HgCl_2$）。

Dan Yao can be classified according to the preparation and color. According to the preparation methods, Dan Yao can be divided into Jiang Dan and Sheng Dan, and according to the color, it can be divided into Red Dan and White Dan. The typical representative are Red-Sheng Dan(HgO)and White-Jiang Dan($HgCl_2$).

四、丹药的制法
18.3.4 The Preparation of Dan Yao

丹药的制法有升法、降法和半升半降法等。

The preparation methods of Dan Yao are Sheng method, Jiang method and Half-Sheng-Half-Jiang method, etc.

升法 系指药料经高温反应，生成物凝结在上方覆盖物内侧面而得到结晶状化合物的炼制法。

Sheng Method Refers to the refining process in which the product condenses in the inner side of the upper covering after the high temperature reaction of the drug material to obtain the crystalline compound.

降法 系指药料经高温反应，生成物降至下方接收器中，冷却析出结晶状化合物的炼制法。

Jiang Method Refers to the refining method in which the product is lowered into the receiver below and the crystalline compound is cooled and precipitated after high temperature reaction of the drug.

半升半降法 系指药料经高温反应，生成的气态化合物，一部分上升凝结在上方覆盖物内，另一部分散落在锅内的炼制法。

Half-Sheng-Half-Jiang Method Refers to the refining process that getting products through high temperature, generated gaseous compounds, partly rising to the overlay and partly fell down into the pot.

五、丹药生产过程中的防护
18.3.5 The Protective Measures During Preparation of Dan Yao

丹药在炼制过程之中会产生大量有毒气体，若此气体不经过净化直接排出，会污染环境，气体泄漏还会使操作人员中毒，因此应注意以下防护措施。

During the preparation process of Dan Yao, a large number of poisonous gas can be produced. If the gas directly discharged without purification, it may cause environment pollution; And the gas leakage will cause the operators poisoning, so attentions should be paid to the following protective measures.

1. 生产丹药的厂房应远离居民区，生产车间应有高效的排风设施及毒气净化回收装置，对车间内空气要进行监测。

(1) The plants of Dan Yao should be far away from residential areas, and production workshops should equipped with efficient ventilation facilities and gas purification recovery units, meanwhile the air in the workshop should be monitored.

2. 烧炼丹药的容器不得有砂眼、裂缝，烧炼全过程应密闭，以防毒气逸出而引起中毒、导致丹药收率低。

(2) There should be no sand holes or cracks in the container for burning alchemy, and the whole clinkering process should be sealed, in case the gas escape and cause poisoning, as well as lead to lower yield coefficient.

3. 操作者必须戴上防护眼镜和防护口罩，操作完毕后及时洗手，操作者还应进行定期体检。

(3) The operator must wear protective glasses and protective mask, wash hands in time after operation.The operator should have regular physical examination..

第四节 烟剂、烟熏剂、香囊（袋）剂

18.4 Fumicants, Fumigants and Sachets

PPT

一、烟剂

18.4.1 Fumicants

烟剂系指将饮片经适宜方法加工后单独或掺入烟丝中，卷制成供点燃吸入用的香烟型固体剂型，也称作药烟，制备时可加入助燃剂，如碳酸钾、氯酸钾、硝酸钾等。

Fumicants refer to the appropriate method after the processing of pieces of Chinese herbal medicine single or mixed with tobacco, made into a kind of cigarette-solid dosage form, for light suction, also known as medicine cigarette. During the preparation process, we can add some combustion improvers, such as potassium carbonate, potassium chlorate and potassium nitrate, etc.

烟剂分为全中药烟剂和含中药烟剂两类，前者如喘息烟一号，后者如华山参药烟。

Fumicants can be divide into two types, the one comprises by all the Chinese herbal medicine, such as Breathing cigarette NO1. the other one comprises by some Chinese herbal medicine, such as Huashanshen medicine cigarette.

全中药烟剂可将饮片切成细丝，加入助燃剂混合均匀，低温干燥后，卷成香烟状，包装，即可。含中药烟剂一般是将饮片用适宜方法提取后所得提取物经含量测定后按一定比例加入烟丝中，若所得提取物量较多，也可部分喷洒使烟丝吸收，其余低温干燥后与烟丝混合均匀按卷烟工艺制备成卷烟，最后分剂量包装，即得。

The preparation processing of fumicants that are just made of TCM, is to cut the slices into filaments, add some combustion improvers, and mix, after drying at a low temperature, roll to cigarettes and pack. To produce the other one which just contain some TCM, the slices should be extracted by using appropriate methods, and after determining the content, inject the extract into filaments in a certain

proportion. If the quantity of extract is enough, the extract also can spray to make the filaments absorb partly, the rest can mix with filaments after drying at low temperature, and roll to cigarettes, packing.

二、烟熏剂
18.4.2 Fumigants

烟熏剂系指借助助燃剂燃烧后产生的烟雾起到杀虫、杀菌和预防、治疗疾病作用的剂型；也有利用艾叶、艾柱等，在穴位灸燃产生的烟雾和温热作用治疗疾病的。

Fumigant refers to the dosage form that can kill insects, kill bacteria and prevent and treat diseases by means of the smog produced by combustion of combustion-promoting agent. There are also the use of mugwort leaves, pillars, and so on, moxibustion at the acupuncture point to produce the smog and heating effect to treat diseases.

不同类型的烟熏剂可采用不同的制备方法。

Different types of fumigants can be prepared by different methods.

1. 灭菌消毒、杀虫烟熏剂的制法 本类烟熏剂除选用具有灭菌杀虫功效的中药外，可酌情添加燃料、助燃剂、稀释剂及冷却剂，混合均匀后插入导火索制成，现已少用。

(1) The preparation of sterilizing and insecticidal fumigant In addition to the traditional Chinese medicine with sterilization and insecticidal effect, this kind of fumigant can be used added as appropriate fuel, accelerant, diluent and coolant, mixed evenly and then inserted into the fuse, is now seldom used.

2. 燃香烟熏剂的制法 制作燃香烟熏剂需要的原料有木粉、中药、黏合剂、助燃剂及其他附加剂等。燃香的制备一般是先将药材粉碎成细粉与其他物料混合均匀后加入一定比例的黏合剂制成软材，再用制药设备压制成直条状或盘卷状，干燥包装，即得。

(2) The preparation of burning fumigant The materials of burning fumigants are wood powder, TCM, adhesive, accelerant and some other additives. The producing process is generally as follow: smash the TCM into fine powder and mixed with other materials, then add some proportion of adhesive to make soft materials, after that pressed them into strips or coils with pharmaceutical equipment, and then dry them for packaging.

三、香囊（袋）剂
18.4.3 Sachets

香囊（袋）剂系指将含有挥发性成分的饮片分装在布制的囊（袋）中或制成荷包状，用于预防、治疗疾病的剂型。目前，临床使用的许多含药枕垫、护膝、护背、护腰、护肩等都属于香囊（袋）剂。

Sachets refer to a kind of dosage that pack TCM slices which contain volatile component into the cloth pouch or bag, used to prevent and treat diseases. At present, many drug pillows, knee pads, back pads, waist pads which are used in clinical, are belong to sachets.

中药香囊（袋）剂制法简单，将饮片粉碎成适宜粒度，分装在布制的囊（袋）中即可。制备时应注意，一般药枕中的中药填充物粉碎成粗粉，香袋中的中药填充物粉碎成细粉。制备囊（袋）的棉布或棉绸要求透气性好、细密、柔软且不漏药粉。

Traditional Chinese medicine sachet agent preparation method is simple, the pieces will be crushed

into appropriate particle size and put into cloth bag. During preparation, some points should be noted. In general, the traditional Chinese medicine fillers in general medicine pillows are crushed into coarse powder, while the traditional Chinese medicine fillers in sachets are crushed into fine powder. The cotton or cotton fabric for preparing the bags requires good permeability, fine density, softness and no leakage of powder.

第五节　离子导入剂与沐浴剂

18.5　Ionphoretic Agent and Bath Agent

PPT

一、离子导入剂

18.5.1　Ionphoretic Agent

（一）含义

(1) Definition

离子导入技术是利用直流电将药物经电极导入皮肤，进入组织或体循环的一种方法。

Ion implantation is a method of using direct current to deliver drugs through electrodes into the skin and into the tissue or systemic circulation.

离子导入剂系指将饮片用适宜方法提取、浓缩、纯化后制成专供离子导入用的药物形式与离子导入系统共同组成的经皮给药制剂。离子导入系统一般由电池、控制线路、电极和贮库四部分组成。

Ionphoretic agent refers to a percutaneous drug delivery preparation composed of a drug form exclusively for ion delivery and an ion delivery system after the preparation is extracted, concentrated and purified by appropriate methods. Ion-delivery system is generally composed of battery, control circuit, electrode and storage.

（二）特点

(2) Characteristics

1. 局部给药疗效好。
2. 药物作用时间长。
3. 出现不良反应少。
4. 兼有局部与全身作用。

① Local administration is effective. ② Long effective time of drug. ③ Less adverse reaction. ④ Have topical and systemic effects.

但在使用过程中应注意：导入时间过长、电流强度过大、电极使用不当等都有可能导致皮肤灼伤。其次，一些恶性血液疾病、皮肤湿疹、重要脏器病变等患者严禁使用，以免病情恶化。

But attentions need to pay: If the import time is too long, current intensity is too large, or electrode improper use may cause skin burns. Meanwhile, Patients who have malignant blood diseases, skin eczema and important viscera lesions, are strictly prohibited to avoid deterioration.

（三）影响离子导入效率的药物因素

(3) The Drug Factors that Influence the Efficiency of Ionphoretic Agent

1. 药物所带的电荷 一般认为，离子导入给药速率与药物所带的电荷成正比。

① **The charge of drug** Generally speaking, the dosing rate of ionphoretic agent is proportional to the charge of drugs.

2. 药物的分子量 一般而言，渗透速率随着药物分子量的增大而减小。

② **The molecular weight of drug** Generally speaking, the penetration rate decreased with the increase of drug molecular weight.

3. 药物浓度 药物浓度高，导入量大，反之则小。但通常情况下，临床采用的制剂中药物含量也不宜过高，一般以 1%~10% 为宜。

③ **The concentration of drug** The higher drug concentration, the larger import quantity, smaller on conversely. But usually, the drug concentration used in clinical is better not too high,1%-10% is appropriate.

4. 贮库溶液的组成 溶液中的其他离子、溶液的 pH 均会显著地影响离子导入效果；渗透促进剂与离子导入剂联合使用，可以有效提高大分子多肽类药物经皮转运效率。

④ **The composition of storage solution** The other ions, pH of the solution will affect the import effect significantly. What's more, osmosis promoter and inophoretic agent used in combination, could improve the efficiency of percutaneous transfer of large-molecule polypeptide drugs effectively.

二、沐浴剂

18.5.2 Bath Agent

沐浴剂是指饮片提取物单独或加入适宜的表面活性剂制成的液体或固体中药剂型。

Bath agent refers to a kind of liquid or solid TCM dosages that made of slice extract solely or with suitable surfactants.

液体沐浴剂一般是将饮片提取物制成每次用量为 10~20ml 的水性或醇性液体制剂，部分沐浴剂还可以添加表面活性剂起到洁肤作用。

Each dosage of liquid bath agent is 10-20ml, and the solvent can be water or alcohol, some liquid bath agent can act cleaning effect by adding surfactants.

固体沐浴剂的制备方法如下：部分药材粉碎成粗粉，其余药材提取浓缩成稠膏，混合后烘干，其中处方中含有的芳香性药物可以直接粉碎成粗粉，也可提取挥发油喷洒在粗粉中，最后将混合物分装在特制纱布包或滤纸袋中，密封后再加一层外包装，即得。

The preparation method of solid bath agent is as follow: some parts of herbs crumbled into coarse powder, the rest of the herbs extracted and condensed into thick paste, dried after mixed, the aromatic herbs can be smashed into coarse powder or extract the volatile oil and sprayed in the powder, finally, packed the mixture in special gauze bag or filter paper bag, added a layer of the outer packing after sealed.

第六节 锭剂、糕剂、钉剂、线剂、条剂、灸剂、熨剂与棒剂

18.6 Pastille, Cake Agent, Nail Agent, Thread Agent, Strip Agent, Moxibustion Agent, Compression Agent and Club Agent

PPT

一、锭剂
18.6.1 Pastille

（一）锭剂的含义
(1) Definition

锭剂系指饮片细粉与适合的黏合剂（或利用药材本身的黏性）制成纺锤形、方形、长方形、圆柱形或块状等不同形状的固体剂型。可供内服或外用。

Pastille is a kind of solid dosages which made of TCM powder with suitable adhesive(or use viscosity of drug itself), it has different shapes, such as spindle-shape, square, rectangular, cylindrical or block, available for internal or external use.

（二）锭剂的制法
(2) Preparation Methods

锭剂的制备方法有捏搓法和模制法两种，具体如下：

There are two kinds preparation methods of pastille: kneading and molding.

1. 捏搓法 先将处方中饮片粉碎成细粉，用糯米糊、蜂蜜或处方规定的其他黏合剂混合均匀，搓条、分割、按规定重量及形状搓捏成型，干燥即得。

① **Kneading** First crushed the slices into fine powder, mixed with adhesives, such as glutinous rice paste, honey or other prescribed adhesive, then rubbed, split, kneaded according to the ruled weight and shape, dried them.

2. 模制法 将处方中药物饮片粉碎成细粉，加入处方规定的黏合剂，混合均匀。先压制成大块薄片，分切成适当大小后，置入锭模中，加模盖压制成一定形状的药锭，剪齐边缘，干燥，即得。也可用压锭机按规定形状及重量压制成锭。

② **Molding** First crushed the slices into fine powder, mixed with adhesives, pressed into large pieces of sheets, cut into appropriate size, then placed in the mold, and cover pressed into a certain shape, cut edge parts and dry. Also can use pastille-pressed machine to made pastilles according to ruled shape and weight.

部分需包衣或打光的锭剂，还应用制法项下规定的包衣材料进行包衣或打光。

Some pastilles which need to be coated or polished should meet the regulations of preparation to choose coating materials.

二、糕剂
18.6.2 Cake Agent

糕剂系指饮片细粉与米粉、蔗糖加水混匀后蒸制而成的块状剂型。糕剂常用于治疗脾胃虚弱、慢性消化不良等疾病。常用的有万应神曲糕、八珍糕等。

Cake agent is a kind of block dosages that made of slice powder, rice flour, sugar and water steamed into cake, which is often used to treat spleen and stomach weakness, chronic indigestion disease and etc. For example, Wanyingshenqu Gao or Bazhen Gao.

三、钉剂
18.6.3 Nail Agent

钉剂系指饮片细粉与糯米粉混匀后加水加热制成软材，按剂量大小分割，搓成细长且一端或两端尖锐的外用固体剂型。钉剂多含有毒性药物或腐蚀性药物，且具有缓释作用。一般供外科插入给药，用于治疗痔疮、瘘管及溃疡等。

Nail agent refers to a kind of solid dosages, which is made by following preparation method: slice powder mixed with glutinous rice flour, and added water, heated to soft materials, split according to dose, then rubbed into slender with one or two ends sharp, for external use. Usually, nail agent contains toxic or corrosive drugs, and has slow-release effect, commonly used for surgical insertion, used in the treatment of hemorrhoids, fistula and ulcer, etc.

四、线剂
18.6.4 Thread Agent

线剂系指将丝线或棉线置药液中先浸后煮，经干燥制成的一种外用剂型。

Thread agent is a kind of external-use dosage, which is made by following process: silk or cotton soak in solution, and cook, then dry.

五、条剂
18.6.5 Strip Agent

条剂系指用桑皮纸黏药膏后搓捻成细条，或用桑皮纸搓捻成条，黏一层面糊，再黏药粉而制成的外用制剂，又称纸捻。条剂主要用于外科插入疮口或瘘管，以引流脓液，拔毒去腐，生肌敛口。

Strip agent refers to the external-use dosage made by rubbing the ointment on mulberry paper and twisting it into fine strips, or twisting it into strips on mulberry paper and sticking a layer of paste and then sticking the powder, also known as paper twisting. Strip agent is mainly used for surgical insertion of wound or fistula to drain pus, extract poison and remove rot, and collect muscle.

六、灸剂
18.6.6 Moxibustion Agent

灸剂系指将艾叶经捣、碾成绒状后，或另加其他药料捻制成卷烟状或其他形状，供熏灼穴位及患部的外用制剂。灸剂按形状可分为艾头、艾柱、艾条三种，按加药与否可分为艾条与含药艾。

Moxibustion agent refers to an external-use dosage that can be used to fumigate acupoints and affected areas, which is made through this process: mugwort leaves are pounded, ground into a pile, or twisted with other ingredients to make a cigarette or other shape grinding. According to the shape, moxibustion can be divided into mugwor thead, mugwort column, mogwor stripe, according to whether contain drug, moxibustion can be divided into mogwort and drug-containing mogwort.

七、熨剂
18.6.7　Compression Agent

熨剂系指将饮片细粉、饮片提取液与经煅制的铁砂混合制成的外用制剂。用时拌醋生热，利用热刺激及药物蒸汽投入熨贴部位达到治疗目的。

Compression agent refers to an external-use dosage made by mixing fine powder or extract with calcined iron sand. Compression agent need be mixed with vinegar to generate heat, the use of thermal stimulation and drug steam into the iron paste site to achieve the purpose of treatment.

岗位对接

八、棒剂
18.6.8　Club Agent

重点小结

棒剂系指将饮片用适宜方法加工后，加入适宜辅料制成的小棒状的外用固体剂型。可直接用于皮肤或黏膜上，起腐蚀、收敛作用，多用于眼科。

Club agent is a kind of solid external-use dosages, made of slice prepared through appropriate process, add suitable auxiliary materials made into small sticks. It can be used directly on the skin or mucous membrane, corrosion, convergence, often used in ophthalmology.

题库

（郑勇凤）

第十九章　药物制剂新技术与新剂型
Chapter 19　New Technologies and New Dosage Forms of Pharmaceutical Preparations

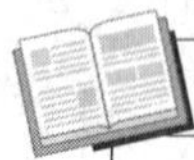

学习目标 ¦ Learning Goals

知识要求：

1. **掌握**　包合物、固体分散体、微囊与微球、脂质体的含义、特点及常用的制备方法，纳米乳、亚微乳、纳米粒的含义与特点，缓释制剂、控释制剂与靶向制剂的含义与特点。

2. **熟悉**　常见的包合材料如环糊精的性质，固体分散体的类型、药物分散状态及常用载体材料，微囊的囊材及质量评价，纳米乳的制备及质量评价，脂质体的组成与分类、质量评价，缓释制剂、控释制剂与靶向制剂的释药机理、分类及制备方法。

3. **了解**　包合物、固体分散体的质量评价、亚微乳及纳米粒的制备，缓释制剂、控释制剂与靶向制剂的研究进展及在中药中的研究现状等。

能力要求：

学会包合物、固体分散体、微囊、脂质体的制备与质量评价，能制备包合物、固体分散体、微囊、脂质体，并进行质量评价。学会缓释、控释制剂和靶向制剂的制备与质量检测方法，认识新剂型的重要性及中药制剂的研究方向。

Knowledge requirements:

1. To master the definitions, characteristics and common preparation methods of inclusion compound, solid dispersion, microcapsule and microsphere, liposome; The definitions and characteristics of nano-emulsion, sub-microemulsion and nanoparticle; The definitions and characteristics of sustained release preparation, controlled release preparation and targeting preparation.

2. To be familiar with the properties of common inclusion materials such as cyclodextrin; types of solid dispersion, drug dispersion and commonly carrier materials; quality evaluation of microcapsules; preparation and quality evaluation of nano-emulsions; classification, composition and quality evaluation of liposomes;drug release mechanism, classification and preparation methods of sustained release preparation, controlled release preparation and targeting preparation.

3. To know the quality evaluation of inclusion compound and solid dispersions; preparation methods of submicroemulsions and nanoparticles; research progress of sustained

release preparations, controlled release preparations and targeting preparations in traditional Chinese medicine.

Ability requirements:

Learn the methods of preparation and quality evaluation of inclusion compound, solid dispersion, microcapsule and liposome, and be able to prepare inclusion compounds, solid dispersions, microcapsules, and liposomes and perform quality evaluation. Learn the methods of preparing and quality evaluation of sustained release, controlled release preparations and targeting preparations. Recognize the importance of new dosage forms and the research direction of traditional Chinese medicine preparations.

第一节 药物制剂新技术

19.1 New Pharmaceutical Technique

PPT

一、包合技术

19.1.1 Inclusion Compounds Technology

（一）含义

(1) The Definition of Inclusion Technology

包合技术是指在一定的条件下，一种分子被包嵌于另一种分子的空穴结构内形成包合物的技术。这种包合物由主分子和客分子组成，又被称为分子胶囊，其主分子即包合材料，具有空穴结构；客分子即药物，被包嵌在主分子空穴结构内。包合是物理过程而不是化学反应，包合物的形成及其稳定性，与主、客分子的立体结构密切相关。

Inclusion technology refers to a technology that one molecule is embedded in the cavity structure of another molecule under certain condition to form an inclusion compound. This inclusion compound is composed of a host molecule and a guest molecule, also known as molecular capsule. The host molecule is the inclusion material which has a hole structure, and the guest molecule is the drug which embedded in the cavity structure of the host molecule. The inclusion process is a physical process rather than a chemical reaction. The formation and stability of inclusion compounds are closely related to the three-dimensional structures of the host and guest molecules.

（二）特点

(2) The Characteristics of Inclusion Technology

1. 增加药物的溶解度 难溶性药物被β-环糊精（β-CD）包合后可形成水溶性包合物，从而提高药物的溶解度。

① Increasing the solubility of the drugs When insoluble drugs are included inside β-cyclodextrin (β-CD), water-soluble inclusion compounds can be formed, which can improve the solubility of drugs.

2. 增加药物的稳定性 易氧化、水解、挥发的药物包合到包合材料的空穴结构中，可使药物与外界环境隔绝，大大增加了药物的稳定性。

② **Increasing the stability of the drugs** The inclusion of drugs which is easy to oxidize, hydrolyze and volatilize can protect drug against the external environment and greatly increase the stability of the drugs.

3. 掩盖药物的不良气味和降低其刺激性 具有不良臭味或较强刺激性的药物经包合后，可掩盖其不良臭味，降低其刺激性。

③ **Concealing the bad smell of the drugs and reducing its irritation** The drugs with bad smell or strong irritation can be embedded to conceal the bad odor and reduce the irritation after inclusion.

4. 调节药物的释药速率 难溶性药物经亲水性材料包合后，可提高其溶出速率；反之，疏水性材料包合水溶性药物后，能降低其溶解度。

④ **Adjusting the release rate of the drugs** The hydrophilic inclusion material can improve dissolution rate of poorly soluble drugs. And the hydrophobic material can reduce the solubility of water-soluble drugs.

5. 使液体药物粉末化 挥发油等液体药物包合后可呈固态粉末状，不仅增加其稳定性，且易于混合和加工成其他剂型，如制成片剂、胶囊剂等。

⑤ **Converting liquid drug into solid powder** Liquid drug such as volatile oil after inclusion can be a solid powder, which can increase the stability of liquid medicine. Besides, the solid powder is easy to mix with other drug, and provides facilitation of preparation formulation, such as tablets, capsules, etc.

6. 提高药物的生物利用度 药物经包合后，可因溶解度的增大或易于通过生物细胞膜而改善吸收，提高药物的生物利用度。

⑥ **Improving the bioavailability of the drugs** The improvement in bioavailability is in part attributed to enhanced solubility of drugs, and in part may be attributed to enhanced bio-membrane’s permeability via the inclusion.

（三）包合物的分类

(3) Classification of Inclusion Compounds

包合物根据主分子的构成可分为单分子包合物、多分子包合物和大分子包合物。根据主分子形成空穴的几何形状，可分为管状包合物、笼状包合物和层状包合物。

According to the composition of the host molecules, inclusion compounds can be divided into single-molecular, multi-molecular, and macromolecular inclusion compounds. According to the 3D structures of the cavity formed by the host molecules, the inclusion complexes can be divided into tubular inclusion compounds, cage inclusion compounds and layered inclusion compounds.

（四）常见的包合材料

(4) Common Inclusion Materials

通常可用环糊精、胆酸、淀粉、纤维素、蛋白质、核酸等作包合材料。目前常用的是环糊精及其衍生物。

Generally, cyclodextrin, cholic acid, starch, cellulose, protein, nucleic acid, etc. can be used as inclusion materials. Cyclodextrin and its derivatives are currently commonly used in preparations.

1. 环糊精（CD） CD 系淀粉经酶解环合后得到的由 6~12 个葡萄糖分子以 1，4- 糖苷键连接而成的环状低聚糖，为水溶性的白色结晶状粉末。常见的有 α、β、γ 三种，分别由 6、7、8 个葡萄糖分子构成。其中以 β-CD 最为常用，其在水中溶解度最小，易从水中析出结晶，且其溶解度随温度升高而增大，如温度在 20℃、40℃、60℃、80℃、100℃时，其溶解度分别为 18.7g/L、

37g/L、80g/L、183g/L、256g/L。

① **Cyclodextrin (CD)** CD, a kind of water-soluble white crystalline powder, is a cyclic oligosaccharide obtained from enzymatic conversion of starch. It is composed of 6-12 glucose molecules linked by 1, 4-glycoside bond. There are three common types including α, β and γ, possessing 6, 7, or 8glucopyranose units, respectively. Among the three CDs, β-CD is the most commonly used material. It has the lowest solubility in water, and it is easy to precipitate crystal from water. As the temperature increases, the solubility of β-CD increases. When the temperature is 20, 40, 60, 80, and 100℃, the corresponding solubility is 18.7, 37, 80, 183, 256g/L, respectively.

2. 环糊精衍生物 近年来β-CD衍生物应用较多，如甲基-β-CD、羟丙基-β-CD、羟乙基-β-CD、葡糖基-β-CD等水溶性衍生物，乙基-β-CD等疏水性衍生物等。

② **Cyclodextrin derivatives** In recent years, β-CD derivatives are widely used, such as methyl-β-CD, hydroxypropyl-β-CD, hydroxyethyl-β-CD, glucosyl-β-CD and other water-soluble derivatives, ethyl-β-CD and other hydrophobic derivatives.

（五）包合物的制备方法

(5) Preparation Methods of Inclusion Compounds

1. 饱和水溶液法 亦称为重结晶法或共沉淀法。系先将β-CD制成饱和水溶液，再以一定比例加入药物，并在适宜温度下搅拌一定时间，直到形成包合物。经静置或冷藏、浓缩、加沉淀剂等使包合物充分析出，滤过、洗涤、干燥，即得。

① **Saturated aqueous solution method** It is also named recrystallization method or coprecipitation method. Firstly, add β - CD into saturated aqueous solution, then add guest drug in a certain proportion, at last stir for a certain time at a suitable temperature until the inclusion compounds is formed. The inclusion compounds can be fully precipitated by standing or cold storage, concentration and addition of precipitants. Finally, the inclusion compounds of β - CD is obtained by filtration, washing and drying.

案例导入 ¦ Case example

案例 19-1 冰片-β-CD 包合物

19-1 The Borneol-β-CD Inclusion Compounds

处方： 冰片 0.66g β-CD 4g

Ingredients: borneol 0.66g β-CD 4g

制法： 取β-CD 4g，溶于100ml 55℃水中，保温。另取冰片0.66g，加乙醇20ml溶解，在搅拌下缓慢滴加冰片溶液于β-CD溶液中，继续搅拌30分钟，冰箱放置24小时，抽滤，蒸馏水洗涤，40℃干燥，即得。

Making Procedure: Take 4g of β-CD, dissolve in 100ml of water at 55℃, keep warm. Take 0.66g of borneol, add 20ml of ethanol to dissolve it, slowly drop borneol solution into β-CD solution under stirring, and continue to stir for 30min. Finally, transfer the solution to the refrigerator and store for 24hours, filter with suction, wash with distilled water, and dry at 40℃.

注解：（1）冰片具有挥发性，制备成β-CD包合物可以防止其挥发散失。

（2）影响饱和水溶液法的因素主要有主客分子投料比、包合温度、包合时间、搅拌方式等。

Notes: ① Borneol is volatile, and the β-CD inclusion compounds can prevent its volatile loss.

② The main factors that affect the saturated aqueous solution method are the ratio of host and guest molecules, inclusion temperature, inclusion time, stirring method, and so on.

思考题：包合物不完全析出时，应如何处理？

Questions: How to deal with incomplete precipitation of inclusion compound in water?

---

2. 研磨法 取β-CD，加入2~5倍量水混合研匀，加入药物（难溶性药物应先溶于有机溶剂中），充分研磨成糊状物，低温干燥，即得。

② **Grinding method** Take β-CD, add 2 to 5 times the amount of water, grind and mix well, then add the drugs (Poorly soluble drugs should be dissolved in organic solvents first), fully grind into a paste, and dry at low temperature to obtain the inclusion compounds.

影响研磨法制备包合物的因素主要有包合时间、溶媒含醇量、药物与β-CD的比例等。

The main factors that affect the preparation of inclusion compounds are the inclusion time, the content of alcohol in the solvent, the ratio of drugs to β – CD, etc.

3. 冷冻干燥法 将药物加入CD的饱和水溶液中，搅拌一定时间，冷冻干燥，即得。该法适用于遇热易分解的药物，所得到的成品疏松、溶解性能好。

③ **Freeze drying method** Added drug to a saturated aqueous solution of CD, stir for a certain time, and freeze-dry to get it. The method is suitable for the thermolabile drugs. The finished products are loose and have good solubility.

4. 喷雾干燥法 将药物分散于CD的饱和水溶液中，搅拌，喷雾干燥，即得。该法适用于难溶性、疏水性药物。

④ **Spry drying method** Disperse the drugs in a saturated aqueous solution of CD, and then stirred and spray-dried to obtain the inclusion compounds. This method is suitable for poorly soluble and hydrophobic drugs.

（六）包合物的物相鉴定

(6) Quality Evaluation of Inclusion Complexes

药物与包合材料是否形成包合物，可根据包合物的性质和结构状态，采用X-射线衍射法、热分析法、红外光谱法、核磁共振法、薄层色谱法、荧光光谱法、紫外分光光度法等进行验证。

Whether the drugs and the inclusion materials form inclusion compounds can be determined by following methods: X-ray diffraction, thermal analysis, infrared spectroscopy, nuclear magnetic resonance, thin layer chromatography, fluorescence spectroscopy, UV spectrophotometry, etc.

二、固体分散技术

19.1.2 Solid Dispersion Technology

（一）含义

(1) Definition of Solid Dispersion Technology

固体分散技术是指药物与载体材料混合制成高度分散的固体分散体的技术。药物与不同载体形成的固体分散体，其溶出速率和程度相差较大。固体分散体作为制剂的中间体，可根据需要进一步制备成片剂、胶囊剂等剂型。

This technology refers to preparing highly dispersive solid dispersion with mixture of drugs and carriers, the dissolution rate and degree of which vary widely with different carriers. Solid dispersions, as intermediate, can be prepared into some dosage forms (e.g., tablets, capsules) as required.

（二）特点

(2) Characteristics of Solid Dispersions

1. 利用不同性质的载体可达到速释、缓释控释的目的 以水溶性材料为载体，可改善难溶性药物的溶解性能，提高溶出速率，从而提高其生物利用度；也可选用难溶性载体制成缓释固体分散体，还可用肠溶性载体材料控制药物在小肠释放。

① Various carriers determine different formulation properties, including immediate-release, extended-release or controlled-release. Water-soluble carriers serve as an effective means of increasing of aqueous solubility, dissolution and bioavailability of hydrophobic drug. Also, water-insoluble carriers are used for sustained-release preparation and enteric-coated carriers are used to ensure that drug is dissolved in the intestine.

2. 提高药物稳定性 因载体材料对药物分子具有包蔽作用。

② Improving drug stability This characteristic is due to the inclusion effect of carriers on drugs.

3. 可使液体药物固体化 液体药物制成固体分散体，不仅提高其稳定性，且利于加工成其他剂型，如片剂、胶囊剂等。

③ Converting liquid drugs to solid state The conversion not only improves drug stability, but also benefits the preparation to other dosage forms (e.g., tablets, capsules).

4. 缺点 固体分散体中药物的分散状态稳定性不高，久贮过程中往往发生老化、溶出速率变慢等现象。

④ Solid dispersions have the disadvantages of reduced physical stability and decreased dissolution rate with aging.

（三）固体分散体的分类

(3) Classifications of Solid Dispersions

1. 按释药特性分类

① Classified by release characteristics

（1）速释型固体分散体 是指用亲水性载体制成的固体分散体。其速释机理为：①药物在固体分散体中可能以分子、胶体、亚稳定态、微晶以及无定形态存在，药物的表面积和分散程度高，有利于药物的溶出和吸收。②亲水性载体材料可提高药物的润湿性。

a. Immediate-release solid dispersions It refers to solid dispersions prepared by hydrophilic carrier. The mechanisms are as follows: Drugs in solid dispersion may exist in molecular, colloidal metastable, microcrystalline and amorphous state, which can improve the dissolution and absorption of drugs with its increased surface area and dispersion. Also, carriers can increase the wettability of drug to avoid precipitation.

（2）缓释、控释型固体分散体 是指用水不溶性或脂溶性载体制成的固体分散体。其释药机制与缓释、控释制剂相同。

b. Extended-release and controlled-release solid dispersions It refers to solid dispersions prepared by hydrophobic carriers. Its mechanisms are same as that of extended-release and controlled-release preparations.

（3）肠溶型固体分散体 是指用肠溶性材料为载体，制成肠道释药的固体分散体。

c. Enteric solid dispersions It refers to solid dispersions prepared by enteric carriers show intestinal-located release performance.

2. 按分散状态分类

② Classified by dispersion state

（1）低共熔混合物 是指药物与载体以适当比例在较低温度下熔融，骤冷固化后形成的固体分散体。药物以微晶状态分散于载体中。

a. Eutectic mixture Drugs and carriers are melt in proper ratio at a low temperature, then a solid dispersion is formed after cooling. Drugs is dispersed in an eutectic mixture in microcrystalline state.

（2）固体溶液　是指药物以分子状态分散于熔融的载体中形成的均相体系，类似于溶液的分散性质。

b. Solid solutions Solid solutions have their drugs dispersed molten carriers in molecular state to form the homogeneous system which is similar to the real solution.

（3）玻璃溶液或玻璃混悬液　是指药物溶于熔融的透明状无定形载体中，骤然冷却，得到质脆透明状态的固体溶液。

c. Glass solutions or glass suspensions This brittle and transparent solid solutions have drugs dissolved in molten amorphous carriers and then cooling.

（4）共沉淀物或共蒸发物　是指固体药物与载体以适当比例形成的非结晶性无定形物。

d. Coprecipitate or co-evaporate It's the amorphous substance formed by solid drugs with carriers in proper ratio.

（四）固体分散体常用的载体材料

(4) Common Carriers

常见的载体材料可分为水溶性、难溶性和肠溶性三大类。既可单一应用，也可联合应用。载体材料应符合以下条件：①生理惰性，无毒。②不与药物发生化学反应，不影响主药的化学稳定性。③不影响药物的药效及含量测定。④使药物得到最佳分散，价廉易得。

Common carriers are divided into water-soluble, insoluble and enteric carriers, which can be used singly or in combination. The characteristics of the carriers are as follows: ① They should be physiological inertia and non-toxic. ② The carrier s shouldn't react with the drug and do not affect the chemical stability of the drugs. ③ They shouldn't affect efficacy and content determination of the drugs. ④ They should enable the drugs to be optimally dispersed, and they are cheap and available.

1. 水溶性载体材料　高分子聚合物（如聚乙二醇类、聚维酮类）、表面活性剂（如泊洛沙姆-188）、有机酸类（如枸橼酸、胆酸等）、糖类与醇类（如蔗糖、山梨醇）等。

① **Water-soluble carriers** They mainly include polymers (e.g., polyethylene glycols, povidones), surfactants (e.g., poloxamer-188), organic acids (e.g., citric acid, cholic acid), carbohydrates (e.g., sucrose), alcohols (e.g., sorbitol), etc.

2. 水不溶性载体材料　主要有纤维素类（如乙基纤维素）、聚丙烯树脂类和脂质类等。

② **Water-insoluble carriers** They mainly include celluloses (e.g., ethyl cellulose), polypropylene resins lipids, etc.

3. 肠溶性载体材料　主要有纤维素类（如醋酸纤维素酞酸酯、羟丙甲纤维素酞酸酯等）、聚丙烯树脂类（如Ⅱ号、Ⅲ号）等。

③ **Enteric carriers** They mainly include celluloses (e.g., cellulose acetate phthalate, hypromellose phthalate), polypropylene resins (e.g., Ⅱ, Ⅲ), etc.

（五）固体分散体的制备方法

(5) Preparations of Solid Dispersions

1. 熔融法　将药物与载体混匀，加热至熔融后，在剧烈搅拌下迅速冷却成固体。制备时必须迅速冷却，以达到较高的过饱和状态，使多个胶态晶核迅速形成，而不至于形成粗晶。该法适用于对热稳定的药物。

① **Melting method** Mix the drugs with the carriers, heat to melt, and rapidly cool to form a solid mass under vigorous stirring. It must be rapidly cooled during preparation to achieve a higher supersaturation state, so that multiple colloidal crystal nucleus can form quickly, rather than forming coarse crystals. It is suitable for thermostable drugs.

案例导入 ¦ Case example

案例 19-2 穿心莲内酯固体分散体

19-2 Andrographolide Solid Dispersion

处方：穿心莲内酯 10g PEG 6000 100g

Ingredients: Andrographolide 10g; PEG 6000 100g

制法：称取 PEG 6000 置 250ml 烧杯中，水浴加热使融化成澄清溶液后，将穿心莲内酯细粉加入其中，搅拌使分散溶解，并迅速放入 –20℃的冰箱中固化，粉碎过 60 目筛，即得。

Making Procedure: Take PEG 6000 and heat to melt, add andrographolide fine powder, mix well, curing at –20℃, pulverize and sift (60 mesh).

注解：穿心莲内酯难溶于水，口服生物利用度低，制成固体分散体后，1 小时体外累积释放达 90%。

Notes: Andrographolide is difficult to dissolve in water and has low bioavailability. After it is made into solid dispersion, its cumulative release *in vitro* reaches 90% at 1h.

思考题：（1）穿心莲内酯 /PEG 固体分散体显著提高穿心莲内酯体外释放的机制是什么？

Questions: ① Andrographolide /PEG solid dispersion can significantly improve the release of andrographolide *in vitro*. What is the mechanism?

（2）为什么在制备过程中要“迅速放入 –20℃的冰箱中固化”？

② Why is it necessary to “curing at –20℃” during the preparation?

2. 溶剂法 也称共沉淀法，将药物与载体共同溶解于有机溶剂中，蒸去溶剂，得到药物在载体中均匀分散的共沉淀固体分散体。常用的有机溶剂为氯仿、无水乙醇、丙酮等。当固体分散体内含有少量溶剂时，易引起药物的重结晶而降低主药的分散度。同时，采用的有机溶剂不同，制备的固体分散体中药物的分散度也不同。本法适用于对热不稳定或易挥发的药物。

② Solvent method It's also called coprecipitation method. The drugs and the carriers are dissolved in organic solvents, and the solvents is evaporated to obtain the uniformly dispersed coprecipitation solid dispersions. Common organic solvents are chloroform, anhydrous ethanol, acetone, etc. When there is a small amount of solvents in a solid dispersion, it is easy to cause the drug's recrystallization and reduce its dispersion. Moreover, the dispersion of drugs in a solid dispersion is different with varying organic solvents. This method is applicable for thermolabile or volatile drugs.

3. 溶剂 - 熔融法 将药物溶于少量溶剂中，再与熔融的载体混合均匀，蒸去有机溶剂，冷却固化，干燥即得。凡适用于熔融法的载体材料皆可采用此法。本法适用于某些液体药物，如鱼肝油，维生素 A、D、E 等，也可用于剂量小于 50mg 的固体药物。

③ Solvent-melting method Dissolve the drugs in a small amount of solvents, and then mix with the melted carriers, and remove the organic solvents by evaporation, solidify by cooling and dried. This method is applicable for any carriers suitable for melting method, and it is suitable for certain liquid drugs (e.g., cod liver oil, vitamin A, D, E, etc.) and solid drugs less than 50mg.

4. 溶剂 - 喷雾（冷冻）干燥法 将药物与载体材料共溶于溶剂中，经喷雾干燥或冷冻干燥，除尽溶剂即得。常用载体材料有 PVP、PEG、纤维素及其衍生物，聚丙烯酸树脂、β-CD、水解明

胶、乳糖及甘露醇等。本法适用于易分解、对热不稳定的药物。

④ **Solvent-spray (freeze) drying method** Dissolve the drugs and carriers in a solvent, and spray-dried or freeze-dried to remove the solvents, and then obtain the products. Common carriers are PVP, PEG, cellulose and its derivatives, polyacrylic acid resin, β-CD, hydrolyzed gelatin, lactose and mannitol, etc. This method is applicable for the decomposable and thermolabile drugs.

5. 研磨法 将药物与载体材料混合后，强力持久地研磨一定时间，即得。本法不需要溶剂，而是借助机械力降低药物的粒度，或使药物与载体材料以氢键结合形成固体分散体。研磨时间长短因药而异。常用的载体材料有微晶纤维素、乳糖、PEG、PVP 等。

⑤ **Grinding method** The drugs and carriers are blended together and subjected to grinding in a lasting intensity. This method doesn't require the solvents, but relies on mechanical forces to reduce the particle size of the drugs or to combine the drugs with the carrier by hydrogen bonding. The grinding time varies with drug. Common carriers include microcrystalline cellulose, lactose, PEG, PVP, etc.

（六）固体分散体的质量评价

(6) Quality Evaluation of Solid Dispersion

固体分散体中药物在载体材料中的分散状态是质量评价的主要指标。常用的物相鉴定方法包括热分析法、X- 射线衍射法、红外光谱法、核磁共振法、薄层色谱法、荧光光谱法、紫外分光光度法，以及溶解度与溶出速率测定等。

The dispersion state of drugs in solid dispersions is the main index of quality evaluation. Common methods for phase identification include thermal analysis, X-ray diffraction, infrared spectroscopy, nuclear magnetic resonance, thin layer chromatography, fluorescence spectrometry, ultraviolet spectrophotometry, and the determination of solubility and dissolution rate, etc.

三、微囊与微球的制备技术

19.1.3 Microencapsulation Technology and Microspheres Technology

（一）微囊与微球的含义

(1) The Definition of Microencapsulation and Microspheres Technology

微囊是指固态或液态药物被辅料包封形成的微小胶囊，制备微囊的技术称为微型包囊技术，简称微囊化。微球是指药物溶解或分散在载体材料中形成的骨架型微小球状实体。微囊与微球的粒径通常在 1~250μm 之间，均属于微米级。根据临床不同给药途径和用途，可将微囊、微球进一步制成片剂、胶囊剂、注射剂等剂型。

Microencapsules are tiny capsules formed by solid or liquid drugs enclosed by excipients. The technology of preparing microcapsules is called microencapsulation. Microspheres are tiny spherical entities formed by dissolving or dispersing drugs in carrier materials. The diameter of microcapsules and microspheres is ranging from 1 to 250 μm, and both of them belong to micron scale. According to different Clinical drug delivery routes and uses Microcapsules and microspheres can be further prepared into tablets, capsules, injections, etc.

（二）微囊与微球的特点

(2) The Characteristics of Microencapsules and Microspheres

药物微囊化或制成微球后，可提高药物的稳定性、掩盖药物的不良气味、防止药物在胃内失活或减少对胃的刺激性、使液态药物固态化、减少复方药物的配伍变化、延缓或控制药物释放、使药物具有靶向性，以及提高活细胞和疫苗的生物相容性和稳定性等。

Microcapsules and microspheres can improve the stability of drugs, mask taste and odor of some drugs, prevent the drugs from intragastric inactivation or reduce gastric irritation of drugs. Besides, they can also convert liquid drugs into solid powders, reduce the incompatibility of compound drugs, play a sustained-release or controlled-release, or targeting effect, and improve biocompatibility and stability of living cells and vaccines.

（三）微囊与微球的组成与结构

(3) Composition and Structure of Microcapsules and Microspheres

微囊由囊心物及囊材组成，微囊是典型的药库膜壳型结构（“囊心 - 囊材”结构），囊心物包括被包封的药物和附加剂（稳定剂、稀释剂等）等辅料。微球具有典型的基质骨架型结构。药物在微球中的分散状态通常为 3 种情况：溶解在微球内，以结晶状态镶嵌在微球内，被吸附或镶嵌在微球表面。常见的微囊囊材和微球骨架材料有以下几种。

Microcapsules are composed of core substances and carrier materials, which have typical core-shell structures. The core substances include the encapsulated drugs (solid or liquid) and additives such as stabilizer, diluent and etc. Microspheres are solid spheres with a typical matrix framework structure. The dispersion state of drugs in microspheres is usually in three forms: dissolving in microsphere, embedding in microspheres with crystalline state and being adsorbed or embedded on the surface of microspheres. The common framework materials of microcapsules and microspheres are as follows.

1. 天然高分子材料 这类材料无毒，成膜性及成球性较好，可在体内生物降解。常用的有明胶、阿拉伯胶、海藻酸盐、壳聚糖、蛋白类、淀粉等。

① **Natural polymer materials** These materials are usually non-toxic with good formability. They can be biodegraded *in vivo*. Commonly used are gelatin, gum arabic, alginate, chitosan, protein and starch, etc.

2. 半合成高分子材料 这类材料毒性小、黏度大，成盐后溶解度增大，易水解，不宜高温处理，需临用时现配。常用的有纤维素衍生物，如羧甲基纤维素、纤维醋法酯、甲基纤维素、乙基纤维素、羟丙甲纤维素、丁酸醋酸纤维素、琥珀酸醋酸纤维素等。

② **Semisynthetic polymeric materials** These materials usually have characteristics of low toxicity, high viscosity and high solubility by salification. In addition, they are easy to hydrolysis and not suitable for high temperature treatment. It is necessary to prepare just before use. Cellulose derivatives are commonly used among them such as carboxymethyl cellulose, cellulose acetate, methyl cellulose, ethyl cellulose, hypromellose, acetate-butyrate cellulose, succinic-acetate cellulose, etc.

3. 合成高分子材料 这类材料无毒，成膜性及成球性好，化学稳定性高，可用于注射。常用的有聚酯、聚合酸酐、聚氨基酸、聚乳酸 - 聚乙二醇嵌段共聚物及羧甲基葡聚糖等。

③ **Synthetic polymeric materials** These materials are usually non-toxic with good formability and high chemical stability. They can be used for injection. Polyanhydrides, polyamino acids, polylactic acid-polyethylene glycol block copolymers and carboxymethyl dextran are commonly used.

（四）微囊与微球的制备

(4) Microencapsulation and Microspheres Techniques

1. 微囊的制备方法 微囊的制备方法按其制备原理可分为物理化学法、化学法、物理机械法等三大类，见表 19-1。

① **Microencapsulation techniques** According to the preparation principle, microencapsulation techniques can be divided into three categories: physicochemical method, chemical method and physical mechanical method (Table 19-1).

表 19-1　微囊的制备方法

分类	常见的制备方法
物理化学法	凝聚法（单凝聚法、复凝聚法）、溶剂 - 非溶剂法、液中干燥法
化学法	界面聚合法、辐射交联法
物理机械法	喷雾干燥法、空气悬浮法

Table 19-1　Preparation of Microcapsules

Classification	Common preparation methods
physicochemical method	Coacervation (Simple coacervation, Complex coacervation), Solvent -nonsolvent, In-Liquid drying
Chemical method	Interfacial polymerization，Radiation crosslinking
Physical mechanical method	Spray-drying, Air suspension

（1）单凝聚法　将囊心物分散于囊材的水溶液中，加入凝聚剂，如电解质［Na_2SO_4，$(NH_4)_2SO_4$ 等］或强亲水性非电解质（乙醇、丙醇等），使囊材凝聚并包封囊心物而形成微囊。主要包括囊材液的配制、药物的混悬或者乳化、凝聚成囊、胶凝固化、洗涤、干燥等工艺过程。以明胶为囊材的单凝聚法制备工艺流程见图 19-1。

a. Simple coacervation　Disperse the core substances in the aqueous solution of the carrier material, add coagulants, such as electrolyte [Na_2SO_4, $(NH_4)_2SO_4$, etc.] or strong hydrophilic non-electrolyte (ethanol, propanol, etc.) to make the carrier materials agglomerate and encapsulate the core substances. The process of simple coacervation generally includes the preparation of carrier material solutions, suspension or emulsification of drugs, coacervation, solidification of coacervate, washing and drying. Preparation process of gelatin capsule by simple coacervation is shown in Figure 19-1.

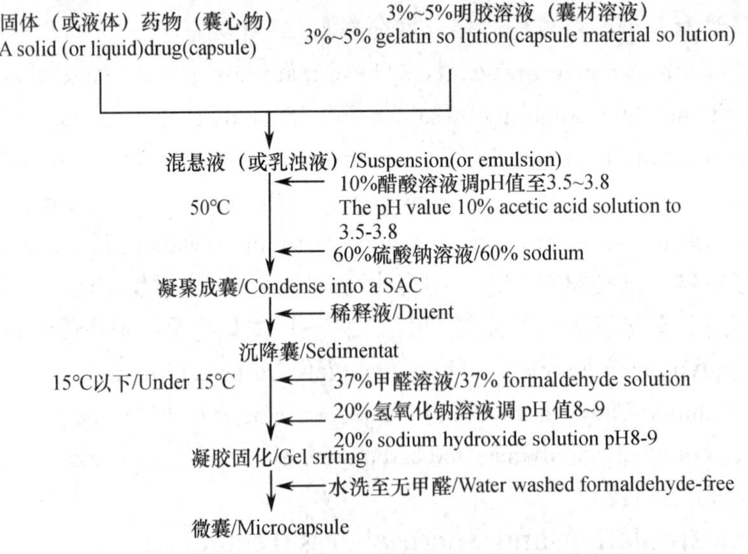

图 19-1　单凝聚法的制备过程

Figure 19-1　Preparation Process of Simple Coacervation

①囊材液的配制　称取适量囊材，加水配成适宜浓度的溶液。单凝聚法常见囊材有明胶、纤维醋法酯（CAP）、甲基纤维素、聚乙烯醇等。

Preparation of carrier materials solution　Weigh appropriate amount of carrier materials, add water to prepare appropriate concentration of solution. The commonly used carrier materials of simple coacervation include gelatin, cellulose acetate, methyl cellulose, polyvinyl alcohol, etc.

②药物的混悬或乳化 单凝聚法的药物一般要求难溶于水，如果药物是固体，则将其微粉化，分散于囊材溶液中形成混悬液；如果为液体，则将其加入囊材液中制成乳浊液。

Suspension or emulsification of drugs Simple coacervation method generally requires drugs to be dissolved in water. If the drug is solid, it will be micronized and dispersed in the polymer solution to form a suspension. If the drug is liquid, add it into the polymer solution to form a emulsion.

③凝聚成囊 在混悬液（或乳浊液）中加入凝聚剂，使囊材包裹囊心物凝聚成微囊。常用凝聚剂包括：强亲水性非电解质如乙醇、丙酮、丙醇等，强亲水性电解质如硫酸钠、硫酸铵、硫酸铝等。电解质中的阴离子对高分子胶凝起主要作用，常见的阴离子胶凝作用次序为：SO_4^{2-}>$C_6H_5O_7^{3-}$>$C_4H_4O_6^{2-}$> CH_3COO^->Cl^-。

Coacervation Add coacervation agents into the suspension or emulsion to make the carrier materials surround the core materials and form microcapsules. The commonly used coacervation agents include: strong hydrophilic non-electrolyte such as ethanol, propanol, acetone, etc, and strong hydrophilic electrolyte, such as sodium sulfate, ammonium sulfate, aluminum sulfate and etc. The anions of electrolyte play a major role in polymer gelation. The most common anions are SO_4^{2-}, followed by Cl^-. Furthermore, SCN^- can prevent the gelation. The common order of anionic gelation is:

$$SO_4^{2-}>C_6H_5O_7^{3-}>C_4H_4O_6^{2-}>CH_3COO^->Cl^-$$

高分子物质的凝聚往往是可逆的，在某些条件下出现凝聚，当这些条件改变或消失，可发生解凝聚现象。利用这种可逆性在制备过程中可多次重复凝聚，直到微囊形状满意为止，再固化形成不可逆的微囊。

The coacervation of polymer materials is usually reversible. Coacervation occurs under certain conditions. When these conditions change or disappear, decohesion can occur. This reversibility can be used to repeatedly agglomerate during the preparation process until the shape of the microcapsules is satisfactory, and then solidified to form irreversible microcapsule.

影响高分子囊材胶凝的因素有囊材浓度、温度、电解质及凝聚剂种类等。

The factors that affect the gelation of polymer materials are the concentration of material, temperature, electrolyte, coagulant, etc.

④胶凝固化 凝聚囊的固化应根据囊材性质而定，如采用CAP做囊材，可加酸固化（CAP不溶于强酸介质），海藻酸盐加氯化钙固化，蛋白质加热或用醛固化，如明胶做囊材时，常用醛类固化，明胶与甲醛发生胺缩醛反应。

Solidification of coacervate The solidification of the coacervate should be determined by the properties of the carrier materials. If CAP is used as the carrier material, acid can be used to solidify, because CAP is insoluble in strong acid medium. Besides alginate can be solidified with calcium chloride and protein can be heated or solidified with aldehyde. When gelatin is used as encapsulation material, aldehyde is usually used to solidify, and the reaction of gelatin and formaldehyde is amine acetal.

⑤洗涤、干燥 微囊经过固化处理后，滤过，用水洗至微囊表面无甲醛，60℃干燥，即得。

Washing and drying Filter and wash the microcapsules with water until there is no formaldehyde on the surface of the microcapsule, then dry at 60℃.

（2）复凝聚法 利用两种具有相反电荷的高分子材料作囊材，将囊心物分散在囊材的水溶液中，在一定条件下，相反电荷的高分子材料互相交联后溶解度降低，自溶液中凝聚析出成囊，这种凝聚也是可逆的。主要包括囊材液的配制、药物的混悬或乳化、凝聚成囊、胶凝固化、洗涤、

干燥等工艺过程。以明胶 - 阿拉伯胶为囊材的复凝聚法工艺流程见图 19-2。

b. Complex coacervation This process involves two polymer carrier materials with opposite charges. The core substance is dispersed in the aqueous solution of the polymer material. Under certain condition, the solubility of the polymer material with opposite charges decreases after cross-linking, then the material coagulate from the solution and the microcapsule is formed. This coacervation is also reversible. The process of complex coacervation includes the preparation of carrier materials solution, suspension or emulsification of drugs, coacervation, solidification of coacervate, washing and drying. The complex coacervation process with gelatin-gum arabic as the capsule material is shown in Figure 19-2.

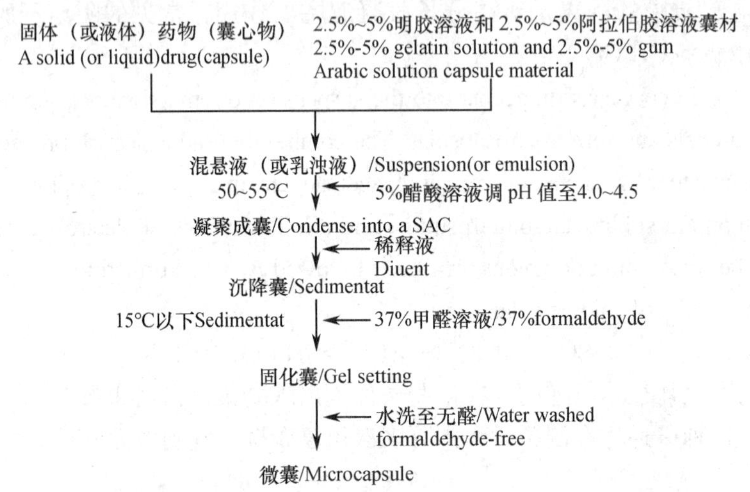

图 19-2 复凝聚法制备工艺流程图

Figure 19-2 Preparation Process of Complex Coacervation

①囊材液的配制 复凝聚法常用的囊材为明胶和阿拉伯胶，两者与水组成囊材液，囊材液的凝聚条件可用图 19-3 示意，其中 K 代表复凝聚的区域，也就是能形成微囊的低浓度明胶和阿拉伯胶混合溶液，P 代表曲线以下明胶和阿拉伯胶溶液既不能混溶也不能形成微囊的区域，H 代表曲线以上明胶和阿拉伯胶溶液可以混溶成均相的区域，A 点代表 10% 明胶、10% 阿拉伯胶和 80% 水的混合溶液。必须加水稀释，沿着 A → B 方向到 K 区域才能产生凝聚。

Preparation of carrier materials solution Gelatin and arabic gum are commonly used in complex coacervation. The preparation of carrier materials aqueous solution is shown in Figure 19-3. K represents the complex coacervation region, in which the mixed polymers solution of gelatin and gum arabic can form microcapsule. P represents the region below the curve where gelatin and gum arabic can neither be mixed nor form microcapsule. H represents the region above the curve where gelatin and gum arabic solutions can be miscible into a homogeneous phase, and A represents the mixed solution of 10% gelatin, 10% gum arabic, and 80% water. Water must be added to dilute the condensation along the A → B direction to the K region.

②药物的混悬或乳化 难溶性药物分散或乳化于囊材液中，并保持温度 50~55℃。

Suspension or emulsification of drugs Insoluble drugs is dispersed or emulsified in the polymer solution at a temperature of 50-55℃.

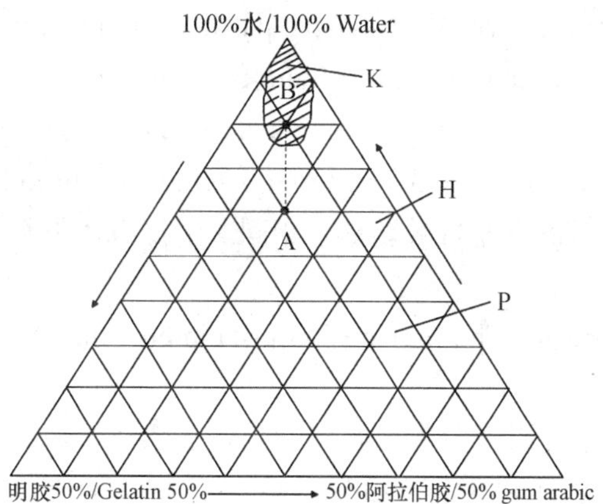

图 19-3 明胶、阿拉伯胶在 pH 值 4.5 用水稀释时的复凝聚三元相图

Figure 19-3 Ternary Phase Diagram of Complex Coacervation of Gelatin and Gum Arabic at pH 4.5 Diluted with Water

③凝聚成囊 pH 值小于等电点时明胶带正电荷（pH 4.0~4.5 时明胶带的正电荷多），而阿拉伯胶带负电荷，因电荷互相吸引而交联，凝聚成微囊。

Coacervation When the pH value is below the isoelectric point, gelatin has a positive charge (when the pH value is 4.0-4.5, the positive charge of gelatin is more), while the gum arabic has negative charge in aqueous solution. When two polymer materials are mixed, cross-link happen due to the attraction of electric charge and agglomerate into microcapsules.

④胶凝固化 将微囊溶液在搅拌下放冷，然后在不断搅拌下急速降温至 15℃以下，加入 37% 甲醛溶液，调 pH 值 8~9，固化。

Solidification of coacervate Stir the microcapsule solution until below 15℃, then add 37% formaldehyde solution and adjust pH to 8-9 by 20% sodium hydroxide solution.

⑤洗涤、干燥 同单凝聚法。

Washing and drying The specific operation is the same as that of single coacervation method.

（3）界面缩聚法 又称界面聚合法，是在分散相（水相）与连续相（油相）的界面上发生单体的聚合反应。

c. Interfacial polycondensation It is also called interfacial polymerization, monomer polymerization occurs at the interface of dispersed phase (water phase) and continuous phase (oil phase)

（4）辐射交联法 是将明胶或 PVP 在乳化状态下，经 γ 射线照射发生交联，再处理制得粉末状微囊。

d. Radiation crosslinking Gelatin or PVP are crosslinked by γ-ray irradiation in emulsification state, and then treated to prepare powder microcapsules.

（5）喷雾干燥法 先将囊心物分散在囊材溶液中，再用喷雾法将此混合物喷入惰性热气流使液滴收缩成球形，进而干燥即得微囊。

e. Spray–drying First, disperse the core substance into the carrier materials solution, and then spray the mixture into the inert hot air stream by spray method to shrink the droplets into spheres, finally the microcapsules can be obtained by drying.

（6）空气悬浮法 应用流化床的强气流将芯材微粒（滴）悬浮于空气中，通过喷嘴将调成适当黏度的囊材溶液喷涂于微粒（滴）表面，提高气流温度使囊材溶液中的溶剂挥发，囊材析出而成囊。

f. Air suspension Suspend the core substances particles/droplets in the air by strong air flow in a fluidized bed, and spray the solution of carrier materials with proper viscosity on the surface of the particles/droplets by a nozzle, so as to increase the air flow temperature to volatilize the solvent in the solution of the carrier materials, and the carrier material is separated out to form capsules.

2. 微球的制备 微球的制备原理与微囊基本相同。根据载体材料和药物性质不同可采用不同的制备方法。

② **Microspheres techniques** The preparation principle of microsphere is basically the same as that of microcapsules.

（1）加热固化法 该法主要用于白蛋白微球的制备，系将含药白蛋白水溶液与食用油乳化成W/O型乳浊液，将此乳浊液滴注到高温（130~180℃）的棉子油中，搅拌，固化，分离，洗涤得微球。加热固化法会导致热敏性药物分解，不适于热敏性药物微球的制备。

a. Heat curing This method is mainly used for the preparation of albumin microspheres. The aqueous solution containing albumin and edible oil is emulsified into W/O emulsion. The emulsion is dripped into cottonseed oil at high temperature (130-180℃). Then, microspheres can be collected after stirring, solidifying, separating and washing. This method can lead to the decomposition of thermosensitive drugs, so it isn't suitable for the preparation of thermosensitive drug microspheres.

（2）化学交联法 利用载体材料所具有的氨基易与其他活性基团发生反应的特点，与交联剂所具有的活性基团发生缩合反应，形成网状或者体形结构，最终固化形成微球。该法主要选用明胶、淀粉、壳聚糖等作为载体材料，微球成品具有良好的圆整度和包合率，稳定性好，且在水中具有较好的分散性。

b. Chemical cross-linking The amino group of the carrier materials is easy to react with other active groups. It condenses with the active groups of the crosslinker to form a network or body structure, and finally solidifies to form microspheres. In this method, gelatin, starch and chitosan are used as carrier materials. The microsphere has good roundness, inclusion rate, stability, and good dispersibility in water.

（3）溶剂挥发法 先将药物与载体材料组成挥发性有机相，加至含乳化剂的水相中搅拌乳化，形成O/W型乳状液，抽真空或加热挥发除去有机溶剂，过滤，即得微球。该法主要用于以聚乳酸和聚乳酸-羟基乙酸共聚物为载体材料的微球制备。

c. Solvent evaporation Volatile organic phase is composed of drugs and carrier materials, which is added into the water phase containing emulsifier to form O/W emulsion. The organic solvent is removed by vacuuming or heating volatilization, and the microsphere is obtained by filtering. This method is mainly used for the preparation of microspheres with polylactic acid and polylactic acid-hydroxyacetic acid copolymer which are used as carriers.

（4）喷雾干燥法 将药物与载体材料的混悬液或溶液，经喷嘴喷入干燥室，同时送入干燥室的热空气流使雾滴中的水分快速蒸发、干燥，即得微球。该法具有操作简便、一步成球、包封率高、粒径均匀等优点。

d. Spray-drying The suspension or solution of drugs and carrier materials is sprayed into a drying chamber by a nozzle. At the same time, the hot air flows into the drying chamber to make the water into the droplets. This process enable evaporation and drying quickly, and then microspheres is obtained. The method has the advantages of easy operation, one-step balling, high entrapment rate and uniform particle size, etc.

（五）微囊与微球的质量评价

(5) Quality Evaluation of Microcapsules and Microspheres

1. 形态、粒径及粒径分布 可采用光学显微镜或扫描、透射电子显微镜观察微囊与微球的形态，通常呈圆整球形或椭球形，表面光滑或粗糙。粒径及其分布测定方法包括筛析法、显微镜法、超速离心法、沉降法、库尔特计数法、吸附法、激光衍射法等。

① **Shape, particle size, particle size distribution** The shape of microcapsules and microspheres can be observed by light microscopy or scanning and transmission electron microscope, which is usually spherical or ellipsoidal, with a smooth or rough surface. The determination methods of particle size and its distribution include sieve analysis, microscope, ultra-speed centrifugation, sedimentation method, coulter counting, adsorption and laser diffraction.

2. 包封率和载药量 对于粉末状微囊（球），可以仅测量载药量；对于混悬于液体介质中的微囊（球），可将其分离后进行测定，并计算其载药量和包封率。

② **Entrapment efficiency and drug loading** For powder microcapsules /microspheres, only drug loading can be measured. But for those microcapsules /microspheres suspended in liquid medium, the drug loading and entrapment efficiency can be calculated after separation.

$$载药量 = 微囊（球）中所含药物量 / 微囊（球）的总质量 \times 100\% \quad (19\text{-}1)$$

$$\text{Drug loading} = \text{The amount of drugs contained in the microcapsule/The total weight of the microcapsule} \times 100\% \quad (19\text{-}1)$$

$$包封率 = 系统中包封的药量 / 系统中包封与未包封的总药量 \times 100\% \quad (19\text{-}2)$$

$$\text{Envelopment efficiency} = \text{The amount of encapsulated drug in the system / The total amount of encapsulated and unencapsulated drugs in the system} \times 100\% \quad (19\text{-}2)$$

3. 药物的释放速率 微囊（球）中药物的释放速率可采用现行版《中国药典》中规定的桨法测定，亦可采用试样置薄膜透析管内按转篮法进行测定，或采用流池法测定。

③ **Drug release rate** The drug release rate in microcapsule/microsphere can be determined by oar method which is adopted in the current *Chinese Pharmacopoeia*. Besides, rotating basket and flow-through cell method can also be used.

4. 有害有机溶剂残留量 生产过程中引入有害溶剂时，应按现行版《中国药典》相关规定检测。凡未规定限度者，可参考人用药品注册的国际技术要求（ICH），否则应制定有害有机溶剂残留量的测定方法与限度。

④ **Limit Test of harmful organic solvent** The introduction of harmful solvent in production process should be in accordance with the current *Chinese Pharmacopoeia*. Those who do not set limits, can refer to the international technical requirements for registration of medicine for human use. Otherwise, the determination method and limit of harmful organic solvent residue should be established.

5. 突释效应或渗漏率 在体外释放试验时，表面吸附的药物会快速释放，称为突释效应，开始 0.5 小时内的释放量要求低于 40%。若微囊与微球产品分散在液体介质中贮藏，应检查渗漏率，可由式（19-3）计算：

⑤ **Burst release effect and leakage rate** *In vitro* release test, the drugs adsorbed on the surface will be released rapidly, which is called burst release effect. The release amount within the first 0.5h should be less than 40%. If microcapsules/microspheres product is stored in a liquid medium, the leakage rate should be checked and calculated from the following formula（19-3）:

$$渗漏率 = 产品贮存一定时间后渗漏到介质中药量 / 产品在贮存前包封药量 \times 100\% \quad (19\text{-}3)$$

$$\text{Leakage rate} = \text{The amount of product that leaks into the medium after storage for a certain period of time / The amount of drug that the product encapsulated before storage} \times 100\% \quad (19\text{-}3)$$

四、纳米乳与亚微乳的制备技术

19.1.4 Nano-Emulsion and Sub-Microemulsion Preparation Technology

（一）含义

(1) Definition of Nano-Emulsion and Sub-Microemulsion

纳米乳是由水相、油相、乳化剂和助乳化剂按适当比例形成粒径为 10~100nm，低黏度、各向同性的热力学和动力学稳定的透明或半透明体系。粒径 100~1000nm 的为亚微乳。

Nano-emulsion is a transparent or semitransparent system with a particle size of 10-100nm, low viscosity, isotropy thermodynamic and dynamic stability, which is formed by water phase, oil phase, emulsifier and co-emulsifier in proper proportion. The particle size of 100-1000nm is sub-microemulsion.

近年来，纳米乳技术发展迅速，出现了自微乳化药物传递系统，是由油相、乳化剂和助乳化剂组成，外观均一透明，在环境温度及温和搅拌条件下，遇水自微乳化成 O/W 型、粒径小于 100nm 的乳剂。

In recent years, with the rapid development of nano-emulsion technology, self -microemulsion drug delivery system (SMEDDS) has emerged. SMEDDS is visually homogeneous, transparent system, and it is composed of oil phase and emulsifier, which can spontaneously form o/w microemulsion with minimal agitation at room temperature while meeting water.

（二）特点

(2) Characteristics of Nano-Emulsion and Sub-Microemulsion

1. 可提高难溶性药物的溶解度与生物利用度 纳米乳粒径小，药物分散度高，可提高药物溶解度，且可促进药物吸收。

① **Improving the solubility and bioavailability of insoluble drugs** Nano-emulsion has small particle size and a very finely subdivided dispersed phase, which can improve the solubility and absorption of drugs.

2. 可经口服、注射或皮肤实现多种途径给药 黏度低，注射时不会引起疼痛，不会引起变态反应和脂肪栓塞。

② **Achieving various routes of administration including oral, injection or transdermal permeation** Nano-emulsion has low viscosity, so it doesn't cause pain, allergy and fat embolism when injected.

3. 稳定性好，易于制备和保存 属热力学稳定体系，可以滤过、热压灭菌，离心后不分层。

③ **Good stability and easy preparation and preservation** Nano-emulsion is a thermodynamic stability system, so it can be filtered, autoclaved, and centrifuged without delamination.

4. 缓释和靶向作用 如油包水型纳米乳可延长水溶性药物的释放时间，起到缓释作用；纳米乳可改变某些药物的体内分布，具有一定靶向性。

④ **Sustained-release and targeted effect** For example, w/o nano-emulsion can be used to prolong the release time of water-soluble drugs and play a role of sustained-release. Nano-emulsion can change the distribution of some drugs *in vivo* and have certain targeting effect.

（三）纳米乳的制备

(3) Preparation of Nano-Emulsions

选择合适的油相、乳化剂及助乳化剂，并确定各组分的最佳比例，是制备纳米乳的关键环节。一般可通过实验并结合绘制相图来进行。一般可将乳化剂及其用量固定，水、油、助乳化剂三个组分占正三角形的三个顶点，滴定法恒温制作相图，找出纳米乳相形成区域（图 19-4），从而确定纳米乳中各组分的用量。只要纳米乳处方选择适当，将各组分按比例混合即可制得纳米乳，无需做很大的功，且与各组分加入次序无关。

In the preparation of nano-emulsions, the key steps are to select the appropriate oil phase, emulsifier and co-emulsifier, and to determine the optimal ratio of each components. Generally, it can be performed by experiment and drawing phase diagram. In general, the emulsifier and its dosage can be fixed, and the three components of water, oil and emulsifier are the three vertices of the equilateral triangle. The phase diagram can be made by titration at constant temperature to find out the nano-emulsion formation region (as shown in Figure 19-4), so as to determine the amount of each components in the nano-emulsions. As long as the formula of the nano-emulsions is properly selected, the nano-emulsions can be prepared by mixing the components in proportion, which does not need to do much work, and has nothing to do with the order of adding components.

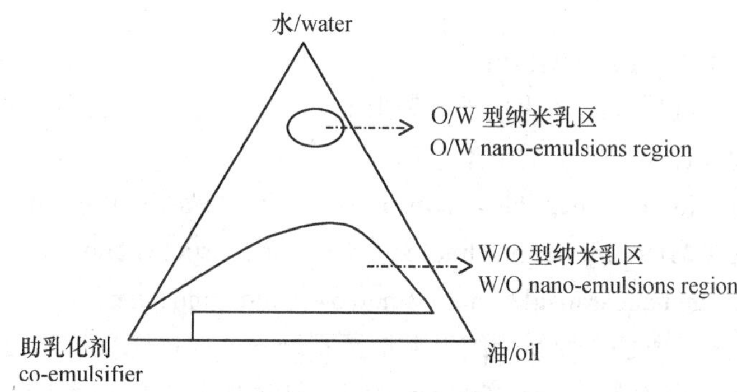

图 19-4 纳米乳伪三元相图

Figure 19-4 Pseudo Ternary Phase Diagram of Nano-Emulsions

（四）亚微乳的制备

(4) Preparation of Sub-Microemulsions

一般采用两步高压乳匀法制备亚微乳，即将药物与其他油溶性成分溶于油相中，将水溶性成分溶于水中，然后将油相和水相加热到一定温度，置组织捣碎机或高剪切分散乳化机中混合，在一定温度下制成初乳。初乳迅速冷却，高压乳匀机乳匀 2 次，滤去粗乳滴与碎片，调节 pH 值，高压灭菌，即得。

Generally, sub-microemulsions is prepared by a two-step high-pressure homogenization method. That is, dissolve the drugs and other oil-soluble components in the oil phase, and dissolve the water-soluble components in water, and then heat the oil phase and the water phase to a certain temperature, mix in a tissue masher or a high-shear dispersion machine to form colostrum at a certain temperature. And then, cool the colostrum rapidly. Homogenize the colostrum with the high-pressure homogenizer twice. Filter the coarse liquid drops and fragments, adjust the pH value, and sterilize the colostrum under high pressure to obtain sub-microemulsion.

制备静脉用亚微乳的关键是如何选择高效低毒的附加剂，并在确保亚微乳稳定的情况下，尽量减少附加剂用量。为避免造成毛细管阻塞，亚微乳的粒径应小于微血管内径（4μm 左右）。若药物或其他成分易于氧化，则制备的各步都应在氮气下进行；如药物对热不稳定，则采用无菌操作。

The key to the preparation of intravenous sub-microemulsions is how to select high efficiency and low toxicity additives, and how to reduce the amount of additives to ensure the stability of sub-microemulsions. To avoid capillary obstruction, the particle size of sub-microemulsion should be smaller than the diameter of microvascular (about 4μm). If the drugs or other ingredients are susceptible to

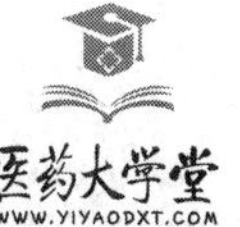

oxidation, each steps of the preparation should be performed under nitrogen. If the drugs is not stable to heat, aseptic operation should be adopted.

（五）纳米乳和亚微乳的质量评价

(5) Quality Evaluation of Nano-Emulsions and Sub-Microemulsions

纳米乳和亚微乳的质量评价主要包括乳滴粒径及其分布、药物含量、稳定性等检测。

The quality evaluation of nano-emulsions and sub-microemulsions mainly includes the detection of droplet size and its distribution, drug content and its stability, etc.

五、纳米粒的制备技术

19.1.5 Nanoparticle Preparation Technology

（一）含义

(1) Definition of Nanoparticles

纳米粒是指药物或与载体经纳米化技术分散形成的粒径小于 500nm 的固体粒子。纳米粒可分为膜壳药库型的纳米囊和骨架实体型的纳米球。

Nanoparticles refers to solid particles with particle size less than 500nm which is formed by dispersing the drugs and carriers by nanotechnology. The nanoparticles can be divided into two types: membrane-shell drug storage nano-capsules and framework solid nanospheres.

20 世纪 90 年代，又出现了一种新型纳米粒给药系统——固体脂质纳米粒（SLN），系以高溶点脂质材料为载体制成，其粒径在 50~1000nm 之间。SLN 既具有纳米粒的物理稳定性高、药物泄漏少、缓释性好的特点，同时毒性低、易于大规模生产，而且对亲脂性药物载药量比较高，不使用有机溶剂，因此是极有发展前途的新型给药系统的载体。

In the 1990s, a new type of nanoparticle drug delivery system, solid lipid nanoparticles (SLN), was developed. It is made of high solubility point lipid material with the particle size ranging from 50 to 1000 nm. Not only does it have the characteristics of high physical stability of nanoparticle, less drug leakage, and good sustained release, but also SLN has low toxicity and is easy to produce on a large scale. Moreover, SLN has high drug loading for lipophilic drug and does not use organic solvent. Therefore, SLN is a promising carrier for new drug delivery system.

（二）特点

(2) The Characteristics of Nanoparticles

纳米粒作为药物载体，其主要特点包括：①靶向性纳米粒经静脉注射，一般被巨噬细胞摄取，主要分布于肝（60%~90%）、脾（2%~10%）和肺（3%~10%），少量进入骨髓。纳米粒经表面修饰，也可发挥主动靶向作用。②缓释药物，从而延长药物的作用时间。③提高药物生物利用度，减少给药剂量，从而减轻毒副作用。④保护药物、提高药物稳定性，可避免多肽等药物在消化道的失活等。

As a drug carrier, the main characteristics of nanoparticles include: ① Targeting After intravenous injection, nanoparticles is generally absorbed by macrophages, mainly distributed in the liver (60%-90%), spleen (2%-10%) and lung (3%-10%), and a small amount of them enter the bone marrow. Nanoparticles can also play an active targeting role after surface modification. ② Slow release drugs, thus prolonging the action time of drug. ③ Improving the bioavailability of the drugs, reducing the dosage of drugs, so as to reduce the side effect. ④ Protecting the drugs and improving the stability of the drug. Nanoparticle can avoid the inactivation of peptide and other drugs in the digestive tract.

（三）制备方法

(3) Preparation Methods of Nanoparticles

1. 乳化 - 溶剂挥发法 将含高分子材料和药物的油相，分散于含乳化剂的水相中，制成 O/W 型乳状液，油相中的有机溶剂被蒸发除去，即得纳米粒。

① Emulsification-solvent evaporation method Disperse drugs in the water phase, and add into oil phase containing polymer materials to prepare o/w emulsions, and remove the organic solvents in the oil phase by evaporation to obtain nanoparticles.

2. 乳化聚合法 将单体分散于水相乳化剂中的胶束内或乳滴中，遇 OH^- 或其他引发剂分子发生聚合，胶束及乳滴作为提供单体的仓库，乳化剂对相分离的纳米粒也起防止聚集的稳定作用，聚合反应终止后，经分离呈固态，即得。

② Emulsion polymerization method Disperse monomer in the micelles or emulsion droplets in the aqueous phase emulsifier, and polymerize with the presence of OH^- or other initiator molecules. Micelle and emulsion droplets serve as monomer storehouses, and emulsifier also plays a stabilizing role in preventing aggregation of phase separated nanoparticle. After the polymerization reaction is terminated, they are obtained in a solid state after separation.

案例导入 ¦ Case example

案例 19-3 紫杉醇聚氰基丙烯酸正丁酯纳米粒

19-3 Paclitaxel Poly Butyl Cyanoacrylate Nanoparticles

处方：紫杉醇（PTX）16.5mg 氰基丙烯酸正丁酯（BCA）0.1ml 大豆卵磷脂 100mg 右旋糖 100mg

Ingredients: Paclitaxel (PTX) 16.5mg; n-Butyl cyanoacrylate (BCA) 0.1ml; Soy lecithin 100mg; Dextran 100mg

制法：称取 100mg 右旋糖酐和 100mg 大豆卵磷脂，加入 10ml 蒸馏水，超声溶解，然后用稀盐酸（0.1mol/L）调 pH 值为 3.0，加入紫杉醇溶液，然后在室温搅拌（600r/min），滴加入 0.1ml BCA（加入一定量丙酮稀释，稀释比例为 1∶4），搅拌 4 小时，然后用 NaOH 溶液（0.1mol/L）调 pH 值为 7.0，继续搅拌 30 分钟，减压抽滤后用 0.45μm 滤膜过滤，得到乳白色的浑浊液，滤过，洗涤，干燥，即得。

Making Procedure: Weigh 100mg dextran and 100mg soybean lecithin, add 10mL distilled water, and sonicate until dissolve. Then adjust the pH value to 3.0 with dilute hydrochloric acid (0.1mol/L), add the paclitaxel solution, and stir at room temperature (600r/min), add 0.1 mL BCA dropwise (dilute with a certain amount of acetone, the dilution ratio is 1∶4), and stir for 4h. Then adjust the pH value to 7.0 with NaOH solution (0.1mol/L), continue to stir for 30min. After suction filtration under reduced pressure, filter through a 0.45μm filter to obtain a milky turbid liquid, and then filter, wash and dry.

注解：（1）以聚氰基丙烯酸正丁酯（PBCA）为载体，其最大优点在于聚合过程简单，所生成的聚合物在生物体内可降解，对人体组织基本无毒。

Notes: ① Taking poly butyl cyanoacrylate (PBCA) as the carrier, the greatest advantage is that the polymerization process is simple, the resulting polymer is degradable in the body, and is basically non-toxic to human tissue.

（2）介质 pH 值，表面活性剂和空间稳定剂（常用右旋糖酐 70）的种类、用量、BCA 用量、滴加速度、药物性质和浓度等都对粒径、包封率、表面电位等有影响。

② The pH value of the medium, the type and amount of surfactant and space stabilizer (dextran 70 in common use), the amount of BCA, the drop acceleration, the nature and concentration of the drug all have influence on the particle size, encapsulation efficiency and surface potential.

思考题：影响乳化聚合法的因素有哪些？

Questions: What are the factors that affect the emulsion polymerization?

（四）纳米粒的质量评价

(4) Quality Evaluation of Nanoparticles

主要包括纳米粒的形态与粒径分布、包封率与渗透率、再分散性、突释效应、有机溶剂残留量等检测。

It mainly includes the detection of morphology and particle size distribution of nanoparticles, encapsulation rate and permeability, redispersion, burst release effect and residual organic solvent.

六、脂质体的制备技术

19.1.6 Liposomes Preparation Technology

案例导入

（一）含义

(1) The Definition of Liposomes

脂质体是将药物包封于类脂质双分子层内而形成的微小囊泡。其粒径大小可从几十纳米到几十微米，双分子层厚度约 4nm。脂质体一般由磷脂和胆固醇构成，脂质体的结构示意图见图 19-5。脂质体根据其结构中所包含的双分子层磷脂膜的层数可分为单室脂质体和多室脂质体。

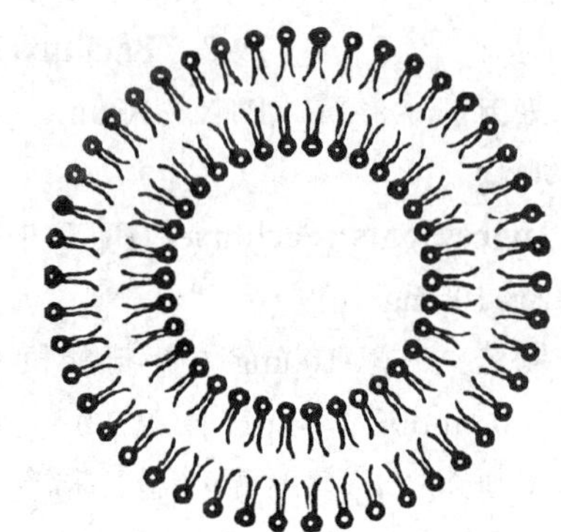

图 19-5 脂质体的结构示意图

Figure 19-5 Structure Diagram of Liposome

Liposomes is composed of small vesicles formed by drugs encapsulated in a lipid-like bilayer. Size of liposomes ranging from tens of nanometers to tens of microns and the thickness of the bilayer is about 4nm. Liposomes is generally composed of phospholipid and cholesterol. The structure of liposomes is shown in Figure 19-5. According to the number of bilayer molecular phospholipid membrane layers contained in their structure, liposomes can be divided into single-compartment liposomes and multi-compartment liposomes.

（二）特点

(2) The Characteristics of Liposomes

1. 靶向性 脂质体能选择性分布于某组织和器官，增加药物对淋巴系统的定向性，提高药物疗效，减少剂量，降低毒性。

① **Targeting** Liposomes can be selectively distributed in specific tissues and organs, increase the targeting of the drugs to the lymphatic system and drug efficacy, reduce the dosage and toxicity of drugs.

2. 细胞亲和性与组织相容性 脂质体结构与生物膜相似，对正常细胞和组织无损害和抑制作用，有细胞亲和性与组织相容性，可增强被包载药物透过细胞膜的能力，从而增强疗效。

② **Cell affinity and histocompatibility** The structure of liposomes is similar to biofilm, and it has no damage and inhibitory effect on normal cells and tissues. Liposomes has cell affinity and histocompatibility, which can enhance the ability of the encapsulated drugs to penetrate the cell membrane, and improve therapeutic effect.

3. 缓释性 将药物包封于脂质体内，可减少肾排泄和代谢而延长药物在血液中的滞留时间，使药物在体内缓慢释放，从而延长药物作用时间。

③ **Sustained-release and long-lasting** Liposomes also has the effects of reducing drug metabolism and renal excretion in kidney, prolonging the residence time of drug in the blood. Thereby the duration of effective drugs can be prolonged.

4. 降低药物毒性 药物被脂质体包封后，主要被网状内皮系统的巨噬细胞所摄取，且在肝、脾和骨髓等单核巨噬细胞较丰富的器官中浓集，而在心、肾中含量较低，降低了药物的毒性。

④ **Reducing toxicity of drugs** Drug-loaded liposomes is mainly consumed by macrophages of the reticuloendothelial system, and it is preferentially delivered in organs which riches in monocytes such as liver, spleen, and bone marrow. Decreased distribution in the heart and kidney can help minimize drug toxicity to tissues.

5. 提高药物稳定性 将一些易氧化或者对酶不稳定的药物包封于脂质体中，因其受到脂质体双分子层膜的保护，故提高了药物的稳定性。

⑤ **Improving drug stability** Some drugs that are easily oxidized or unstable to enzyme are entrapped in liposomes, bilayer membrane of liposomes can improve stability of these drugs.

（三）脂质体的性质

(3) Properties of Liposomes

1. 相变温度 脂质体膜的物理性质与介质温度有密切关系。当升高温度时，脂质双分子层中酰基侧链从有序排列变为无序排列，这种变化会引起脂膜物理性质的一系列变化，可由“胶晶”态变为“液晶”态，膜的横切面和流动性增加，双分子层厚度减小，这种转变时的温度称为相变温度。当达到相变温度时，因膜的流动性增加，脂质体内药物释放速率增大。

① **Phase transition temperature** The physical properties of liposome membrane are closely related to the temperature of the medium. When the temperature increases, the acyl side chain in the lipid bilayer changes from ordered to disordered form. This transform will cause a series of physical changes of the lipid film, such as transition from colloid to crystalline. Thus, the cross section and the fluidity of the membrane increase, the thickness of the bilayer decrease. The temperature at this transition is called the phase transition temperature. When the phase transition temperature reaches a threshold, the drug release rate in the liposomes increases with the increase of membrane fluidity.

2. 荷电性 含磷脂酸、磷脂酰丝氨酸等酸性脂质的脂质体荷负电，含十八胺等碱基（胺基）脂质的脂质体荷正电，不含离子的脂质体显电中性。脂质体表面电性对其包封率、稳定性、靶器官分布及对靶细胞作用影响较大。

② **Charge ability** Liposomes containing acidic lipid, such as phosphatidic acid (PA) and phosphatidylserine (PS) are negatively charged. Liposomes containing base (amine) groups is positively charged, such as octadecylamine. Ion-free liposomes shows electrically neutral. The surface electrical property of liposomes has a great influence on its encapsulation efficiency, stability, target organ distribution, and effects on target cell.

（四）脂质体制备方法

(4) Preparation of Liposomes

1. 薄膜超声法 将磷脂、胆固醇等脂质及脂溶性药物溶于氯仿或其他有机溶剂中，然后将溶

液在烧瓶中旋转蒸发，脂质在瓶内壁形成薄膜；将水溶性药物溶于磷酸盐缓冲液中，加至烧瓶中不断搅拌水化，即得。

① **Thin-film ultrasound** Dissolve lipids such as phospholipid, cholesterol, and fat-soluble drug in chloroform or other organic solvents, then evaporate the solution under reduced pressure in a flask. The lipid forms a film presented on the inner wall of the flask. Dissolve water-soluble drugs in a phosphate buffer solution, then add the solution into the above flask, continuously stir to hydrate and obtain liposomes.

2. 注入法 将磷脂、胆固醇等类脂物质和脂溶性药物溶于有机溶剂中，然后将其缓慢注入到搅拌下的恒温磷酸盐缓冲液（可含水溶性药物）中，搅拌挥尽有机溶剂，即得多孔脂质体。其粒径较大，不宜静脉注射。也可高压乳匀或超声得到单室脂质体。

② **Injection method** Dissolve lipid substance such as phospholipid, cholesterol, and fat-soluble drug in organic solvent, and then slowly inject them into a constant temperature phosphate buffer solution (which contain water-soluble drug) under stirring. Macroporous liposome is obtained by stirring and volatilizing the organic solvent. The liposome is not suitable for intravenous injection because its large particle size. Single-compartment liposome can also be obtained by high pressure homogenization or ultrasound.

3. 冷冻干燥法 将磷脂超声处理高度分散于缓冲盐溶液中，加入冻结保护剂（如甘露醇、葡萄糖等）冷冻干燥后，再将干燥物分散到含有药物的缓冲盐溶液或其他水性介质中，即得脂质体。该法适合于对热敏感的药物。

③ **Freeze drying method** The liposomes is obtained by dispersing phospholipid in buffer salt solution, adding freeze-protected agents (eg, mannitol, glucose, etc.) to freeze-drying, and then dispersing the dried products into buffer salt solution or other aqueous media containing drugs. The method is suitable for heat-sensitive drugs.

4. 逆相蒸发法 将磷脂等膜材溶于有机溶剂中，加入待包封的药物水溶液，超声形成 W/O 乳状液，减压除去有机溶剂，达到胶态后滴加缓冲液，旋转蒸发制得水性混悬液，通过分离除去未包入的游离药物，即得大单室脂质体。该法适合于水溶性药物及大分子生物活性物质。

④ **Reverse phase evaporation method** Dissolve phospholipid and other membrane materials in organic solvent, add aqueous solution of the drugs, sonicate to form w/o emulsion. Remove the organic solvent under reduced pressure, drop buffer after reaching the colloidal state, rotate evaporation to prepare the aqueous suspension, and remove the free drugs by separation to obtain large single-compartment liposome. This method is suitable for water-soluble drugs and macromolecular bioactive substances.

5. pH 梯度法 根据弱酸、弱碱药物在不同 pH 介质中的解离不同，通过控制脂质体膜内外 pH 梯度，使药物以离子形式包封于脂质体的内水相中。

⑤ **pH gradient method** According to the different dissociation of weak acid and weak base drugs in different pH media, the drugs is encapsulated in the internal aqueous phase of the liposomes in ionic form by controlling the pH gradient inside and outside the liposome membrane.

（五）影响脂质体载药量的因素

(5) Factors Affecting Drug Loading

1. 药物溶解度 极性药物在水中溶解度越大，在脂质体水层中的浓度则越高。非极性药物的脂溶性越大，体积包封率越高，水溶性与脂溶性都小的药物体积包封率较低。

① **Drug solubility** The greater the solubility of a polar drug in water is, the higher concentration in the liposome aqueous layer is. The larger space of the water layer is, the more polar drugs can

be encapsulated. The greater the lipid solubility of non-polar drug is, the higher the entrapment efficiency is. The drugs with low water solubility and fat solubility usually presents lower entrapment efficiency.

2. 脂质体的粒径大小　当类脂质的量不变时，类脂质双分子层的空间体积越大，则载药量越多。

② **Particle size of liposomes**　When the amount of the lipidoid is constant, the larger volume of the lipidoid bilayer is, the more drugs will be loaded.

3. 脂质体电荷　当相同电荷的药物包封于脂质体双层膜中，同电荷相斥致使双层膜之间的距离增大，可包封更多亲水性药物。

③ **Liposome charge**　When drug with the same charge is encapsulated in the liposome bilayer membrane, the distance between bilayers increases due to charge repulsion, which is good for encapsulating more hydrophilic drugs.

4. 处方组成　药脂比、类脂质膜材的投料比、类脂质种类对包封率、载药量都有影响，如增加胆固醇含量，可提高水溶性药物的载药量。

④ **Prescription composition**　The ratio of drug-lipid, the ratio of lipid-like membrane materials, and the type of lipids have effects on the encapsulation rate and drug loading. For example, increasing the cholesterol content can increase the drug loading of water-soluble drugs.

（六）脂质体的质量评价

(6) Quality Evaluation of Liposomes

主要包括脂质体的形态、粒径与分布，包封率，渗漏率，主药含量，体外释放度，脂质体氧化程度及有机溶剂残留量等。

It mainly includes morphology, particle size and its distribution of liposomes, encapsulation efficiency, leakage rate, the content of the drug, the release *in vitro*, the degree of liposome oxidation, and the residual amount of organic solvent, etc.

PPT

第二节　药物制剂新剂型

一、缓控释制剂

（一）含义

1. 缓释制剂　系指在规定释放介质中，按要求缓慢地非恒速释放药物，其与相应普通制剂比较，给药频率比普通制剂减少一半或有所减少，且能显著增加患者依从性的制剂。缓释制剂中药物释放主要为一级速度过程。

2. 控释制剂　系指在规定释放介质中，按要求缓慢地恒速释放药物，其与相应普通制剂比较，给药频率比普通制剂减少一半或有所减少，血药浓度比缓释制剂更加平稳，且能显著增加患者依从性的制剂。控释制剂中药物释放主要为零级或接近零级速度过程。

（二）特点

与普通制剂相比，缓控释制剂主要具有以下特点：

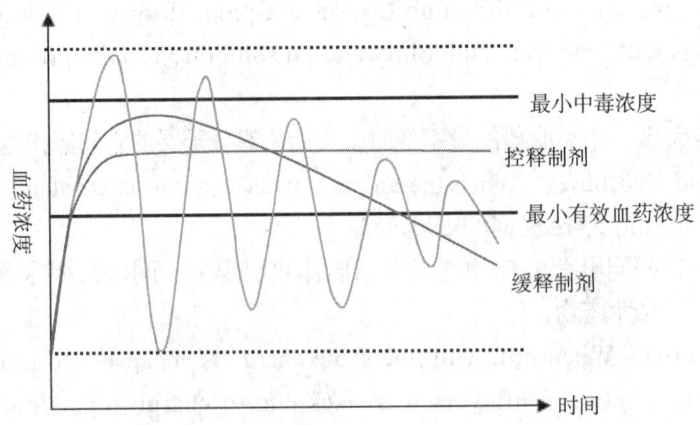

图 19-6 缓控释制剂与普通常规制剂的血药浓度 - 时间图

1. 药物治疗作用持久、毒副作用低、用药次数显著减少。

2. 药物可缓慢地释放进入体内，血药浓度的“峰谷”波动小，可避免超过治疗血药浓度范围的毒副作用，又能使药物保持在有效浓度范围（治疗窗）之内以维持疗效。

缓控释制剂也有其局限性，①临床应用中对剂量调节的灵活性较低，临床应用中如遇某些特殊情况，往往不能立刻停止治疗。②缓控释制剂的生产工艺较复杂，制备设备较昂贵。

有些药物不适宜制成普通缓控释制剂，①一般生物半衰期（$t_{1/2}$）很短（小于 1 小时）或很长（大于 24 小时）。因为 $t_{1/2}$ 很短时，需要很大剂量才能制成一个缓释制剂，使用不方便。$t_{1/2}$ 很长，则无须制成缓控释制剂。②单次服用剂量很大（大于 1g）。③药效剧烈、溶解度小、吸收无规律或吸收易受影响的药物；④在肠中需在特定部位主动吸收的药物。例如维生素 B_2 有效吸收部位在小肠上段，在结肠仅 9%，不宜制成缓释制剂。

（三）缓控释制剂的组成

1. 缓释制剂的组成 理想的缓释制剂，一般包含速释与缓释两部分药物。速释部分是指释放速度快，能迅速建立起治疗所需的最佳血药浓度的那部分药物，缓释部分是指释放速度较慢或恒速，能较长时间维持最佳血药浓度的那部分药物。

有些缓释制剂的速释部分与缓释部分同时释药，有些缓释制剂中的速释部分与缓释部分间隔释药。不论是同时释药还是间隔释药，缓释制剂在体内的血药浓度是速释和缓释两部分药物之和。因此，速释与缓释两种组分的比例以及缓释部分的释药速度直接关系到制剂的质量、用药疗效及安全。

2. 控释制剂的组成 根据释药机理不同，控释制剂通常包括以下 4 个部分。

（1）药物贮库　是贮存药物的部位，将药物溶解或混悬分散于聚合物中，药物剂量应符合治疗要求，满足预期恒速释药的需要。

（2）控释部分　使药物以预定的速度恒速释放，如包衣控释片上的微孔膜。

（3）能源部分　供给药物能量，推动药物由贮库中释放出来。

（4）传递孔道　药物分子通过孔道释出，同时兼具控释作用，如不溶性骨架片。

（四）缓释、控释制剂的释药原理

缓释、控释制剂的释药原理主要有控制溶出、扩散、溶蚀或扩散与溶出相结合，也可以利用渗透压或离子交换机制，从而达到缓释控释的目的。

1. 溶出原理 药物的释放受溶出度的限制，溶出速度慢的药物显示出缓释作用。根据 Noyes-Whitney 溶出速率方程［式（19-4）］，可通过降低药物的溶出度，增大药物粒径，以降低药物的溶出速率，使药物缓慢释放，达到缓释作用。

$$dc/dt = KS(C_s - C) \tag{19-4}$$

式中，dc/dt 为溶解速度，K 为溶解速率常数，S 为表面积，C_s 为药物的饱和溶解度，C 为药物的浓度。

具体有以下几种方法：①制成溶解度小的盐或酯；②与高分子化合物生成难溶性盐；③控制药物粒子大小。

2. 扩散原理 降低药物的扩散速率，可控制药物从制剂中扩散出来进入体液的速度，延缓药物的吸收，达到缓释、控释目的，可以通过以下几种方法来实现：①用水不溶性材料包衣。②制成微囊；③以水不溶性材料为骨架制成不溶性骨架制剂。④增加黏度以降低扩散速度。

3. 溶蚀与扩散、溶出相结合 溶蚀型缓控释制剂，不仅药物可以从骨架中扩散出来，骨架本身也处于溶蚀过程。

溶胀型缓控释制剂，药物溶于具有膨胀性的聚合物中，水进入骨架，药物溶解并从膨胀的骨架中扩散出来，释药速度取决于聚合物的膨胀速度、药物的溶解度和骨架中可溶部分的量。

4. 渗透压原理 渗透压作为驱动力，可以均匀恒速地释放药物，实现零级释放。以单室口服渗透泵片为例说明其原理和构造：片芯由水溶性药物和水溶性聚合物或其他辅料制成，外面用水不溶性聚合物包衣，制成半透膜，水可以渗透进入膜内，但药物不能渗出，然后用激光或适宜的方法在半透膜一端壳顶打一个细孔。其释药过程为：片剂口服后胃肠道的水分通过半透膜进入片芯，药物溶解成饱和溶液，膜内外渗透压差较大，药物由细孔持续流出，流出量与渗透进入膜内的水量相等，直到片芯药物溶解完为止。

胃肠液中离子不会进入半透膜，故渗透泵片的释药速率与 pH 无关，在胃中和肠中的释药速率相等。片芯的处方、半透膜的厚度和渗透性，以及释药孔的直径，是影响渗透泵片释药的关键。

5. 离子交换作用 离子交换树脂是由水不溶性交联聚合物组成，在其侧链上有可供交换的阴离子和阳离子基团，带电荷的药物可结合于树脂上。载药树脂制成口服制剂，药物与胃肠液中的离子交换后释放出来，其交换及扩散过程如下：

树脂$^{+}$ – 药物$^{-}$ + X^{-} ⟶ 树脂$^{+}$ – X^{-} + 药物$^{-}$　　树脂$^{-}$ – 药物$^{+}$ + Y^{+} ⟶ 树脂$^{-}$ – Y^{+} + 药物$^{+}$

式中，X^{-} 和 Y^{+} 为消化道内的离子，交换后，游离的药物从树脂中扩散出来。离子交换树脂的组成、交联度、酸碱度、孔隙率和溶胀度对药物释放速率有显著影响。

（五）缓控释制剂的类型及制备方法

1. 骨架型缓控释制剂

（1）骨架片

亲水凝胶骨架片　以亲水性高分子材料作为骨架材料，与药物混匀后直接压片或湿法制粒压片。骨架片遇水后骨架膨胀，形成的凝胶屏障可以控制药物的溶出和释放。常用的骨架材料有：羟丙甲纤维素、壳聚糖、海藻酸钠、卡波姆、甲基纤维素、羟乙基纤维素、羧甲基纤维素钠和聚羧乙烯等。

案例导入 ¦ Case example

案例 19-4　穿心莲总内酯亲水凝胶骨架片

处方：穿心莲 羟丙基甲基纤维素　羧甲基淀粉钠　十二烷基硫酸钠　乳糖　硬脂酸镁

制法：穿心莲药材用 10 倍量 95% 乙醇回流提取 2 次，每次 1 小时，合并提取液，减压回收浓缩，得到浓缩液，加入活性炭，热处理 30 分钟，趁热抽滤，浓缩至无醇味，得到水溶液，经乙酸乙酯萃取，浓缩至有微量黄色结晶析出，放置，抽滤，得黄色粉末，晾干。按处方量称取过 80 目筛的主药和辅料，主药辅料 1∶1，片重 3g，采用等量递加法混匀，加入适量无水乙醇作为润湿剂制软材，过 20 目筛制粒，于 60℃干燥 2 小时，再过 18 目筛整粒，干颗粒中加入适量硬脂

酸镁，混匀，压片，控制该片硬度在8.0~10.0kg/cm^2，即得。

注解：穿心莲总内酯为难溶于水的药物，实验考察了3种羟丙甲纤维素（HPMC）型号：K4M, K100LV, E50LV，黏度K4M>K100LV>E50LV，随着HPMC的相对分子量的增加，HPMC的黏度变大，HPMC的分子链变长，形成的凝胶层不容易溶蚀，导致药物的释放速率降低，不太适宜水难溶性药物的溶解。因而制备时选择低黏度的E50LV羟丙甲纤维素较适宜。

思考题：穿心莲总内酯骨架片的释药机制是什么？

溶蚀性骨架片　由不溶解但可溶蚀的蜡质材料制成。骨架片通过孔道扩散与溶蚀控制药物的释放，除骨架材料外，常添加一些致孔剂来调节释药速度。常用骨架材料有：蜂蜡、硬脂酸、巴西棕榈蜡、氢化植物油和单硬脂酸甘油酯等。常用致孔剂有聚维酮、聚乙二醇和表面活性剂等。

不溶性骨架片　由不溶于水或水溶性很小的高分子聚合物与药物混合均匀后制得。药物通过骨架中极细的孔径通道缓慢向外扩散而释放，而骨架始终保持原形，最后随粪便排出体外。常用骨架材料有：聚乙烯、乙基纤维素、聚丙烯等。

案例导入

（2）胃滞留片　根据流体动力学原理设计，由药物与低密度亲水性高分子材料及其他辅料混合压制成片。口服后长时间漂浮于胃液之上，既延缓药物的释放又延长其在胃内滞留的时间，改善药物的吸收，提高生物利用度。

常用亲水高分子材料有：羟丙甲纤维素、羟丙纤维素、羟乙基纤维素、羟甲基纤维素钠、甲基纤维素、乙基纤维素等。为了提高胃内滞留时间，还需加入疏水性、相对密度小的蜡类、脂肪醇类、脂类辅料。

（3）生物黏附片　药物与具有生物黏附作用的辅料混合制成的片剂，能黏附于生物黏膜，缓慢释放药物并由黏膜吸收以达到治疗目的。常用的辅料有卡波普、羟丙基纤维素、羧甲基纤维素钠以及壳聚糖等。

（4）骨架型小丸　采用骨架材料与药物混合，或再加入一些其他辅料，如调节释药速率的辅料PEG类、表面活性剂等，经适当方法制成小丸，即为骨架型小丸。

2. 膜控型缓控释制剂　膜控型缓控释制剂是指用包衣材料对片剂、颗粒、小丸等进行包衣，以控制药物的溶出和扩散而制成的缓控释制剂。控释膜通常为一种半透膜或微孔膜。包衣材料包括肠溶材料和水不溶性高分子材料。根据膜的性质和需要可加入致孔剂、抗黏剂等物质。膜控型缓控释制剂主要有微孔膜包衣片、膜控释小片、肠溶膜控释片和膜控释小丸等。

3. 渗透泵型控释制剂　由药物、半透膜材料、渗透压活性物质和推动剂等组成。常用的半透膜材料有醋酸纤维素、乙基纤维素等。渗透压活性物质起调节药室内渗透压的作用，其用量多少与零级释药时间长短有关，常用的有乳糖、果糖、甘露醇、葡萄糖等。推动剂能吸水膨胀，产生推动力，将药物层的药物推出释药小孔，常用的有分子量为1万~36万的PVP等。此外，还可加入助悬剂、黏合剂、润滑剂等。

渗透泵片一般由片芯和包衣膜两部分组成，按照结构特点有单室渗透泵片和双室渗透泵片之分，如图19-7所示。半透膜的厚度、孔径、片芯的处方以及释药小孔的直径，是制备渗透泵片剂的关键。

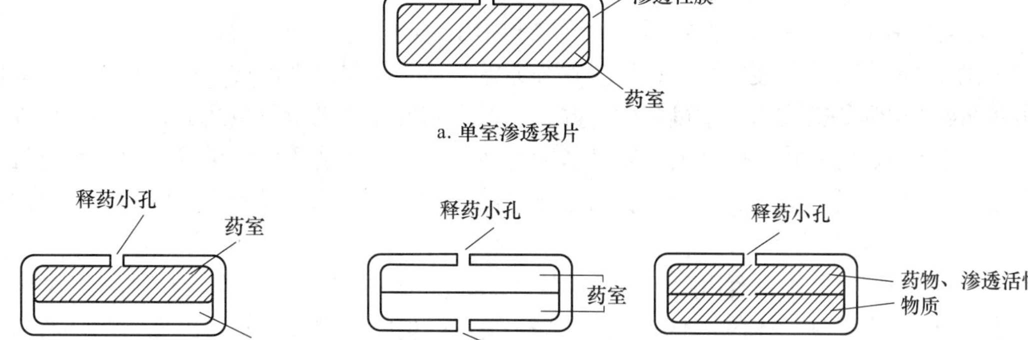

图 19-7 渗透泵片结构示意图

（六）体内外评价方法

1. 体外释放度试验 本试验在模拟体内消化道条件下（如温度、介质 pH、搅拌速率等），对制剂进行药物释放速率试验，最后制定出合理的体外药物释放度，以监测产品的生产过程与对产品进行质量控制。

（1）仪器 除另有规定外，缓释、控释制剂的体外药物释放度试验可采用溶出度测定仪进行。

（2）温度 缓释、控释制剂模拟体温应控制在 37℃ ± 0.5℃。

（3）释放介质 以脱气的新鲜纯化水为常用释放介质，或根据药物的溶解特性、处方要求、吸收部位，使用稀盐酸（0.001~0.1mol/L）或 pH 值 3~8 的磷酸盐缓冲液，对难溶性药物不宜采用有机溶剂，可加少量表面活性剂（如十二烷基硫酸钠等）。

释放介质的体积应符合漏槽条件。

（4）释放度取样时间点 体外释放速率试验应能反映受试制剂释药速率的变化特征，且能满足统计学处理的需要，释药全过程的时间不应低于给药的间隔时间，且累积释放百分率要求达到 90% 以上。除另有规定外，通常将释药全过程的数据作累积释放百分率 - 时间的释药曲线图，制订出合理的释放度检查方法和限度。

缓释制剂从释药曲线图中至少选出 3 个取样时间点，第一点为开始 0.5~2 小时的取样时间点，用于考察药物是否有突释，第二点为中间的取样时间点，用于确定释药特性，最后取样时间点，用于考察释药是否基本完全。此 3 点可用于表征体外缓释制剂药物释放度。

控释制剂除以上 3 点外，还应增加 2 个取样时间点，此 5 点可用于表征体外控释制剂药物释放度，释放百分率的范围应小于缓释制剂，如果需要，可以再增加取样时间点。

多于一个活性成分的产品，要求对每一个活性成分均按以上要求进行释放度测定。

（5）工艺的重现性与均一性试验 应考察 3 批以上、每批 6 片（粒）产品批与批之间体外药物释放度的重现性，并考察同批产品 6 片（粒）体外药物释放度的均一性。

（6）释药模型的拟合 缓释制剂的释药数据可用一级方程和 Higuchi 方程等拟合，即：

$$\ln(1 - M_t/M_\infty) = -Kt \text{（一级方程）} \quad (19\text{-}5)$$

$$M_t/M_\infty = Kt^{1/2} \text{（Higuchi 方程）} \quad (19\text{-}6)$$

控释制剂的释药数据可用零级方程拟合，即：

$$M_t/M_\infty = Kt \text{（零级方程）} \quad (19\text{-}7)$$

式中，M_t 为 t 时间的释药量，M_∞ 为 t_∞ 时间的释药量，M_t/M_∞ 为 t 时间的累积释放百分率，拟合时以相关系数（r）最大而均方差（MSE）最小的拟合效果最好。

2. 体内生物利用度与生物等效性研究 生物利用度是指活性物质从药物制剂中释放并被吸收后，在作用部位可利用的速度和程度，通常用血浆浓度 - 时间曲线来评估。如果含有相同活性物质的两种药品药剂学等效或药剂学可替代，并且它们在相同摩尔剂量下给药后，生物利用度（速度和程度）落在预定的可接受限度内，则被认为生物等效。在生物等效性试验中，一般通过比较受试药品和参比药品的相对生物利用度，根据选定的药动学参数和预设的接受限，从而对两者的生物等效性做出判定。

缓释、控释制剂进行生物利用度与生物等效性试验，按照《中国药典》进行研究。

3. 体内 - 体外相关性 体内 - 体外相关性指由制剂产生的生物学性质或由生物学性质衍生的参数（如 t_{max}、C_{max} 或 AUC）与同一制剂的物理化学性质（如体外释放行为）之间，建立了合理的定量关系。

缓释、控释制剂要求进行体内外相关性的试验，它应反映整个体外释放曲线与血药浓度 - 时间曲线之间的关系。只有当体内外具有相关性，才能通过体外释放曲线预测体内情况。

体内外相关性可归纳为三种：①体外释放曲线与体内吸收曲线上对应的各个时间点应分别相关，这种相关简称点对点相关，表明两条曲线可以重合；②应用统计矩分析原理建立体外释放的平均时间与体内平均滞留时间之间的相关，由于能产生相似的平均滞留时间可有很多不同的体内曲线，因此体内平均滞留时间不能代表体内完整的血药浓度 - 时间曲线；③将一个释放时间点（$t_{50\%}$、$t_{90\%}$）与一个药物动力学参数（AUC、C_{max} 或 t_{max}）之间单点相关，只说明部分相关。

缓释、控释制剂体内外相关性，系指体内吸收相的吸收曲线与体外释放曲线之间对应的各个时间点回归，得到直线回归方程的相关系数符合要求，即可认为具有相关性。

二、迟释制剂

迟释制剂系指在给药后不立即释放药物的制剂，包括肠溶制剂、结肠定位制剂和脉冲制剂等。

（一）肠溶制剂

肠溶制剂系指在规定的酸性介质中不释放或几乎不释放药物，而在要求的时间内，于 pH 为 6.8 的磷酸缓冲液中大部分或全部释放药物的制剂。

（二）结肠定位制剂

结肠定位制剂系指在胃肠道上部基本不释放、在结肠内大部分或全部释放的制剂，即一定时间内在规定的酸性介质与 pH 6.8 的磷酸盐缓冲液中不释放或几乎不释放，而在要求的时间内，于 pH 7.5~8.0 的磷酸盐缓冲液中大部分或全部释放的制剂。

案例导入 ¦ Case example

案例 19-5　白头翁（汤）结肠定位缓释片

处方： 白头翁汤干浸膏 421.31mg　丙烯酸乙酯 - 甲基丙烯酸酯共聚物 26.892mg　聚丙烯酸树脂 Eudragit S100 41.25mg　邻苯二甲酸二乙酯（DEP）2.5mg　微晶纤维素 0.9mg　滑石粉 7.15mg

制法： 一部分白头翁汤干膏粉用适量的 95% 乙醇制粒，过 16 目筛，低温（60℃）干燥，用 14 目筛整粒制成速释颗粒，另一部分白头翁汤干膏粉，用聚丙烯酸树脂（加 95% 乙醇溶解）胶体液混合制粒，过 16 目筛，低温（60℃）干燥，用 14 目筛整粒制成缓释颗粒，将速释颗粒和缓

释颗粒混合，加入 0.2% 的滑石粉和微晶纤维素，混匀，压片，包结肠衣（Eudragit S100、DEP、滑石粉），使包衣增重 10%，即得。

用法与用量：口服。1 次 4 片，1 日 2 次。

注解：①白头翁（汤）结肠定位缓释片由白头翁汤改剂型而来，以方中有效成分白头翁皂苷 B_4 和盐酸小檗碱为评价指标，采用桨法测定 2 个指标成分的累积溶出率，结果表明，药物在胃液及小肠液中基本不释放，且在结肠持续释药 12 小时，累积释放量超过 90%。

②方中丙烯酸乙酯 - 甲基丙烯酸酯共聚物为缓释辅料；聚丙烯酸树脂 Eudragit S100 为包衣材料，当 pH>7.0 时，包衣层开始溶解，释药部位在结肠；微晶纤维素为黏合剂；邻苯二甲酸二乙酯（DEP）在包衣工艺中作为增塑剂，滑石粉作为润滑剂。

思考题：查阅相关资料，说明包衣增重是怎么计算的？

（三）脉冲制剂

脉冲制剂系指不立即释放药物，而在某种条件下（如在体液中经过一定时间或一定 pH 或某些酶作用下）一次或多次突然释放药物的制剂。

三、前体药物

将一种具有药理活性的母体药物进行化学修饰（如导入另一种载体基团或与另一种作用相似的母体药物相结合），形成一种新的化合物。进入机体后，经生物转化成母体药物呈现疗效，这种可逆的母体衍生物称为前体药物，多在抗癌药、脑部位和结肠部位中给药。

除可以制备靶向制剂外，前体药物还有以下特点：产生协同作用，扩大临床应用范围；改善药物的溶解度和吸收，提高血药浓度；延长药物的作用时间，或使药物达到靶向性；降低药物的毒副作用；增加药物的稳定性等。前体药物常用的制备方法有酸碱反应法、复分解反应法、钡盐沉淀法、离子交换法及络合法等。

四、靶向制剂

（一）含义

靶向制剂系指采用载体将药物通过循环系统浓集于或近靶器官、靶组织、靶细胞和细胞内结构的一类新制剂。

（二）特点

与普通制剂相比，靶向制剂可使药物浓集于靶组织、靶器官和靶细胞，提高药物对“靶”的指向性；提高疗效，降低药物对于正常细胞的毒性；减少药物用量；增加药物的稳定性等。

（三）分类

按药物的分布水平，靶向制剂可以分为三级：一级靶向制剂，系指药物到达特定的器官或组织；二级靶向制剂，系指药物到达特定的细胞；三级靶向制剂，系指药物到达细胞内的特定部位。

按靶向给药的机制，靶向制剂可以分为被动靶向制剂、主动靶向制剂、物理化学靶向制剂三类。

1. 被动靶向制剂　被动靶向制剂系指载药微粒通过正常生理过程选择性地积集、运送至肝、脾、肺等器官，而达到靶向作用目的的制剂。常见的载体有脂质体、微囊与微球、纳米粒、乳剂等。

（1）脂质体　脂质体是一种定向药物载体，进入血液循环后，可选择性地分布于富有巨噬细胞的网状内皮组织，并改变被包封药物的体内分布。将脂质体表面进行修饰，可延长脂质体在体内的循环时间，回避吞噬系统或具有主动寻靶的功能。

（2）微囊与微球　微囊与微球在体内的分布与粒径大小和给药方式有密切关系。药物制成微囊或微球的主要特点是发挥缓释长效和靶向作用。

（3）纳米粒　纳米粒的靶向性主要与其粒径大小及表面的化学性质密切相关。有些纳米粒具有在肿瘤中集中的倾向，可以作为抗癌药物的载体。

（4）乳剂　乳剂对淋巴系统有亲和性。乳剂在体内的靶向性与乳滴粒径、表面电荷、处方组成及给药途径等因素有关。

2. 主动靶向制剂　主动靶向制剂包括经过修饰的药物载体和前体药物两大类制剂。前者是用修饰的药物载体作为“导弹”，将药物定向地运送到靶区浓集发挥药效。后者是将药物修饰成前体药物，在特定靶区被激活而发挥作用。

（1）表面修饰的载药微粒　载药微粒经表面修饰后，减少或避免被单核 - 巨噬细胞识别，有利于靶向除肝脾以外的缺少单核 - 巨噬细胞系统的组织；利用抗体修饰，可制成定向于细胞表面抗原的免疫靶向制剂；载体表面结合细胞特异性配体，可使微粒导向具有特异受体的细胞。主动靶向制剂通过修饰的药物微粒载体来实现，主要包括修饰脂质体、免疫脂质体、修饰微球、修饰微乳、修饰纳米粒等。

（2）前体药物靶向制剂　前体药物靶向制剂是前体制剂与靶向制剂的有机结合，通过前体药物产生靶向性。

3. 物理化学靶向制剂　物理化学靶向制剂系指应用某些物理化学方法使药物在特定部位发挥药效的靶向给药系统。常用的物理化学方法包括磁性、温度、电场和 pH 值等。

（1）磁性靶向制剂　采用体外磁响应导向药物至靶部位的制剂称为磁性靶向制剂，主要用作抗癌药物的载体。磁性制剂包括磁性微球、磁性微囊、磁性纳米粒、磁性脂质体、磁性片剂、磁性胶囊等。

（2）栓塞靶向制剂　动脉栓塞是通过插入动脉的导管将栓塞物输送到靶组织或靶器官的医疗技术，通过阻断靶区的供血和营养，致靶区肿瘤细胞坏死，栓塞制剂含有的抗肿瘤药释放产生治疗作用，起到栓塞和靶向化疗的双重作用。

（3）热敏靶向制剂　利用外部热源对靶区进行加热，使靶组织局部温度稍高于周围未加热区，实现载体中药物在靶区内释放的一类制剂。

（4）pH 敏感靶向制剂　疾病状态会改变病理组织的 pH，利用 pH 差异，选择合适的载体材料即可将药物选择性地靶向到特定位置。

（四）靶向性评价

药物的靶向性是靶向给药系统的重要评价指标，可以由以下三个参数衡量。

1. 相对摄取率

$$r_e=(AUC_i)_p/(AUC_i)_s \quad (19\text{-}8)$$

式中，AUC_i 是由浓度 - 时间曲线求得的第 i 个器官或组织的药物浓度 - 时间曲线下面积，下标 p 和 s 分别表示试验药物制剂浓度和药物浓度。r_e 大于 1 表示药物制剂在该器官或组织具有靶向性，r_e 越大，靶向效果越好；r_e 等于或小于 1 表示无靶向性。

2. 靶向效率

$$t_e=(AUC)_{靶}/(AUC)_{非} \quad (19\text{-}9)$$

式中，t_e 值表示药物制剂或药物浓度对靶器官的选择性。t_e 值大于 1 表示药物对靶器官比非靶器官有选择性，t_e 值越大，选择性越强。

3. 峰浓度比

$$C_e=(C_{max})_p/(C_{max})_s \qquad (19\text{-}11)$$

式中，C_{max} 为峰浓度，每个组织或器官中的 C_e 值表示药物制剂改变药物分布的效果，C_e 值越大，表明改变分布的效果越明显。

（桂双英　孙　黎）

岗位对接

重点小结

题库

第二十章　中药制剂的稳定性

Chapter 20　The Stability of TCM Preparations

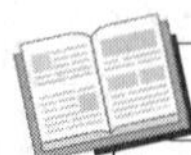

学习目标 | Learning Goals

知识要求：

1．**掌握**　影响中药制剂稳定性的因素及提高稳定性的方法。

2．**熟悉**　中药制剂稳定性的考察方法及有效期的求解。

3．**了解**　研究中药制剂稳定性的意义；包装材料对中药制剂稳定性的影响。

能力要求：

能够掌握并解释药物制剂制备和储存中药物不稳定因素及稳定化方法。

Knowledge requirements:

1. To master the factors affecting the stability of TCM preparations and the methods to improve the stability.

2. To be familiar with the methods investigating stability of TCM preparations and the solution of validity period.

3. To know the significance of studying the stability of TCM preparations, and the effects of packaging materials on the stability of TCM preparations.

Ability requirements:

To be able to grasp and explain the unstable factors and stabilization methods in preparation and storage of pharmaceutical preparations.

第一节　概述

20.1　Overview

一、中药制剂稳定性的研究意义

20.1.1　Significance of Research on the Stability of TCM Preparations

安全有效、稳定可控是对药物制剂的基本要求，而稳定性是保证有效和安全的基础。中药制剂的稳定性是指中药制剂从制备到使用，其化学、物理及生物学特性发生变化的速度和程度。

Safety, effectiveness, stability and controllability are the basic requirements for pharmaceutical preparations, and stability is the basis to ensure effectiveness and safety. The stability of TCM preparations refers to the speed and degree of changes in the chemical, physical and biological characteristics of TCM preparations.

不同环境下（如温度、湿度、光照、包装材料等）对中药制剂进行稳定性研究，探讨环境因素对中药制剂稳定性的影响及其变化规律，以认识和预测制剂的稳定趋势，为生产、包装、贮存、运输条件的确定和有效期的制定提供科学依据，对保障药品临床应用的安全和有效是非常重要的。因此，我国《药品注册管理办法》规定，新药申请必须呈报有关稳定性研究的资料。

It is very important to study the stability of TCM preparations in different environments (such as temperature, humidity, light, packaging materials, etc.) for ensuring the safety and effectiveness of clinical application of drugs. It provides a scientific basis for the determination of production, packaging, storage, transportation conditions and the formulation of expiration dates by exploring the influence of environmental factors on the stability of TCM preparations and its changing rules. Therefore, China's "Provisions for Drug Registration" stipulates that new drug applications must submit data on stability studies.

随着科技的进步，中药新制剂、新剂型不断出现，社会和公众对药品质量的要求越来越高。为了提高中药制剂的质量，保证其疗效与安全，提高中药新药研究、制剂生产、质量控制和临床应用的科学性和先进性，获得更好的社会效益和经济效益，必须重视中药制剂的稳定性研究。

With the advancement of science and technology, new preparations and dosage forms of TCM are constantly appearing, and the public is increasingly demanding high-quality medicines. It is essential to pay attention to the stability of TCM, which may benefit new drug research, preparation production, quality control, and clinical application. Sound social and economic benefits will be achieved simultaneously.

二、中药制剂稳定性的研究内容
20.1.2 Research Contents on the Stability of TCM Preparations

中药制剂稳定性变化的主要内容包括化学稳定性、物理稳定性和生物学稳定性。化学稳定性变化是指由于水解、氧化、聚合、分解等化学降解反应，引起药物的含量（或药效）、色泽产生变化等。物理稳定性变化主要指制剂的物理性状发生变化，如固体制剂的吸湿，乳剂的分层、破裂，液体制剂的浑浊、沉淀，片剂的崩解度、溶出度的改变等。生物学稳定性变化一般是指制剂由于受微生物的污染，而导致的腐败、变质。各种变化可单独发生，也可同时发生，一种变化可以成为诱因，导致另一种变化的发生。

The main contents on stability changes of TCM preparations include chemical stability, physical stability and biological stability. Changes in chemical stability refer to the chemical degradation reactions such as hydrolysis, oxidation, polymerization and decomposition, which causes the change in drug content (or drug effect) and color. Changes in physical stability refer to the conversion of physical properties, such as moisture absorption of solid preparations, delamination and cracking of emulsions, turbidity and precipitation of liquid preparations, changes in disintegration and dissolution of tablets, etc. Changes in biological stability refer to the deterioration caused by microbial contamination. Changes can occur individually or simultaneously, and one change can be the cause of another.

稳定性研究具有阶段性特点，不同阶段有不同的目的。一般始于制剂的临床前研究，贯穿制剂研究与开发的全过程，在制剂上市后还要继续进行稳定性研究。

Stability research is characterized by stages, and different stages have different purposes. Generally, it starts from the pre-clinical research of preparations, covers the whole process of preparation research and development, and continues after approval for market.

第二节 影响中药制剂稳定性的因素及提高稳定性的方法

20.2 Factors Affecting the Stability of TCM Preparations and Methods for Improving the Stability

PPT

一、影响中药制剂稳定性的因素

20.2.1 Factors Affecting the Stability of TCM Preparations

1. 药物化学降解及其影响因素 药物的化学降解反应级数有零级、一级、二级及分数级等。多数制剂的分解可按零级、一级和伪一级反应处理。零级、一级反应药物浓度随时间变化的方程分别为：

(1) Chemical degradation of drugs and the affecting factors The grades of chemical degradation reactions of drugs include zero order, first order, second order and fractional order. The decomposition of most preparations can be treated as zero-order, first-order and pseudo-first-order reactions. The equations of zero-order and first-order describe drug concentration changes as follows:

$$C=-kt+C_0 \quad （零级反应，zero-order reaction） \tag{20-1}$$

$$\lg C=\frac{kt}{2.303}+\lg C_0 \quad （一级反应，first-order reaction） \tag{20-2}$$

式中，C_0 为初始浓度，t 为时间，C 为经过 t 时间后反应物的浓度，k 为反应速度常数。

In the formula, C_0 is initial concentration, t is time, C is reactant concentration after specific (t) time, k is reaction rate constant.

影响药物化学降解反应速度的因素有药物浓度、温度、pH、水分、光线、溶剂等。

Factors affecting the chemical degradation reaction rate of drugs include drug concentration, temperature, pH value, moisture, light, and solvent.

在制剂稳定性研究中，将药物含量降低 50% 所需的时间称为半衰期，用 $t_{1/2}$ 表示；药物含量降低 10% 所需的时间称为有效期，用 $t_{0.9}$ 表示。一级反应的有效期和半衰期按以下公式计算。

In the study of preparation stability, the required time for a 50% reduction in drug content is called half-life and expressed as $t_{1/2}$. The required time for a 10% reduction in drug content is called validity period and is expressed in $t_{0.9}$. The validity period and half-life of the first-order reaction are calculated according to the following equations.

$$t_{0.9}=-\frac{0.1054}{k} \tag{20-3}$$

$$t_{1/2}=-\frac{0.693}{k} \tag{20-4}$$

由式（20-1）和式（20-2）可知，一级反应的有效期和半衰期与制剂中药物的初始浓度无关，而与速度常数 k 值成反比。

In terms of equations 20-1 and 20-2, the validity period and half-life of the first-order reaction are independent of the initial concentration of the drug in the preparation, but are inversely proportional to the value of k.

2. 药物的化学降解类型 药物的化学降解反应有水解、氧化、异构化、聚合、脱羧等途径，其中水解、氧化是主要的降解途径。

(2) Chemical degradation types of drugs The chemical degradation reactions of drugs include hydrolysis, oxidation, isomerization, polymerization and decarboxylation. Among them, hydrolysis and oxidation are the main degradation pathways.

（1）易水解的药物结构类型 ①酯类药物：具有酯键结构的药物较易水解，相对分子质量小的脂肪族酯类极易水解，几乎无法制成稳定的液体制剂，如亚硝酸乙酯。有些酯类药物则比较稳定，如阿托品，可以制成水溶液注射剂。酯类药物制成水溶液时要特别注意 pH 的调节。一般而言，溶液碱性愈强，水解愈快，如穿心莲内酯在 pH 为 7 时内酯环水解极其缓慢，在偏碱性溶液中则水解加快；当 pH 接近 10 时，不仅内酯环开环转变成穿心莲酸，而且二萜双环可能发生双键移位、脱水、异构化、树脂化等反应，抗炎解热的疗效降低。②酰胺类药物：一般较酯类药物难水解，如青霉素等。③苷类药物：苷类药物在酶或酸碱的作用下产生水解。水解的难易程度与构成苷类药物的糖、苷元的种类以及苷元和糖连接的方式有关。如强心苷易水解，故常以浓度较高的乙醇为溶剂，其注射液多采用水与乙醇、丙二醇或甘油等为混合溶剂。洋地黄酊多采用 70% 乙醇浸出。

a. Types of easily hydrolyzed drugs ① Ester drugs: Aliphatic esters with low molecular mass are easily hydrolyzed and can hardly be made into stable liquid preparations, such as ethyl nitrite. While some ester drugs are stable, such as atropine, which can be made into aqueous injection. High attention should be paid to the adjustment of pH value when making aqueous solution of ester drugs. In general, the more alkaline solution is, the faster drugs will hydrolyze. For example, the lactone ring of andrographolide hydrolyzes very slowly when the pH value is 7, but the hydrolysis is accelerated in the alkaline solution. When the pH value is close to 10, not only does the lactone ring open to andrographolic acid, but also the diterpene ring may undergo double bond translocation, dehydration, isomerization, resinization and other reactions, and the anti-inflammatory antipyretic effect is reduced accordingly. ② Amide drugs: Amides are more difficult to hydrolyze than esters, such as penicillin. ③ Glycoside drugs: Glycosides are hydrolyzed by an enzyme or acidity-alkalinity. The degree of hydrolysis is related to the types of sugar and aglycones, and the connections between aglycones and sugars. For example, cardiac glycosides are easy to hydrolyze, so ethanol with higher concentration is often used as the solvent. Water and ethanol, propylene glycol, or glycerin are often used as the mixed solvent for the injection. Digitalis tincture is mostly extracted by 70% ethanol.

（2）易氧化的药物结构类型 ①具有酚羟基或潜在酚羟基的有效成分，如黄芩苷等；②含有不饱和碳链的油脂、挥发油等，在光线、氧气、水分、金属离子以及微生物等影响下，都能产生氧化反应。

b. Types of easily oxidized drugs ①Active components with phenolic hydroxyl or potential phenolic hydroxyl, such as baicalin. ②Oils and volatile oils containing unsaturated carbon chains can be oxidized under the influence of light, oxygen, moisture, metal ions and microorganisms

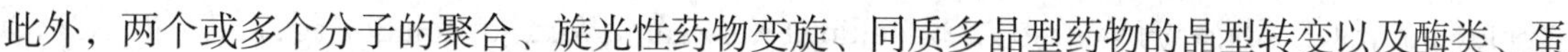

此外，两个或多个分子的聚合、旋光性药物变旋、同质多晶型药物的晶型转变以及酶类、蛋

白质类药物的变性，亦是药物变质的原因。

In addition, the polymerization of two or more molecules, optical rotation of drugs, crystal transformation of homogeneous polycrystalline drugs and denaturation of enzymes and proteins are also the causes of drug deterioration.

3. 影响中药制剂稳定性的因素

(3) Factors affecting the stability of TCM preparations

（1）处方因素　①pH 的影响。液体制剂通常在某一特定的 pH 范围内比较稳定。酸或碱是催化剂，可使溶液中不同反应的速度增大。以 H^+ 或 OH^- 为催化剂的反应，称为专属酸、碱催化反应。在酸、碱催化反应中，pH 通过对反应速度常数 k 的影响而影响制剂的稳定性。反应速度常数 k 随着介质 pH 变化而变化，其数值可通过动力学实验加以测定。通过不同条件下化学反应的 lg$k$ 值，可以计算药物最稳定的 pH。②溶剂、基质及其他辅料的影响。对于易水解的药物，有时采用非水溶剂如乙醇、丙二醇、甘油等使其稳定，有时要加入表面活性剂，利用所形成胶束的屏障作用而延缓水解。

a. The composition of preparation　①The influence of pH value. Liquid preparations are usually relatively stable within a specific pH range. Acidity or alkalinity is a catalyst that increases the rate of different reactions in a solution. The reaction with H^+ or OH^- as catalyst is called exclusive acid and base catalysis. In acid and alkaline catalytic reactions, the pH value changes the stability of the preparations by affecting the reaction rate constant k, and the value of k can be determined by kinetic experiments. The most stable pH value of the drug can be calculated by the lg$k$ value of the chemical reaction under different conditions. ② The influence of solvents, matrix and other excipients. Easily hydrolyzed drugs can be stable by using non-aqueous solvents such as ethanol, propylene glycol, glycerol, and adding surfactants to form a barrier of micelles.

案例导入 ¦ Case example

案例 20-1　银黄口服液

20-1　Yinhuang Oral Liquid

处方： 金银花提取物（以绿原酸计）12g　黄芩提取物（以黄芩苷计）24g　单糖浆 适量　水 适量

Ingredients: Lonicerae Japonicae Flos extract (calculated as chlorogenic acid) 12g; Scutellaria extract (calculated as baicalin) 24g; Moderate syrupus simplex and water

功能与主治： 清热解毒，消炎。用于上呼吸道感染，急性扁桃体炎，咽炎。

Functions and indications: Clean heat and toxic, anti-inflammatory. It can be used for upper respiratory tract infections, acute tonsillitis, pharyngitis.

制法： 以上二味，分别加水适量使溶解，黄芩提取物再用 8% 氢氧化钠溶液调节 pH 至 8，滤过，滤液与金银花提取物溶液合并，用 8% 氢氧化钠溶液调节 pH 至 7.2，煮沸 1 小时，滤过，加入单糖浆适量，加水至近全量，搅匀，用 8% 氢氧化钠溶液调节 pH 至 7.2，加水至 1000ml，滤过，灌封，灭菌，即得。

Making Procedure:Add the appropriate amount of water to dissolve the Lonicerae Japonicae Flos extract and Scutellaria extract. Adjust the pH value of Scutellaria extract to 8 by using 8% sodium hydroxide solution. Then combine the filtration with the Lonicerae Japonicae Flos extract, and adjust the pH value to 7.2 by 8% sodium hydroxide solution. After boiling for 1h, filter the solution and add appropriate amount of syrupus simplex and water. Adjust pH value to 7.2 by adding 8% sodium hydroxide solution again. Finally, add water to

1000ml, filter, encapsulate, and sterilize to obtain the drug.

用法与用量：口服。一次 10~20ml，一日 3 次，小儿酌减。

Usage and dosage: For oral administration, 10-20ml per time, three times a day. Reduce the dosage in children

注解：pH 的影响：银黄口服液中的主要有效成分为绿原酸和黄芩苷，绿原酸在碱性溶液中易水解，黄芩苷在酸性溶液中易沉淀析出。因此，应对制剂的 pH 进行调整，使溶液中 pH 既保证绿原酸不水解，又不使黄芩苷产生沉淀。

Notes: The main active ingredients in Yinhuang oral liquid are chlorogenic acid and baicalin. Chlorogenic acid is easily hydrolyzed in alkaline solution, and baicalin is easily precipitated in acidic solution. Therefore, the pH value of the preparation should be adjusted to prevent chlorogenic acid hydrolyzation and baicalin precipitation.

研究表明，当 6.0<pH<7.5 时，绿原酸含量较稳定。当 pH>8 时，绿原酸含量随着加热时间的延长急剧下降；当 pH>7.0 时，药液澄清度较好；当 pH<6.5 时，随着加热时间的延长药液澄清度变差，且有沉淀析出。综合以上因素，应选择 pH 在 7.0~7.5 为最佳，在该条件下，既能保证药液的澄清度，又能防止绿原酸的水解。

Studies have shown that when pH value is in the range of 6.0-7.5, the chlorogenic acid content is relatively stable. When pH value >8.0, the chlorogenic acid content decreases sharply with the extension of the heating time; when pH value >7.0, the clarity of the liquid is better; when pH value <6.5, the precipitate appears in liquid. Based on the above facts, it is best to control the pH value in the range of 7.0-7.5.

思考题：制备银黄口服液的关键技术点包括哪些方面？

Questions: What are the key technical points of preparing Yinhuang Oral Liquid?

（2）制剂工艺　同种药物的不同剂型，乃至同种剂型的不同工艺，其稳定性差异较大。应根据药物性质，结合临床需要，设计合理的剂型和制剂工艺，以提高制剂的稳定性。

b. Preparation process　The stability of the drug is different due to various dosage forms of the drug and distinct preparation processes. In order to improve the stability of the preparation, a suitable dosage form and preparation process should be designed according to the nature of the drug and the clinical needs.

（3）贮藏条件　①温度：反应速度常数 k 值通常随温度升高而增大，但对不同药物的影响程度可能不同。根据 Van't Hoff 经验规律，温度每升高 10℃，反应速度则增加 2~4 倍。因此，在中药制剂提取、浓缩、干燥、灭菌过程中，都必须考虑温度对药物稳定性的影响。②光线：药物暴露在日光下，可引起光化反应。如因光线照射酚类药物可产生氧化反应，酯类药物可产生水解反应，挥发油可产生聚合反应等。对光敏感的制剂，应选用适宜的遮光容器包装。③氧气和金属离子：氧是引起中药制剂自氧化反应的根本原因；微量的铜、铁、锌等金属离子对自氧化反应有显著的催化作用。④湿度和水分：固体药物暴露于湿空气中，表面吸附水分，也可产生化学反应。这种反应是在固体吸水后表面形成的液膜中进行的，而吸水的程度与药物的性质和空气的相对湿度有关。⑤包装材料：要注意玻璃、塑料、橡胶和金属等包装材料与药物制剂相互作用而引起的稳定性变化。

c. Storage conditions　①Temperature: The k value usually increases with temperature, but the incidence may vary from drug to drug. According to Van't Hoff empirical rule, for every 10℃ increase in temperature, the reaction rate increases by 2-4 times. Therefore, the influence of temperature on drug stability must be considered in the process of extraction, concentration, drying and sterilization of TCM preparations.②Light: A drug exposed to sunlight can cause a photochemical reaction. Such as phenolic drugs undergo oxidation, ester drugs undergo hydrolysis, and volatile oils undergo polymerization. Light-sensitive preparations should be packaged in suitable light-blocking containers.③Oxygen and metal ions: Oxygen is the primary cause of autooxidation. Trace copper, iron, zinc and other metal ions have a significant catalytic effect on auto-oxidation.④Moisture: A chemical reaction may also occur when a solid drug is exposed to wet air, absorbing water on its surface. This reaction is carried out in the liquid film formed on the surface of the solid drug. The degree of water absorption is related to the nature of the drug and the relative humidity of the air.⑤Packaging materials: The interaction of packaging materials such as glass, plastic, rubber and metal with pharmaceutical preparations may also cause changes in drug stability.

（4）制剂的包装与贮藏要求　制剂的包装与贮藏是制剂稳定性的重要保障，包装与贮藏条件应根据制剂稳定性试验的影响因素及其考察结果，参照下列相关规定，选用不同包装和贮藏条件。

d. The requirements of packaging and storage　The packaging and storage of the preparation is an important guarantee for the stability of the preparation. The following relevant provisions can be used as a reference when selecting different packaging and storage conditions.

遮光：用不透光的容器包装，例如棕色容器或黑色包装材料包裹的无色透明、半透明容器。

Shading: colorless transparent containers wrapped in opaque packaging.

密封：将容器密封，以防止尘土及异物进入。

Seal: seal the container to prevent dust and foreign matter.

熔封或严封：将容器熔封或用适宜的材料严封，以防止空气与水分的侵入并防止污染。

Heat sealed: seal the container by melting or using appropriate material to prevent air and water.

阴凉处：贮藏温度不超过 20℃。

Cool place: the storage temperature is not exceeding 20℃.

凉暗处：在避光条件下贮藏且温度不超过 20℃。

Cool and dark: store in dark condition with temperature not exceeding 20℃.

冷处：贮藏温度为 2~10℃。

Cold place: the storage temperature is in the range of 2-10℃.

常温：贮藏温度为 10~30℃。

Normal temperature: the storage temperature is in the range of 10-30℃.

二、提高中药制剂稳定性的方法
20.2.2 Methods for Improving the Stability of TCM Preparations

1. 延缓药物水解的方法
(1) Methods for delaying drug hydrolysis

（1）调节 pH　一般药物在适宜 pH 时较稳定。可通过实验找出药物最稳定的 pH，然后用酸、碱或适当的缓冲剂调节，使溶液维持在最稳定的 pH 范围内。

① *Adjusting the pH value:* In general, drugs are stable at an appropriate pH value. The most suitable pH value of the drug can be found through experiments. Then the solution can be adjusted with an acidity, an alkalinity or an appropriate buffer to maintain the most stable pH value range.

（2）降低温度 降低温度可使水解反应减慢。在提取、浓缩、干燥、灭菌、贮存过程中，可以适当降低温度，以减少水解的发生。特别是某些热敏性药物。

② *Reducing the temperature:* Especially for some heat-sensitive drugs, the temperature can be appropriately lowered to reduce the occurrence of hydrolysis in the process of extraction, concentration, drying, sterilization and storage,

（3）改变溶剂 在水溶液中很不稳定的药物，可用乙醇、丙二醇、甘油等极性较小的溶剂，以减少药物水解。

③ *Changing the solvent:* Ethanol, propylene glycol, glycerol and other less polar solvents can be used to reduce hydrolysis of the drugs which are unstable in aqueous solution.

（4）制成干燥固体 对于极易水解的药物，可制成干燥的固体，如注射用无菌粉末等。并尽量避免与水分的接触。

④ *Making dry solid:* Highly hydrolytic drugs can be made into dry solids. such as sterile powder for injection, and try to avoid contacting with water.

案例导入 ¦ Case example

案例 20-2 穿心莲片
20-2 Chuanxinlian Tablet

处方：穿心莲 1000g 辅料 适量

Ingredients: Andrographis Herba 1000g; Appropriate amount excipient

功能与主治：清热解毒，凉血消肿。用于感冒发热，咽喉肿痛，口舌生疮，顿咳劳嗽，泄泻痢疾，热淋涩痛，痈肿疮疡，毒蛇咬伤。

Functions and indications: Clean heat and toxic, cool blood to reduce swelling. It can be used for cold, fever, sore throat, sore tongue, cough, diarrhea and dysentery, and snake-bites.

制法：取穿心莲，用 85% 乙醇热浸提取 2 次，每次 2 小时，合并提取液，滤过，滤液回收乙醇，浓缩至适量，干燥，加辅料适量，制成颗粒，干燥，压制成 1000 片（小片）或 500 片（大片），包糖衣或薄膜衣，即得。

Making Procedure: Extract Andrographis Herba with 85% ethanol twice, 2h for each time, and combine the filtrate. Then recover ethanol from the filtrate, concentrate to an appropriate amount, dry, and add an appropriate amount of excipient to make granules. The dried granules are compressed into 1000 tablets (small tablets) or 500 tablets (large tablets). Finally, coat with sugar or film.

用法与用量：口服，一次 2~3 片（小片），一日 3~4 次；或一次 1~2 片（大片），一日 3 次。

Usage and dosage: For oral administration, 2-3 tablets (small tablets) per time, 3-4 times a day; 1-2 tablets (large tablets) per time, 3 times a day.

注解：制法中包衣对提高制剂稳定性十分重要。如未包衣，穿心莲片在贮存过程中吸湿之后，易发生水解开环，降低药效。穿心莲内酯的水解反应如图 20-1 所示。

Notes: Coating is very important for the stability of the preparation. If not coated, the lactone ring in andrographolide molecular may open after moisture absorption, resulting in reduction of efficacy.

The hydrolysis reaction of andrographolide is shown in Figure 20-1.

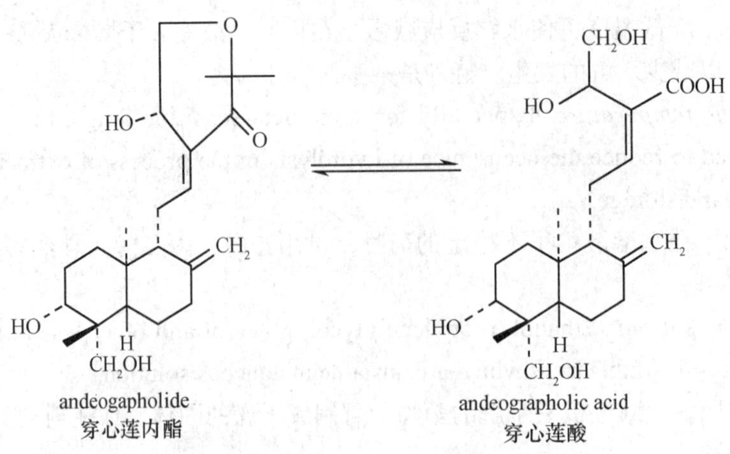

图 20-1　穿心莲内酯水解图

Figure 20-1　Hydrolytic Diagram of Andrographolide

2. 防止药物氧化的方法

(2) Methods to prevent drug oxidation

（1）降低温度　在制备和贮存过程中，应适当降低温度，以减少药物的氧化。

① *Reducing the temperature:* During the preparation and storage process, the temperature should be lowered appropriately to reduce the oxidation of the drug.

（2）避光　在制备的全部过程中，应严格避免日光的照射，成品用棕色玻璃容器包装，避光贮藏。

② *Avoiding light:* During the whole process of preparation, the sunlight should be strictly avoided. The finished drugs should be packed in a brown glass container.

（3）驱逐氧气　可采取加热煮沸法驱逐溶液中的氧气或通入惰性气体（N_2、CO_2 等）驱逐溶液上部空气中的氧气。

③ *Expelling oxygen:* The oxygen in the solution can be removed by heating and boiling. The inert gas (N_2, CO_2, etc.) can be introduced to remove oxygen from the upper air of the solution.

（4）添加抗氧剂　药物的氧化降解通常为自动氧化降解，因此，在驱逐氧气的同时，还应加入抗氧剂。

④ *Using antioxidants:* The oxidative degradation of drugs is usually automatic. Therefore, antioxidants should be added while expelling oxygen.

（5）控制微量金属离子　制备过程中应尽可能减少金属离子的带入，必要时在制剂成品中可加入金属离子络合剂。

⑤ *Reducing trace metal ions:* During the preparation process, metal ions should be removed as much as possible. When necessary, metal ion complexing agent can be added into the preparation.

（6）调节 pH　适宜的药液 pH，可延缓药物的氧化。因此，对于容易氧化变质的药物，须调节药液的 pH 在最稳定的范围内。

⑥ *Adjusting the pH value:* For drugs that are easily oxidized and deteriorated, the pH value of the solution must be adjusted to the most stable range, which can delay the oxidation of the drug.

第三节 中药制剂的稳定性考察方法

20.3 Methods to Test the Stability of TCM Preparation

中药制剂稳定性试验的目的是考察影响中药制剂稳定性的因素在不同环境下随时间变化的规律，为药品的生产、包装、贮存、运输条件提供科学依据，同时通过试验建立药品的有效期。

The purpose of the stability test is to investigate how the quality of TCM preparation varies with time under the influence of many environmental factors. It provides scientific basis for the production, packaging, storage and transportation conditions of drugs. And the validity period of drugs can also be established through tests.

一、中药制剂稳定性考察要求

20.3.1 Requirements for the Stability of TCM Preparation

1. 稳定性试验包括影响因素试验、加速试验和长期试验。影响因素试验用 1 批制剂进行，加速试验与长期试验要求用 3 批制剂进行。

(1) Stability tests includes affecting factor test, accelerated test and long-term test. The affecting factor test is conducted with 1 batch of preparations, and the accelerated test and the long-term test require 3 batches of preparations.

2. 制剂应为放大工艺产品，其处方与工艺应与大生产一致。药物制剂如片剂、胶囊剂，每批放大试验规模，片剂至少应为 10000 片，胶囊剂至少应为 10000 粒。大体积包装的制剂如静脉输液，每批放大规模的数量至少应为各项试验所需总量的 10 倍。特殊品种、特殊剂型所需数量，根据情况另定。

(2) The process of the preparation should be consistent with the industrial production. For tablets and capsules, the scale of the experiment for each batch should be at least 10,000. For large-volume packaged preparations such as injections for intravenous infusion, the scale of the experiment for each batch should be at least 10 times of the total amount required for the test.

3. 制剂质量标准应与临床前研究、临床试验和规模生产所使用的制剂质量标准一致。

(3) The quality standard of the preparation should be consistent with the quality standard of the preparation used in preclinical research, clinical trials and industrial scale production.

4. 加速试验与长期试验所用制剂的包装应与上市产品一致。

(4) The packaging of the preparations used in the accelerated test and long-term test should be consistent with the listed products.

5. 药物稳定性试验应采用专属性强、准确、精密、灵敏的药物分析方法。

(5) The analysis methods which are specific, accurate, precise and sensitive should be used in stability tests.

6. 对最初通过验证的 3 批规模生产产品仍需进行加速试验和长期试验。

(6) Accelerated and long-term tests are still required for the initial 3 batches of approved mass production products.

二、中药制剂稳定性考察项目

20.3.2 Testing Items of the Stability of TCM Preparation

稳定性试验的考察项目因剂型不同而不同，常用剂型的考察项目见表 20-1。

The testing items of stability vary with different dosage forms. The testing items of commonly used dosage forms are shown in Table 20-1.

表 20-1 制剂稳定性考察项目

剂型	稳定性试验主要考核项目
片剂	性状、鉴别、含量、崩解时限（溶出度、释放度）
胶囊剂	外观、鉴别、含量、崩解时限（溶出度、释放度）、水分，软胶囊检查内容物有无沉淀
注射剂	性状、鉴别、含量、pH、可见异物、无菌
栓剂	性状、鉴别、含量、融变时限
软膏剂	性状、均匀性、鉴别、含量、粒度
乳膏剂	性状、均匀性、鉴别、含量、粒度、分层现象
糊剂	性状、均匀性、鉴别、含量、粒度
凝胶剂	性状、均匀性、鉴别、含量、粒度、乳剂应检查分层现象
眼用制剂	若为溶液，应考察性状、可见异物、含量、pH；若为混悬剂，应考察粒度、再分散性；洗眼剂应考察无菌；眼用丸剂应考察粒度与无菌
丸剂	性状、鉴别、含量、溶散时限
糖浆剂	性状、鉴别、含量、澄清度、相对密度、pH
口服溶液剂	性状、鉴别、含量、澄清度
口服乳剂	性状、鉴别、含量、分层现象
口服混悬剂	性状、鉴别、含量、沉降体积比、再分散性
散剂	性状、鉴别、含量、粒度、外观均匀度
气雾剂	泄漏率、每瓶主药含量、每瓶总揿次、每揿主药总含量、雾滴分布
喷雾剂	每瓶总吸次数、每吸喷量、每吸主药含量、雾滴分布
颗粒剂	性状、鉴别、含量、粒度、溶化性（溶出度、释放度）
贴剂	性状、鉴别、含量、释放度、黏附力
冲洗剂、洗剂、灌肠剂	性状、鉴别、含量、分层现象（乳状型）、分散性（混悬型），冲洗剂应考察无菌
搽剂、涂剂、涂膜剂	性状、鉴别、含量、分层现象（乳状型）、分散性（混悬型），涂膜剂应考察成膜性
耳用制剂	性状、鉴别、含量，耳用散剂、喷雾剂与半固体制剂分别按相关剂型要求检查
鼻用制剂	性状、pH、鉴别、含量，鼻用散剂、喷雾剂与半固体制剂分别按相关剂型要求检查

Table 20-1 Testing Items of the Stability of TCM Preparation

Dosage form	Main inspection items in stability test
Tablet	Character, identification, content, disintegration time (dissolution, release)
Capsule	Character, identification, content, disintegration time (dissolution, release), moisture. It is essential for soft capsule to check precipitation
Injection	Character, identification, content, pH value, visible foreign body, asepsis
Suppository	Character, identification, content and melting time
Ointment	Character, uniformity, identification, content and particle size
Cream preparation	Character, uniformity, identification, content, particle size, stratification
Paste	Character, uniformity, identification, content and particle size
Gel	Properties, uniformity, identification, content, particle size. Emulsion should be examined for stratification
Eye ophthalmic preparation	The characters, visible foreign matter, content and pH value should be investigated for solution. The particle size and redispersibility should be investigated for suspension. Eye lotion should be examined for asepsis. Eye pills should be examined for size and asepsis
Pill	Character, identification, content and dissolution time
Syrup	Character, identification, content, clarification, relative density, pH value
Oral solution	Character, identification, content and clarification
Oral emulsion	Character, identification, content and stratification
Oral suspension	Character, identification, content, settling volume ratio, redispersibility
Powder	Character, identification, content, particle size and appearance uniformity
Aerosol	Leakage rate, main drug content per bottle, total lifts per bottle, main drug content per lift, distribution of fog drops
Spray	Total times of suction, spray amount per suction, content of main drug per suction, distribution of fog drops
Granules	Character, identification, content, particle size, solubility (dissolution, release)
Patch	Character, identification, content, release and adhesion
Lotion, enema	Character, identification, content, stratification (emulsion type), dispersion (suspension type). Lotion should be investigated for asepsis
Liniment, paints, coating agent	Characteristics, identification, content, stratification (emulsion type), dispersion (suspension type). Coating agent should be investigated for film-forming
Ear preparation	Character, identification, content. Ear powder, spray and semi-solid preparation should be checked according to the relevant dosage form
Nasal preparation	Character, pH value, identification, content. Nasal powder, spray and semi-solid preparation should be checked according to the relevant dosage form

三、中药制剂稳定性考察方法

20.3.3 Methods for Testing the Stability of TCM Preparation

（一）影响因素试验

(1) Affecting Factor Test

影响因素试验是在剧烈条件下进行的试验，其目的是探讨药物的稳定性、了解影响其稳定性的因素及所含成分的变化情况。为制剂处方设计、工艺筛选、包装材料和容器的选择、贮存条件的确定、有关物质的控制提供依据，并为加速试验和长期试验应采用的温度和湿度等条件提供参考。

Affecting factor test is conducted under severe conditions. The purpose is to explore the stability of the drug, to understand the factors that affect the stability and the changes of the contained ingredients. This provides a basis for formulation design, process screening, selection of packaging materials and containers, determination of storage conditions, and control of related substances. It also provides a reference for the temperature and humidity conditions that should be adopted for accelerated testing and long-term testing.

1. 高温试验 将供试品开口置于适宜的洁净容器中（一般样品摊成≤5mm 厚的薄层，疏松样品摊成≤10mm 厚的薄层），60℃下放置 10 天，分别于第 5 天、第 10 天取样，按照稳定性试验重点考察项目进行检测。若供试品标示成分含量低于规定限度，则在 40℃下同法进行试验。如 60℃温度下无明显变化，则不必进行 40℃试验。

① High temperature test Put the open products in a suitable clean container for 10 days at 60℃. The general sample is amortized into a thin layer ≤5mm, while the loose sample is amortized into a thin layer ≤10mm. Test the samples which were taken on day 5 and day 10 respectively according to the key items of stability test. If the content of the labeled components of the test products is below the prescribed limit, the test should be performed with the same method at 40℃. However, if there is no obvious change at 60℃, it is unnecessary to conduct test at 40℃.

2. 吸湿试验

② Moisture absorption test

（1）高湿度试验 供试品开口置于恒湿设备中（一般样品摊成≤5mm 厚的薄层，疏松样品摊成≤10mm 厚的薄层），在温度 25℃、相对湿度 92.5% ± 5% 条件下（KNO_3 饱和溶液，相对湿度 92.5%，25℃，）放置 10 天，于第 5 天、第 10 天取样，按照稳定性试验重点考察项目进行检测，同时准确称量试验前后供试品的重量，以考察供试品的吸湿潮解性能。若吸湿增重在 5% 以上，则应在 25℃、相对湿度 75% ± 5% 下同法进行试验；若吸湿增重在 5% 以下，且其他考察项目符合要求，则不再进行此项试验。

a. High humidity test Put the open products in a constant humidity equipment for 10 days at 25℃, relative humidity 92.5%±5%. The general sample is amortized into a thin layer ≤5mm, while the loose sample is amortized into a thin layer ≤10mm. Test the samples which were taken on day 5 and day 10 respectively according to the key items of stability test. At the same time, weigh the sample accurately before and after the test, so as to investigate the hygroscopicity of the sample. If the hygroscopic weight increasement is more than 5%, the test should be performed with the same method at 25℃ and relative humidity of 75%±5%. If the hygroscopic weight gain is less than 5% and other inspection items meet the requirements, the test will not be conducted.

（2）药物的引湿性试验 取干燥的具塞玻璃称量瓶（外径 50mm，高 15mm）于前一天置于适宜的 25℃ ± 1℃恒温干燥器（下部放置氯化铵或硫酸铵饱和溶液）或人工气候箱（设定温度为

5℃ ± 1℃，相对湿度为 80% ± 2%）内，精密称重（m_1）。取供试品适量，置上述称量瓶中并平铺于称量瓶内，供试品厚度一般约为 1mm，精密称重（m_2）。将称量瓶敞口，并与瓶盖同置于上述恒温恒湿条件下 24 小时。盖好称量瓶，精密称重（m_3），计算增重百分率：

b. Hygroscopicity test Weigh a dry glass bottle with glass stopper (external diameter 50mm, height 15mm) and put them into the appropriate 25℃±1℃ constant temperature dryer (with the saturated solution of ammonium chloride or ammonium sulfate in the lower part), or artificial climate box (5℃±1℃, relative humidity of 80%±2%) on the previous day, and weigh precisely (m_1). Take the appropriate amount of the test sample, place and lay it flat in the above weighing bottle. The thickness of the sample is generally about 1mm, and is weighed precisely (m_2). Open the weighing bottle and place it with the cap for 24h under the above constant temperature and humidity conditions. Then, cover the weighing bottle and weigh it precisely (m_3). Calculate the percentage of hygroscopic weight increasement according to the formula below:

$$\text{增重百分率（Percentage gain，\%）} = \frac{m_3 - m_2}{m_2 - m_1} \times 100\% \qquad (20\text{-}5)$$

引湿性特征描述与引湿增重的界定如下：

The description of hygroscopicity and the definition of weight increasement due to hygroscopicity are as follows:

潮解：吸收足量水分形成液体。

Deliquescence: The liquid has formed by absorbing enough water.

极具引湿性：引湿增重不小于 15%。

Strong hygroscopic: Weight increasement due to hygroscopicity is not less than 15%.

有引湿性：引湿增重小于 15% 且不小于 2%。

Hygroscopicity: Weight increasement due to hygroscopicity is more than 2% and less than 15%.

略有引湿性：引湿增重小于 2% 且不小于 0.2%。

Slightly hygroscopic: Weight increasement due to hygroscopicity is more than 0.2% and less than 2%.

无或几乎无引湿性：引湿增重小于 0.2%。

No hygroscopic: Weight increasement due to hygroscopicity is less than 0.2%.

（3）湿度加速试验 为探讨固体制剂的吸湿性，可在各种湿度条件下测定其吸湿速度和平衡吸湿量，进一步获得供试样品的临界相对湿度（CRH）。

c. Accelerated humidity test Measure the moisture absorption rate and equilibrium moisture absorption of the solid preparation under various humidity conditions to obtain the critical relative humidity (CRH) of the test sample.

平衡吸湿量是样品于一定相对湿度下，达到平衡状态以后的吸湿量。经不同时间连续测定，样品吸湿量如不再变化，即达吸湿平衡。在一定温度下，变更不同的相对湿度，测定各湿度下的平衡吸湿量。以平衡吸湿量对相对湿度作图，即为吸湿平衡图。从吸湿平衡图上可求得药物的 CRH。不同的药物有其相应的 CRH 值，可用 CRH 值作为吸湿性大小的指标。即 CRH 值越大，越不易吸湿；CRH 值越小，越易吸湿。

The equilibrium moisture absorption refers to the state that the moisture absorption of the sample does not change along with measuring continuously at different times. At a certain temperature, the equilibrium moisture absorption can be measured at different relative humidity. The hygroscopic equilibrium figure takes the equilibrium moisture absorption as the Y-axis and the relative humidity as the X-axis. The CRH of the drug can be obtained from the hygroscopic equilibrium figure. Different drugs have different CRH values, which can be used as an indicator of hygroscopicity. That is, the larger CRH value, the less hygroscopicity, and the smaller CRH value, the easier hygroscopicity.

案例导入 | Case example

案例 20-3　8 种颗粒的吸湿平衡曲线

20-3　Hygroscopic Equilibrium Figures of 8 Granules

某地区生产 8 种可溶性颗粒剂，于 37℃分别测定其平衡吸湿量，绘制吸湿平衡图，如图 20-2 所示。

Measure the equilibrium moisture absorption of 8 soluble granules at 37℃, plot hygroscopic equilibrium as Figure 20-2.

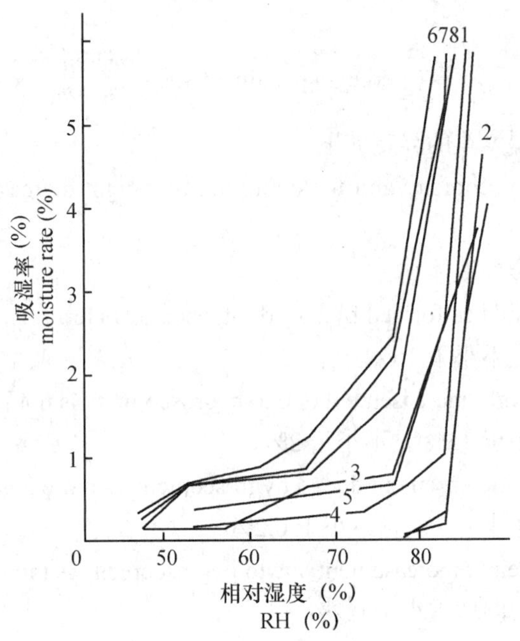

图 20-2　8 种颗粒吸湿平衡图

Figure 20-2　Hygroscopic Equilibrium of 8 Particles

1. 小儿化痰止咳颗粒剂　2. 复合维生素 B 颗粒剂　3. 伤风止咳颗粒剂　4. 止咳枇杷颗粒剂　5. 脾舒宁颗粒剂　6. 感冒灵颗粒剂　7. 复方感冒灵颗粒剂　8. 板蓝根颗粒剂

1. Xiao er Huatan Zhike granules; 2. Compound vitamin B granules; 3. Shangfeng Zhike granules; 4. Zhike Pipa granules; 5. Pishuning granules; 6. Ganmaoling granules; 7. Compound Ganmaoling granules; 8. Banlangen granules

注解：如图 20-2 所示，每一种颗粒剂的吸湿平衡曲线，均由下端平缓部分及上端几乎与纵坐标平行的陡直部分组成，当提高相对湿度至某一值时，吸湿量迅速增加，此时的相对湿度即为 CRH。吸湿是含干浸膏中药固体制剂的特性。应针对具体制剂，选择适宜的防潮措施。

以下几种防潮措施可供参考：①减少制剂原料，特别是中药干浸膏中水溶性杂质。例如采用水醇法除去胶质、黏液质、蛋白质、淀粉等，常可降低吸湿性。②加入适宜的辅料（如吸收剂），对降低吸湿有一定效果。此前可通过湿度加速试验筛选辅料，例如乳糖可静滴丹参颗粒剂的吸湿百分率，将生脉成骨胶囊原料用微晶纤维素制成颗粒也可减低吸湿性。③采用防潮包衣和防湿包装。如鸢都感冒颗粒上喷Ⅵ号胃溶聚丙烯酸树脂，其吸湿性明显降低。

Notes: The hygroscopic equilibrium curve of each granule is composed of the flat part at the lower end and the steep part at the upper end which is almost parallel to the vertical coordinate. When the relative

humidity raises to a certain value, the moisture absorption increases rapidly, and the relative humidity at this point is defined as CRH. Hygroscopicity is the characteristic of TCM solid preparation containing dry extract. Suitable moisture-proof measures should be selected for specific preparations. ① Decrease the hygroscopicity of dry extract by reducing the water-soluble impurities. For example, use water extraction and alcohol precipitation method to remove colloid, mucus, protein, starch, etc. ② It can reduce hygroscopicity by adding appropriate auxiliary materials (such as absorbent). Before then, screen the auxiliary materials through the accelerated humidity test. For example, lactose can reduce the percentage of hygroscopicity of Danshen granules, microcrystalline cellulose can reduce the percentage of hygroscopicity of Shengmaichenggu capsules. ③The moisture-proof coating and moisture-proof packaging can significantly reduce the hygroscopicity. For example, the No. Ⅵ gastric-soluble polyacrylate is sprinkled on the Yuandu Ganmao granules.

---

3. 强光照射试验　供试品置装有日光灯的光照箱或其他适宜的光照容器内，于照度为4500lx ± 500lx 条件下放置 10 天，于第 5 天、第 10 天取样检测。试验中应注意控制温度，与室温保持一致，并注意观察供试品的外观变化。

③ **Strong light test**　Put the test products in a light box or other light container equipped with a fluorescent lamp for 10 days under the condition of illumination of 4500lx ± 500lx. Test the samples which were taken on day 5 and day 10 respectively. During the test, it should keep consistent with the room temperature and observe the change of appearance of the sample.

光照稳定性变化的指标，液体制剂可测定其有效成分的含量变化，也可以利用其吸收度的变化，反映其变色程度；固体制剂表面层的变化，可应用漫反射光谱法测定其反射率的改变。

The discoloration degree of liquid preparation can be reflected by measuring the contents change of its active component or by the change of its absorbance. The reflectivity of surface layer of solid preparation can be determined by diffuse reflectance spectrometry.

对光敏感的制剂，应选用适宜的遮光容器包装，使其免受光线照射。无色玻璃无遮光性能，而棕色玻璃对于波长 290~450nm 的光线，具有良好的遮光性能，并且随着玻璃厚度的增加，透光率降低。橙色和褐色软胶囊囊壳也有较好的遮光性能，可增加对光敏感药物的稳定性。

Light-sensitive preparations should be packaged in appropriate light-blocking containers to protect them from light exposure. Colorless glass has no shading performance, while brown glass has good shading performance for light with the wavelength of 290-450nm, and the light transmittance decreases with the increase of glass thickness. In addition, the orange and brown soft capsules also have better shading properties, which can increase the stability of light-sensitive drugs.

4. 其他试验　根据药物的性质必要时应设计其他试验，探讨 pH、氧及其他条件（如冷冻等）对药物稳定性的影响。

④ **Other tests**　Other tests should be designed to investigate the effects of pH value, oxygen and other conditions (such as freezing) on the stability of the drug.

（二）长期试验

(2) Long-Term Test

长期试验在接近药品的实际储存条件下进行，其目的是为制定药品的有效期提供依据。

Long-term trials are conducted under conditions close to the actual storage of the drug and are intended to provide the basis for determining the expiry date of the drug.

试验方法：取市售包装的供试品制剂 3 批，在温度 25℃ ± 2℃、相对湿度 60% ± 10% 或在温

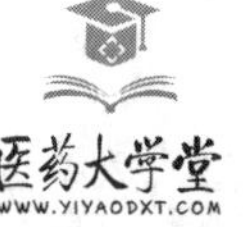

度 30℃ ± 2℃，相对湿度 65% ± 10% 的条件下放置 12 个月。分别于第 0、3、6、9、12 个月取样，按稳定性考察项目进行检测。12 个月后仍需要观察的，分别于 18 个月、24 个月、36 个月取样进行检测。将结果与 0 月药品比较以确定药品的有效期。申报生产时，应继续考察其稳定性，据此确定有效期。由于实测数据的分散性，一般应按 95% 可信限进行统计分析，得到合理的有效期。如 3 批统计分析结果差别较小，则取其平均值为有效期。若差别较大，则取其最短的为有效期。数据分析结果很稳定的药品，不做统计分析。

Methods: Place 3 batches of commercially packaged test preparations for 12 months at 25℃ ± 2℃ and relative humidity 60% ± 10%, or 30℃ ± 2℃ and relative humidity 65% ± 10%. Take the samples at 0, 3, 6, 9 and 12 months respectively, and test them according to the stability items. If the sample is still need observation after 12 months, it should be taken at 18 months, 24 months and 36 months respectively for detection. The results are compared with 0 month to determine the expiry date of the drug. Due to the dispersion of the measured data, statistical analysis should be performed according to the 95% confidence limit to obtain a reasonable period of validity. If the statistical analysis difference of the 3 batches is small, the average value should be adopted to evaluate validity period. If the difference is large, then select the shortest time as the reference for validity evaluation. The drugs with stable data analysis need no statistical analysis.

对温度敏感的药物，长期试验可在 6℃ ± 2℃条件下放置 12 个月，按照上述时间要求进行检测，12 个月以后，仍需要按规定继续考察，制定在低温贮存条件下的有效期。

Temperature-sensitive drugs can be carried out at 6℃ ± 2℃ for 12 months. After 12 months, it is still necessary to continue the investigation in accordance with the regulations to establish the period of validity under low temperature storage conditions.

对采用半通透性容器包装的中药制剂，长期试验应在 25℃ ± 2℃、相对湿度 40% ± 5%，或 30℃ ± 2℃，相对湿度 35% ± 5% 条件下进行。

Preparations packed in semi-permeable containers should be investigated under the conditions of 25℃ ± 2℃, relative humidity 40% ± 5%, or 30℃ ± 2℃, relative humidity 35% ± 5%.

（三）加速试验

(3) Accelerated Test

加速试验的目的是为了加速药物的化学或物理变化，考察制剂的稳定性，为制剂处方设计、工艺条件、质量控制、包装材料、运输和储存提供必要的参考依据。

The purpose of accelerated testing is to accelerate chemical or physical changes in the drug and to investigate the stability of the preparation.

1. 加速试验法 取市售包装的供试品制剂 3 批，在温度 40℃ ± 2℃、相对湿度 75% ± 5% 条件下放置 6 个月。试验期间第 1、2、3、6 个月末分别取样一次，按该剂型的稳定性考察项目进行检测。

① Accelerated test method Place 3 batches of commercially packaged test preparations for 6 months at 40℃ ± 2℃ and relative humidity 75% ± 5%. Take the samples at the end of 1, 2, 3 and 6 months respectively, and test them according to the stability items.

在上述条件下，如 6 个月供试品检测不符合质量标准相关规定，则应在中间条件（30℃ ± 2℃、相对湿度 65% ± 5%）下进行加速试验，试验时间为 6 个月。

If the 6-month sample does not meet the relevant provisions of the quality standard, the accelerated test should be carried out under the intermediate conditions (30℃ ± 2℃, relative humidity 65% ± 5%) for another 6 months.

溶液剂、注射剂等含水性介质的制剂可以不要求相对湿度，其他条件同上。

The relative humidity may not be required in the test conditions of preparations containing aqueous media such as solution and injection.

对温度敏感的药物（预计只能在 4~8℃内保存使用），其加速试验可在 25℃ ± 2℃、相对湿度 60% ± 5% 条件下进行，试验时间为 6 个月。

Temperature-sensitive drugs (which can only be stored and used within 4-8℃) can be performed under the conditions of 25℃ ± 2℃ and relative humidity 60% ± 5% for 6 months.

乳剂、混悬剂、软膏剂、乳膏剂、糊剂、凝胶剂、眼膏剂、栓剂、气雾剂、泡腾片、及泡腾颗粒的加速试验条件为温度 30℃ ± 2℃，相对湿度 65% ± 5%，时间为 6 个月。

Emulsions, suspensions, ointments, creams, pastes, gels, eye ointments, suppositories, aerosols, effervescent tablets, and effervescent particles should be tested under 30℃ ± 2℃ and relative humidity 65% ± 5% for 6 months.

对于包装在半透明容器中的药物制剂，如低密度聚乙烯制备的输液袋、眼用制剂容器，则应在温度 40℃ ± 2℃，相对湿度 25% ± 5% 条件下进行试验。

Preparations packed in semi-permeable containers such as infusion bag and eye preparation container prepared by low density polyethylene should be investigated under the conditions of 40℃ ± 2℃, relative humidity 25% ± 5%.

需要冷冻保存的药品可不进行加速试验。

Drugs that require cryopreservation are not subject to accelerated testing.

2. 经典恒温法　经典恒温法的理论依据是 Arrhenius 指数规律，其对数形式为：

② **Classical constant temperature method**　The theoretical basis of the classical constant temperature method is Arrhenius exponential law, whose logarithmic form is as follows:

$$\lg K = -\frac{E}{2.303RT} + \lg A \qquad (20\text{-}6)$$

以 $\lg K$ 对 $1/T$ 作图，称作 Arrhenius 图，如图 20-3 所示，直线的斜率 $K = -E/(2.303R)$，由斜率得出室温时的速度常数 $K_{25℃}$，由 $K_{25℃}$ 可求出分解 10% 所需的时间 $t_{0.9}$ 或室温储存若干时间以后残留的浓度。

As shown in figure 20-3, the slope of the line is $K = -E/(2.303R)$. Then, obtain the velocity constant $K_{25℃}$ at room temperature in terms of the slope. Finally, according to $K_{25℃}$, calculate the time required for decomposition of 10% ($t_{0.9}$) and the residual concentration after storage at room temperature for some time.

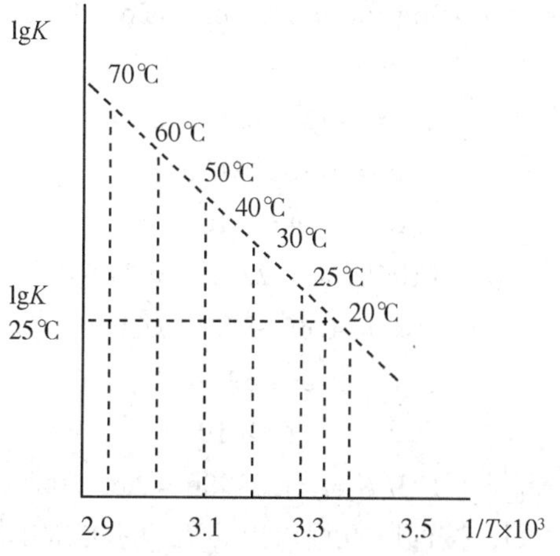

图 20-3　Arrhenius 图

Figure 20-3　Arrhenius Figure

具体试验内容包括以下步骤：①预实验确立反应制剂稳定性的指标成分及含量测定方法；②选定4~5个试验加速温度和间隔取样时间，测定不同温度加速试验条件下，不同取样中指标成分的含量，经 $\lg C\text{–}t$ 图解确定为一级反应后，再经线性回归，求出各温度下的反应速度常数；③经 $\lg K\text{–}1/T$ 图解法，得出25℃时 K 值；④计算25℃时药物分解10%所需的时间。

The specific steps are as follows: ①Establish the method of determining the index composition and content of the preparation stability by pre-test.②Determine the contents of index components in different samples under 4-5 different temperatures. Then identify the first order reaction by $\lg C\text{-}t$ diagram. And the reaction velocity constant at each temperature is obtained by linear regression. ③Obtain the $K_{25℃}$ by $\lg K$ - $1/T$ graphical method.④Calculate $t_{0.9}$ via $K_{25℃}$.

案例导入 ¦ Case example

案例 20-4　加速试验测定制剂稳定性

20-4　The Stability of Preparation Determined by Accelerated Test

某药物制剂在40℃、50℃、60℃、70℃四个温度下进行加速试验，测得加速温度下不同时间的药物浓度，确定为一级反应，用线性回归法求出反应速度常数，结果如表20-2所示。

A pharmaceutical preparation was subjected to accelerated tests at four temperatures of 40℃, 50℃, 60℃, and 70℃. It is determined as the first-order reaction by measuring drug concentration at different times. Reaction rate constant can be calculated by linear regression. The results are shown in Table 20-2.

表 20-2　温度与速度常数表

Table 20-2　Constant Table of Temperature and Velocity

t（℃）	$1/T\times10^3$	$K\times10^3$（h^{-1}）	$\lg K$
40	3.193	2.66	−4.575
50	3.094	7.94	−4.100
60	3.001	22.38	−3.650
70	2.9114	56.50	−3.248

将上述数据（$\lg K$ 对 $1/T$）进行一元线性回归，得回归方程：

The above data is calculated by using the linear regression method of one variable to obtain the equation:

$$\lg K = -4765.98/T + 10.64$$

$$E = 91302.69\text{J/mol}$$

$$K_{25℃} = -4.6\times10^{-6}\text{h}^{-1}$$

$$t_{0.9} = 0.105/K_{25℃} = 22198\text{h} = 2.65\ 年$$

$$\lg K = -4765.98/T+10.64$$

$$E = 91302.69\text{J/mol}$$

$$K_{25℃} = -4.6\times10^{-6}\text{h}^{-1}$$

$$t_{0.9} = 0.105/K_{25℃} = 22198\text{h} = 2.65\text{ years}$$

根据 $\lg K$ 对 $1/T$ 进行线性回归，按回归方程求出 $\lg K_{25℃}$ 的95%单侧可信限置信区间：$\lg K_{25℃}\pm z$。其中：

According to the regression equation, the 95% unilateral confidence limit confidence interval of $\lg K_{25℃}$ was obtained: $\lg K_{25℃} \pm z$.

$$z = t_{N-2} \cdot s \cdot \sqrt{\frac{1}{N} + \frac{(X_0 - \overline{X})^2}{\sum (X_i - \overline{X})^2}} \tag{20-7}$$

式中，$t_{N\text{-}2}$ 是概率为0.05，自由度 N–2 的 t 单侧分布值，N 为组数。$s = \sqrt{\frac{Q}{N-2}}$；$Q = L_{yy} - bL_{xy}$；b 为直线的斜率；L_{yy} 为 y 的离差平方和；L_{xy} 为 xy 的离差平方和；$L_{yy} = \sum y^2 - \frac{1}{N}(\sum y)^2$；$L_{xy} - \frac{1}{N}(\sum x)(\sum y)$；$X_0$ 为给定自变量；$\overline{X}$ 为自变量 X 的平均值。

In the formula, $t_{N\text{-}2}$ is the t unilateral distribution value of probability 0.05, degree of freedom N-2, and N is the number of groups. $s = \sqrt{\frac{Q}{N-2}}$; $Q = L_{yy} - bL_{xy}$; b is the slope of the line; L_{yy} is the sum of the square deviations of y; L_{xy} is the sum of the squares of the deviations of xy; $L_{yy} = \sum y^2 - \frac{1}{N}(\sum y)^2$; $L_{xy} - \frac{1}{N}(\sum x)(\sum y)$; X_0 is the given independent variable; $\overline{X}$ is the average value of the independent variable X.

为了方便计算，列出 t 分布的单侧临界值，见表 20-3。

表 20-3　t 分布单侧临界值表（P=0.05）

Table 20-3　Unilateral Critical Values of t Distribution

N–2	1	2	3	4	5	6	7	8
t 值	6.31	2.92	2.35	2.13	2.02	1.94	1.89	1.86

3. 简化法　鉴于经典恒温法实验及数据处理工作量大、费时等缺点，出现了一些简化的方法。其理论是基于化学动力学原理和 Arrhenius 指数定律。如减少加速试验温度数的方法（温度系数法、温度指数法），或减少抽样次数（初匀速法、单测点法），或简化数据处理的方法（$t_{0.9}$ 法，活化能估算法）等。尽管简化法的准确性可能有不同程度的降低，但对结果预测仍有一定的参考价值。下面对几种主要方法进行介绍：

③ **The simplified method**　Because of the shortcomings of the classical thermostatic method and data processing, some simplified methods have appeared. The theory is based on chemical kinetics and Arrhenius exponential law. Although the accuracy of the simplified method may be reduced to some extent, it still has some reference value for the prediction of results.

（1）$t_{0.9}$ 法　经典恒温试验所得数据，也可以用 $t_{0.9}$ 法处理。由于不同温度下的 K 值和 $t_{0.9}$ 成反比关系，根据 Arrhenius 指数定律，若测得各温度下药物分解 10% 所需时间，由 $\lg t_{0.9}$ 代替 $\lg K$ 对 $1/T$ 作图或进行线性回归得一直线，直线外推至室温，即可求出室温下的 $t_{0.9}$。用图解法则不用求出 K 值，可在加速试验温度的 $\lg C$ 对 t 所作直线上，在 lg90=1.9542 处作 t 轴的平行线，该平行线与各温度下的 $\lg C$-t 直线交点所对应的 t 值就分别为各温度下的 $t_{0.9}$ 值。用回归法要通过各加速温度下的 K 值，进而求算出各温度下的 $t_{0.9}$，仍需要对每个加速温度下做一系列不同时间的取样分析，从中找出相应的 $t_{0.9}$。实际工作量也并未减少，只是数据处理简单化。若药物分解在 10% 以内时，用 $\lg C$-t 直线规律或 C-t 直线规律处理差别不大，这种情况下，不知反应级数也可采用 $t_{0.9}$ 法。

a. $t_{0.9}$ methods　The data obtained from the classical constant temperature method can also be processed by $t_{0.9}$ methods. K value at different temperature is inversely proportional to $t_{0.9}$. According to Arrhenius exponential law, if the time required for drug decomposition of 10% at each temperature is

measured, a straight line can be drawn from lg $t_{0.9}$ instead of lg$K$. The straight line can be extrapolated to room temperature to obtain the $t_{0.9}$ at room temperature. In the graphic method, the line is made by lg$C$ to t, the parallel line of the t-axis is made at lg90 = 1.9542. The t value corresponding to the intersection of the parallel line and the lg$C$-t line at each temperature is respectively the $t_{0.9}$ value at each temperature. In order to calculate the $t_{0.9}$ at each temperature through the K value at each acceleration temperature by the regression method, it is still necessary to do a series of sampling analysis at each acceleration temperature at different times to find the corresponding $t_{0.9}$. The actual workload is not reduced, but the data processing is simplified. If the drug decomposition is within 10%, there is no significant difference in the treatment with lg$C$-t linear rule or C-t linear rule. In this case, it can also be used by the $t_{0.9}$ methods with unknown reaction order.

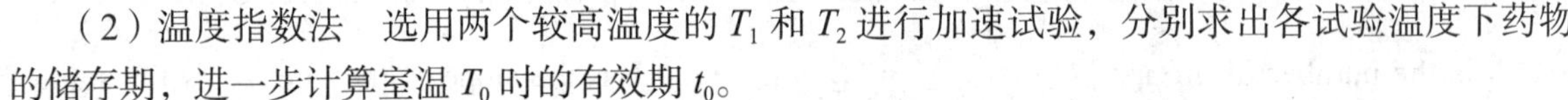

（2）温度指数法　选用两个较高温度的 T_1 和 T_2 进行加速试验，分别求出各试验温度下药物的储存期，进一步计算室温 T_0 时的有效期 t_0。

案例导入

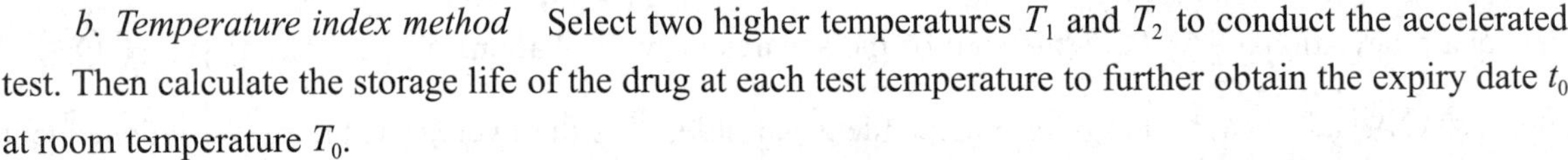

b. Temperature index method　Select two higher temperatures T_1 and T_2 to conduct the accelerated test. Then calculate the storage life of the drug at each test temperature to further obtain the expiry date t_0 at room temperature T_0.

$$t_0 = t_1\left(\frac{t_1}{t_2}\right)^{\alpha} \tag{20-8}$$

其中 t_1 和 t_2 分别为温度为 T_1、T_2 时的储存期，α 为温度指数。

t_1 and t_2 are the storage periods when the temperature is T_1 and T_2, α is temperature index.

$$\alpha = \frac{T_2(T_1 - T_0)}{T_0(T_2 - T_1)} \tag{20-9}$$

为了使 α 等于整数，可以按照表 20-4 选择 T_1、T_2。

To make α equal to the integer, T_1 and T_2 can be selected according to Table 20-4.

表 20-4　温度指数法的选用温度（T_0=25℃）

Table 20-4　The Choice of Temperature Index Method

T_1（℃）	T_2（℃）	α
82.1	100	4
71.2	90	3
59.5	80	2
45.9	70	1
41.5	60	1

（3）初均速法　该法是以反应试验初速度 V_0 代替反应速度常数 k，按 Arrhenius 定律外推得室温有效期，其表达式为：

c. Initial average velocity method　In this method, the initial reaction speed V_0 replaces the reaction speed constant k. The room temperature validity period can be extrapolated according to Arrhenius law, and the expression is:

$$\lg V_{0i} = \frac{E}{2.303RT_i} + \lg A' \tag{20-10}$$

式中，V_{0i} 为温度 T_i 时药物分解的初均速度。

V_{0i} is the initial mean velocity of drug decomposition at temperature T_i.

$$V_{0i}=\frac{C_0-C_1}{t_i} \tag{20-11}$$

C_0 为药物的初始浓度；C_i 为药物在 T_i 时，经历时间 t_i 后 剩余浓度；$i=1$，2，…n。

C_0 is the initial concentration of the drug; C_i is the residual concentration after the drug experiences time t_i when it is in T_i; $i = 1, 2, ... n$.

试验选取数个加速温度 T_i，在各温度下加热样品至一定时间 t 后测定药物浓度 C_i，将浓度和时间数据带入式（20-11）中，求出各温度下药物分解的初均速度 V_{0i}。然后以 $\lg V_{0i}$ 对 $1/T_i$ 做线性回归的直线方程。由直线方程可计算出反应活化能和室温下的有效期。

Select a number of accelerating temperatures T_i for the experiment, and determine the drug concentration C_i after the samples were heated at each temperature to a certain time t. Substitute the concentration and time data into equations 20-11 to obtain the initial mean velocity V_{0i} of drug decomposition at each temperature. Then calculate the activation energy of the reaction and the expiration date at room temperature from the linear equation with linear regression of $1/T_i$ with $\lg V_{0i}$.

案例导入 ¦ Case example

案例 20-5 初均速法预测人参茎叶皂苷的有效期

20-5 Predicted the Validity of Ginserg Stem and Leaf Faponins by Initial Average Velocity Method

利用初均速法预测人参皂苷的有效期。

The validity of Ginserg Stem and Leaf Faponins is predicted by initial average velocity method.

表 20-5 初均速法预测人参皂苷的有效期相关数据

Table 20-5 Related Forecast Data

温度（Temperature, ℃）	$1/T\times10^{-3}$	T(h)	含量（%）	V_{0i}	$\lg V_{0i}$
60	3.003	10	96.3	0.370	−0.4318
65	2.959	9	93.7	0.700	−0.1549
70	2.915	8	91.2	1.100	0.0414
75	2.847	7	88.8	1.600	0.2041
80	2.833	6	86.1	2.317	0.3649
85	2.793	5	83.5	3.280	0.5159
90	2.755	4	81.9	4.525	0.6556

回归分析计算，以 $\lg V_{0i}$ 对 1/（$T\times10^{-3}$）得回归方程：$\lg V_{0i}=12.4327$，$4.2633\times1/(T\times10^{-3})$，$R=0.996$，$t_{0.9}^{25℃}=t_{0.9}^{25℃}=11058.7\text{h}=460.78\text{d}$。

四、中药制剂稳定性试验应注意的问题

20.3.4 Problems Requiring Attention Regarding the Stability of TCM Preparations

1. 正确选择稳定性考核指标。中药制剂稳定性考察应选择能反映一定治疗活性的，特别是其中不稳定的成分作为考察指标，如蛇胆川贝液中的胆酸和贝母碱、养血止痛丸中的丹参酮、咽喉

清水蜜丸中的橙皮苷和冰片等。在复方制剂中测定两种或两种以上成分的，应选择其中较不稳定的有效成分作为制定有效期的依据，如银黄微型灌肠剂按绿原酸和黄芩苷计，有效期分别为 1.99 年和 3.82 年，因此确定其有效期为 2 年。

(1) Select appropriate stability assessment indicators: The stability of TCM preparations should be determined by selecting ingredients which can reflect certain therapeutic activity, especially unstable ones. Such as the cholic acid and fritillary base in Shedanchuanbei Oral Liquid, the tanshinone in Yangxue Zhitong pill, the hesperidin and borneol in the Yanhouqing water-honeyed pill. If two or more components are determined in a compound preparation, the less stable active component should be selected as the basis for determining the period of validity. For example, chlorogenic acid and baicalin in Yinhuang microenema have a validity of 1.99 years and 3.82 years respectively, so their validity is determined to be 2 years.

2. 选择专属性强、灵敏度高的测定方法。若质量标准规定的含量测定方法，由于降解产物的干扰不能准确测定有效成分的含量变化时，应考虑选择灵敏度高、专属性强的含量分析方法。如何首乌中二苯乙烯苷在 310nm 波长处有最大吸收，但其降解产物在该波长处的吸收不仅不降，反而随着加热时间成线性增加，因此，以分光光度法难以考察二苯乙烯苷的降解情况，宜采用高效液相色谱法。

(2) Select the methods with strong specificity and high sensitivity: When the interference of degradation products cannot accurately determine the change of the content of the active ingredient, the method with high sensitivity and strong specificity should be considered. For example, the maximum absorption of stilbene glycoside in Polygonum Multiflori Radix is at the wavelength of 310nm, but the absorption of its degradation products at this wavelength would increase linearly with the heating time. Therefore, HPLC should be used to investigate the degradation of stilbene glycosides instead of spectrophotometry.

3. 注意适用范围。以 Arrhenius 指数定律为基础的加速试验法，只适用于活化能在 41.84~125.52kJ/mol 的热分解反应。由于光化反应的活化能只有 8.37~12.55kJ/mol，温度对反应速度影响不大，不宜采用热加速反应。某些多羟基药物，活化能高至 209~292.6kJ/mol，温度升高，反应速度急剧增加，用热加速试验预测室温的稳定性没有实际意义。

(3) The scope of application: The accelerated test method based on Arrhenius exponential law is only applicable to thermal decomposition reactions with activation energy of 41.84-125.52kJ/mol. Since the activation energy of photochemical reaction is only 8.37-12.55kJ/mol, the temperature has little influence on the reaction speed, so the thermal acceleration reaction is not suitable. The activation energy of some polyhydroxy drugs is as high as 209-292.6kJ/mol. Their reaction speed increases sharply when the temperature increases. Therefore, it is of no practical significance to predict the stability of room temperature by thermal acceleration test.

4. 稳定性加速试验。其要求加速过程中反应级数和反应机理均不改变。Arrhenius 指数定律是假设活化能不随着温度变化而提出的，试验中只考虑温度对反应速度的影响，因此其他条件应保持恒定。同时，加速试验预测只能用于所研究的制剂，不能任意推广到同一药物的其他制剂。

(4) Accelerated test of stability: It requires that the reaction series and mechanism remain unchanged during the process of acceleration. Arrhenius exponential law is proposed on the assumption that activation energy does not vary with temperature. In the experiment, only the influence of temperature on reaction rate is considered, other conditions should be kept constant. At the same time, the accelerated test

prediction can only be applied to the studied preparations, and cannot be arbitrarily extended to other preparations of the same drug.

5. 加速试验预测有效期，应与留样观察结果对照，才能确定产品实际有效期。

(5) Compare with the retained samples to determine the actual validity period of the product in the predicted validity period of accelerated test.

6. 上述加速试验方法用于均相系统，一般能得出一个满意的结果。而对于非均相系统，如乳状液、混悬液等，在升温后可能改变物理状态，不宜运用 Arrhenius 定律。

(6) The above accelerated test method is applied to homogeneous system. However, for heterogeneous systems, such as emulsion and suspension, the physical state may change after heating up, so it is not suitable to apply Arrhenius law.

中药复方制剂的质量难以用一两个成分的含量来代表制剂的全部质量含义，所测定的某一成分在许多情况下并不意味着该成分是在临床治疗上起主要作用，只是配合原料、工艺等质量管理起着质量指标的作用，因此运用质量标准中的含量测定内容作为稳定性研究手段，在一些情况下不一定能够全面反映出产品的稳定性真实情况，在制定有效期时仅作为参考。也有用加速试验后考察制剂药效学指标变化判断中药制剂稳定性的报道。

It is difficult to use the content of one or two components to represent the total quality of a compound preparation. In many cases, a component measured does not mean that the component plays a major role in clinical treatment, but only plays a role as a quality indicator in combination with quality management such as raw materials and processes. Therefore, the content determination in the quality standard is only used as a reference when formulating the validity period. It is also useful to evaluate the stability of TCM preparations by studying the change of pharmacodynamics index after accelerated test.

第四节　包装材料对制剂稳定性的影响

20.4　The Effect of Packaging Materials on the Stability of Preparation

PPT

药品包装材料是指药品生产企业生产的药品和医疗机构配制的制剂所使用的直接接触药品的包装材料和容器。药品通常储存于室温环境下，受各种环境的影响，如光、热、水分、空气等，选择适宜的包装材料可减小这些环境因素对制剂稳定性的影响。因此，药品的包装设计既要考虑外界环境因素对制剂稳定性的影响，又要注意包装材料与药物制剂相互作用而引起的稳定性变化。

Pharmaceutical packaging materials refer to the packaging materials and containers that are directly in contact with pharmaceutical preparations produced by pharmaceutical manufacturers and prepared by medical institutions. Drugs are usually stored at room temperature. Appropriate packaging materials can reduce the impact of these environmental factors such as light, heat, moisture, air, etc. on the stability of the formulation. Therefore, the drug packaging design should not only consider the influence of the external environment on the stability of the drug, but also pay attention to the stability changes caused by the interaction between the packaging material and the drug.

理想的药物包装材料应该满足以下几点：①自身性质稳定，不产生毒副产物的产生；②良好

的阻隔性，能隔绝药物免受周围环境的影响；③与药物不相溶性，不影响其质量，气味，颜色等；④能适应碰撞、加热等特殊要求；⑤便于运输、储存和使用。

The ideal drug packaging material should meet the following requirements:

(1) The packaging material is stable in property and does not produce toxic by-products.

(2) The packaging material has good barrier properties and can isolate the drug from the surrounding environment.

(3) The packaging material is incompatible with the drug and does not affect the quality, smell, and color of the drug.

(4) The packaging materials can meet special requirements such as collision and heating.

(5) The packaging materials are easy to transport, store and use.

中药制剂的包装材料通常有玻璃、塑料、橡胶和金属等，下面简要介绍几种主要包装材料。

The packaging materials of TCM preparations usually include glass, plastic, rubber and metal.

一、玻璃

20.4.1 Glass

药用玻璃包装材料具有化学性质较为稳定，空气和水分阻隔性好，价廉易得等优点，广泛使用于注射液、口服液及外用制剂等剂型中。其对制剂稳定性的影响主要有四个方面：①释放碱性离子，影响药液的 pH；②容易脱落产生不溶性玻璃碎片；③透光；④含有氧化物，易使药物氧化、分解。

Glass used in pharmaceutical packaging materials has the advantages of stable chemical properties, good barrier, cheap and easy to get. It is widely used in injection, oral liquid and external preparations. The influence of glass material on the stability of the preparation mainly includes four aspects:

(1) The glass material will release alkaline ions, affecting the pH value of the drug solution.

(2) The glass material is easy to fall off insoluble glass fragments.

(3) The glass material is transparent.

(4) The glass material contains oxide which making the drug oxidation, decomposition.

玻璃主要成分是二氧化硅，辅以钠、钾、钙、镁、铝、硼、铁等元素的氧化物改变其理化性能。低硼硅酸盐玻璃（中性玻璃）有较好的化学性质，可以用作近中性或弱酸性的注射液的容器；含锆元素的玻璃则具有更稳定的化学性质，抗酸碱，适用于酸性或碱性的药物制剂；而普通的钠钙玻璃，其中 Na^+ 含量较高，容易与药物水溶液中的 OH^- 结合，生成 NaOH，从而影响药物的 pH；同时，NaOH 会与玻璃表面的 SiO_4 作用产生 SiO_2 微粒，因此这种材质的玻璃不能用于注射液，只能包装一般的口服液等剂型。普通钠钙玻璃的“脱片”现象需要引起高度的重视。

The main composition of glass is silica, supplemented by sodium, potassium, calcium, magnesium, aluminum, boron, iron and other oxides to change its physical and chemical properties. Low borosilicate glass (neutral glass) has good chemical properties and can be used as a container for near neutral or weak acid injection. Glass containing zirconium is more stable and is suitable for acidic or alkaline pharmaceutical preparations. However, ordinary soda-lime glass has a high content of Na^+, which is easy to combine with OH^- in drug aqueous solution to form NaOH, thus affecting the pH value of the drug. At the same time, NaOH will interact with SiO_4 on the glass surface to produce SiO_2 particles. Therefore, this kind of glass cannot be used for injection, and can only be used to package oral liquid. The phenomenon

of "disconnection" of ordinary soda-lime glass should be paid much attention.

棕色玻璃能阻挡小于 470nm 的光线透过，常用于对光敏感的药物制剂，但是应该关注其中的氧化铁容易脱落进入制剂的现象。

Brown glass can block the passage of light less than 470nm. It is often used in photosensitive pharmaceutical preparations. But it should be concerned that the iron oxide in the glass which is easy to fall off and enter the preparation.

另外，玻璃易碎、笨重、冻干炸裂等问题也需要给予考虑。

In addition, it should be considered that the glass is fragile, bulky, freeze-dried and cracked.

二、塑料
20.4.2 Plastic

塑料具有材质轻、可塑性强、有韧性、不易破碎、便于运输、在输液过程中不需补充空气而避免空气污染药液等优点，广泛用于输液、注射液、胶囊剂、丸剂等剂型。其对制剂稳定性的影响主要有两个方面：①透过性：外界的空气、水分等能透过塑料进入包装内部，容易引起药物的氧化、水解、吸潮等反应，而内部的水分、气体等也能透过包装，造成挥发油逸散，乳剂脱水甚至破裂变质等物理学和化学变化。②泄漏与吸附：塑料中的物质可以泄漏到溶液中，高分子材料会吸附药物，降低药物主要成分的含量。

Plastic has the advantages of light material, strong plasticity, toughness and easy transportation. It does not need to add air during the infusion process, which can avoid air pollution. Plastic packaging is widely used in infusion, injection, capsule and pill. The influence of plastic material on the stability of the preparation mainly includes two aspects:

(1) Permeability: The air and water from the outside can enter the package through the plastic and easily cause the reactions of oxidation, hydrolysis and moisture absorption of the medicine. And the internal water, gas can also go through the packaging, resulting in volatile oil escape, emulsion dehydration and even rupture metamorphism.

(2) Leakage and adsorption: The substance in the plastic can leak into the solution. The polymer material will absorb the drug, reducing the content of the main component of the drug.

常用的塑料有聚乙烯、聚丙烯、聚氯乙烯、聚碳酸酯及聚酰胺等高分子聚合物。塑料中常常加入添加剂，如稳定剂、增塑剂、抗氧剂等。有些添加剂具有毒性，在较长时间之后浸出，严重影响药物的质量。因此，塑料材料不宜用于需要长期保存的药物，特别是化学性质不稳定的药物，且使用前有必要对塑料材料进行物理、化学、生物毒性等试验，以确保使用安全。

Commonly used plastics are polyethylene, polypropylene, polyvinyl chloride, polycarbonate and polyamide polymer. Additives are often added to plastics, such as stabilizer, plasticizer, antioxidant, etc. Some additives are toxic. Therefore, plastic materials should not be used for drugs that need to be kept for a long time, especially unstable chemical properties. Before use, it is necessary to test the physical, chemical and biological toxicity of plastic materials to ensure the safety.

三、橡胶
20.4.3 Rubber

橡胶具有弹性好、遇外力变形后能迅速恢复、易于清洗等优点，广泛应用于制作垫圈、瓶塞、滴头等。但同样存在漏液和吸附的问题，同时，天然橡胶含有异性蛋白和乳胶过敏原，容易引起过敏。

Rubber has the advantages of good elasticity and easy cleaning. It can recover quickly after being deformed by external force. Rubber is widely used to make gaskets, bottle stoppers and drippers. But rubber has problems of leakage and adsorption. At the same time, natural rubber contains foreign proteins and latex allergens, which can easily cause allergies.

橡胶成型过程中加入的硫化剂、填充剂、防老剂等附加剂，与药液长时间接触之后，容易浸出，污染药液，增加毒性，也对药物成分的化学测定造成干扰。

Additives such as vulcanizing agents, fillers, and anti-aging agents added to the rubber are easy to leach out and contaminate the chemical solution. This increases toxicity and also interferes with the chemical determination of drug ingredients.

橡胶可吸附药液中的主药和抑菌剂，使药物的抑菌能力大大降低。若使用环氧树脂涂层，可明显减少上述现象，但是不能消除吸附现象，因此，预先使用抑菌剂浸泡饱和橡胶，能有效地防止橡胶对抑菌剂的吸附，也能防止橡胶成分溶于水中。

Rubber can absorb the main components and bacteriostatic agent in the drug solution, which greatly reduces the bacteriostatic ability of the drug. Epoxy resin coating can significantly reduce the adsorption. Therefore, soaking the saturated rubber with bacteriostatic agent in advance can effectively prevent the rubber from adsorbing the bacteriostatic agent, and also prevent the rubber component from dissolving in water.

四、金属
20.4.4 Metal

金属包装材料遮光性能好，空气及水分阻隔性好，氧化物无毒，加工性能好，耐热耐寒，密闭性好，对药物有良好的保护作用，尤其适用于化学稳定性差的药物。但其抗腐蚀能力差，遇金属离子易发生反应，且成本较高。

Metal packaging material has good lightproof performance, leakproofness and barrier ability. Metal material is heat - resistant and cold - resistant, and its oxide is non-toxic. Metal material has a good protective effect on drugs, especially for drugs with poor chemical stability. However, the corrosion resistance of metal materials is poor and the cost is high.

锡管和铝管常用于眼用制剂或者软膏剂的包装材料。为了保证制剂的稳定性，要求镀层金属且不与药物发生化学反应，并牢固覆盖，不得有微孔、裂隙等。

Tin tubes and aluminum tubes are often used as packaging materials for ophthalmic preparations or ointments. In order to ensure the stability of the preparation, it is required that the coated metal does not react with the drug. And the coated metal should be firmly covered without micropores, cracks.

锡的化学性质稳定，但氯化物和酸性物质能腐蚀锡，在锡的表面涂纤维漆薄层，增加其抗腐蚀性能。汞化物对铝管的腐蚀作用非常强。铝管如包装 pH 为 5.6~8.0 的药物制剂，要在铝管表面涂环氧树脂增加其抗腐蚀性。

Tin is stable, but chloride and acid corrode it. Applying a thin layer of fiber paint to the surface of tin can increase its corrosion resistance. Mercury compounds have a very strong corrosion effect on aluminum tubes. If the pH value of the drug is 5.6-8.0 in aluminum tube, the surface of the aluminum tube should be coated with epoxy resin to increase its corrosion resistance.

目前铝箔的使用越来越广泛，但是其价格成本较高，且铝箔的气孔多，热密封强度差，所以多常用铝塑复合材料。

At present, the use of aluminum foil is more and more widely. But the price of aluminum foil is high, and the thermal seal of aluminum foil is poor due to more pores. Therefore, aluminum-plastic composites are often used.

（刘文龙）

岗位对接

重点小结

题库

第二十一章　中药制剂的配伍变化
Chapter 21　The Compatibility Changes in Traditional Chinese Medicine Preparations

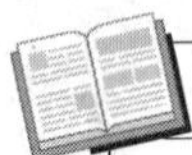

学习目标 | Learning Goals

知识要求：

1. **掌握**　药物制剂配伍变化的概念；药剂学配伍变化的内容；预测制剂配伍变化的实验变化。

2. **熟悉**　药理学配伍变化中制剂在体内的发生相互作用；注射剂配伍变化的分类及其发生原因。

3. **了解**　发生配伍变化后的处理方法。

Knowledge requirements:

1. To master the concept of compatibility changes in pharmaceutical preparations, content of the compatibility changes in pharmaceutics, predictions of the experimental changes of compatibility changes in preparations.

2. To be familiar with the pharmacology changes *in vivo* caused by compatibility of Traditional Chinese Medicine; the classifications and causes of injection compatibility changes.

3. To know the treatment method after compatibility changes.

第一节　概述
21.1　Overview

PPT

一、药物配伍的概念
21.1.1　The Concept of the Medical Compatibility

在药剂生产或临床用药中，有目的、有规则地将两种或两种以上的药物、辅料等配合在一起使用的过程，称为药物配伍。药物配伍应用后在理化性质或生理效应方面产生的变化，称为药物配伍变化。在一定条件下产生的不利于生产、应用和治疗的药物配伍变化，称为药物配伍禁忌。

配伍禁忌为不合理的配伍体现，应当避免产生。

In pharmaceutical production or clinical use, the process in which two or more drugs or excipients are combined under specific guidance for certain purposes is called medical compatibility. The changes in physical and chemical properties or in the physiological effects after medical compatibility are called medicine compatibility changes. The medicine compatibility changes which are not conducive to the production, application and treatment under certain conditions are incompatibility. The incompatibility is an unreasonable embodiment of compatibility and should be avoided.

二、药物配伍应用的目的
21.1.2 The Purposes of the Medical Compatibility Application

复方配伍用药是中医用药的特点和精髓，其目的概括为以下几点：

The compound combination medications are the characters and essences of traditional Chinese medicine, whose purposes can be concluded as follows:

1. 满足临床预防或治疗合并症（兼病或兼证）的需要。

(1) To meet the clinical prevention or treatment of complications (concurrent disease or concurrent syndrome) needs.

2. 发挥协同作用，增强疗效。如“相须”、“相使”配伍。

(2) To develop the synergistic effect and enhance the curative effect, such as the mutual “promotion” and “assistance” of the compatibility.

3. 减少药物不良反应。如用吗啡镇痛时配伍阿托品，可消除吗啡对呼吸中枢的抑制作用及对胆道、输尿管及支气管平滑肌的兴奋作用。中药“相畏”“相杀”配伍可抑制毒副作用或克服药物的偏性。

(3) To adverse the side effects. The mutual “restraint” and “detoxication” can inhibit the side effects or overcome the bias of drugs. Such as compatibility of atropine with morphine analgesia, morphine can eliminate inhibition effect of respiratory center and excitation effect of biliary tract, ureter and bronchial smooth muscle.

4. 减少或延缓耐药性的发生。如磺胺药与甲氧苄氨嘧啶（TMP）、阿莫西林与克拉维酸配伍使用。

(4) To reduce or delay the drug resistance. For example, sulfonamide is used in combination with trimethoprim (TMP), amoxicillin and clavulanic acid.

三、药物配伍变化的类型
21.1.3 The Types of Medical Compatibility Changes

根据配伍变化性质，结合药物的特点，药物配伍变化类型主要有以下几种：

According to the properties of compatibility changes and the characteristics of drugs, the types of medical compatibility changes mainly include the following:

1. 中药学配伍变化 中药学配伍系指根据病情需要和药物性能，在中医药理论指导下，有选择地将两种或两种以上的药物配合在一起运用的配伍方法，其药物配伍会出现一定的相互作用关系，称为中药学配伍变化。中药的“君、臣、佐、使”组方原则和“七情配伍”理论（包括单行、相须、相使、相畏、相杀、相恶和相反）是中医药的主要配伍理论。中药配伍禁忌包括

“十八反”“十九畏”，系指在一般情况下不宜相互配合使用的药物。“相恶”也是临床上一种相对的配伍禁忌。此外，尚有妊娠用药禁忌，服药时的饮食禁忌等。

(1) The compatibility changes of traditional Chinese medicine The compatibility changes in traditional Chinese medicine refer to the compatibility method in which two or more herbs are combined selectively according to the condition and drug properties under the guidance of traditional Chinese medicine theory. The principle of “monarch, minister, assistant and guide” and the theory of “seven relations” (including singular application, mutual promotion, mutual assistance, mutual restraint, mutual detoxitation and incompatibility) are the main compatibility theories of traditional Chinese medicine.

The incompatibilities of Chinese medicine include “eighteen incompatibility” and “nineteen mutual restraints” which refer to drugs that are generally not suitable for combination. The “mutual detoxitation” is also incompatibility in clinic use. Besides, there are pregnancy medication contraindications, medication dietary contraindications, etc.

2. 药剂学配伍变化 系指药物及其制剂进入机体前发生于体外的配伍变化。这种变化是在药剂生产、贮藏及用药配伍过程中发生的配伍变化。根据变化的性质不同，药剂学的配伍变化分为物理的配伍变化和化学的配伍变化。药剂学的配伍变化，有的在较短时间内即可发生，有的则需较长时间才会出现。不利于生产、贮藏，造成使用不便或对治疗有害，而又无法克服的药剂学配伍变化，称为药剂学配伍禁忌。

(2) The compatibility changes in pharmaceutics It refers to the compatibility changes before clinical application. Those changes occur in the process of production, storage or drug compatibility. According to the different properties the changes, pharmaceutical compatibility changes are divided into physical compatibility changes and chemical compatibility changes. Compatibility changes in pharmaceutics can occur either in a short time or over a long period of time. Incompatibility in pharmaceutics refers to changes in pharmacy compatibility that are not conducive to production or storage, causing inconvenience to use or harmful to treatment, but cannot be overcome.

3. 药理学配伍变化 系指两种或两种以上的药物合并或先后使用后，受合用或前后应用的其他药物或内源性物质及食物等的影响，使其药理作用的性质、强度等发生改变的配伍变化，也称为疗效学配伍变化或体内药物相互作用。出现疗效降低或消失，产生毒性反应，甚至危及生命的药理学配伍变化称为药理学配伍禁忌。

(3) The compatibility changes in pharmacology It refers to the changes when two or more drugs are used in combination or changes after successive application of other endogenous substances or foods, which vary the pharmacological effect property or intensity of active components. This compatibility change is also known as therapeutic compatibility changes or drug interaction *in vivo*. The change of pharmacologic compatibility resulting in the decrease or disappearance of efficacy, toxicity, or even life-threatening is called pharmacological incompatibilities.

第二节 药剂学的配伍变化
21.2 The Compatibility Changes in Pharmaceutics

PPT

一、物理的配伍变化
21.2.1 The Physical Compatibility Changes

物理的配伍变化，系指药物配伍后在制备、贮存过程中，发生了物理性质的改变，从而影响制剂的外观或内在质量的变化。药物配伍后的物理变化主要体现在以下三个方面：

The physical compatibility changes refer to the changes of physical properties in the process of preparation and storage after the medical compatibility, which affect the appearance or internal quality of the preparation. The physical changes after the medical compatibility are mainly reflected in the following three aspects:

（一）溶解度的改变
(1) Changes in Solubility

1. 温度改变 温度对药物的溶解度有直接影响。

① **The temperature change** Temperature has direct influence on the solubility of drugs.

2. 药渣吸附 群药合煎时，某些药物成分可被其他药渣吸附，影响其在药液中的溶解量和提取率。

② **Herb residue absorption** Some ingredients can be adsorbed by residues of drugs during the decoction, reducing dissolution and extraction rate of ingredients.

3. 盐析作用 在溶液中加入无机盐类可使某些成分溶解度降低而析出。

③ **Salting-out effects** Adding inorganic salts to the solution can reduce the solubility of some components and increase their precipitation amount.

4. 增溶作用 糊化淀粉对酚性药物会产生增溶作用。

④ **Solubilization** Gelatinized starch can increase the solubility of phenolic drugs.

5. 改变溶剂 不同溶剂的液体配合在一起，常会析出沉淀。

⑤ **Changes of solutions** Solutions composed by different solvents are prone to precipitate substances.

6. 贮藏过程 药液中有效成分或杂质为高分子物质时，在放置过程中，受空气、光线等影响，可使胶体“陈化”而析出沉淀。

⑥ **Storage procedure** When the active components or impurities in the liquid are the macromolecules, the aged colloid can be precipitated under the influence of air or light during the storage.

（二）吸湿、潮解、液化与结块
(2) Hygroscopicity, Deliquescence, Liquefaction and Agglomeration

1. 吸湿与潮解 某些吸湿性很强的药物，如中药的干浸膏、颗粒、某些酶、无机盐类等易发生吸湿、潮解。使用吸湿性强的辅料时，也因吸收水分而使遇水不稳定的药物分解或降低效价。

① **Hygroscopicity and deliquescence** Some highly hygroscopic drugs, such as dry extract of traditional Chinese medicine, particles, some enzymes, inorganic salts, etc., are prone to moisture absorption and deliquescence. When highly hygroscopic excipients are used, the adsorbed moisture also

increase decomposition rate of active components leading to efficacy reduction.

2. 液化 可形成低共熔混合物的药物配伍时，因发生液化而影响制剂的配制。但根据剂型及临床需要，在制备中也可对处方中低共熔混合物的液化现象加以利用，如樟脑、冰片与薄荷脑混合时产生的液化。

② **The liquefaction** Drugs can form low eutectic mixtures while combining, and this liquefaction phenomenon may affect preparation process of drugs. However, the liquefaction phenomenon of the low-eutectic mixture can also be utilized for the production according to the dosage forms and clinical needs, such as the liquefaction when mixing camphor, borneol and menthol.

3. 结块 粉体制剂（如散剂、颗粒剂）可由于药物配伍后吸湿性增加而结块，同时也可能导致药物的分解而失效。

③ **The agglomeration** Powder preparation (such as powder, granule) may agglomerate due to the increase of moisture absorption after drug compatibility, and may also lead to drug decomposition and failure.

（三）粒径或分散状态的改变

(3) Change in Particle Size or Dispersion State

粒径或分散状态的改变可直接影响制剂的内在质量。例如乳剂、混悬剂中分散相的粒径可因与其他药物配伍而变大，分散相聚结、凝聚或分层，导致使用不便或分剂量不准，甚至影响药物在体内的吸收。胶体溶液可因加入电解质或其他脱水剂使胶体分散状态破坏而产生沉淀。某些保护胶体中加入浓度较高的亲水物质如糖、乙醇或强电解质可使保护胶失去作用。

The change of particle size or dispersion state can directly affect the internal quality of preparation. For example, the particle size of the dispersed phase in emulsions and suspensions can be increased due to the compatibility with other drugs, which lead to dispersion, aggregation or stratification, resulting in inconvenience of use or improper dose distribution, and even the low absorption of drugs in the body. Colloidal solutions may be precipitated by the addition of electrolytes or other dehydrating agents which break the colloidal dispersion. The addition of hydrophilic substances such as sugar, ethanol, or strong electrolyte of high concentration to protective colloid can disable its protective effect.

二、化学的配伍变化

21.2.2 The Chemical Compatibility Changes

化学的配伍变化系指药物成分之间发生化学反应而导致药物成分的改变。化学的配伍变化既包括浑浊、沉淀、变色、产气和爆炸等可以观察到的现象，也包括肉眼看不到的许多变化。

The chemical compatibility changes refer to the changes of pharmaceutical ingredients caused by the chemical reactions among medical components. The changes of chemical compatibility not only include visible phenomena, such as the turbidity, precipitation, discoloration and explosion, but also include many invisible ones.

（一）产生浑浊或沉淀

(1) The Generation of Turbidity or Precipitation

与因物理的配伍变化引起的浑浊、沉淀或分层不同，在配制和贮藏过程中若配伍不当，各成分间可能会由于发生化学反应而产生浑浊或沉淀。

Different from the turbidity or precipitation caused by the physical compatibility changes, the turbidity and precipitation caused by chemical reactions are among all the ingredients, if there is any improper compatibility in the preparation or storage.

1. 生物碱与苷类 糖基上含有羧基的苷类或其他酸性较强的苷类与生物碱结合，会产生沉淀。如甘草与含生物碱的黄连、黄柏，吴茱萸、延胡索、槟榔、马钱子共煎可发生沉淀或浑浊。葛根黄酮、黄芩苷等羟基黄酮衍生物及大黄酸、大黄素等羟基蒽醌衍生物在溶液中能与小檗碱生成沉淀。

① The alkaloids and glycosides Glycosides which contain carboxyl or other strong acidic glycosides combining with alkaloids will cause precipitation. For example, precipitation or turbidity may occur when glycyrrhiza decocts with coptis, cortex phellodendri, evodia rutaecarpa, corydalis, areca-nut or semen strychni which contain alkaloids. Hydroxyl anthraquinone derivatives such as radix puerariae flavone and baicalin and hydroxyl anthraquinone derivatives such as rhubarb acid and emodin can precipitate with berberine.

2. 有机酸与生物碱 金银花中含有绿原酸和异绿原酸，茵陈中含有绿原酸及咖啡酸，两药与小檗碱、延胡索乙素等多种生物碱配伍使用，均可生成难溶性的生物碱有机酸盐。

② The organic acids and alkaloids Flos lonicerae contains chlorogenic acid and isochlorogenic acid, and oriental wormwood contains chlorogenic acid and caffeic acid. Insoluble alkaloid organic acid salts will generate when the above two drugs are used in combination with alkaloids such as berberine and tetrahydropalmatine.

3. 无机离子的影响 石膏中的 Ca^{2+} 可与甘草酸、绿原酸、黄芩苷等生成难溶于水的钙盐。以硬水作为提取溶剂时，硬水中含有的 Ca^{2+}、Mg^{2+} 能与一些大分子酸性成分生成沉淀。

③ The influence of inorganic ions Ca^{2+} in gypsum can be combined with glycyrrhizic acid, chlorogenic acid and baicalin, forming calcium salts which are insoluble in water. When hard water is used as extraction solvent, Ca^{2+} and Mg^{2+} contained in hard water will precipitate with some acidic components of large molecular mass.

4. 鞣质和生物碱 大多数生物碱能与鞣质反应生成难溶性的沉淀。如大黄与黄连配伍，汤液苦味消失，并形成黄褐色的胶状沉淀。含鞣质的中药较多，因此在中药复方制剂制备时，应防止生物碱的损失。

④ The tannins and alkaloids Most alkaloids can react with tannins to generate precipitation. Such as the compatibility of rhubarb and rhizome coptidis, the bitterness disappears and colloidal precipitation is formed. As there are many traditional Chinese medicines containing tannins, the loss of alkaloids should be prevented.

5. 鞣质和其他成分结合 ①鞣质能和皂苷结合生成沉淀。如含柴胡皂苷的中药与拳参等含鞣质的中药提取液配伍时可生成沉淀。因此，在制备感冒退热颗粒时，应防止板蓝根、大青叶中的吲哚苷被拳参中的鞣质所沉淀而滤除。②鞣质可与蛋白质、白及胶生成沉淀，使酶类制剂降低疗效或失效。③含鞣质的中药制剂与抗生素（如红霉素、灰黄霉素、氨苄西林等）配伍，可生成鞣酸盐沉淀物，不易被吸收，降低各自的生物利用度。④鞣质与含金属离子的药物（如钙剂、铁剂等）配伍易产生沉淀。

⑤ The tannins and other ingredient components Ⅰ.Tannins can react with saponins to generate the insoluble precipitation. For example, drugs containing Bupleuri Radix saponin can react with tannins of Bistortae Rhizoma to generate precipitation. Therefore, indole glycoside in radix isatidis and folium isatidis should be prevented from being precipitated by tannins in Bistortae Rhizoma when preparing some antipyretics. Ⅱ.Tannins can react with proteins and bletilla striata gum to generate precipitation, lowering the efficacy of enzyme preparation, or even causing failure. Ⅲ.The compatibility of antibiotics and chinese medicine preparations which contain tannins can generate tannate precipitation and is not easy to be absorbed, leading to reduction of bioavailability of antibiotics and chinese medicine

preparations. Ⅳ.The compatibility of tannins and drugs containing metal ions is easy to generate precipitation.

（二）产生有毒物质

(2) The Generation of Toxicity

成分间相互作用产生有毒物质的配伍属配伍禁忌。如含朱砂（主要含 HgS）的中药制剂（如朱砂安神丸、冠心苏合丸、七厘散等）不宜与还原性药物（如碘化物、硫酸亚铁等）配伍，否则会产生有很强刺激性的溴化汞或碘化汞，导致胃肠道出血或发生严重的药源性肠炎。

When a combination of drugs generates toxicity, it is incompatibility. For example, preparations containing cinnabar can not be combined with the reducible ingredients (e.g. iodide, ferrous sulfate, etc.). Otherwise, highly irritating mercury bromide or mercury iodide will be produced, leading to gastrointestinal hemorrhage or severe drug-induced enteritis.

（三）变色

(3) The Discoloration

制剂配伍发生氧化、还原、聚合、分解等反应时，可引起颜色的改变。如多巴胺注射液与碳酸氢钠注射液配伍后逐渐变成粉红至紫色。某些固体药物及其制剂配伍也可发生颜色变化，如碳酸氢钠或氧化镁粉末能使大黄粉末由黄色变为粉红色，氨茶碱或异烟肼与乳糖粉末混合变成黄色，维生素 C 与烟酰胺粉末混合也会产生橙红色。液体制剂的变色反应常与药液的 pH 有关，一般光照、高温、高湿环境中反应更快。分子中有酚羟基的药物与铁盐相遇，使颜色变深。反应式，见图 21-1 所示。

Compatibility of drugs may lead to reactions of oxidation, reduction, polymerization and decomposition, which may cause color changes. When dopamine injection combines with sodium bicarbonate injection, the color will gradually change to pink to purple. Color change can also occur in the compatibility of certain solid drugs and their preparations. For example, sodium bicarbonate or magnesium oxide powders can turn rhubarb powders from yellow to pink, and aminophylline or isoniazid powders will turn yellow when mixing with lactose powders. Vitamin C turns salmon red when mixing with niacinamide powders. The discoloration reaction of liquid preparations is related to the pH values. In general, the reaction will be faster in light, high temperature, high humidity environment. When a drug whose molecule contains phenolic hydroxyl and meets iron salts, the color will darken. The equation is shown in Figure 21-1.

对不影响疗效的配伍变色，可通过加入微量抗氧剂、调 pH 或调整制备、服用方法等予以避免。若产生有毒物质的变色反应，则属于配伍禁忌。

For the discoloration caused by compatibility that does not affect curative effect, it can be avoided by adding trace antioxidant, adjusting pH value and resetting preparation method or administration method. If the combination of drugs triggers toxicity, it is incompatibility.

（四）产气

(4) The Aerogenesis

产气现象一般由化学反应引起。如溴化铵与强碱性药物或利尿药配伍可分解产生氨气；乌洛托品与酸性药物配伍能分解产生甲醛；碳酸盐、碳酸氢盐与酸类药物配伍产生二氧化碳等。

The aerogenesis is usually caused by chemical reactions. For example, ammonium bromide can be decomposed to generate ammonia when combined with strong alkaline drugs or diuretics, etc.

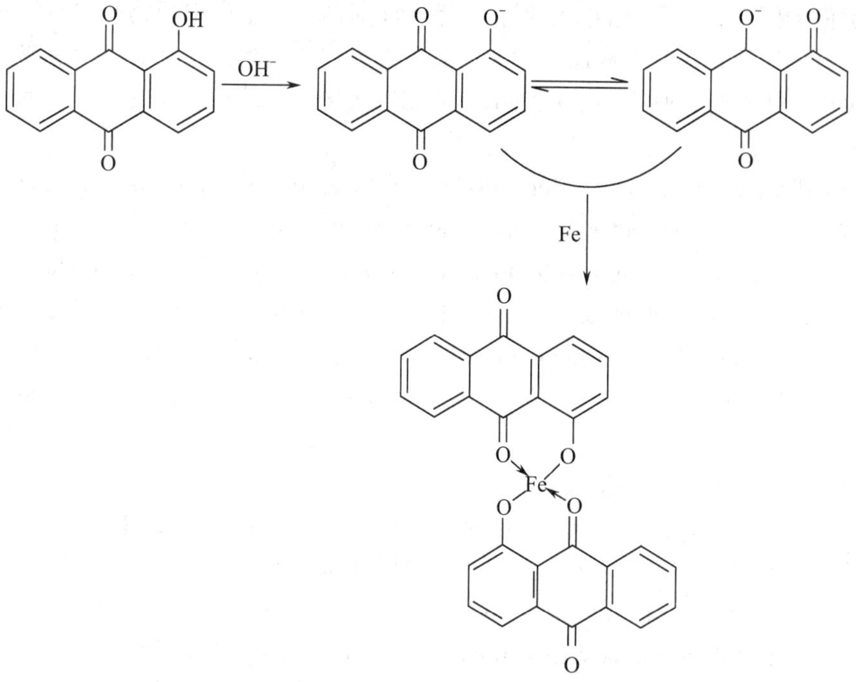

深红色 Crimson

图 21-1 α- 羟基蒽醌变色反应原理

Figure 21-1 The Metachromatism Principle of α-Hydroxy Anthraquinone

（五）发生爆炸

(5) The Explosions

发生爆炸大多由强氧化剂与强还原剂配伍而引起。如火硝与雄黄、高锰酸钾与甘油、氯酸钾与硫、强氧化剂与蔗糖或葡萄糖等药物混合研磨时，均可能发生爆炸。碘与白降汞（$HgNH_2Cl$）混合研磨能产生碘化汞，若有乙醇存在可引起爆炸。

Most explosions are caused by the compatibility of strong reducing agents and strong oxidizing agents. For example, the explosions can be caused by the combinations of potassium nitrate and realgar, potassium permanganate and glycerine, potassium chlorate and sulfur, and the strong oxidant and sucrose or glucose. Mercury iodide will generate when iodine is mixed with $HgNH_2Cl$, which can explode with the presence of ethanol.

三、注射剂的配伍变化

21.2.3 The Compatibility Changes of Injections

临床上将几种药物注射液配伍使用时，特别在输液中添加药物进行静脉滴注的情况是很普遍的。因注射给药的特殊性，为确保临床安全合理用药，掌握注射剂配伍应用的相关理论与知识，对注射剂，特别是中药注射液的合理应用及其安全性、有效性再评价尤为重要。

Clinically, it is common to use injections in combination, especially in intravenous drip. It is particularly important to master the relevant theories and knowledge of the injection compatibility in order to ensure the clinical safety and the rational use of drugs.

（一）注射剂配伍变化的分类

(1) The Classification of the Compatibility Changes in Injections

注射剂的配伍变化同样可分为药理的配伍变化和药剂的配伍变化。药剂的配伍变化，分为可

见的和不可见的配伍变化。可见的配伍变化，系指注射剂由于生产中药物与辅料等的配伍，或将一种注射剂与其他注射剂混合，或加入输液中后出现了浑浊、沉淀、结晶、变色或产气等可见的变化。不可见的配伍变化，则指肉眼观察不到的配伍变化，如某些药物的水解、抗生素的分解和效价下降等。

The compatibility changes of injections can be classified as pharmacological changes and pharmaceutical changes. The pharmacological changes are classified as visible and invisible compatibility changes. Visible compatibility changes refer to the changes such as turbidity, precipitation, crystallization, discoloration or aerogenesis, which can be caused by the compatibility of drugs with excipients or the combinations of injections. The invisible compatibility changes refer to changes that can't be noticed by the naked eyes, such as the hydrolysis of drugs, the degradation of anti-biotic and the decrease of titers, etc.

（二）注射剂产生配伍变化的因素

(2) Factors Affecting the Changes of Injection Compatibility

1. 溶剂组成的改变 当某些含非水溶剂的注射剂与输液配伍时，溶剂组成的改变会使药物析出。

① The changes in solvent compositions When non-aqueous solvents injections are combined with infusions, changes in the compositions of the solvents may lead to drugs precipitate.

2. pH 的改变 注射剂都有各自最稳定的 pH。pH 的改变可能会导致某些药物产生沉淀或加速分解。不同的输液剂均有其一定的 pH 范围，凡混合后导致该输液剂 pH 超出特定范围的注射剂，均不宜与之配伍使用。因此，不但要注意配伍药液的 pH，而且要注意输液特定的 pH 范围。

② The pH values Different injections have their specific pH values to maintain stable state. Thereby, the changes of pH values may lead to the precipitation of some drugs or accelerate the degradation. Meanwhile, infusions can remain stable within a specific pH range. If pH value of infusion exceeds appropriate range of drugs, drugs should not be used in combination. Therefore, attention should be paid not only to the pH value of the compatible solution, but also to the specific pH value range of the infusion.

3. 缓冲容量 缓冲剂抵抗 pH 变化能力的大小称缓冲容量。加入缓冲剂的注射液其 pH 可稳定在一定范围，从而使制剂稳定。但混合后的药液 pH 若超出其缓冲容量，仍可能出现沉淀。如 5% 硫喷妥钠注射液与氯化钠注射液配伍不发生变化，但加入含乳酸盐的葡萄糖注射液则会析出沉淀。

③ The buffer capacity The ability of buffer to resist the change of pH value is called the buffer capacity. Injections with buffers can be stable in a certain pH range. However, when the pH value of the mixed solution exceeds its buffer capacity, drugs may precipitate. For example, the 5% thiopental sodium injection remains stable when combines with sodium chloride injection, but it will precipitate when glucose injection containing lactate is added.

4. 原、辅料的纯度 原、辅料的纯度不符合要求也可引起注射液之间的配伍变化。例如氯化钠原料若含有微量的钙盐，当与含甘草酸、绿原酸等的注射液配合时，往往可与 Ca^{2+} 生成难溶于水的钙盐而出现浑浊。中药注射液中未除尽的高分子杂质在贮藏过程中，或与输液配伍时也会出现浑浊或沉淀。

④ The purity of the raw materials and adjuvants The inconformity of the purity of raw materials and adjuvants to the requirements may also cause the compatibility changes. For example, when sodium chloride raw material contains trace calcium salts, it can form water-insoluble calcium salts when mixing with injections which contain glycyrrhizin, chlorogenic acid, etc., resulting in turbidity. Turbidity or precipitation may also occur in the storage of traditional Chinese medicine injections which contain macromolecule impurities.

$$2C_{39}H_{59}O_{10}(COOH)_3+3Ca^{2+} \rightleftharpoons Ca_3[C_{39}H_{59}O_{10}(COO)_3]_2\downarrow + 6H^+$$

甘草酸 Glycyrrhizic acid　　甘草酸钙 Glycyrrhizic acid calcium

$$2C_{15}H_{17}O_7COOH+Ca^{2+} \rightleftharpoons Ca(C_{15}H_{17}O_7COO)_2\downarrow + 2H^+$$

绿原酸 Chlorogenic acid　　绿原酸钙 Chlorogenic acid calciu

5. 成分之间的沉淀反应　某些药物可直接与输液剂或另一注射剂中的某种成分反应生成沉淀。如含黄芩苷的注射剂遇含小檗碱的注射剂会发生沉淀反应。

⑤ The precipitation among ingredients　Some drugs may generate precipitation with ingredients in injection or infusions. For example, the injection containing baicalin can generate precipitation when it meets the injection containing berberine.

6. 盐析作用　某些呈胶体分散体的注射液，如两性霉素 B 注射剂，若加在含大量电解质的输液中由于胶体分散体的水化膜受到电解质的反离子作用，使 ζ 电位降低，水化膜变薄，使胶体粒子凝聚而产生沉淀。

⑥ The salting-out effects　When colloidal dispersion injection, such as amphotericin B injection, is added into infusion with large amounts of electrolytes, their ζ potential decreases and hydration film turns thin, because the hydration membrane of the colloidal dispersion is negatively ionized by the electrolytes, condensing colloidal particles to generate precipitation.

7. 混合顺序及混合液浓度　改变混合顺序可避免有些药物配伍时产生沉淀。如 1g 氨茶碱与 300mg 烟酸配合，应先将氨茶碱用生理盐水稀释至 1000ml，再慢慢加入烟酸可得澄明溶液。若先将两种药物配制的浓溶液混合再稀释则会析出沉淀。药物配伍后沉淀物的产生，与其浓度和配制时间也有关。

⑦ The mixing order and the concentration of the mixture The change of mixing order may avoid precipitation in the compatibility of some drugs. For example, dissolve 1g aminophylline in 1000 mL normal saline, and then gradually add 300 mg niacin to get a transparent solution. If two concentrated solutions are mixed directly without dilution, precipitation will occur. The precipitation caused by compatibility is related to the concentration and the mixing time.

第三节　药理学的配伍变化

21.3　The Pharmacological Compatibility Changes

PPT

药理学的配伍变化是指药物配伍使用后，使药理作用的性质和强度发生变化，产生协同作用、拮抗作用、不良反应。

The pharmacological compatibility changes refer to changes in the property and intensity of pharmacological effects, resulting in synergistic effects, antagonistic effects or adverse reaction.

一、协同作用
21.3.1 The Synergistic Effects

协同作用系指两种以上药物合并使用后，使药物作用增加。协同作用又可分为相加作用和增强作用。相加作用为两药合用的作用等于两药作用之和。增强作用又称为相乘作用，表现为两药合用的作用大于两药作用之和。药物的协同作用在临床上具有重要意义。例如：红花与当归、川芎配伍应用后可增强抗凝作用，提高对血栓性疾病的治疗效果。

The synergistic effects refer to the improvement on curative effects of drugs after compatibility. The synergistic effects can be divided into additive and reinforcing effects. The additive effect means that the combined effect of drugs is equal to the sum of their respective effects. The reinforcing effect is also called multiplication effect, which represents that the combined effect of drugs is stronger than the sum of their respective effects. The synergistic effects of drugs are very important in clinic. For example, the compatibility of afflower and angelica sinensis or ligusticum wallichii can enhance their therapeutic effect of thrombotic diseases.

二、拮抗作用
21.3.2 The Antagonistic Effects

拮抗作用系指两种以上药物合并使用后，使作用减弱或消失，多数情况下不宜配伍使用。如藿香正气水、消炎解毒片、蛇胆川贝散与乳酶生合用，可使乳酸菌被灭活，引起药效下降。含蛋白质及其水解物的中成药珍珠丸、清热解毒丸等不宜与小檗碱同服，因其所含蛋白质等成分水解生成的多种氨基酸可拮抗小檗碱的抗菌作用。但在临床上有时将有拮抗作用的药物有意识地配伍使用，以纠正主药的副作用和突出主药的主要作用。

The antagonistic effects refer to the efficacy reducing or losing after combination of drugs, which represents incompatibility in most of the cases. For example, the combination of Huoxiangzhengqi liquid, Anti-inflammatory tablets, Shedanchuanbei powders and biofermin can inactivate the lactic acid bacteria, weakening the efficacies of drugs. Sometimes, drugs with antagonistic effects are combined in clinic for certain purposes, such as to avoid the side effects or strengthen the major effects of principal drug.

三、产生不良反应
21.3.3 The Adverse Reactions

某些药物配伍后，能产生毒性或副作用等不良反应，则不宜配伍使用或应慎用。例如抗癌药石蒜含石蒜碱，与大剂量维生素 C 配合使用时，能增强石蒜碱的毒性，故不宜配伍使用。

Some drugs compatibilities which may generate toxicity or side effects should not be compatible use or should be used with caution. For example, the toxicity of lycoris containing lycorine can be enhanced when it is combined with large amounts of vitamin C. Therefore, it is not suitable for compatibility.

四、制剂在体内发生的相互作用
21.3.4 The *in vivo* Interactions of the Preparations

药物制剂在体内发生的相互作用，主要表现在体内吸收及分布、代谢与排泄过程所发生的协同作用、拮抗作用或毒副作用。

The interaction of drug preparation *in vivo* is mainly manifested as the synergistic, antagonistic or side effects during absorption, distribution, metabolism and excretion.

（一）吸收过程的相互作用

(1) The Interactions in the Absorption Process

制剂在吸收部位发生物理化学反应，包括由于温度、pH、水分、金属离子等作用引起的结构性质改变，以及由于药物的溶解度、解离度、胃肠道蠕动的变化，影响药物制剂的崩解时间、溶出速度、吸收速度和程度等。例如：元胡止痛片中含有生物碱，与强心苷类同服时，前者可使胃排空延迟，胃肠蠕动减慢，增加了强心苷的吸收。

Physical and chemical reactions of the preparations occur at the absorption sites, including the structural changes caused by temperature, pH values, moisture, metallic ions, as well as the changes caused by the drug solubility, dissociation degree and gastrointestinal peristalsis, which influence the disintegration time, dissolution rate, absorption rate and degree of preparations. For example, when the Yuanhu painkillers which contain alkaloids are used with cardiac glycosides, the former can delay the gastric emptying and slow the gastrointestinal peristalsis, enhancing the absorption of cardiac glycosides.

（二）分布过程的相互作用

(2) The Interactions in the Distribution Process

药物吸收进入血液循环后，大多数与血浆蛋白或组织蛋白结合，而药物只有在游离状态下才具有药理活性，结合了蛋白的药物会暂时失去活性。药物与蛋白的结合是个可逆的过程，随着体内药物不断被消除，结合药物又被释放出来，发挥疗效。而药剂配伍对分布的影响最常见的正是对药物与蛋白结合的影响，我们称为置换作用，即一种药物减少了另一种药物与蛋白的结合。当两种药物在蛋白质某一结合位置上进行竞争时，亲和力强的药物将亲和力弱的药物置换出来，被置换的药物其游离型浓度显著增加。

When drugs are absorbed into the blood, most of them bind to plasma proteins or histones. However, the pharmacological activities of drugs only exist when they are in free state. Once drugs are combined with proteins, the activities temporarily lose. The most common distribution influence of preparations compatibility lies in the combination of drugs and proteins which is called the substitution effect, indicating one drug reducing the binding of the other to the proteins. When two drugs competing at a certain binding position of the protein, the drug with strong affinity replaces the drug with weak affinity, and the free state concentration of the replaced drug increases significantly.

（三）代谢过程的相互作用

(3) The Interactions in the Metabolism Process

药物在体内受药酶的作用发生的配伍变化，分为酶促作用或酶抑作用。当药物重复使用或与其他药物合并应用时，药物代谢被加快的现象，称为酶促作用，反之则称为酶抑作用。

The effects of enzymes on drug compatibility can be divided into enzymatic action and enzymatic inhibition. When drugs are used repeatedly or in combination with others, the phenomenon that metabolism of drugs be accelerated is called enzymatic action. If metabolism slows down, it is called enzyme inhibition.

（四）排泄过程的相互作用

(4) The Interactions in the Excretion Process

药物一般以原型药物或代谢物通过肾脏、肝胆系统、呼吸系统及皮肤汗腺分泌等途径排出体外，并大多以肾脏排泄为主。一些弱酸或弱碱类药物均可在肾小管分泌时产生相互竞争而发

生变化。

Generally, drugs can be excreted through kidney, liver, respiratory system and sweat glands in form of prototype or metabolites, and most of them are excreted by the kidney. Some weak acid or weak base drugs may change when they compete at kidney tubules.

此外，药物在作用部位或作用环节也可能产生相互竞争，而使其中某一种药物的疗效增强或减弱。

In addition, drugs may compete with each other, which enhances or weakens the efficacy of them.

总之，药物之间相互作用的机制是非常复杂的，有些目前尚不清楚，有待进一步研究。在目前的临床应用中，中药制剂之间以及中药制剂与西药制剂之间的配伍越来越多，在应用时应根据病情需要酌情处理，并注意避免因配伍引起的不良反应及毒副作用。

In summary, the mechanisms of drug interactions are complex, and some of them remain unclear and need further study. Clinically, there are more and more traditional Chinese medicines compatibilities and traditional Chinese medicine preparations and western preparations compatibilities. The application should be careful according to the needs of patients, and the adverse and side effects caused by compatibility should be paid enough attentions and be avoid.

第四节 预测配伍变化的实验方法

21.4 Experimental Methods for Predicting Compatibility Changes

PPT

药物制剂产生配伍变化的情况往往较为复杂，判断配伍药物之间是否产生配伍变化首先可根据配伍药物的相关知识（如药物的理化性质、药理作用；药物制剂的配方、工艺、附加剂等；临床用药的对象、剂量、浓度、医师用药的意图等）进行分析研究，必要时通过实验预测，力求解决药物配伍后相关的“变化”问题（如有无外观上的变化及其变化产物；有无观察不到的变化，有无新物质生成；药物的效价、毒性、药理学作用和动力参数有无变化），以及产生变化的原因及影响变化的因素等。

The compatibility changes of pharmaceutical preparations are complicated. To determine whether compatibility changes exist in compatible drugs, first of all, it is necessary to review relevant knowledge of the compatible drugs, to predict through experiments when necessary. In order to solve the problem of “change”, reasons and factors affecting the change should be analyzed.

判断两种药物之间是否产生配伍变化一般应从两方面进行：①根据药物的理化性质、药理性质及其配方、临床用药的对象、剂量、用药意图等，结合易产生配伍变化的因素进行分析；②通过实验观察作出合理的判断。

The judgement of whether there is a compatibility change between two drugs is made from the following two aspects: ① To analyze the factors that cause the compatibility changes according to the physical, chemical and pharmacological properties of drugs as well as the formulations, the clinical objects, dosages, medication intention, etc; ② To make a reasonable judgment through experiment and observation.

预测制剂配伍变化的一般实验方法如下。

General experimental methods for predicting the compatibility changes of preparations as follows.

（一）可见的配伍变化实验方法

(1) Experimental Methods of Visible Compatibility Changes

一般是将两种注射液混合均匀，在一定时间内，肉眼观察有无浑浊、沉淀、结晶、变色、产气等现象。

Generally, two injections are mixed evenly, and the phenomena such as turbidity, precipitation, crystallization, color changes and aerogenesis can be observed by the naked eyes in a certain period of time.

（二）测定注射剂变化点的 pH

(2) Determination of the pH Values at the Variation Point of Injection

许多注射剂的配伍变化是由 pH 改变引起的，所以测定注射液变化点的 pH，可作为预测配伍变化的依据之一。

Many compatibility changes of injections are caused by the changes of pH values, so the determination of pH values at the variation point of injection can be used as one of the facts to predict compatibility changes.

（三）稳定性试验

(3) The Stability Tests

临床输液时间往往较长，如将稳定性差的药物添加到输液中，因受 pH、光线或其他成分的影响，其含量或效价往往下降较快，有的甚至产生毒性成分。一般认为若在规定时间内（如 6 小时、24 小时等）药物含量或效价降低超过 10% 者，属于不稳定药物，应进行稳定性试验。

Clinically, infusion time is relatively long. When a drug with poor stability is added to infusion, its content or titer could drop rapidly due to the influences of pH value, light or other ingredients, and even generate toxic components. It is generally believed that if the drug content or titer is reduced more than 10% within a specified period of time, it could be listed as an unstable drug and stability test should be conducted.

（四）成分鉴定与含量测定

(4) The Component Identifications and the Content Tests

药剂配伍后产生物理或（和）化学变化，可用紫外光谱、薄层色谱、高效液相色谱等方法，鉴定分解产物或产生的沉淀成分及其含量。

If physical or (and) chemical changes generate after the combination of drugs, methods such as ultraviolet spectrum, thin layer chromatography and high performance liquid chromatography can be used to identify the components and contents changes.

（五）药理学、药效学实验及药物动力学参数的测定

(5) Pharmacology, Pharmacodynamics Experiments and Determination of Pharmacokinetic Parameters

药剂配伍后是否产生疗效的变化常须进行药理学或药效学实验。如果药物配伍应用后药物动力学参数发生变化，则说明存在着药理学或药效学上的相互作用或配伍变化。

Pharmacologic or pharmacodynamic experiments are often required to determine whether there are changes in therapeutic efficacy after drug compatibility. If the pharmacokinetic parameters change, it indicates that there are pharmacological or pharmacodynamic compatibility changes.

第五节 配伍变化的处理原则与方法

21.5 The Handling Principles and Methods of the Compatibility Changes

一、处理原则

21.5.1 The Handling Principles

为减少或避免药物制剂之间发生配伍变化，处理原则如下。

In order to reduce or avoid the compatibility changes in pharmaceutical preparations, the handling principles are listed as follows:

1. 审查处方，了解用药意图 审查处方，如发现疑问，应先与医师或处方者联系，了解用药意图，明确必需的给药途径。根据具体对象与条件，结合药物的物理、化学和药理等性质，确定剂型，判定或分析可能产生的不利因素和作用，对剂量和用法等加以审查，或确定解决方法，使药剂能更好地发挥疗效。

(1) The prescription review, the knowledge of the medication intention Review prescriptions and, if in doubt, contact the physician or prescriber to understand the medication intention and identify the necessary route of administration. According to specific objects and conditions, combining with the physical, chemical and pharmacological properties of the drug, determine the dosage form and possible adverse factors. Review the dosage and usage, and determine the solution, so that to improve drug efficacy.

2. 制备工艺和贮藏条件的控制 控制温度、光线、氧气、痕量重金属是延缓水解和氧化反应的基本条件。制备与使用药物制剂，均应注意药物之间，或药物与附加剂之间可能产生的物理、化学或药剂学、药理学的配伍变化。

(2) The controls over the preparation technology and storage conditions Controlling temperature, light, oxygen and trace heavy metals are the basic requirements to retard hydrolysis and oxidation reactions.

During preparation and usage, attention should be paid to the physical, chemical, pharmaceutical and pharmacological compatibility changes that may occur in drugs or additives.

二、药剂学配伍变化的处理方法

21.5.2 The Handling Method of the Pharmaceutical Compatibility Changes

减少或避免药物制剂之间发生配伍变化，在剂型设计和制剂工艺条件等选择时就应严格控制，而调配时首先应认真审查处方，了解用药意图。药剂学的配伍变化，一般可按下列方法进行处理。

In order to reduce or avoid compatibility changes in pharmaceutical preparations, dosage form design and preparation process conditions should be strictly controlled. When dispensing, the prescription should be carefully reviewed to understand the medication intention. Compatibility changes in pharmacy can generally be treated as follows:

1. 改变调配次序 调配时的混合次序可能影响某些药液成品的质量，改变调配次序可克服一些不应产生的配伍禁忌。如制备碳酸镁、枸橼酸、碳酸氢钠溶液型合剂时，应将枸橼酸溶于水，并与碳酸镁混合溶解后，再将碳酸氢钠溶入。若碳酸氢钠先与枸橼酸混合耗尽酸液，则不能配成溶液剂。

(1) The changes of the blending orders The blending order may affect the quality of products. Changing the blending order can overcome some incompatibility

Such as the preparation of solution of magnesium carbonate, citric acid, bicarbonate sodium. Citric acid should be dissolved in water first, and then mix it with magnesium carbonate. Finally, dissolve bicarbonate sodium. If acid is exhausted when blending bicarbonate sodium and citric acid, they cannot be mixed in a solution.

2. 调整溶剂或使用附加剂 使用混合溶剂或适当增加溶剂用量，可有效地防止或延缓溶液剂析出沉淀。必要时可添加增溶剂或助溶剂。

(2) The adjustments of solvents or the uses of additives With the use of mixed solvents or by the increase of the solvent dosages, the precipitation may be effectively prevented. The solubilizers or cosolvents can be added if necessary.

3. 调节药液 pH pH 与很多药物的溶解度和稳定性有关，因此，应调节溶液 pH 在适宜的范围内。

(3) The adjustments of the solutions' pH values The pH values are related to the solubility and stability of many drugs. Therefore, the pH values of solutions should be adjusted within a proper range.

4. 改变剂型或改变有效成分 根据药物制剂产生配伍变化和临床用药要求，某些药物可设计制成其他适宜剂型，而调剂时征得医师同意，可改换成药效、用法与原成分类似的药物。

(4) The changes of the dosage forms or the effective components According to the compatibility changes of pharmaceutical preparations and the clinical medication requirements, some medicines can be designed to other proper dosage forms, and the compounding should be permitted by the doctors to replace the medicines with similar efficacies, uses and components.

5. 控制贮存条件 有些药物在使用过程中，会由于贮存条件，如温度、空气、水分、光线等环境因素影响而加速沉淀、变色或分解，对于此类药物一般应在密闭、避光条件下，贮于棕色瓶中。每次发出的药量也应适宜。更应注意控制某些要求冷藏的制剂的贮存条件。

(5) The controls over the storage conditions The precipitation, discoloration or degradation of some drugs may be accelerated during use and these changes are influenced by the storage conditions and environmental factors, such as the temperature, air, moisture and light, etc. For drugs that are susceptible to external influences, they should be stored in brown bottles under closed, dark conditions. What's more, dosage of these drugs should also be verified for each dispensing. Besides, more attention should be paid to the storage conditions of preparations that require refrigeration.

总之，在制剂的生产、贮存和使用过程中，可能发生药物制剂的配伍变化或配伍禁忌。为避免因药物制剂配伍不当而造成的内在质量问题，应制定合理的处方和制备工艺，一旦发生药物制剂的配伍变化或配伍禁忌，应认真分析原因，从制剂处方、剂型、工艺和贮存条件等环节入手，寻找解决办法。

In short, the compatibility of pharmaceutical preparations may change during production, storage and use. In order to avoid internal quality problems caused by improper compatibility of pharmaceutical

岗位对接

重点小结

题库

preparations, reasonable prescriptions and preparation processes should be formulated. Once the compatibility of preparation changes or incompatibility happen, it is necessary to carefully analyze the reason in detail including preparation prescriptions, dosage forms, processes and storage conditions, and then find out the solutions.

（王　芳）

第二十二章　生物药剂学与药物动力学在中药制剂中的应用

Chapter 22　Application of Biopharmaceutics and Pharmacokinetics in the Preparations of Chinese Medicine

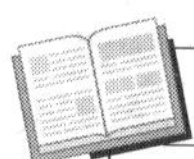

学习目标 ┆ Learning Goals

知识要求：

1. **掌握**　生物药剂学和药物动力学的概念及研究内容，药物的体内过程。
2. **熟悉**　药物动力学参数的意义，影响中药制剂疗效的因素。
3. **了解**　中药制剂生物利用度和药物动力学的应用和研究进展。

能力要求：

清楚药物在体内处置的基本过程，学会药物（中药）动力学研究的方法。

Knowledge requirements:

1. **To master** the concepts and contents of biopharmaceutics and pharmacokinetics, the *in vivo* behavior of drugs.

2. **To be familiar with** the significance of pharmacokinetic parameters, and factors affecting the efficacy of Chinese medical preparations.

3. **To know** the application of bioavailability and pharmacokinetics of Chinese medical preparations.

Ability requirements:

Learn the *in vivo* behavior of drugs, and how to investigate the pharmacokinetics of drug (Chinese medicine).

PPT

第一节 生物药剂学概论

22.1 Introduction to Biopharmaceutics

一、生物药剂学的含义与研究内容

22.1.1 Concept and Contents of Biopharmaceutics

生物药剂学是研究药物及其制剂在体内吸收、分布、代谢与排泄的过程，阐明药物的剂型因素、机体生物因素和药物疗效之间相互关系的科学。生物药剂学的研究目的主要是正确评价药剂质量、设计合理的药物剂型和制剂工艺以及为临床合理用药提供科学依据，保证用药的安全性与有效性。

Biopharmaceutics is a science that studies the behavior of absorption, distribution, metabolism, and excretion of drugs and their preparations in the body, and clarifies the interrelationships between dosage factors, biological factors and drug efficacy. Biopharmaceutics aims to evaluate the quality of pharmaceuticals, design reasonable pharmaceutical dosage forms and preparation processes, and provide scientific basis for rational clinical use of drugs to ensure their safety and efficacy.

生物药剂学是20世纪60年代发展起来的药剂学新分支。作为一门体内的药剂学，它与医药学中的一些其他学科，如药理学、生物化学等有着密切联系，在内容上互相渗透和补充，共同研究药物及其他生理有效物质与机体的关系。生物药剂学的研究内容主要包括以下几个方面：

Biopharmaceutics is a new branch of pharmaceutics developed in the 1960s. As an *in vivo* pharmacology, it is closely related to some other disciplines in medicine, such as pharmacology and biochemistry. They penetrate and complement each other in contents, and jointly studies the relationship between drugs and the body. The contents of biopharmaceutics mainly include the following aspects:

1. 药物剂型因素的研究 ①研究剂型、制剂处方和工艺对药物体内过程的影响；②研究新剂型、新的给药途径和方法；③研究药物理化性质与其体内处置的关系；④根据机体的生理功能设计缓控释制剂和靶向给药系统。

(1) Studies on the factors of drug dosage forms ① Study the effects of dosage forms, formulations, and preparation processes on the *in vivo* behavior of drugs; ② Study new dosage forms, new routes and methods of administration; ③ Study the relationship between the physical properties of drugs and their *in vivo* disposal; ④ Design slow and controlled release preparations and targeted drug delivery systems.

2. 药物制剂质量评价的研究 为制剂提供新的、更为合理的评价方法，例如测定方法与装置的改进。

(2) Researches on quality evaluation of pharmaceutical preparations Provide new and more reasonable evaluation methods for preparations, such as improvement of measurement methods and devices.

3. 药物及其制剂体内过程的研究 包括药物（含中药）及其制剂进入体内后的吸收、分布、代谢与排泄研究。

(3) Studies on the *in vivo* behavior of drugs and their preparations including the absorption, distribution, metabolism and excretion of drugs (including Chinese medicine) and their preparations after entering the body.

4. 生物药剂学研究方法的探索 建立模拟体内处置的体外模型和开发以药物理化性质预测其体内吸收的方法等。

(4) Exploration of biopharmaceutical research methods Establish *in vitro* models that simulates the *in vivo* disposition, and develop methods to predict the absorption of drugs based on their physicochemical properties.

二、药物的体内过程

22.1.2 The in *vivo* Behavior of Drugs

1. 药物的跨膜转运 药物在体内的处置首先要通过细胞膜，跨细胞膜转运的速度直接影响药物的体内过程。细胞膜主要是由按照一定规律排列的脂质、蛋白质及少量糖类等化学成分构成。药物跨细胞膜转运的方式主要有被动转运和主动转运，此外，还有膜动转运等方式（图 22-1）。

(1) Transmembrane transport of drugs Drugs need to pass through the cell membrane to enter and exit the bloodstream, and the speed of transport across cell membranes directly affects their efficacies. Cell membranes are mainly composed of chemical components such as lipids, proteins, and small amounts of sugars arranged in accordance with a certain regularity. There are three modes of drug transport across cell membranes: passive transport, active transport, and membrane transport (Figure 22-1).

细胞外 Extracellular
被动转运
Passive diffusion
简单扩散
Simple diffsion
易化扩散
Facilitaed diffusion
主动转运
active diffusion
蛋白质
Proteins
转运体
Transporters
ATP
ADP+Pi
磷脂双层
Phospholipid bilayer
细胞内Intracellular

图 22-1 药物主要的跨膜转运机制示意图

Figure 22-1 Schematic Diagram of Drug Transmembrane Transport Action

（1）被动转运 是指生物膜两侧的药物顺着浓度梯度（由高浓度侧向低浓度侧）或电化学梯度进行的跨膜转运，不消耗能量。被动转运又包括简单扩散和易化扩散。①简单扩散：即药物仅在浓度梯度的驱动下，顺浓度梯度转运的过程，也称为被动扩散；②易化扩散：指借助于细胞膜上的转运体，顺浓度梯度转运的过程，也称为促进扩散。

① *Passive transport* It refers to the transmembrane transport of drugs along the concentration gradient (from the high concentration side to the low concentration side) or the electrochemical gradient without consuming energy. Passive transport includes simple diffusion and facilitated diffusion. a. Simple diffusion: Transporting drugs only under the driving of a concentration gradient, also known as passive

diffusion; b. Facilitated diffusion: Transporting drugs along a concentration gradient with the help of transporters on the cell membrane, also called promote diffusion.

（2）主动转运　药物借助细胞膜上的特异性载体，由低浓度侧向高浓度侧的转运过程，需要能量。主动转运可出现饱和及竞争抑制现象。

② *Active transport*　Drugs require energy to transfer from a low concentration side to a high concentration side by means of a specific carrier on the cell membrane. Active transport can be saturated and competitively inhibited.

（3）膜动转运　通过细胞膜的主动变形，将药物摄入细胞内或从细胞内释放到细胞外的转运过程。膜动转运包括向细胞内摄入的入胞作用和排出细胞外的出胞作用。

③ *Membrane dynamic transport*　A behavior of transporting a drug into or released from a cell through the active deformation of cell membrane.

2. 药物的体内过程　药物的体内过程包括吸收、分布、代谢和排泄。其中，分布、代谢和排泄过程称为处置，代谢和排泄过程又称为消除。药物的体内过程会影响血药浓度的变化，从而影响药效（图 22-2）。

(2) The *in vivo* behavior of drugs　The *in vivo* behavior of drugs include absorption, distribution, metabolism, and excretion. Among them, the behavior of distribution, metabolism and excretion are called disposition, and the behavior of metabolism and excretion are also called elimination. The *in vivo* behavior of a drug will affect its concentration in blood, thus affecting the efficacy (Figure 22-2).

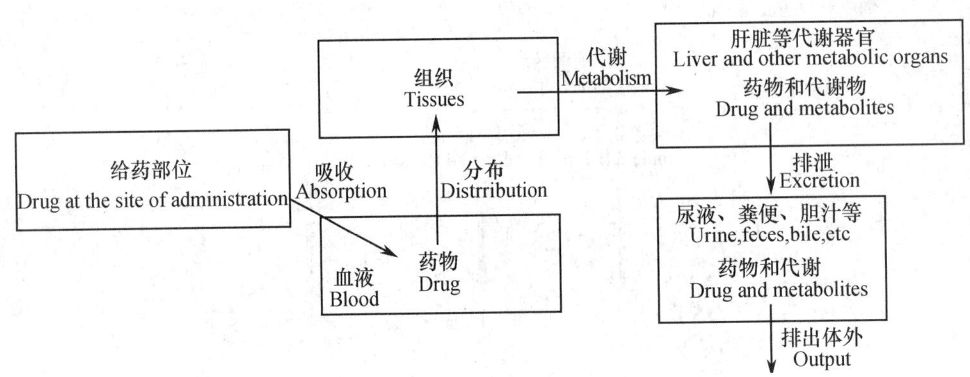

图 22-2　药物的体内过程

Figure 22-2　*In vivo* Behavior of Drugs

（1）吸收　吸收是指药物从用药部位进入体循环的过程。除血管内给药不存在吸收外，其他给药途径均存在吸收过程。根据吸收部位不同，吸收可分为胃肠道吸收和非胃肠道吸收。

① *Absorption*　Absorption is the transfer of a drug from its site of administration to the bloodstream. Except for intravascular administration (absorption is complete), drug delivery by other routes results in only partial absorption. Absorption can be divided into gastrointestinal absorption and parenteral absorption.

①胃肠道吸收　口服给药因方便，且多数药物能在胃肠道充分吸收，是最常用的给药途径。小肠由于吸收面积大且肠道内适宜的酸碱度对药物解离影响小，故是药物吸收的主要部位。一般而言，水溶性药物吸收快。大多数药物在胃肠道内以简单扩散的方式被吸收，一部分在肝脏代谢转化后，与原型一起经血液到达相应的组织器官发挥作用，最终经肾脏从尿中排出或经胆汁从粪便排出。此外，一些药物还可在消化道其他部位被吸收，例如硝酸甘油可经口腔黏膜吸收，阿司

匹林可经胃黏膜吸收。

a. Gastrointestinal absorption Oral administration is convenient, and most drugs can be fully absorbed in the gastrointestinal tract, therefore, it is the most commonly used route of administration. The small intestine is the main site for drug absorption due to its large absorption area and the appropriate pH. In general, water-soluble drugs are absorbed more quickly. Most drugs are absorbed in the gastrointestinal tract by simple diffusion, some of them are metabolized in the liver before reach the corresponding tissues, finally excreted into the urine via the kidney or into the feces via bile. In addition, some drugs can be absorbed in other parts of the digestive tract. For example, nitroglycerin can be absorbed through the oral mucosa, aspirin can be absorbed through the gastric mucosa.

②非胃肠道吸收 非胃肠道吸收包括注射部位吸收和肺部吸收等。注射部位的吸收速率取决于注射部位的血流量，血流量越大则吸收越快。此外，注射途径和药物分散状态不同，药物的吸收速率也不同。除关节腔内注射及局部麻醉药外，注射给药一般产生全身作用。静脉注射药物直接进入血液循环，无吸收过程。肺部吸收是指挥发性或气体性药物通过肺上皮细胞或器官黏膜吸收，可避免首过消除。

b. Parenteral absorption Parenteral absorption includes absorption at the injection site, lung, etc. For injection absorption, the absorption rate depends on the blood flow at the injection site. The greater the blood flow, the faster the absorption. In addition, it also depends on the injection route and dispersion state of the drug. With the exception of intra-articular injections and local anesthetics, injections generally have systemic effects. Drugs enter the blood circulation directly after intravenous administration, without absorption. Lung absorption refers to the absorption of volatile or gaseous drugs through lung epithelial cells or organ mucosa, which can avoid first pass elimination.

（2）分布 分布是指药物进入体循环后向各组织、器官或者体液转运的过程。影响药物分布的因素主要有：①药物的性质：脂溶性大的药物分布到组织器官的速度快；②组织器官的血流量和血管透过性：脑、心、肝、肾等组织器官血管丰富且血流量大，故药物浓度较高，有利于发挥药效，但也易引起这些组织器官的损伤；③药物与血浆蛋白的结合率：药物与血浆蛋白（主要是白蛋白）结合后往往无活性，不易透过毛细血管壁，故影响药物的分布与药效；④血脑屏障、血胎屏障转运：极性小而脂溶性大的药物较易通过。

② *Distribution* Distribution refers to the behavior by which a drug transport to various tissues, organs or body fluids after entering the systemic circulation. The main factors affecting the distribution of a drug are: a. The physicochemical properties of drugs: The fat-soluble drug is distributed to tissues and organs more quickly; b. The blood flow and vascular permeability: Brain, heart, liver, kidney and other tissues are rich in blood vessels are conducive to distribution; c. Drug and plasma protein binding rate: Drugs and plasma proteins (mainly albumin) are often combined without activity, and not easy to penetrate the capillary wall, so the binding affects the distribution and efficacy of drugs; d.Blood-brain barrier and blood-fetal barrier transport: Drugs with small polarity and large fat solubility are easier to pass.

（3）代谢 代谢是指药物在体内多种药物代谢酶作用下所经历的化学结构的转变，又称为生物转化。代谢往往会使药物的水溶性增大，利于排出体外，故使进入全身血液循环的有效药量明显减少，药效降低。代谢主要发生在富含药物代谢酶的肝脏中。此外，肠也参与药物的代谢。药物在体内的代谢主要分为Ⅰ相反应和Ⅱ相反应两个阶段。Ⅰ相代谢反应包括氧化、去甲基化和水解反应等，主要由细胞色素 P450 酶（Cytochrome P450, CYPs）介导。Ⅱ相代谢反应是结合反应，是指药物或其Ⅰ相代谢物与内源性物质如葡萄糖醛酸结合，使水溶性进一步加大，最终排出体

外。典型的Ⅱ相代谢酶包括葡萄糖醛酸转移酶（UDP-glucuronosyltransferases, UGTs）、磺酸转移酶（Sulfotransferases, SULTs）和谷胱甘肽 -S- 转移酶（Glutathione-S-transferase, GSTs）等。

③ *Metabolism* Metabolism refers to the transformation of the chemical structure of a drug under the catalysis of various drug-metabolizing enzymes in the body, also known as biotransformation. Metabolism tends to increase the water solubility of the drug and facilitates its excretion. Therefore, the amounts of the drugs that enter the systemic circulation are usually significantly reduced. Metabolism occurs mainly in the liver, which is rich in drug-metabolizing enzymes. In addition, the intestine is also involved in drug metabolism. The metabolism of drugs is mainly divided into two phases: phase I reaction and phase II reaction. Phase I metabolic reaction includes oxidation, demethylation, and hydrolysis reactions, which are mainly mediated by cytochrome P450 enzymes (CYPs). Phase II metabolic reaction is a conjugation reaction, which means that the drug or its phase I metabolite is combined with an endogenous substance, such as glucuronic acid to further increase the water solubility. Typical phase II metabolic enzymes include UDP-glucuronosyltransferases (UGTs), sulfotransferases (SULTs), glutathione-S-transferases (GSTs), etc.

影响药物代谢的因素主要包括：①药剂学因素：如给药途径、剂量、剂型和联合用药等。②生理因素：如性别、年龄、种族、饮食和疾病等。

Factors affecting drug metabolism include: a.Pharmaceutical factors: such as the route of administration, dose, dosage form and combination medication. b.Physiological factors: such as gender, age, race, diet and disease.

（4）排泄　排泄是指药物或其代谢产物排出体外的过程。药物及其代谢物最主要的排泄途径是肾排泄，其次是胆汁途径，也可由乳汁、唾液、呼吸和汗腺等排泄。

④ *Excretion* Excretion is the behavior by which drugs or their metabolites are excreted from the body. The main excretion route of drugs and their metabolites is renal excretion, followed by bile route, breast milk route, saliva route, respiratory route and sweat glands route.

第二节　药物动力学概论

22.2 Introduction to Pharmacokinetics

PPT

一、药物动力学的含义与研究内容

22.2.1 Concept and Contents of Pharmacokinetics

药物动力学是应用动力学原理与数学处理方法，定量研究药物在体内吸收、分布、代谢和排泄等过程动态变化的科学，亦称为“药动学”“药物代谢动力学”和“药代动力学”。

Pharmacokinetics is a science that describes the dynamic changes in the absorption, distribution, metabolism, and excretion of drugs in the body.

药物动力学研究是新药临床前期和Ⅰ期临床研究的内容，主要揭示机体对药物的处置规律及这些处置对药物疗效和毒性的影响，研究内容主要包括：

Pharmacokinetic research is a part of pre-clinical and phase I clinical studies of new drugs. It mainly reveals the disposition of drugs and the impact of these disposition on drug efficacy and toxicity. The

contents include:

1. 建立药动学数学模型，找出体内药物及其代谢产物的量（浓度）与时间之间的函数关系，求算出药动学参数。

(1) Establish a mathematical model of pharmacokinetics, find out the relationship between the amount (concentration) of drugs and their metabolites in the body and time, and calculate the pharmacokinetic parameters.

2. 应用药动学参数设计临床给药方案，进行治疗药物监测，从而达到最佳的药物治疗，使毒副反应降至最低，为开展临床药学提供科学依据。

(2) Apply pharmacokinetic parameters to design a clinical dosing regimen and perform therapeutic drug monitoring to achieve the best treatment effect, minimize the side effects and toxicity, and provide a scientific basis for clinical pharmacy.

3. 指导剂型改造，开发新剂型，例如缓控释制剂的开发与研究。

(3) Guide the formulation reform and develop new dosage forms, such as the sustained and controlled release preparations.

4. 开展生物利用度和生物等效性研究，其是新剂型特别是口服制剂的重要研究内容。

(4) Carry out researches on bioavailability and bioequivalence, which are important for develop new dosage forms, especially oral preparations.

5. 研究中药的活性成分、活性组分，单方或复方在体内的动态变化规律。

(5) Investigate the dynamic changes of the active ingredients of Chinese medicine *in vivo*.

二、药物动力学常用术语
22.2.2 Commonly used Terms in Pharmacokinetics

1. 隔室模型 药物进入体内后，各部位的药物浓度始终在不断变化，这种变化虽然复杂，但仍服从一定规律。隔室模型亦称房室模型，是经典的药物动力学模型。隔室模型是将整个机体按动力学特性划分为若干个独立的隔室，把这些隔室串联起来构成一种足以反映药物动力学特征的模型，包括单室模型、双室模型和多室模型。隔室的划分具有抽象性、相对性和客观性（图 22-3）。

(1) Compartment model After the drug enters the body, its concentration in each tissue is constantly changing. Although the change is complicated, it still obeys a certain law. The compartment model, also known as the atrioventricular model, is a classic pharmacokinetic model. The model divides the entire body into several independent compartments according to the kinetic characteristics, including single compartment model, two compartment model and multi compartment model. The division of compartments is abstract, relative and objective (Figure 22-3).

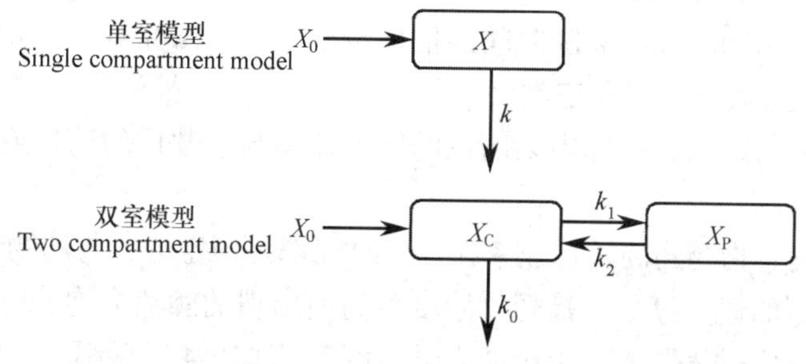

图 22-3 隔室模型示意图

Figure 22-3 Schematic of the Compartment Models

在单室模型中，X_0 为给药剂量，X 为体内药量，k 为一级消除速率常数；在双室模型中，X_0 为给药剂量，X_C 和 X_P 分别为中央室和外周室的药量，k_0 为药物从中央室消除的一级速率常数，k_1 为药物从中央室向外周室转运的一级速率常数，k_2 为药物从外周室向中央室转运的一级速率常数。

In the single compartment model, X_0 is the administered dose, X is the amount of drug in the body, and k is the first-order elimination rate constant. In the dual-compartment model, X_0 is the administered dose, X_C and X_P are the amount of drug in the central compartment and peripheral compartment, respectively, K_0 is the first-order rate constant for drug elimination from the central compartment, k_1 is the first-order rate constant for drug transport from the central compartment to the peripheral compartment, and k_2 is the first-order rate constant for drug transport from the peripheral compartment to the central compartment.

（1）单室模型　单室模型把机体视为由一个单元组成，即药物进入体循环后迅速分布，于组织、器官和体液中达到动态平衡的“均一”状态，此时的机体可以看作一个隔室。

① *Single compartment model*　The single compartment model considers the body as a unit, that is, the drug is rapidly distributed after entering the systemic circulation, and reaches a “uniform” state of dynamic equilibrium in tissues, organs and body fluids. At this time, the body can be regarded as a compartment.

（2）双室模型　双室模型把机体看成由药物分布速度不同的两个隔室单元组成，其中一个称为中央室，由血流丰富的组织器官（如心、肺、肝和肾等）组成，药物在中央室迅速达到分布平衡；另一室为周边室，由血液供应不丰富的组织器官（如肌肉和皮肤等）组成，药物在周边室分布较慢。

② *Two compartment model*　The two compartment model considers the body to be composed of two compartment units with different drug distribution speed. One of them is called the central compartment, which is composed of organ rich in blood flow (such as heart, lung, liver, and kidney). The compartment quickly reaches the distribution equilibrium; the other compartment is the peripheral compartment, which is composed of tissues and organs (such as muscle and skin) that are not rich in blood supply, the drug is distributed slowly in the peripheral compartment.

（3）多室模型　若周边室中又有一部分组织、器官或细胞内药物的分布特别慢，还可以从中划分出隔室，称为多室模型。

③ *Multi compartment model*　If there are some drugs in the peripheral compartment that are particularly slow in distribution, new compartments can also be divided from peripheral compartment, called a multi compartment model.

2. 药物转运的速度过程

(2) Speed process of drug transport

药物进入体内后，药物量和浓度随时间的推移不断变化，研究该变化就涉及速度过程。通常将药物体内转运的速度过程分为以下三类。

（1）一级速率过程　即药物在体内某部位的转运速率与该部位的药量或血药浓度的一次方成正比的速率方程。

（2）零级速率过程　指药物的转运速率在任何时间都是恒定的，与药物量或浓度无关。

（3）受酶活力限制的速率过程　指药物浓度较高而出现的酶活力饱和时的速率过程，也称为“Michaelis-Menten 型速度过程”或“米氏动力学过程”（图 22-4）。米氏动力学过程可以用米氏方程表示：

After the drug enters the body, the amount and concentration of the drug continuously change over time, which involves the speed process. The speed process of drug transport in vivo is usually divided into the following three categories. ① First-order rate process: Drug transport rate is directly proportional to its dose or blood concentration. ② Zero-order rate process: Drug transport rate is constant at any time, regardless of the amount or concentration of the drug. ③ Rate process limited by enzyme activity: Rate process when the enzyme activity is saturated at higher drug concentrations, and it is also called "Michaelis-Menten rate process" (Figure 22-4), described by the Michaelis-Menten equation:

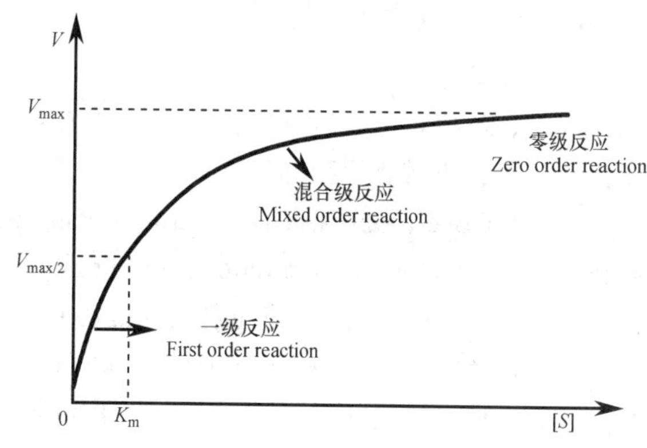

图 22-4　米氏动力学过程

Figure 22-4　Michaelis-Menten Kinetics

$$V=\frac{V_{max}\times[S]}{K_m+[S]} \tag{22-1}$$

式中，V 是药物反应速率，$[S]$ 为底物浓度，V_{max} 是酶被底物饱和时的反应速度，K_m 是米氏常数。由公式可知，K_m 是达到 $1/2V_{max}$ 时的底物浓度，只由酶的性质决定，而与酶的浓度无关。在底物浓度较低时，反应相对于底物是一级反应；当底物浓度处于中间范围时，反应相对于底物是混合级反应；当底物浓度增加时，反应由一级反应向零级反应过渡。

In the above formula, V is the transport rate, $[S]$ is the substrate concentration, V_{max} is the transport rate of substrate when the enzyme is saturated, and K_m is the Michaelis-Menten constant, which is determined only by the property of the enzyme. When the substrate concentration is low, the reaction is a first-order reaction; when the substrate concentration is in the middle range, the reaction is a mixed-level reaction; when the substrate concentration is increased, the reaction changes from a first-order reaction to a zero-order reaction.

3. 药物动力学常用参数

(3) Common parameters of pharmacokinetics

（1）速度常数　速度常数是描述药物转运（消除）快慢的动力学参数，常用 K 表示。根据质量作用定律：

① *Velocity constant*　Velocity constant is a kinetic parameter describing the speed of drug transport (elimination). According to the law of mass action:

$$\frac{dX}{dt}=-KX^n \tag{22-2}$$

式中，dX/dt 为药物转运的速率，X 为体内药量，K 为转运速率常数，n 为转运级数。当 $n=1$ 时，K 为一级速度常数，以"时间的倒数"为单位，如 1/h；当 $n=0$ 时，K 为零级速度常数，以"浓度 / 时间"为单位。速度常数越大，转运（消除）速度越快。

In the above formula, dX/dt is the rate of drug transport, X is the amount of drug in the body, K is the constant of the transport rate. The larger the speed constant, the faster the transport (elimination) speed.

（2）表观分布容积（V）　指体内药量与血药浓度间相互关系的一个比例常数。即：

② *Apparent distribution volume (V)*　It refers to a proportionality constant between the amount of drug in the body and the concentration of drug in blood, which is:

$$V = \frac{X}{C} \tag{22-3}$$

式中，X 和 C 分别为体内药量和血药浓度。表观分布容积反映药物的分布情况，不代表体液真正的容积，不具有直接的生理意义。

In the above formula, X is the drug amount in the body, C is the drug concentration in blood. The apparent distribution volume reflects the distribution of the drug, does not represent the true volume of body fluids, and has no physiological significance.

（3）清除率（Cl） 指机体或消除器官在单位时间内清除药物的速度或效率。清除率的单位是"体积 / 时间"。单位时间所清除的药物量等于清除率与血药浓度的乘积。

③ *Clearance (Cl)* It refers to the speed of the body or elimination organs to clear the drug in a unit time. The unit of clearance is "volume/time". The amount of drug removed per unit time is equal to the product of clearance rate and drug concentration in blood.

（4）达峰时间（t_{max}） 指单次服药以后，血药浓度达到峰值所需的时间。在这个时间点，血药浓度最高。

④ *Peak time* (t_{max}) It refers to the time required for the blood concentration to reach its peak after a single dose. At this point in time, the blood concentration is the highest.

（5）达峰浓度（C_{max}） 药物吸收后，血药浓度的最大值称为达峰浓度。

⑤ *Peak concentration* (C_{max}) After drug absorption, the maximum concentration in blood is called peak concentration.

（6）药 - 时曲线下面积（AUC） 是以时间为横坐标，药物浓度或体内药量为纵坐标绘制的曲线下的面积。药时曲线下面积反映药物在体内吸收的总量。

⑥ *Area under the concentration-time curve (AUC)* AUC is the area under the curve drawn with time as the abscissa and drug concentration or the amount of drug in the body as the ordinate. The AUC reflects the total amount of drug absorbed in the body.

（7）生物半衰期（$t_{1/2}$） 指生物体内药物量或血药浓度减少一半所需的时间，又称为消除半衰期。生物半衰期是药物从体内消除速度快慢的指标，与药物的性质和消除器官的功能有关。

⑦ *Biological half-life* ($t_{1/2}$) It refers to the time required to reduce the amount of drug or blood concentration in the body by half, and is also called elimination half-life. Biological half-life is an indicator of how fast a drug is eliminated from the body, and is related to the properties of the drug and the function of the elimination organ.

三、生物利用度与生物等效性
22.2.3 Bioavailability and Bioequivalence

1. 生物利用度与生物等效性的含义 生物利用度和生物等效性是衡量制剂质量和疗效差异的重要指标。

(1) Meaning and contents of bioavailability and bioequivalence Bioavailability and bioequivalence are important indicators to evaluate the quality and efficacy of preparations.

生物利用度是指制剂中药物被吸收进入体循环的速度与程度，常用 F 表示。生物利用度可分为绝对生物利用度与相对生物利用度。绝对生物利用度是以静脉注射制剂为参比标准，获得药物吸收进入体循环的相对量，通常比较二者的 AUC。相对生物利用度则是以非静脉途径给药的制剂为参比制剂获得的药物吸收进入体内的相对量。

Bioavailability (F) refers to the speed and degree of drug absorption into the systemic circulation, which can be divided into absolute bioavailability (F_a) and relative bioavailability (F_r). Fa and Fr are the relative amount of drug absorbed into the systemic circulation based on intravenous and non- intravenous preparations as reference standard, respectively.

$$\text{绝对生物利用度 } F\ (F_a) = \frac{AUC_t \cdot X_{iv}}{AUC_{iv} \cdot X_t} \times 100\% \tag{22-4}$$

$$\text{相对生物利用度 } F\ (F_r)\ F = \frac{AUC_t \cdot X_r}{AUC_r \cdot X_t} \times 100\% \tag{22-5}$$

式中，脚注 t 为试验制剂，iv 和 r 分别为静脉注射参比制剂和非静脉注射参比制剂，X 为给药剂量。

In the above formula, footnote t is the test preparation, iv and r are the intravenous and non-intravenous reference preparations, respectively. *AUC* is the area under the concentration-time curve, X is the dose.

生物等效性是指在同样试验条件下，试验制剂和对照标准制剂中药物的吸收程度和速度的统计学差异。当某些药物制剂吸收速度的差别没有临床意义时，吸收程度相同也可以认为生物等效。生物等效性已经成为国内外药物仿制和移植品种的重要评价内容，也是药物制剂开发中最有价值的评价指标。

Bioequivalence refers to the statistical difference in the degree and rate of drug absorption between the test preparation and the standard preparation under the same conditions. Some pharmaceutical preparations have the same degree of absorption but different rates can also be considered bioequivalent. Bioequivalence has become an important evaluation index of domestic and foreign drug imitation, transplantation varieties, and development of pharmaceutical preparations.

2. 生物利用度与生物等效性的研究方法 生物利用度和生物等效性的数据应用体内（药物动力学、药效学或临床研究）和体外方法来评价，在某些情况下，可只进行体外研究。

(2) Research methods of bioavailability and bioequivalence Bioavailability and bioequivalence data should be evaluated using the *in vivo* (pharmacokinetic, pharmacodynamic or clinical studies) and *in vitro* methods.

血药浓度法是生物利用度研究的最常用方法。受试者分别给予受试制剂和参比制剂，测定血药浓度，计算 AUC、C_{max} 和 t_{max} 等参数，估算生物利用度。当原型药物及其代谢产物大部分（70% 以上）经尿排泄，且排泄量与吸收量比值（肾排泄率）恒定时，可以采用尿药浓度法。但尿药浓度法误差大，尿样收集时间长，故应用较少。此外，还有一些其他方法，如药理效应法和同位素标记法等也可用于生物利用度的研究。

The blood concentration method is the most commonly used method for bioavailability research. The drug concentration in blood are measured after participants were given test preparations and reference preparations, respectively. Parameters such as AUC, C_{max} and t_{max} are calculated to estimate bioavailability. When the most of drugs and their metabolites (more than 70%) are excreted in urine, and the ratio of excretion to absorption (renal excretion rate) is constant, the urine concentration method can be used. However, the urine concentration method is rarely used due to its low accuracy and a long time to collect urine samples. In addition, there are other methods, such as pharmacological effect method and isotope labeling method, which can also be used in bioavailability research.

生物等效性的研究方法主要包括：①药物动力学法：即采用药动学研究获得药动学参数，经

统计学分析比较 AUC、C_{max} 和 t_{max} 等参数是否有统计学差异，从而判断两制剂是否等效；②药效学研究法：即采用可分级定量（痊愈、显效、进步、无效）的药效学指标进行比较；③临床对照试验：是较为直接的评价方法，指在药物临床试验中，给予患者两种制剂后，观察药物的疗效和不良反应等进行评价。该法所需的样本量较大，检测指标不够灵敏，试验周期长且成本高；④体外研究法：FDA 规定具有高溶解性、高渗透性、溶出快速和辅料不影响吸收的非窄指数口服制剂可采用体外溶出度比较法证明生物等效。该法经济简单，省去了大量繁琐的体内研究工作。

The research methods of bioequivalence mainly include: ① Pharmacokinetic method: Pharmacokinetic parameters are obtained by pharmacokinetic research, and whether the parameters such as AUC, C_{max} and t_{max} are statistically different between the two preparations; ② Pharmacodynamics research method: that is, the use of quantifiable (healing, markedly effective, progressive, ineffective) pharmacodynamic indicators for comparison; ③ Clinical controlled trial: It is a more direct evaluation method, refers to the clinical trials after the patients were given the two preparations, the efficacy and adverse reactions of the drugs were evaluated. This method requires a large sample size, sufficient detection sensitivity, plenty of time and high costs; ④ *In vitro* research method: The non-toxic oral preparations with high solubility, high permeability, rapid dissolution, and excipients that do not affect absorption, can be proved to be bioequivalent by the method of *in vitro* dissolution comparison.

第三节 中药制剂的生物药剂学与药物动力学研究

22.3 Biopharmaceutics and Pharmacokinetics in Chinese Medical Preparations

PPT

生物药剂学与药物动力学研究对中药制剂的开发、生产和临床应用具有重要的指导意义。由于中药制剂的有效成分复杂，故体内过程的研究难度较大。自 20 世纪 70 年代以来，中药制剂的生物药剂学与药物动力学研究取得了较快的发展。

Biopharmaceutical and pharmacokinetic studies have important guiding significance for the development, production and clinical application of Chinese medical preparations. Due to the complexity of the effective ingredients in Chinese medical preparations, the study of their *in vivo* behavior is difficult. Since the 1970s, biopharmaceutical and pharmacokinetic research of Chinese medical preparations has made rapid progress.

一、中药制剂的生物药剂学与药物动力学研究意义

22.3.1 Significance of Research on Biopharmaceutics and Pharmacokinetics of Chinese Medical Preparations

伴随着中药药剂学的不断发展，研究表明许多口服中药制剂中的有效成分生物利用度较低，极大地限制了其临床应用。为提高疗效和方便患者用药，中药不断被研发成各种制剂，而提高中药制剂的生物利用度也一直是中药新药研发中亟待解决的问题。中药制剂的生物药剂学与药物动力学研究在解决以上科学问题中发挥着关键作用，对中药制剂的发展有着重要意义。主要体现在

以下方面：

Chinese medicine has been continuously developed into various preparations. However, the clinical applications of Chinese medical preparations are greatly limited by their low bioavailabilities. Therefore, improving their bioavailability has always been an urgent problem. Biopharmaceuticals and pharmacokinetics study plays a key role in solving this problems and mainly reflected in the following aspects:

1. 通过研究中药及其制剂中有效成分的体内过程，阐明其作用机制。

(1) Study the *in vivo* behavior of active ingredients in Chinese medical preparations.

2. 求算药动学参数，为中药制剂确定合理给药方案和中药配伍设计提供实验依据，从而保证临床用药的安全性与有效性。

(2) Calculate the pharmacokinetic parameters, provide experimental basis for rational drug use, so as to ensure the safety and efficacy of clinical medicine.

3. 优选制剂工艺，为中药剂型改革提供依据。

(3) Optimize the preparation processes, provide the basis for the dosage reform of Chinese medicine.

4. 评价中药制剂的内在质量，从而科学化控制中药制剂的质量。

(4) Evaluate the quality of Chinese medical preparations.

二、中药制剂的生物药剂学与药物动力学发展概况

22.3.2 Overview of the Development of Biopharmaceutics and Pharmacokinetics in Chinese Medical Preparations

由于有效成分复杂，中药制剂的生物药剂学与药物动力学研究较为困难。对于有效成分明确的中药及其制剂，生物药剂学与药物动力学的研究方法与西药基本类似。但许多中药及其复方制剂由于化学结构不明确，或由于是混合物而非单体，有效成分和作用机制不清楚，给研究带来了挑战。目前多用复方或其制剂中的某一种或多种单体成分来代替整方研究体内处置过程，得出的结果与实际情况相比可能有一定偏差。对于有效成分和测定方法不明确的中药，可用生物效应法进行药物动力学研究。即根据体内药量在一定条件下与药效相关，从药效的变化推知不同时间点体内药量的变化。但此法不够精确，只能粗略看出体内药物浓度变化的过程。

Due to the complexity of the active ingredients, it is difficult to study the biopharmaceutics and pharmacokinetics of Chinese medical preparations. For the preparations with clear active ingredients, the research methods are basically similar to western medicine. However, due to the unclear chemical structures of many Chinese medicine, or because they are mixtures rather than monomers, the active ingredients and pharmacodynamic mechanism are unclear. At present, one or more monomer components in the compound (preparations) are often used instead of the whole prescription to study their *in vivo* behavior. The results obtained may be biased compared with the actual situation. For Chinese medicine whose active ingredients are unclear, pharmacokinetic studies can be carried out by biological effect method. That is, according to the amount of drug is related to its efficacy in the body under certain conditions. However, this method is not accurate enough.

随着现代分析仪器和检测技术的改进和完善，越来越多的中药特别是单味中草药的有效成分及其代谢物已明确，为中药及其制剂的生物药剂学与药物动力学研究提供了有力保障，已取得的进展主要包括：

With the improvement of modern analytical instruments and detection technologies, more and more

Chinese medicine, especially the active ingredients and their metabolites, have been identified. These technologies are benefit to the study of biopharmaceutics and pharmacokinetics of Chinese medicine and their preparations. The progress that has been made mainly includes:

1. 阐明了许多中药成分的体内处置特征及机理。采用多种体内外模型，如单向肠灌流模型、细胞模型（如 Caco-2 细胞和 MDCK 细胞等）、中药生物药剂学分类系统和基于生理的药代动力学（PBPK）模型考察或预测了中药及其制剂中有效成分在体内处置的特征，深入评价了药物代谢酶和外排转运蛋白对中药生物利用度和药物间相互作用的影响，从而为改善中药生物利用度和阐释中药复方的配伍机制提供了理论依据。

(1) The characteristics and mechanism of *in vivo* disposition of many Chinese medicine ingredients were clarified. A variety of *in vivo* and *in vitro* models, such as single-pass perfusion model, cell models (Caco-2 cells and MDCK cells, etc.), biopharmaceutical classification system, and physiological-based pharmacokinetic (PBPK) models were used to investigate or predict the *in vivo* behavior of the active ingredients in Chinese medicine and their preparations. These models were also widely used to evaluate the effects of drug metabolizing enzymes and efflux transporters on their bioavailability and drug-drug interactions.

2. 通过开展中药药动学研究，拟合有效成分在体内的药动学参数，为中药的临床合理应用和制定个体化给药方案提供了依据。

(2) By carrying out pharmacokinetic studies and fitting the pharmacokinetic parameters of active ingredients *in vivo*, it provides a basis for the rational application of Chinese medicine and the formulation of individualized drug therapy.

3. 以生物利用度为指标，优选中药制剂工艺或剂型。

(3) Taking bioavailability as an index, optimize the preparation or dosage form of the Chinese medicine.

总之，近年来中药及其制剂的生物药剂学与药物动力学研究取得了较快的发展，但在研究方法及检测仪器方面还需要更大的创新，并需要进一步加强中药复方代谢物的体内处置研究，从而为中药及其制剂的开发和临床合理应用起到指导作用。

In short, the biopharmaceutical and pharmacokinetic research of Chinese medicine and their preparations has made rapid progress in recent years, but greater innovation is still needed in research methods and detection instruments. Additionally, the *in vivo* disposal of metabolites of Chinese medicine needs further exploration.

三、影响药物（中药）制剂疗效的因素
22.3.3 Factors Affecting the Efficacy of Pharmaceutical Preparations

1. 物理化学因素
(1) Physical and chemical factors

（1）药物的解离度与脂溶性　药物的非解离型往往较易透过生物膜吸收。然而，有些非解离型药物口服后的吸收效果仍不佳，主要原因是药物分子的脂溶性较差。药物的脂溶性也并非越大越好，因为脂溶性过强不易于溶解于体液。

① *Dissociation degree and fat solubility of drugs*　Non-dissociated drugs are often more easily absorbed through cell membrane. However, the absorption of some non-dissociated drugs is still not good, mainly due to their poor fat solubility.

（2）溶出度与溶解度　溶出度是指在规定介质中，药物从固体制剂中溶出的速度和程度。溶

解度是在一定条件下，在一定量溶剂中溶解药物的最大量。一般而言，药物必须以单个分子（或离子）与生物膜接触才能吸收进入体循环，药物的吸收通常是从溶液中开始的。因此，对于固体制剂和药物而言，吸收前存在崩解溶出的过程。因此，溶出度和溶解度直接影响着固体制剂中药物的疗效。

② *Dissolution and solubility* The transfer of molecules or ions from a solid preparation into solution is known as dissolution. The extent to which the dissolution proceeds under a given set of experimental conditions is referred to as the solubility. Drug absorption usually begins in solution. Dissolution and solubility directly affect the efficacy of drugs in solid preparations.

（3）粒径　药物粒径越小，比表面积越大，故溶解速度和吸收速度越快，药效也越好。

③ *Particle size* The smaller the particle size of the drug, the larger the specific surface area, so the faster the dissolution rate and the absorption rate, the better the efficacy.

（4）晶型　多晶型在固体药物中是一种常见的现象。不同药物晶型可能具有不同的药效，有些晶型甚至具有毒性，故选择合适的晶型具有重大的药用意义。

④ *Crystal form* Polymorphism is a common phenomenon in solid drugs. Different drug crystal forms may have different pharmacological effects, and some crystal forms are even toxic. Therefore, it is of great medicinal significance to choose the appropriate crystal form.

2. 剂型因素

(2) Dosage factors

（1）剂型与给药途径　剂型的差异会影响药物的溶出、吸收和疗效。常用口服剂型吸收的一般顺序是：溶液剂 > 混悬剂、乳剂 > 散剂 > 胶囊剂 > 片剂 > 丸剂 > 包衣片剂。

① *Dosage form and route of administration* The difference in dosage form will affect the dissolution, absorption and efficacy of the drug. The general order of absorption rate is: solution > suspension, emulsion > powder > capsule > tablet > pill > coated tablet.

不同给药途径中药物吸收的一般顺序是：静脉 > 吸入 > 肌内 > 皮下 > 直肠或舌下 > 口服 > 皮肤。

The general order of drug absorption in different routes of administration is: intravenous > inhalation > intramuscular > subcutaneous > rectal or sublingual > oral > skin.

（2）药用辅料　辅料会改变制剂的溶出速率和吸收速率，从而影响制剂的疗效。如亲水性辅料可以增大疏水性药物的溶出度，疏水性辅料会影响制剂的崩解和溶出。

② *Medical excipients* Excipients will change the dissolution rate and absorption rate of the preparation, thereby affecting the efficacy of the preparation. For example, hydrophilic excipients can increase the dissolution of hydrophobic drugs. Hydrophobic excipients can affect the disintegration and dissolution of the formulation.

（3）制剂工艺　提取精制、制备工艺和成型工艺等会影响药物制剂中有效成分的含量、分散状态和溶出等，从而影响制剂疗效。特别是在固体中药制剂的工艺中，粉碎、提取、分离除杂、浓缩、干燥及工艺条件等因素均会影响中药制剂疗效的发挥。

③ *Preparation processes* Extraction and refining, preparation process and molding process will affect the content, dispersion state and dissolution of active ingredients in pharmaceutical preparations, thus affecting their efficacies. Especially in the process of solid preparations of Chinese medicine, factors such as pulverization, extraction, removal of impurities, concentration drying and process conditions are closely related to their efficacies.

3. 生物因素

(3) Biological factors

（1）首过效应　首过效应是指某些药物经胃肠道给药，在尚未吸收进入血循环之前，在肠黏膜和肝脏被代谢，而使进入血循环的原形药量减少的现象，也称为首关效应或第一关卡效应。肝肠首过效应使进入体循环的药量减少，故药效降低。

① *First pass effect*　First pass effect refers to the phenomenon that drugs are metabolized in the intestinal mucosa and liver after oral administration, before being absorbed into the blood circulation. The first pass effect reduces the amount of drug entering the systemic circulation, thereby reduces the efficacy.

（2）用药部位的生理状态　机体生理条件如性别、年龄、种族、疾病、胃肠道 pH、胃排空速度、血流和饮食等因素均会影响药物在用药部位的吸收，从而影响制剂的疗效。

② *Physiological status of medication site*　Physiological conditions such as gender, age, race, disease, gastrointestinal pH, gastric emptying speed, blood flow, and diet will affect the absorption and efficacy of the drug.

（3）药物相互作用　药物相互作用是指一种药物的作用被同时应用的另一种药物所改变。近年来，临床上联合应用多种药物治疗患者疾病的现象日益增多。这些药物同时服用后，由于药物间相互作用，有的产生协同作用，增强疗效，也有的产生拮抗作用，使疗效降低，甚至产生毒性。

③ *Drug-drug interaction*　Drug-drug interaction is that in which the efficacy of one drug is altered by another. In recent years, the clinical application of multiple drugs to treat diseases has increased. Due to the interaction between the drugs after taking these drugs at the same time, some produce synergistic effects and enhance the curative effect, while others produce antagonistic effects, which reduce the curative effect and even produce toxicity.

岗位对接

4. 其他　除了以上因素，原料药的质量也是影响药物（中药）制剂疗效的重要因素。特别是中药制剂，中药材的种类、质量和炮制技术等都会影响其疗效。中药制剂由于组成成分多，而且绝大多数的中药制剂都是以复方发挥疗效，很难确定单一的有效成分。因此，合理制定完善的质量标准是提高中药制剂疗效的关键。

重点小结

(4) Other　In addition to the above factors, the quality is also an important factor affecting the efficacy of the drug (Chinese medicine) preparations. All of the type, quality and preparation process will affect the efficacy of Chinese medical materials. Reasonable formulation of quality standards is the key to improving the efficacy of Chinese medical preparations.

题库

（刘中秋）

参考文献

[1] 傅超美，刘文 . 中药药剂学［M］. 2 版 . 北京：中国医药科技出版社，2018.
[2] 方亮 . 药剂学［M］. 8 版 . 北京：人民卫生出版社，2016.
[3] 冯年平 . 中药药剂学［M］. 北京：科学出版社，2017：255-263.
[4] 张兆旺 . 中药药剂学［M］. 2 版 . 北京：中国中医药出版社，2017.
[5] 杨明 . 中药药剂学［M］. 10 版 . 北京：中国中医药出版社，2016.
[6] 刘建平 . 生物药剂学与药物动力学［M］. 5 版 . 北京：人民卫生出版社，2016：165-167.
[7] 王建，傅超美 . 中药学专业知识［M］. 6 版 . 北京：中国医药科技出版社，2012.
[8] 张兆旺 . 中药药剂学习题集［M］. 北京：中国中医药出版社，2003.
[9] 张炳盛 . 中药药剂学习题集［M］. 北京：中国中医药出版社，2016：188-195.
[10] Kevin Taylor，Michael Aulton. Aulton's Pharmaceutics［M］. 5th Edition. Amsterdam：Elservier，2017：126-199，465-467，476-485.
[11] 徐芳芳，石伟，张晖，等 . 穿心莲总内酯亲水凝胶骨架片的制备及体外释药机制研究［J］. 中国中药杂志，2015，40（01）：79-83.